The Handbook of Language in Public Health and Healthcare

Blackwell Handbooks in Linguistics

This outstanding multi-volume series covers all the major subdisciplines within linguistics today and, when complete, will offer a comprehensive survey of linguistics as a whole.

The Handbook of Child Language
Edited by Paul Fletcher & Brian MacWhinney

The Handbook of Phonological Theory, Second Edition
Edited by John A. Goldsmith, Jason Riggle, & Alan C. L. Yu

The Handbook of Sociolinguistics
Edited by Florian Coulmas

The Handbook of Phonetic Sciences, Second Edition
Edited by William J. Hardcastle & John Laver

The Handbook of Morphology
Edited by Andrew Spencer & Arnold Zwicky

The Handbook of Japanese Linguistics
Edited by Natsuko Tsujimura

The Handbook of Contemporary Syntactic Theory
Edited by Mark Baltin & Chris Collins

The Handbook of Language Variation and Change, Second Edition
Edited by J. K. Chambers & Natalie Schilling

The Handbook of Historical Linguistics
Edited by Brian D. Joseph & Richard D. Janda

The Handbook of Language, Gender, and Sexuality, Second Edition
Edited by Susan Ehrlich, Miriam Meyerhoff, & Janet Holmes

The Handbook of Second Language Acquisition
Edited by Catherine J. Doughty & Michael H. Long

The Handbook of Bilingualism and Multilingualism, Second Edition
Edited by Tej K. Bhatia & William C. Ritchie

The Handbook of Pragmatics
Edited by Laurence R. Horn & Gregory Ward

The Handbook of Applied Linguistics
Edited by Alan Davies & Catherine Elder

The Handbook of Speech Perception
Edited by David B. Pisoni & Robert E. Remez

The Handbook of the History of English
Edited by Ans van Kemenade & Bettelou Los

The Handbook of English Linguistics
Edited by Bas Aarts & April McMahon

The Handbook of World Englishes
Edited by Braj B. Kachru, Yamuna Kachru, & Cecil L. Nelson

The Handbook of Educational Linguistics
Edited by Bernard Spolsky & Francis M. Hult

The Handbook of Clinical Linguistics
Edited by Martin J. Ball, Michael R. Perkins, Nicole Muller, & Sara Howard

The Handbook of Pidgin and Creole Studies
Edited by Silvia Kouwenberg & John Victor Singler

The Handbook of Language Teaching
Edited by Michael H. Long & Catherine J. Doughty

The Handbook of Language Contact
Edited by Raymond Hickey

The Handbook of Language and Speech Disorders
Edited by Jack S. Damico, Nicole Muller, & Martin J. Ball

The Handbook of Computational Linguistics and Natural Language Processing
Edited by Alexander Clark, Chris Fox, & Shalom Lappin

The Handbook of Language and Globalization
Edited by Nikolas Coupland

The Handbook of Hispanic Sociolinguistics
Edited by Manuel Diaz-Campos

The Handbook of Language Socialization
Edited by Alessandro Duranti, Elinor Ochs, & Bambi B. Schieffelin

The Handbook of Intercultural Discourse and Communication
Edited by Christina Bratt Paulston, Scott F. Kiesling, & Elizabeth S. Rangel

The Handbook of Historical Sociolinguistics
Edited by Juan Manuel Hernandez-Campoy & Juan Camilo Conde-Silvestre

The Handbook of Hispanic Linguistics
Edited by Jose Ignacio Hualde, Antxon Olarrea, & Erin O'Rourke

The Handbook of Conversation Analysis
Edited by Jack Sidnell & Tanya Stivers

The Handbook of English for Specific Purposes
Edited by Brian Paltridge & Sue Starfield

The Handbook of Spanish Second Language Acquisition
Edited by Kimberly L. Geeslin

The Handbook of Chinese Linguistics
Edited by C.-T. James Huang, Y.-H. Audrey Li, & Andrew Simpson

The Handbook of Language Emergence
Edited by Brian MacWhinney & William O'Grady

The Handbook of Korean Linguistics
Edited by Lucien Brown & Jaehoon Yeon

The Handbook of Speech Production
Edited by Melissa A. Redford

The Handbook of Contemporary Semantic Theory, Second Edition
Edited by Shalom Lappin & Chris Fox

The Handbook of Classroom Discourse and Interaction
Edited by Numa Markee

The Handbook of Narrative Analysis
Edited by Anna De Fina & Alexandra Georgakopoulou

The Handbook of English Pronunciation
Edited by Marnie Reed & John M. Levis

The Handbook of Discourse Analysis, Second Edition
Edited by Deborah Tannen, Heidi E. Hamilton, & Deborah Schiffrin

The Handbook of Bilingual and Multilingual Education
Edited by Wayne E. Wright, Sovicheth Boun, & Ofelia Garcia

The Handbook of Portuguese Linguistics
Edited by W. Leo Wetzels, Joao Costa, & Sergio Menuzzi

The Handbook of Translation and Cognition
Edited by John W. Schwieter & Aline Ferreira

The Handbook of Linguistics, Second Edition
Edited by Mark Aronoff & Janie Rees-Miller

The Handbook of Technology and Second Language Teaching and Learning
Edited by Carol A. Chapelle & Shannon Sauro

The Handbook of Psycholinguistics
Edited by Eva M. Fernandez & Helen Smith Cairns

The Handbook of Dialectology
Edited by Charles Boberg, John Nerbonne, & Dominic Watt

The Handbook of Advanced Proficiency in Second Language Acquisition
Edited by Paul A. Malovrh & Alessandro G. Benati

The Handbook of the Neuroscience of Multilingualism
Edited by John W. Schwieter

The Handbook of Historical Linguistics
Ediited by Richard D Janda, Brian D Joseph & Barbara S Vance

The Handbook of Asian Englishes
Kingsley Bolton, Werner Botha, & Andy Kirkpatrick

The Handbook of Language in Public Health and Healthcare
Pilar Ortega, Glenn Martínez, Maichou Lor, & A. Susana Ramírez

The Handbook of Language in Public Health and Healthcare

Edited by

Pilar Ortega
Accreditation Council for Graduate Medical Education
IL, USA

Glenn Martínez
University of Texas at San Antonio
TX, USA

Maichou Lor
University of Wisconsin-Madison
WI, USA

A. Susana Ramírez
University of California-Merced
CA, USA

WILEY Blackwell

Copyright © 2024 by John Wiley & Sons, Inc. All rights reserved.

Published by John Wiley & Sons, Inc., Hoboken, New Jersey.
Published simultaneously in Canada.

No part of this publication may be reproduced, stored in a retrieval system, or transmitted in any form or by any means, electronic, mechanical, photocopying, recording, scanning, or otherwise, except as permitted under Section 107 or 108 of the 1976 United States Copyright Act, without either the prior written permission of the Publisher, or authorization through payment of the appropriate per-copy fee to the Copyright Clearance Center, Inc., 222 Rosewood Drive, Danvers, MA 01923, (978) 750-8400, fax (978) 750-4470, or on the web at www.copyright.com. Requests to the Publisher for permission should be addressed to the Permissions Department, John Wiley & Sons, Inc., 111 River Street, Hoboken, NJ 07030, (201) 748-6011, fax (201) 748-6008, or online at http://www.wiley.com/go/permission.

Trademarks: Wiley and the Wiley logo are trademarks or registered trademarks of John Wiley & Sons, Inc. and/or its affiliates in the United States and other countries and may not be used without written permission. All other trademarks are the property of their respective owners. John Wiley & Sons, Inc. is not associated with any product or vendor mentioned in this book.

Limit of Liability/Disclaimer of Warranty
While the publisher and author have used their best efforts in preparing this book, they make no representations or warranties with respect to the accuracy or completeness of the contents of this book and specifically disclaim any implied warranties of merchantability or fitness for a particular purpose. No warranty may be created or extended by sales representatives or written sales materials. The advice and strategies contained herein may not be suitable for your situation. You should consult with a professional where appropriate. Further, readers should be aware that websites listed in this work may have changed or disappeared between when this work was written and when it is read. Neither the publisher nor authors shall be liable for any loss of profit or any other commercial damages, including but not limited to special, incidental, consequential, or other damages.

For general information on our other products and services or for technical support, please contact our Customer Care Department within the United States at (800) 762-2974, outside the United States at (317) 572-3993 or fax (317) 572-4002.

Wiley also publishes its books in a variety of electronic formats. Some content that appears in print may not be available in electronic formats. For more information about Wiley products, visit our web site at www.wiley.com.

Library of Congress Cataloging-in-Publication Data
Names: Ortega, Pilar, editor. | Martínez, Glenn A., 1971– editor. | Lor, Maichou, editor. | Ramírez, Susana (A. Susana), editor.
Title: The handbook of language in public health and healthcare / edited by Pilar Ortega, Accreditation Council for Graduate Medical Education, IL, United States, Glenn Martínez, University of Texas at San Antonio, OH, United States, Maichou Lor, University of Wisconsin-Madison, WI, United States, A. Susana Ramírez, University of California, CA, United States.
Description: First edition. | Hoboken, New Jersey : Wiley-Blackwell, [2024] | Series: Blackwell handbooks in linguistics | Includes bibliographical references and index.
Identifiers: LCCN 2023041642 (print) | LCCN 2023041643 (ebook) | ISBN 9781119853817 (cloth) | ISBN 9781119853831 (adobe pdf) | ISBN 9781119853848 (epub)
Subjects: LCSH: Communication in public health–Handbooks, manuals, etc. | Communication in medicine–Handbooks, manuals, etc.
Classification: LCC RA423.2 .H358 2024 (print) | LCC RA423.2 (ebook) | DDC 610.1/4–dc23/eng/20231003
LC record available at https://lccn.loc.gov/2023041642
LC ebook record available at https://lccn.loc.gov/2023041643

Cover Design: Wiley
Cover Image: © Merve Ozkaya/Getty Images

Set in 10/12pt Palatino by Straive, Pondicherry, India

To all my students and patients, for being the best teachers.
Para mis estudiantes y pacientes, por ser quienes mejor nos enseñan.
PO

To Sandra for showing me the meaning of care.
GM

To Mao and Pao Lor.
ML

To my mom.
ASR

Contents

Editor Biographies	xi
Contributor Biographies	xiii
Endorsement	xix
Preface	xxi
Acknowledgments	xxv

Part I Theory, History, and Context: Language in Public Health and Healthcare 1

1 Are We Overlooking Language? An Applied Linguistics Perspective on the Role of Language as a Social Determinant of Health 3
   STEFANIE HARSCH AND MARICEL G. SANTOS

2 Sociolinguistics, Public Health, and Healthcare 25
   DALIA MAGAÑA

3 A Critical Overview of Illness Narratives: Sociolinguistic, Literary, and Graphic Perspectives 43
   ROXANA DELBENE

4 Anthropological Linguistics, Health, and Healthcare 59
   MILENA A. MELO, CARLA PEZZIA, WILLIAM J. ROBERTSON, AND K. JILL FLEURIET

5 Applied Linguistics, Public Health, and Healthcare 77
   HOLLY E. JACOBSON

Part II Language Interpretation and Translation in Public Health and Healthcare 97

6 Recognizing and Addressing Language Discordance 101
   ALLISON SQUIRES

7 The Role of Healthcare Interpreters 117
   ELAINE HSIEH

8 Healthcare Translation for Patients 137
   WIOLETA KARWACKA

9 Health Literacy and Plain Language 155
   SUAD GHADDAR

Part III	**Language Concordance in Public Health and Healthcare**	**175**
10	Language Concordance in Clinical Care ALICIA FERNÁNDEZ AND FRANCINE RÍOS-FETCHKO	179
11	Language Concordance as Interactional Concordance in Multilingual Clinical Consultations CAROLINE H. VICKERS AND RYAN A. GOBLE	189
12	Assessing Clinician Language Skills UTE KNOCH AND JASON FAN	215
13	Setting Standards for Clinician Language Use in Patient Care JOHN D. COWDEN	231
14	Current Gaps and Future Directions in Language Concordance Research and Policy GEORGE S. CORPUZ, DAVID A. CHIRIKIAN, AND LISA C. DIAMOND	255
Part IV	**Pedagogy of Medical Language Education**	**277**
15	Second Language Acquisition for Healthcare Purposes KAROL J. HARDIN	281
16	Centering Translanguaging for Inclusive Health Communication: Implications for Healthcare Professional Education JOSH PRADA AND ROBYN WOODWARD-KRON	305
17	Dedicated Medical Spanish Courses and Crosslinguistic Healthcare Communication Skills MARCO A. ALEMÁN AND ALEJANDRA ZAPIÉN-HIDALGO	325
18	Medical Language Programs to Enhance Engagement with Diverse Communities in the United States and Around the World ROSE L. MOLINA AND JENNIFER KASPER	349
19	Clinical Communication Skills Training in Minoritized Languages CARMEN PÉREZ-MUÑOZ AND TIFFANY M. SHIN	367
20	Faculty Development in Medical Language Education MÓNICA B. VELA AND ADRIANA C. BLACK MOROCOIMA	387
Part V	**Mass Communication and Health: Theory, Research, and Application with and for Linguistically Diverse Populations**	**403**
21	Mass Media and Health Research in, with, and for Linguistically Diverse Populations KATHARINE J. HEAD AND KATHERINE E. RIDLEY-MERRIWEATHER	407
22	Health Information Seeking among Linguistically Diverse Populations in the United States CHRISTINE SWOBODA, PRITI SINGH, A. SUSANA RAMÍREZ, AND NALEEF FAREED	429
23	Entertainment-Education as Linguistic Duality in Practice SURUCHI SOOD AND RACHAEL HAILESELASSE	445
24	Graphic Medicine and Visual Communication Techniques for Public Health and Healthcare in Linguistically Diverse Settings MK CZERWIEC, Q. JANE ZHAO, ISA ÁLVAREZ, AND PILAR ORTEGA	469

25 Social Media and Health in Linguistically Diverse Communities:
   An Examination of Overlooked Populations and Understudied Platforms   493
   ANNA GAYSYNSKY, KATHRYN HELEY, AND WEN-YING SYLVIA CHOU
26 Urgent Communication During Public Health Crises: Reaching
   Linguistically Diverse Populations   511
   VICTORIA LEDFORD, A. SUSANA RAMÍREZ, AND XIAOLI NAN

Glossary   533
Index   541

Editor Biographies

Pilar Ortega, MD, MGM, is Vice President, Diversity, Equity, and Inclusion at the Accreditation Council for Graduate Medical Education and Clinical Associate Professor of Emergency Medicine and Medical Education at the University of Illinois College of Medicine in Chicago, Illinois, United States. Dr. Ortega co-founded the National Association of Medical Spanish and the Medical Organization for Latino Advancement and holds a master's degree in graphic medicine.

Glenn Martínez, PhD, MPH, is Dean of the College of Liberal and Fine Arts and Professor of Spanish, Bicultural/Bilingual Studies, and Public Health at the University of Texas at San Antonio in San Antonio, Texas, United States. Dr. Martínez's research focuses on the sociolinguistics and applied linguistics of Spanish-speaking communities in the United States and along the United States–Mexico border.

Maichou Lor, PhD, RN, is Assistant Professor at the University of Wisconsin-Madison School of Nursing in Madison, Wisconsin, United States. Dr. Lor's research focuses on reducing health disparities through improving health communication between clinicians and patients, specifically patients with low health literacy and/or non-English language preference, beginning with the Hmong population. She is a board member of the National Council on Interpreting in Health Care.

A. Susana Ramírez, PhD, MPH, is Associate Professor of Public Health Communication at the University of California, Merced, in Merced, California, United States. As an infodemiologist, Dr. Ramírez applies communication science to advance public health goals. She is an internationally recognized expert in media, inequality, and health.

Contributor Biographies

Marco A. Alemán, MD, is Professor in the Department of Internal Medicine and Director of CAMPOS (Comprehensive Advanced Medical Program of Spanish) at the University of North Carolina School of Medicine in Chapel Hill, North Carolina, United States.

Isa Álvarez, BA, is a graduate of the University of Chicago in the History, Philosophy, and Social Studies of Science and Medicine (HIPS) with a focus on reproductive health. She is currently a post-baccalaureate pre-medical student at Washington University in St. Louis, Missouri, United States.

Adriana C. Black Morocoima, MPH, MAT, is Director of Health Affairs, Diversity, Equity, and Inclusion at both the Office of the Vice Chancellor for Health Affairs and the Office of the Vice Chancellor for Diversity, Equity, and Engagement at the University of Illinois in Chicago, Illinois, United States.

David A. Chirikian, MS, BS, is a medical student at California Northstate University in Elk Grove, California, United States.

Wen-Ying Sylvia Chou, PhD, MPH, is Program Director in the Health Communication and Informatics Research Branch of the National Cancer Institute, Rockville, Maryland, United States.

George S. Corpuz, BA, BS, is a medical student at Weill Cornell Medicine in New York, New York, United States.

John D. Cowden, MD, MPH, is Professor of Pediatrics and Director of the Culture and Language Coaching Program at Children's Mercy Kansas City, Kansas City, Missouri, United States.

MK Czerwiec, RN, MA, is a nurse, cartoonist, educator, co-founder of the field of graphic medicine, and artist-in-residence in the Department of Medical Humanities & Bioethics at the Feinberg School of Medicine, Northwestern University, Chicago, Illinois, United States.

Roxana Delbene, PhD, DMH, MS, has a doctoral degree in Hispanic linguistics from the University of Pittsburgh, a master's degree in narrative medicine from Columbia University, and recently completed a doctorate in medical humanities from Drew University. She is interested in an interdisciplinary approach to the study of health communication that combines the methodological approaches of sociolinguistics with the medical/health humanities.

Lisa C. Diamond, MD, MPH, is Associate Attending Physician in the Immigrant Health and Cancer Disparities Service of the Departments of Medicine and Psychiatry and Behavioral Sciences and the Hospital Medicine Service of the Department of Medicine at Memorial Sloan Kettering Cancer Center in New York, New York, United States.

Jason Fan, PhD, is Associate Professor, Deputy Director, and Principal Senior Research Fellow at the Language Testing Research Centre (LTRC), University of Melbourne in Melbourne, Australia.

Naleef Fareed, PhD, MBA, is Associate Professor of Biomedical Informatics in the College of Medicine at the Ohio State University, Columbus, Ohio, United States.

Alicia Fernández, MD, is Professor of Medicine and Associate Dean of Population Health and Health Equity at the University of California, San Francisco (UCSF) School of Medicine. She is the Founding Director of the UCSF Latinx Center of Excellence and directs the Latinx and Immigrant Health Research Program at the UCSF Center for Vulnerable Populations in San Francisco, California, United States.

K. Jill Fleuriet, PhD, is Professor of Anthropology and Associate Dean for Faculty Success in the College of Liberal and Fine Arts at the University of Texas at San Antonio, in San Antonio, Texas, United States.

Anna Gaysynsky, MPH, is Senior Communications Specialist at ICF Next. In that role, she provides support to the Health Communication and Informatics Research Branch of the National Cancer Institute, Rockville, Maryland, United States.

Suad Ghaddar, PhD, is Assistant Professor in the Department of Health and Biomedical Sciences, College of Health Professions, University of Texas Río Grande Valley, in Edinburg, Texas, United States. Her research centers on understanding the causal pathways through which health literacy contributes to health disparities in minoritized Texas-Mexico border communities.

Ryan A. Goble, PhD, is Academic Program Specialist and the Wisconsin Intensive Summer Language Institutes (WISLI) coordinator for the South Asia Summer Language Institute (SASLI) and the Less Commonly Taught Languages Career Fair in the Language Program Office at the University of Wisconsin-Madison Language Institute in Madison, Wisconsin, United States.

Rachael HaileSelasse, MA, is a doctoral student in the Department of Community Health and Prevention at the Dornsife School of Public Health, Drexel University, Philadelphia, Pennsylvania, United States.

Karol J. Hardin, PhD, is Professor of Spanish in the Department of Modern Languages and Cultures, Director of Spanish for Health Professions, and Affiliated Faculty in the Department of Medical Humanities at Baylor University in Waco, Texas, United States.

Stefanie Harsch, PhD, is a postdoctoral scholar at the University Freiburg, conducts health literacy research and intervention projects worldwide, such as in Afghanistan, Germany, and sub-Saharan Africa. As an adult educator, health educator, and second language trainer, she enjoys working with migrants, adults with low literacy skills, and cancer patients to improve their agency and health.

Katharine J. Head, PhD, is Associate Professor in the Department of Communication Studies and Director of the PhD Graduate Program in Health Communication at Indiana University-Purdue University, Indianapolis, Indiana, United States.

Kathryn Heley, PhD, MPH, is Cancer Prevention Fellow in the Health Communication and Informatics Research Branch of the National Cancer Institute, Rockville, Maryland, United States.

Elaine Hsieh, PhD, JD, is Professor and Chair of the Department of Communication Studies, University of Minnesota-Twin Cities, in Minneapolis, Minnesota, United States. An award-winning author, Fulbright Scholar, and National Institutes of Health (NIH)-funded researcher, Dr. Hsieh has published extensively to examine the intersections of culture, language, health, and medicine in interpersonal and cross-cultural contexts.

Holly E. Jacobson, PhD, is Associate Professor of Linguistics at the University of New Mexico in Albuquerque, New Mexico, United States. Her research focuses on health discourse, intercultural communication in healthcare settings, and health literacy. She has contributed to quantitative and qualitative studies exploring language and health funded by private, state, and federal agencies, including the National Institutes of Health (NIH). She has been an NIH Senior Research Fellow at the National Institutes on Minority Health and Health Disparities (NIMHD). Dr. Jacobson has geared her research agenda toward advancing our understanding of language as a social determinant of health.

Wioleta Karwacka, PhD, is Translator and Assistant Professor at the Division of Translation Studies, University of Gdańsk, Poland. Her research focuses on medical translation and eco-translation. She has authored articles, book chapters, and conference papers on various aspects of medical translation and medical terminology.

Jennifer Kasper, MD, MPH, is Assistant Professor of Pediatrics and Global Health and Social Medicine and Chair of the Faculty Advisory Committee on Global Health at Harvard Medical School in Boston, Massachusetts, Unted States. She also serves on the President's Council of Doctors for Global Health.

Ute Knoch, PhD, is Director of the Language Testing Research Centre at the University of Melbourne in Melbourne, Australia.

Victoria Ledford, PhD, is Assistant Professor in the School of Communication and Journalism at Auburn University in Auburn, Alabama, United States.

Dalia Magaña, PhD, is Associate Professor of Spanish Linguistics at the University of California, Merced in Merced, California, United States. Her research focuses on improving healthcare communication with Spanish speakers and developing intentional language pedagogy.

Milena A. Melo, PhD, is Assistant Professor of Anthropology at the University of Texas Río Grande Valley in Edinburg, Texas, United States.

Rose L. Molina, MD, MPH, is Lawrence Director of Professionalism, Humanism, and Health Equity, Medical Language Program Director, and Assistant Professor of Obstetrics, Gynecology, and Reproductive Biology at Harvard Medical School in Boston, Massachusetts, United States.

Xiaoli Nan, PhD, is a Distinguished Scholar-Teacher and Professor of Communication Science at the University of Maryland, College Park, Maryland, United States, where she directs the Center for Health and Risk Communication.

Carmen Pérez-Muñoz, PhD, is Assistant Teaching Professor in the Department of Spanish at Wake Forest University and Associate Director of the MAESTRO (Medical Applied Education in Spanish through Training, Resources, and Overlearning) Program at Wake Forest School of Medicine in Winston-Salem, North Carolina, United States.

Carla Pezzia, PhD, is Associate Professor of Global Health and Health Disparities in the Department of Biology at the University of Dallas in Dallas, Texas, United States.

Josh Prada, PhD, is Assistant Professor of Applied Linguistics and Multilingualism in the Center for Language and Cognition at the University of Groningen in Groningen, the Netherlands.

Katherine E. Ridley-Merriweather, PhD, is Communication, Recruitment, and Outreach Manager of the Biospecimen Collection and Banking Core at the Indiana University Simon Comprehensive Cancer Center, Indianapolis, Indiana, United States.

Francine Ríos-Fetchko, BA, is Research Data Analyst at the University of California, San Francisco Latinx Center of Excellence in San Francisco, California, United States.

William J. Robertson, PhD, is Assistant Professor of Anthropology at the University of Memphis in Memphis, Tennessee, United States.

Maricel G. Santos, PhD, is Professor of English at San Francisco State University in San Francisco, California, United States. Dr. Santos explores the role of adult learners as change agents in health equity work. She was a 2008–2013 Fellow with the Research Infrastructure in Minority Institutions (RIMI) program, National Center for Minority Health and Health Disparities, National Institutes of Health.

Tiffany M. Shin, MD, is Assistant Professor in the Department of Pediatrics and director of the MAESTRO (Medical Applied Education in Spanish through Training, Resources, and Overlearning) Program at Wake Forest School of Medicine in Winston-Salem, North Carolina, United States.

Priti Singh, PhD, is a postdoctoral scholar at the Ohio State University, Columbus, Ohio, United States.

Suruchi Sood, PhD, is Director of Communication Science at the Johns Hopkins Center for Communication Programs, Baltimore, Maryland, United States.

Allison Squires, PhD, RN, FAAN, is Associate Professor and Director of the Global Consortium for Nursing and Midwifery Studies (www.gcnms.org) at New York University's Rory Meyers College of Nursing, New York, United States. Her domestic line of research focuses on improving health services for immigrant populations.

Christine Swoboda, PhD, MS, is a research scientist in the Department of Family and Community Medicine in the College of Medicine at The Ohio State University, Columbus, Ohio, United States.

Mónica B. Vela, MD, is Professor of Medicine in the Department of Medicine and the Department of Medical Education and Director of the Hispanic Center of Excellence at the University of Illinois College of Medicine in Chicago, Illinois, United States. She is also Associate Editor at the *Journal of the American Medical Association Network Open*.

Caroline H. Vickers, PhD, is Professor in the Department of English and Associate Dean of Graduate Studies at California State University, San Bernardino, California, United States.

Robyn Woodward-Kron, PhD, is Professor of Healthcare Communication and Director of Research and Research Training in the Department of Medical Education at Melbourne Medical School in Melbourne, Australia.

Alejandra Zapién-Hidalgo, MD, MPH, is Assistant Professor of Family and Community Medicine and Director of the Bilingual Medical Spanish and Distinction Track at the University of Arizona Health Sciences College of Medicine in Tucson, Arizona, United States.

Q. Jane Zhao, MSc, is a medical researcher, health policy PhD student at the University of Toronto, graduate of the Narrative Medicine master's degree from Columbia University, and burgeoning cartoonist based in Toronto, Canada.

At its very core, the delivery of equitable healthcare is centered on the paramount importance of the exchange of correct information via language concordance – including the language nuances, customs, and cultural meanings that add to the subtext of the conversation. This handbook offers a comprehensive analysis with well-written chapters that function as guidepost for such. The authors have done their diligence in identifying gaps with language incongruence and offer thoughtful frameworks on how best to enhance our current healthcare system and how best to prepare the next generation of healthcare workers. Each chapter reviews and distills what has been studied on relevant and important related topics. Collectively, the chapters in this handbook answer the call of a national imperative: As our population demographics continue to change, healthcare workers will be required to think differently in a pluralistic-facing society that is more than ever, multilingual and multicultural.

Antonia Coello Novello, MD, MPH, DrPH

Preface

What happens when an infodemiologist-public health expert, a nurse-scientist, a language professor-dean, and a physician-educator enter a videoconference? In our case, the outcome was this volume, *The Handbook of Language, Public Health and Healthcare*. Bringing together interdisciplinary voices and international perspectives, our collaboration has yielded what we hope will be a useful reference for scholars across the many fields of study that are impacted by and explore the impact of language and health.

The Handbook of Language in Public Health and Healthcare provides a comprehensive overview of the theory, history, and leading research pertaining to language and health. This volume uniquely addresses interprofessional topics related to the theory, linguistic analysis, education, assessment, clinical application, and public health implications of language in health. Authors explore both individual patient-clinician encounters and also look beyond the examination room to explore systemic issues in healthcare, education, and society. Importantly, the book relies on the perspectives of a diverse group of contributing authors and editors, whose collective expertise spans multiple continents and numerous professional domains, including linguistics, sociology, medicine, nursing, interpreting, and translation, among others.

This *Handbook* is organized in five sections. We have divided the book into sections that, first, provide a theoretical framework for the field of language and healthcare (Part I), and then more deeply explore focused ways in which the field has evolved. These areas include interpreting and translation (Part II), patient-clinician language concordance (Part III), the pedagogy of medical language education to enhance language-appropriate care (Part IV), and mass communication (Part V).

In Part I, edited by Glenn Martínez, we begin by providing a broad overview of theory, history, and context of linguistics in public health and healthcare. An introductory chapter by Stefanie Harsch and Maricel Santos traces independent developments in linguistics and public health that have resulted in the intersections of language, population health, and healthcare. Four additional chapters flesh out key theoretical concepts and demonstrate their application to the interdisciplinary understanding of language, health, and healthcare. Chapter 2 focuses on sociolinguistics as a key methodological approach for understanding language in healthcare in Spanish-speaking populations in the United States. Chapter 3 focuses on pragmatics and narrative theory as a methodological source for understanding illness narratives with a focus on Latin America and Spain. In Chapter 4, Milena Melo, Carla Pezzia, William Robertson, and Jill

Fleuriet draw on anthropological linguistic methods to explore health in border regions. Drawing on the theorizations of Bruno Latour, they apply border theory to case studies from the Texas-Mexico borderlands, the Guatemalan Highlands, and Chicago. Finally, Holly Jacobson provides theoretical insights at the intersection of applied linguistics, sociolinguistics, and anthropological linguistics, and the relevance of that intersection on public health.

Part II, edited by Maichou Lor, examines language interpretation and translation in public health and healthcare. In this section, we present evidence for the benefits and proper use of strategies to facilitate communication with linguistically diverse populations in language discordant scenarios. The section begins with a discussion on key issues that contribute to language-discordant situations in healthcare settings and an overview of the strategies to address the communication needs of linguistically diverse groups. Each subsequent chapter focuses on a specific strategy. In Chapter 6, Allison Squires provides a brief history of medical interpreting and methods for identifying linguistically diverse patients who would benefit from language assistance in healthcare settings. In Chapter 7, Elain Hsieh presents the different types of medical interpreting and the roles of medical interpreters in healthcare delivery, and synthesizes the impact of distinct types of medical interpreting on patient outcomes. Chapter 8 focuses on the translation of healthcare information to patients. Wioleta Karwacka emphasizes the translation of medical instructions for linguistically diverse patients across the care continuum. The section concludes with a chapter on health literacy. In Chapter 9, Suad Ghaddar provides an overview of health literacy in linguistically diverse patients, including existing clinical health literacy assessments. Efforts to improve health literacy among linguistically diverse populations, including plain language and other interventions, are also reviewed.

In Part III, edited by Pilar Ortega and Glenn Martínez, we focus on language concordance in public health and healthcare. We begin by describing language concordance and the competent use of language skills in healthcare settings. In Chapter 10, Alicia Fernández and Francine Ríos-Fetchko present a conceptual framework for how the term language concordance has historically been applied in healthcare and analyze how researchers currently identify whether a clinical encounter is language-concordant or -discordant. In Chapter 11, Caroline Vickers and Ryan Goble deconstruct what is meant by language concordance and challenge existing perspectives that normalize monolingualism and view multilingualism as foreign or "other." In Chapter 12, Ute Knoch and Jason Fan discuss tools for assessing clinicians' communication skills in a language different from that of their medical training, paying special attention to how evaluating language proficiency for clinical contexts differs from general language proficiency tools, how instruments should be validated for this purpose, and standard-setting for passing thresholds. Next, John Cowden further explores the concept of setting standards for clinician practice in multiple languages in Chapter 13, including issues related to existing proficiency examinations, self-assessment options, and considerations for progressive review of skills and maintenance of certification. The section concludes with Chapter 14 in which George Corpuz, David Chirikian, and Lisa Diamond identify current gaps in language concordance work and outline the types of research needed to advance the field.

Part IV of the Handbook, edited by Pilar Ortega, turns to the pedagogy of medical language education. The section begins with a discussion of medical language learners: Who are they, and what are their language education needs? In Chapter 15, Karol Hardin presents a linguistic perspective on pedagogy for second language acquisition for healthcare purposes and addresses issues in distinguishing learner proficiency level in healthcare language courses. The next chapter addresses individuals with multilingual skills. In Chapter 16, Josh Prada and Robyn Woodward-Kron define the concept of heritage learner and discuss the relevance of this population of learners in the medical language classroom. In addition, this chapter reviews evidence for the incorporation of translanguaging into medical language pedagogy. In Chapter 17, Marco Alemán and Alejandra Zapién-Hidalgo focus on medical Spanish education and the similarities and differences between educational initiatives that target specific competencies in medical Spanish compared to those that target more general cross-linguistic such as caring for minoritized communities of any language and determining one's limitations in a particular language. In Chapter 18, Rose Molina and Jennifer Kasper share examples of medical language programs in multiple languages, with a focus on international partnerships and global impact. Carmen Pérez-Muñoz and Tiffany Shin then present an overview of guidance on teaching clinical skills for communicating with patients who prefer non-dominant languages in Chapter 19. They describe how to create medical language programs that focus on patient needs and are institutionally structured in a way that promotes program sustainability and effectiveness. The section ends with a focus on faculty development. In Chapter 20, Mónica Vela and Adriana Black Morocoima describe issues in faculty development and institutional leadership for developing and teaching medical language courses.

In the fifth and final section of the Handbook, Part V, edited by Susana Ramírez, we move beyond the clinical setting to examine the global health information environment and consider the role played by the mass media in communicating health information to linguistically diverse populations. We begin this section with a historical perspective on mass communication in health. In Chapter 21, Katharine J. Head and Katherine Ridley-Merriweather trace the development of mediated interventions for public health in the context of communicable disease prevention, the shift to considering the influence of the information environment on patients' knowledge and behaviors, through the current focus on information seeking behaviors and misinformation effects. In Chapter 22, Christine Swoboda, Priti Singh, Susana Ramírez, and Naleef Fareed present a conceptual framework to examine critical issues in health information seeking behaviors and outcomes among linguistically diverse populations. In Chapter 23, Suruchi Sood and Rachael HaileSelasse explore the dynamic relationship between linguistic diversity and entertainment-education strategies that promote social and behavioral change. They briefly review the modern histories and definitions of both linguistic diversity and entertainment-education, describing the organic cross-influence between the two disciplines. Intervention examples from the field illustrate current practices and provide overall guidance on ways to integrate linguistic diversity and entertainment-education. Chapter 24 specifically explores the use of graphic medicine (comics) as a strategy for communicating with linguistically diverse populations. MK Czerwiec, Jane Zhao, Isa Álvarez, and Pilar Ortega situate the emergence of graphic medicine within the context of narrative medicine, sharing examples of comics developed for health education and then proposing graphic medicine as a tool to improve public health messaging, patient-clinician communication, and clinician wellness among healthcare students and professionals from linguistically diverse backgrounds. Chapter 25 examines the health implications of social media use. Anna Gaysynsky, Katherine Heley, and Sylvia Chou discuss the importance of studying social media use in linguistically diverse populations, highlight the potential benefits and harms of social media use for these populations, and outline future directions for research and practice. This section closes with a reflection on communication during times of public health crises. In Chapter 26, Victoria Ledford, Susana Ramírez, and Xiaoli Nan present COVID-19 as a case study highlighting the urgent need for effective communication to linguistically diverse populations especially in situations of public health crises.

In addition to the substantive chapters, we provide a glossary of essential terms in the study and practice of language in public health and healthcare. Most of the glossary terms are used throughout the volume. In some cases, we have included some terms in the glossary that we consider problematic and have intentionally avoided throughout the Handbook. In the glossary, we provide a description and rationale for why we recommend avoiding certain terms or usages and propose alternatives.

The Handbook for Language in Public Health and Healthcare's innovative approach was made possible thanks to the contributions of an interdisciplinary group of scholars with a *depth* and *breadth* of professional and personal perspectives in language, health, and healthcare. In addressing theory, history, and practice as related to patient-clinician communication, education, assessment, research, and mass public health communication about language, we not only discuss issues and gaps but also present actionable strategies that have the potential to improve the health and healthcare of linguistically diverse populations worldwide.

Acknowledgments

We thank Valerie Burnett for her assistance with developing the glossary.

Part I Theory, History, and Context: Language in Public Health and Healthcare

Introduction to Part I

Glenn Martínez

This section opens a window on multiple interactions and interstices between the scientific study of language, healthcare, and public health. The goal of the section is to demonstrate how a variety of approaches within the fields of linguistics and applied linguistics have interacted with healthcare and public health and to shed light on the ways in which theoretical approaches to language inform and enrich public health and healthcare practices. Many of the themes discussed in this section including health literacy, graphic medicine, the social determinants of health, and language concordance will be treated more fully in later sections of this volume. The present section seeks to highlight the ways in which linguistics and applied linguistics interact with and inform these themes.

The section opens with Chapter 1 by Stefanie Harsch-Oria and Maricel Santos. In this chapter, Harsch-Oria and Santos provide an applied linguistics perspective on language in public health and healthcare with a focus on two key areas of focus: language as a social determinant of health and health literacy. The authors approach these two focus areas from the optic of language teachers in adult education settings. This framing allows the authors to peel back the often unstated assumptions about language that are settled into health literacy and language as a social determinant of health research and practice. The authors conclude by exposing six myths about language and healthcare while at the same time exemplifying the underlying theoretical perspectives of applied linguistic scholarship.

Chapter 2 reviews sociolinguistic studies that shed light on language, public health, and healthcare. After introducing the field of sociolinguistics and its turn from a focus

---

The Handbook of Language in Public Health and Healthcare, First Edition.
Edited by Pilar Ortega, Glenn Martínez, Maichou Lor, and A. Susana Ramírez.
© 2024 John Wiley & Sons, Inc. Published 2024 by John Wiley & Sons, Inc.

on distribution to a focus on mobility, Dalia Magaña shows how sociolinguistic research informs efforts to promote health equity with a particular focus on Spanish-speaking communities in the United States. Her approach covers issues related to languages in contact during the clinical encounter, the role of language in COVID-19 health communication, and issues around language access in the wider health delivery system. The chapter concludes by offering practical advice for working against language prestige, promoting local language, and creating more equitable healthcare for minoritized language speakers.

Chapter 3 extends the focus on sociolinguistics to the analysis of illness narratives across multiple genres including oral, written, and graphic. Roxana Delbene draws on theoretical insights from sociolinguistics, literary studies, and graphic medicine to shed light on our understanding of illness narratives as they emerge in their local context and as they circulate in different contexts. She begins by tracing the development of thinking around illness narratives and pointing out different traditions rooted in testimonial narrative and pathography. She proposes a communicative-oriented view of illness narratives that considers the target audience, the message, and the communicative intent in order to glean the intrinsic value of each genre. Her approach draws on the key applied linguistics notion of communicative affordances as a way of grasping the import of illness narratives across traditions.

Chapter 4 provides a linguistic anthropological lens to language, public health, and healthcare to shed light on bordering and debordering practices in health through a multiple case study approach. Melo, Fleuriet, Pezzia, and Robertson contend that language is a key operator in boundary-making and that geopolitical, social, political, and economic borders are made and remade through linguistic practice. Using three case studies focusing on undocumented patients with end-stage renal disease in South Texas, indigenous Maya struggling with addiction in the Guatemala highlands, and LGBTQ patients with anal cancer in Chicago, the authors draw on Bruno Latour's bordering theory to highlight the role of performative, communicative practices in healthcare settings in reinscribing, rejecting and creating boundaries between people, objects and bodily conditions that shape health and healthcare experiences.

Finally, Chapter 5 brings an applied linguistics perspective to key issues in public health and healthcare such as health literacy and plain language. Holly Jacobson traces the history of applied linguistic incursions into public health and outlines the various methodologies that have borne fruit in this endeavor. The chapter highlights the contributions of conversational analysis, interactional sociolinguistics, discourse analysis, first and second language acquisition, and text and genre analysis to these efforts. Together, these five chapters lay out key theoretical insights that inform the intersection of language, public health, and healthcare. Applied linguistics, sociolinguistics, and anthropological linguistics have a long history of engagement with public health and healthcare. In this section, readers will appreciate this history of engagement and glean the theoretical insights that enrich our understanding of language in public health and healthcare.

1 Are We Overlooking Language? An Applied Linguistics Perspective on the Role of Language as a Social Determinant of Health

STEFANIE HARSCH
AND MARICEL G. SANTOS

Introduction

In this chapter, we examine the power of language in healthcare and public health communication from our perspective as applied linguists and language educators. We begin by recalling the words of linguist James Gee, "In socially situated language use one must simultaneously say the "right" thing, do the "right" thing, and in such saying and doing also express the "right" beliefs, values, and attitudes" [1] (p. 168). Without a doubt, understanding the socially situated expectations of language use in the healthcare context is essential to our ability as patients and caregivers to advocate for ourselves and navigate healthcare systems. Language can contribute to both healing and harm: our ability to understand our healthcare options and access quality care lies, in part, on our ability to engage in productive, meaningful conversations with clinical providers. We are especially concerned that the lack of understanding about language can lead to dangerous assumptions about language users, including minoritized groups that do not speak the dominant language of the healthcare system.

In this chapter, we invite you to explore the complexities of language, and in so doing, to consider new possibilities for the way we communicate and interact in healthcare settings. We hope that exploring applied linguists' views on language in healthcare is akin to trying out a new pair of glasses. While we do not claim that the glasses of applied linguistics offer the only or best perspectives, we argue that they can help to sharpen our view of language use and communication in health and public health settings with linguistically minoritized groups, including migrant and refugee communities.

The Handbook of Language in Public Health and Healthcare, First Edition.
Edited by Pilar Ortega, Glenn Martínez, Maichou Lor, and A. Susana Ramírez.
© 2024 John Wiley & Sons, Inc. Published 2024 by John Wiley & Sons, Inc.

We begin this chapter by sharing a bit about ourselves as applied linguists to provide context for our thinking about language in healthcare. We then address two areas of scholarship – social determinants of health and health literacy (HL) – to highlight how research can challenge and at times reinforce deficit assumptions on language and language users. We also show how debates in these areas reveal competing views on language – as an individual trait versus a social phenomenon – which has implications for the way we think about the underlying causes of health outcomes. The heart of our chapter is organized around six persistent assumptions (we will refer to them as myths) about language and language users that arguably make it hard for applied linguists and clinical/public health researchers to find common ground. Interdisciplinary collaboration is vital to tackling health disparities [2–4], but without shared background knowledge on language, language use, and language communities, potential collaborators are not likely to understand each other or readily agree on intervention priorities. We hope this chapter provides readers with an opportunity to fuel their curiosity and reflection about language, with the ultimate goal of supporting stronger interdisciplinary collaborations that promote health equity in multilingual communities.

Who we are

Our insights are anchored in nearly three decades of experience working in community-based adult language education, as classroom teachers, teacher trainers, and HL experts, primarily in the United States and Germany. We work in a variety of settings that serve large numbers of immigrant and refugee adults, including community centers, church basements, public schools, workplaces, or public libraries. These settings have proven to be strategic venues to work with immigrant and refugee communities who are often considered hard to reach [5, 6]. While there are important differences in funding structures and enrollment requirements between Germany and the United States, a common denominator is that programs are organized in response to local identities and integration needs in a particular country, region, or locale [7, 8].

Additionally, we focus on adult learners, and thus our pedagogical mandate is to ensure a strong connection between classroom learning and adults' real-world communicative needs. As we highlight throughout this chapter, adult learners' everyday healthcare needs and experiences represent an essential contextual resource for planning language teaching and learning: the significance of this contextualized approach, indeed, distinguishes adult learning from child learning [9]. We are particularly passionate about working with adult language learners who are in the process of becoming print-literate and have completed little-to-no formal education, a relatively understudied sector of the adult learner population both in applied linguistics and public health [10, 11]. For this population, a contextualized approach is imperative as it can reveal areas of learner competence and social practice that do not show up in conventional measures of proficiency, such as vocabulary or reading tests. We strongly identify as teachers who view people's efforts to stay well and live well as *a lifelong learning process* that builds on what we learn in formal classrooms, in informal (everyday) settings (e.g., navigating a patient portal on our laptop while sitting at our kitchen table), and through social interaction.

Based on our classroom work with immigrant and refugee learners, we argue that it is unproductive to treat language learning and HL learning as separate domains [12]. We also worry that this false divide assumes that adult learners can simply absorb new skills, practices, and knowledge with little attention to the role that language and context play in meaning-making processes [13]. An alternative view sees learning as arising from the "sum of all interactions" [14] across contexts (classrooms, clinics, communities, etc.). From this view, all of us (whether we work in applied linguistics or health) play a role in the way our learners/patients make meaning. We all bear responsibility for understanding the linguistic demands of our healthcare systems and addressing sources of linguistic inequities.

In sum, we have seen first-hand that critical interrogation of the linguistic demands of healthcare language opens new possibilities for interventions aimed at dismantling linguistic inequities in healthcare. Some readers may wonder, *hold on, are you asking healthcare professionals to think like an applied linguist or even a language teacher?* Clearly, healthcare providers rightfully must consider themselves first and foremost in the role of protecting and maintaining good health [15]. At the same time, when we say we want our patients to understand their healthcare choices, what do we really mean? Clearly, our expectations for "understanding" extend beyond simply the patient "doing" a healthcare task or "knowing about" the task. Understanding is an active process of meaning-making, and the role of language as the medium for that meaning-making cannot be ignored [13, 16]. Critical reflection on the linguistic demands of healthcare has prepared us to integrate health topics and healthcare navigation skills into our classroom teaching. With this chapter, we signal our hope that practitioners across disciplines view this kind of critical praxis as a collectively owned responsibility.

Exploring perspectives on language and health

We now turn our attention to perspectives on language and health in two research domains: the work on social determinants of health, and the work in HL. These domains have helped to shape the conceptualization of language in healthcare, at times helping to bring complexity to the linguistic demands of our healthcare systems, and other times reinforcing narrow views on language and language users.

Language as a social determinant of health

Understanding the link between language and health relies on an understanding of health and the factors that contribute to differences in people's health outcomes. According to the World Health Organization (WHO), "health is a state of complete physical, mental, and social well-being and not merely the absence of diseases and infirmity" [17]. This definition of health is both comprehensive and radical as it aims for complete well-being. Using this definition as the ultimate goal, we immediately notice that people's health status worldwide is far from "complete" and moreover, there are immense differences in health status, and certain groups are worse off than others. The reasons for these differences are manifold and lie in the genetic makeup of the individual person, the individual health behavior, but also the life context of respective social and environmental determinants of health [18]. The social and environmental determinants of health are all nonmedical influences on health such as income, education, housing, social inclusion, and structural barriers and opportunities. The United States Department of Health and Human Services (HHS) defines social determinants of health (SDOH) as "the conditions in the environment where people are born, live, learn, work, play, worship, and age that affect a wide range of health, functioning, and quality-of-life outcomes and risks." [19]. Although genetics and health behavior play a role in health, long-term studies showed that two-thirds or even three-quarters of all health differences between people are due to social determinants of health [20, 21].

While the WHO has long acknowledged the role of contextual factors in health outcomes (e.g., as prerequisites of health in the Ottawa Charter [18]), Michael Marmot's studies on health inequalities initiated the specific focus on the various social determinants of health [22]. The WHO Commission on Social Determinants of Health does not list language or literacy as separate determinants but stresses their important role in education, early childhood development, and understanding the healthcare needs of indigenous peoples and other minoritized groups [23]. The United States HHS, however, gives language and literacy skills a more prominent role and considers them part of the SDOH "education access and quality" [19].

This prominent role of SDOH in health challenges us to look not only at a person's physical constitution and behavior but also at the dynamic interaction with various sociodemographic characteristics, such as language background or communication skills. The SDOH framework prompts us not to exclusively focus on a patient's language skills but also on the conditions that enable or constrain the deployment of those skills. The focus on SDOHs also challenges us to reconsider the ways we develop these language skills in informal and formal learning settings and how we can ensure equitable access to learning resources and opportunities for linguistically minoritized children and adults.

But what then do we know about the relationship between language and health? Empirical evidence points to various concrete examples here, such as research on language concordance, that is, when a patient and the healthcare provider speak the same language and/or share the same linguistic resources. Language concordance has been shown to lead to greater trust, patient questions, and shared decision-making, as well as better quality of care and less confusion and frustration [24–26]. Studies also report that people labeled as "limited English proficient" are less likely to receive adequate treatment and preventive health services, have lower vaccination rates, are less likely to participate in health-promoting activities, have more extended hospital stays, and have less often a full informed consent documentation [27–31]. These examples show how language and literacy are fundamental in health communication, decision-making processes, behavior, and consequently health outcomes. To improve health and health communication, one can therefore either focus on an outcome and develop interventions geared at bringing about that outcome, or one can focus on the antecedent "upstream" conditions – the social determinants of health – that foundationally constrain or support well-being.

Given the pervasive influence of language, researchers label language a "super social determinant of health" [3]. Despite this undeniable great influence, we argue that at least three further thoughts are necessary to be taken into account. First, these results are often based on linear association and neglect other factors that can mediate or moderate this association, for example, language preferences, use, and intersubjective processes [3]. Second, these findings rarely analyze the status quo and discuss whether it is fair and equal or whether it contributes to the reproduction of these inequalities and work counter to our best efforts to intervene. And third, the social determinants of health perspective even challenge us to ask how society and educational offers can be used to avoid these preventable health disparities from occurring.

Views on language in health literacy research

In 2004, a seminal report, *Health Literacy: A Prescription to End Confusion*, defined health literacy (HL) as "the degree to which individuals have the capacity to obtain, process, and understand basic health information and services needed to make appropriate health decisions" [32]. In HL research, language has often been regarded as the key barrier to an individual's ability to function in these critical areas of healthcare navigation, which in turn can impact the quality of the health communication, treatment, and health outcomes [33, 34]. Further, the coupling of "linguistic minority status" with low HL is tied to a sizable empirical base [12, 35, 36]. Linguistically minoritized groups, newcomer groups, and people speaking another language than the prioritized language tend to be associated with lower HL levels, poor health outcomes, and inadequate comprehension of health knowledge [37].

Language and literacy scholars have rejected the conflation of "low literacy" with people's intelligence, educational potential, or quality of life, emphasizing that any evaluation of a learner's skills cannot be separated from the social meanings and values placed on specific language and literacy practices [38, 39]. The social view on literacy emphasizes the language experiences and needs of people and communities in real-world contexts of use, a paradigmatic shift that has contributed to new thinking in many areas, such as the role of language education in schools, the assessment of proficiency, debates about linguistic norms and standards, specialized uses of language in acts of translation/interpretation, to the protection of disappearing languages, as well as the interrogation of monolingual biases in the assessment of language-related disabilities [40–47].

Over the past several decades, significant amounts of research have focused on the measurement of HL levels, and the association between low HL levels and poor health outcomes [48–54], but relatively less on exploring the contexts of use and the meaning-making strategies used by individuals with low print literacy or beginning English skills (e.g., seeking out help from others), their sources of resilience, and problem-solving skills [55–57]. This latter micro-view has been described as the *social practice view on health literacy* [58–60], "a framework for understanding how the social contexts, purposes shape health literacy skills, and relationships within which reading, writing, math, or speaking skills are put to use" [59]. This social view does not discount the importance of an individual's language and literacy skillset but rather emphasizes what multilinguals actually *do* with language in specific healthcare contexts; moreover, the social view seeks to understand how our ability to be well and live well is a function of the quality of our social connections with our healthcare system and providers.

Healthcare providers and public health specialists have endeavored to compensate for low HL by focusing on improving language access: for example, such as providing interpreters and language mediators, and translating material into migrants' and minorities' languages [33, 61–63]. These strategies are effective in enabling people to better access health information, but they often fail to account fully for the social conditions that enable people to feel safe, welcomed, and heard in their healthcare encounters. In this regard, Don Nutbeam's three-part HL framework usefully accounts for ways that individuals access health information (functional HL), as well as their ability to manage communication with different kinds of healthcare providers (interactive HL), and their ability to use their skills to problem-solve and advocate for themselves (critical HL) [64].

Despite the existence of policies regulating access to interpreters and translated materials, we see the need for more attention to linguistic encounters in healthcare; in other words, the healthcare contexts in which language is put to use such as when bilingual patients interact with monolingual providers, or when bilingual patients work across languages to make sense of oral and written health information. We see the need for greater curiosity about the ways that HL is a translingual competence, referring to the ways that multilinguals routinely draw on knowledge and skills across languages to navigate our healthcare system [65–67]. Accordingly, we also see value in re-thinking HL within the sociolinguistic realities of particular countries (e.g., as a monolingual or multilingual country, a country with one or multiple dominant languages). For example, while English is the major and dominant language in the healthcare sector in the United States, other countries use two or more languages in healthcare encounters (e.g., English, Swahili, and local languages in Kenya). Moreover, while written health information is very relevant in the United States, oral communication of health information (e.g., through community health workers or radio) can be of far greater importance in countries with high illiteracy rates, such as Afghanistan.

We value the scholarly work on social determinants of health and HL that has elevated awareness of the linguistic demands of healthcare. We also suggest that insights from applied linguistics can offer some course-correcting commentary on the characterizations of language itself and language users from minoritized backgrounds. If we are to take seriously the premise that language shapes health outcomes, we (regardless of discipline) will need to develop a deeper awareness and knowledge base about the role of language in healthcare and health communication.

Re-thinking six myths about language in healthcare

Reflecting on our decades of interdisciplinary work as adult educators, we have selected six popular myths about language in healthcare and public health debates. For each myth, we present empirical evidence and ideas of how language teaching responds to these challenges and introduce concepts that are already long-established in applied linguistics but have yet to gain ground in healthcare and public health. We apply the concepts and insights to healthcare and public health contexts and thus demonstrate the practical implications of interdisciplinary research and action. By unpacking these myths, we hope to help practitioners in applied linguistics, healthcare, and public health (re)discover the contributions of each discipline to health equity and renew their commitment to interdisciplinary work.

One note of caution: we have somewhat exaggerated the myths to illustrate the different approaches in applied linguistics as distinguished from public health. We also acknowledge that many health professionals do not hold these assumptions in the strongest terms and that there is a wide spectrum between the myth and the path taken in language teaching and health communication. Through this exaggeration, we would like to raise awareness of the inadequacy of these myths and invite you to discover alternative approaches and apply them in your everyday professional life.

Myth #1: Migrants and people with low literacy will always have low language and health literacy levels

We begin by examining the frequent characterization of language and literacy levels, and by extension, HL levels, in migrant communities as "low" [6]. Concerns about inadequate skill levels prompt efforts to adapt the language, involve a translator if necessary, and make communication as easy as possible [63]. These well-intentioned responses often perpetuate the assumption that "low-skilled" is an immutable characteristic of migrants and people who do not speak the dominant language. This assumption can obscure the fact language and literacy skills shift across the lifespan, and language and literacy learning are lifelong enterprises [68]. This myth can be found in public health reports, such as the WHO report "health literacy solid facts" that states that "[m]igrants generally score lower on literacy and health literacy measures" [37] or the Robert Koch Report on women's health that reports lower HL for migrant women [69]. In addition, the reliance on cross-sectional studies of HL makes it hard to appreciate how our HL skills evolve as we age and experience different healthcare circumstances [60].

In our classrooms, we strive to embrace a lifelong learning perspective on skill development [70]. We work with language learners whose skills dynamically emerge as they experience and engage with new situations for using language, for example, at work, in healthcare, and in their children's schools [60, 71]. Two examples derived from German-as-a-second-language courses focused on literacy acquisition illustrate this development. A female student of Iraqi origin was working on improving her vocabulary related to health and children because she was strongly motivated to take care of her children. In another course, two students of Syrian origin approached us to make a phone call to the family doctor; instead of calling for them, we practiced common communication patterns when calling a doctor. The student called the doctor on her own, on speakerphone, so that the teacher could support if necessary. The learner was all smiles when she successfully made the call and later supported other students to make calls themselves.

The "low-skilled" attribution often fails to reveal the multifaceted nature of language development, referring to the idea that learners need to be competent with an increasingly complex array of modalities (spoken, written, digital, visual, audio, gestural, and spatial) for different communicative purposes and audiences (e.g., describing symptoms to a nurse in a clinic visit, navigating a patient portal, seeking a second opinion). In language education courses, we know that the language skills of learners are quite heterogeneous and do not develop unilaterally across these modalities and domains. We work with immigrants whose oral communication skills are better developed than their written skills. These people's abilities would not adequately be captured in a single written skills assessment, and the conclusion drawn would be far from what the person can actually do and express.

The "low-skilled" myth also distracts from the learning conditions that are essential to increasing confidence and competence with new skills. Skilled language teachers understand that language can be continuously developed through meaningful practice opportunities. In language courses, we use pedagogical strategies to foster language development, such as:

- using real-world materials so learners see the relevance of new skills to their own lives [72, 73],
- problem-posing dialogue that invites learners to connect new knowledge and learning goals with prior experience [67, 74],
- scaffolding opportunities for learners to transition from imitative to independent use of skills [75, 76],
- an emphasis on reflection that supports learner awareness of their own learning strategies and progress [77], and
- frequent opportunities to give and get feedback, from teachers and peers [78–80].

These pedagogical strategies aim to close skills gaps and support new practices that lead to meaningful differences in our ability to thrive in the real world.

Myth #2: Written information is reliable information

Written communication is so ubiquitous today that for many of us, a world without print is unimaginable. Suppose you wake up one day and all printed forms of language have disappeared – no books, forms, labels, and signs; you would frantically grab your phone, only to discover there are no text feeds or news chyrons helping you to make sense of the chaos. That thought experiment reminds you how much we rely on printed information to make sense of – indeed, to impose order on – our everyday environments. We may not read in detail every label on the products we buy, or every word on the forms we sign, but the fact that such labels and forms exist affords us some sense of security that what we are buying or signing is legitimate. Although technology has migrated much of our communication experiences onto digital platforms and repositories, we continue to live in a world where physical printed artifacts, like your Covid-19 vaccination card, official forms of identification, or financial forms (e.g., loan agreements), carry authoritative weight. This conferral of authority and legitimacy to the printed word is not a universal fact about language itself [46], but rather these properties reflect the tremendous social, political, and economic power of written communication in many modern-day contexts [38, 39, 81].

We say "many" because there are people in the world whose lives are not print-mediated as described in the above scenario. For example, over 773 million adults are not print-literate [82]. In United States adult education, we have seen an increase in the number of adult learners with limited print literacy (in any language) and minimal to no prior schooling in publicly-funded programs [83], which reflects patterns in cross-border migration from countries where schooling is not a given. In Germany, the last literacy study revealed that 12.1% of all adults (6.2 million) have limited literacy; among these, 47.4% do not have German as their first language [84]. Another 20.5% of the adult population has challenges writing correctly. For many of these adults, the challenges of navigating a new linguistic environment, including healthcare, are complex and onerous. Their human stories are already part of the public imagination – recently resettled refugees, women in particular, with no access to school while in exile; adults who arrive as unaccompanied minors with interrupted schooling histories; and adults who, after residing in the new country for several years, develop sufficient oral English skills but cannot read/write well in any language [83, 85, 86]. The literacy experiences of these populations remain unaccounted for in HL research [10, 87]. Because these subpopulations sources tend to be lumped under broadly applied labels "low skilled," "limited English proficient," or "low educated," we have yet to account for the diversity of experiences that give rise to HL competence [88]. Moreover, if we treat familiarity with print-communication practices as a primary indicator of ability, we are likely to overlook important sources of resilience and strategies (e.g., use of trusted helpers, assistive technologies, and oral communication) deployed by adults with emergent literacy skills.

A growing body of applied linguistics studies on these subpopulations should kick-start a research agenda on HL practices among adult language learners with emergent print literacy. For example, Leong [10] has documented important shifts in desired autonomy among refugee and immigrant women, who recently arrived in Calgary, Canada, as they navigated healthcare bureaucracies around insurance enrollment or specialist referrals. In another study of women who had recently immigrated to Canada,

Wall [57] documents the cultivation of social and cultural capital (as well as structural barriers to access) in response to "documentation-heavy lives" (p. 57). Studies of visual graphic interpretation, such as iconic images like speech bubbles [89] and multimodal assessment designs [90], among adults with emergent print literacy lay important groundwork for more inclusive research designs in HL.

The bias toward written communication is reinforced by the fact that there is often no distinction between what we think of as written communication and written communication in the dominant language of healthcare. Consider this scenario: adult literacy teachers were asked to describe their students' "literacy levels," and for the students in their English-as-a-Second-Language (ESL) classes, the teachers "would answer (. . .) as if the question were being asked about being literate in English (. . .) despite the explicit re-quest to comment on the students' literacy levels in both their native languages and in English" [91]. Moreover, the ESL learner participants in the study "often described themselves as nonliterate or low literate," even though some read and wrote in their first language but could not read in English very well (p. 90).

Martinez [92] documents a similar bias toward English literacy – or what he aptly describes as the "deliteracization of Spanish" – in United States healthcare. In this study, several Spanish-English bilingual patients described interactions in which the medical provider provided an oral translation in Spanish of written medical directives in English because no print version in Spanish was available. Patients felt the brief oral translations in Spanish served as a "surrogate" version of the more extensive medical information available only in printed English. Martinez observes that portrayal of Spanish as the "nonliterate language" has both ideological and practical consequences: we see the "ubiquitous privileging of English literacy" (p. 356), which leads to the "fractured and non-reinforced transmission of health information" (p. 357) to the patient. Particularly concerning about both examples is the potential for bilingual speakers to view their own bilingualism through the "dominant gaze" [93] of English-based literacy. What may appear on the surface to ensure linguistic access, in fact, serves to reinforce the elevated status of English as the desired language of healthcare communication.

A coordinated research agenda on adult emergent, bilingual/biliterate populations is fundamental to our understanding of what it means to be *print-literate* in our healthcare communication landscape. We share Alterr Flores' [90] concerns that any new knowledge about bilingual, emergent adult readers' "unexpected ways of making meaning (. . .) may not be valued by text designers or other such people in power" (n.p.). We call attention to mantras from two leading applied linguists: "Get literacy off the page" from literacy expert Patsy Egan [94], and "put English in the backseat" from bilingualism expert Alison Phipps [95]. We appeal to readers to adopt both mantras in their HL research and practice: by getting HL "off the page" and "putting English in the backseat," we open up new avenues in thinking about HL as a socially-situated, multilingual, and multimodal phenomenon.

Myth #3: Sending information is enough

This myth originates from mass media communication and the belief that the provision of written information leads to people reading, understanding, and ultimately using it. This assumption implicitly underlies mass media health communication and the creation of brochures, as well as many clinical encounters. However, numerous studies have repeatedly shown that this causal relationship is not always present and is much more complex. A greater focus should be placed on the actual ability of individuals in response to the linguistic demands of health information. This focus has recently been taken up in the HL debate, with HL scholars and health promotion specialists critically examining the interdependence of patients' skills, the skills of those who create health materials, and the demands of the healthcare environment [36, 64, 96–99]. The expertise of applied linguistics with the study of language in context can be particularly useful in developing strategies for facilitating engagement with health information and improving skills.

Overall, the assumption that providing information leads to successful uptake follows outdated, wrong learning theories. Applied linguistics (with adults) shows that both listening and reading are not passive but active processes in which the listener/reader draws on their linguistic and content knowledge to understand the presented information [58, 100, 101]. Likewise, the process of understanding is not a passive intake but an active construction process. As an action model, applied linguistics further describes this process by highlighting different steps such as *input, intake, output, and uptake*. Input refers to any information such as *language that encodes meaning* [102] provided by teachers, instructors, and media. Intake is the reception of what is presented, whereby the process from input to intake is influenced by selection, emotional filters, and whether the information presented can be linked to any previous knowledge and making a form-meaning connection, etc. [103–105]. Output is what the individual has learned and can proactively produce [106]. Lastly, uptake refers to processing information, which is often facilitated through corrective feedback [107, 108]. Applying the knowledge on input, intake, output, and uptake results in better learning as it is absorbed through different channels and better processed by transferring it to other modes.

We offer two insights for health professionals. First: turning from the mere presentation of information toward developing and facilitating interactive tasks that help patients/learners to engage with the information in multiple ways. While the teach-back method, which is part of the core HL method repertoire, already turns the gaze away from the mere presentation of information to a higher activity of the individual, it should not be assumed that the mere repetition of information (understood as output) has already stimulated a process of understanding. It may also be merely due to the individual's ability to reproduce heard speech. Activities that imply a deeper engagement with what is heard are instructions such as "Repeat it in your own words," "How would you explain it to your partner?", "Please try to describe it to a child." Another core component is *building background*, or the practice of introducing important words or concepts before engaging with a topic or a text [109]. Thus, learners are not confused and distracted by unknown words and can follow the topic easily. *Building background* can be linguistic or content-related, for example, by introducing that stroke is called apoplexy or using the example of a key that fits exactly into a lock (key-lock-principle) to explain the mechanism behind the screening for viruses. It is important to make sure that these words or concepts are not just presented but that the learner actively uses them with known and unknown contexts [110].

Myth #4: The bilingual patient is two monolingual patients in one

We draw inspiration from bilingualism researcher Francois Grosjean, who in 1989 cautioned, "Neurolinguists, beware! The bilingual is not two monolinguals in one person!" [111]. Grosjean demonstrates that people's confusion of what constitutes a "bilingual" stems from flawed thinking about the nature of language itself and a "monolingual bias," the assumption that monolingualism is the normative, prevalent condition in the world and that what monolinguals do with language is the best reference point against which all other language use profiles can be understood. We invite readers to consider the extent to which this "monolingual bias" pervades our interactions in healthcare, particularly with linguistically minoritized groups.

Most people describe language users in terms of the number of languages they know: monolinguals know one, bilinguals know two, and multilinguals know two or more. Yet the number of languages tells us very little about how well a person speaks each language they know and the different contexts of use. A "perfectly balanced bilingual" is described as someone who can pass for a "native speaker" in either language. The idea that someone can pass as "native" in all circumstances sets up an untestable illusion: Can they schedule a Covid-19 booster equally well in both languages? Can the person express pain or tell a joke equally well in both languages? Can they write a dissertation in both languages? These questions illustrate that bilingualism is more productively characterized as being able to use different languages in meaningful ways, based on the contexts of desired/expected use.

A related reality check is that bilinguals develop mastery in their languages that reflects their communicative purposes and in response to situational demands. Imagine a bilingual patient whose first language is Spanish and has acquired English as an additional language, largely over several years of living in the United States. The person handles communication needs in English, with no difficulty, when picking up a prescription from the local pharmacy or scheduling a vaccination appointment via their smartphone; the person opts to communicate in Spanish when talking to an advice nurse about their child's painful ear infection. Finally, when searching online for information about administering the Covid-19 vaccine to young children, the person checks multiple social media sources, in English and Spanish, and joins a Twitter feed where they chat in English and Spanish with people around the world, of varying proficiency levels in the two languages. The "monolingual bias" perpetuates several deficit-oriented claims about this person's language use: *communicating in two languages is inefficient and time-consuming; having to choose between language is confusing; when you can't understand something in the dominant language of English, you just fall back on your first language; it's confusing to manage all that information in two languages.* Here, mythic thinking is evident in the assumption that "bilingualism" results in difficulty, confusion, and messiness in healthcare, and "monolingualism" is the easier condition for communication. (If this were true, monolinguals would never have communication problems, and that's just simply false!)

Let us also consider the person's choice to communicate in Spanish when talking to the advice nurse in this scenario. The "monolingual bias" accentuates the idea that the person is unable to communicate their concerns in English so thus must revert to Spanish. The myth-busting counter-claim is that the person chooses the best language to express worry and urgency, and ultimately to ensure the child gets better. This alternative characterization is grounded in a growing body of studies on the emotional life of bilinguals [112–114], suggesting that emotions manifest with different forces, in different languages. Thus, it is quite human for bilinguals to choose the language that best fits the intended emotion. Sadly, the "monolingual bias" tends to strip this basic human function from our characterization of bilingual meaning-making.

Efforts to dismantle monolinguistic bias is now referred to as the "multilingual turn" in the study of language and language users [115]. Now that language is widely regarded as a social determinant of health, to what extent are we seeing signs that the world of healthcare is experiencing its own "multilingual turn," in its research, policies, and patient interactions? On the one hand, we see evidence of missed opportunities to lift up multilinguality in healthcare: for example, in a study of health and public safety professions, Alarcón et al. [116] found that "fluent bilinguals receive lower average wages than monolingual English speakers, despite their added linguistic asset" (p. 156). On the other hand, we applaud innovation in university training programs. For example, Martínez and Schwartz [117] highlight the benefits of service learning for heritage language speakers volunteering in a health clinic at the United States–Mexico border. Bilingual students helped to translate nutrition educational materials and interpret during diabetes education classes. Students gained important insight into the intermingling of standard and nonstandard varieties of Spanish in clinical interactions and deepened their respect for local varieties of Spanish.

We hope readers of this volume will be part of the cadres of practitioners who advance research on bi/multilingual HL competence: we lack funding streams for this kind of exploratory work, and we lack measures (see myth #6) for documenting multicompetence in healthcare navigation. We also lack the conceptual frameworks and terminology (e.g., keywords used in database searches) for documenting HL as a multilingual phenomenon [59]. These problems could be productively and creatively addressed through cross-disciplinary exchange between researchers of bilingualism and HL.

Myth #5: Reducing language complexity will ensure comprehension and empower people

Communication and dissemination of health information is not an end in and of itself in public health and healthcare but serves to empower people to make and implement health-related decisions and shape their lives in a health-promoting manner. However, migrants often report that they have difficulty understanding the information due to language barriers. Language complexity can be a tremendous obstacle in health communication and in engaging with health information [58, 60]. To simplify understanding, researchers, health professionals, and other practitioners have developed strategies and best practices. The most prominent recommendation to reduce complexity for migrants and nonmigrants is creating health material in plain language [118, 119]. This strategy can reduce cognitive load and facilitate understanding and processing of information (see psycholinguistically informed models of language acquisition) and thus comprehension (see Nutbeam's functional HL [64]). However, health education and literacy interventions focus on simplifying the language with the expectation that people will better understand information and consequently are empowered to improve their health [120]. Much criticism can be directed at this assumption. To support or reject the claim that comprehension leads to empowerment, we first need to clarify what is meant by comprehension, empowerment, and their relationship. While the concept of comprehension is widely theorized in applied linguistics [121], the concept tends to be relatively under-examined in health promotion. Applied linguistics models reveal a multitude of factors influencing comprehension, at the level of the text (e.g., the text's ease of processing) and the individual level (e.g., the degree to which the reader engages in strategic comprehension processes). Moreover, comprehension models often illustrate the complex context-dependent nature of the comprehension process: individuals need to apply specific competencies across a variety of text types (genres), modalities, and purposes. But even if comprehension has occurred, it does not imply that the person will use the knowledge to act or ultimately "gain greater control over decisions and actions affecting their health." [122] (p. 14). The latter refers to empowerment in health promotion and is reflected in acts of agency and self-determination (e.g., expressing needs, decision-making, questioning strategies, and cocreating policies and services to improve health). The focus on empowerment shifts attention beyond strengthening individual capacities to influencing determinants of health. If we seek to empower people, our HL strategy needs to move beyond text comprehension and support individuals in understanding the complex influence of social determinants on their health and the possibilities for influencing them.

By solely focusing on reducing linguistic complexity, we simplify access to information but miss the opportunity to empower people beyond promoting comprehension skills. Our role as language educators is to develop people's agency with newly acquired language skills, in diverse contexts, including healthcare [79]. Drawing on Paolo Freire's words, to learn to "read the word and the world" [123] means that we learn to navigate the linguistic demands of our healthcare system even as we critically question the system that imposes those linguistic demands on linguistically minoritized communities. To what extent then does reducing linguistic complexity empower people to express their healthcare needs and desires and to advocate for themselves (cf. critical HL [64])? As applied linguists, we would like to see more research and interventions that link linguistic simplifications to patient empowerment outcomes, not only indicators of patient compliance (e.g., following instructions, accepting medical advice) typically reflected functional HL definitions. Tracing the impact of linguistic simplifications to shifts in power dynamics between patients and providers (e.g., in terms of trust, patient-centeredness, and provider humility) seems foundational to the goals of health promotion and health equity [18, 124].

As a concrete recommendation, health professionals can look for opportunities to stimulate engagement with information. Language teachers focus on *message abundancy* in their teaching – the "amplifying and enriching" of meaning in the learning context, "so that students do not get just one opportunity to come to terms with the concepts involved, but in fact may construct their understanding on the basis of multiple clues and perspectives encountered in a variety of class activities" [125] (p. 196). In the healthcare context, both the presentation of information and the stimuli/activities for the active engagement can support multimodal meaning-making: using pictures, films, texts, and various modes of presentation. Furthermore, it is necessary to invite people to apply but even change the information in various modes (what Merrill Swain describes as "reformulation"). An effective method is "see it, do it, and teach it once," in which the individual first observes an action (or process), then performs it under the guidance of another, and lastly teaches it to others [126]. This method facilitates acquisition of new skills and increased independence with those skills. Moreover, health professionals can consider pedagogical models such as the content and language integrated learning approach (CLIL) [127] or language-sensitive health communication frameworks [128]; these models place a strong emphasis on supporting engagement with complex words and concepts, not through replacement with "simpler" words or concepts, but by giving equal priority to language learning and content learning.

Myth #6: Assessing reading is a useful proxy for assessing literacy

Well-established definitions of HL project a broad understanding of competence to include knowing, doing, and problem-solving (e.g., Nutbeam's [64] three-part focus on functional, interactive, and critical HL). Moreover, our understanding of what skilled HL looks like is closely tied to the demands of specific health contexts [129]. This insight has led to a proliferation of *literacy* attributions: for example, *digital HL, health insurance literacy, genetic literacy, cancer HL, and immigrant adolescent HL* [130]. The use of written and spoken forms of communication in healthcare is hardly new, but the digital transformation of healthcare has only expanded the possibilities around modalities (e.g., speaking with a doctor in person, chatting with a chatbot, asynchronous email communication, and remote interpretation) and genres encountered in everyday healthcare interactions (e.g., consent forms, e-health records, advance directives, and patient support blogs). The health communication landscape, replete with these many *literacies*, often overwhelms even the most savvy among us; navigating that landscape requires far more than good reading skills. For these reasons, the reliance on measures that assess reading in a health context stands out as an area most critically in need of innovative reform. We argue that greater understanding about the contextualized nature of language/literacy, and specifically the variation in language use (e.g., the routine use of more than one language in meaning-making among bilinguals, see myth 4), is an essential key to turning the dial in any measurement reform.

In an appeal for renewed clarity about the alignment of conceptualizations and measurements of HL competence, we offer two insights from applied linguistics. One, any measure of ability is *de facto* a measure of language [131]. In other words, we cannot take for granted the decisions we are making *about* language when we design and administer measures of competence: the kinds of questions we ask, the way those questions are asked, the modality through which we present the questions (online, orally, in print), in what languages, and our expectations about what constitutes a "correct" answer all shape our perceptions of the competence we are hoping to measure [132]. Underperformance on a test thus may reflect lack of competence, or lack of familiarity with the linguistic features of measures, or both. Two, we must recognize the power of our judgments of other people's abilities, whether this takes place formally (e.g., via screener questionnaires or as part of research protocols) or informally, such as in the course of a clinical encounter, we endeavor to quickly take stock as to whether someone understands what we just told them (e.g., in "teach back" moments). In schools, teacher judgments can weightily shape learning pathways for linguistically minoritized learners, such as whether a learner advances to the next grade, is able to access accelerated coursework, or is referred to special education services. In healthcare, judgments about literacy can play an important function in specifying a patients' communication needs: who among linguistically minoritized patients is able to manage the communicative expectations of the healthcare environment, and who needs more support? Fillmore and Snow [133] cede that, while "sorting" learners according to ability levels may help us differentiate support strategies and resources for linguistically diverse groups, the ethical soundness of these judgments can be undermined by the reliance on assessments of limited or questionable validity.

Pleasant's [134] scoping review demonstrates that efforts to conceptualize HL as a socially situated phenomenon have by far outpaced efforts to generate measures that meaningfully document that situatedness: "theoretical understandings and methods of measuring the complex social construct of health literacy have experienced a continual evolution that remains incomplete" (p. 1481) – a reality that largely reflects the kind of research on HL most consistently funded and disseminated over the past 30 plus years. Against this funding/publishing backdrop, our calls for an elevation of applied linguistic expertise in HL measurement feel rather desperate and overidealized. At the same time, we choose to focus on specific areas where positive change is evident. We look to innovative university degree programs that support exchange between preprofessionals in language education and health professions, through cross-disciplinary coursework [135] or service learning opportunities [136]: these efforts may help to ensure the next generation of practitioners has the expertise to support linguistically equitable assessments of HL. We also look to research that adds to the measurement of socially situated HL. For example, Hohn and Rivera [137] explore the nature of *collective efficacy* around health-related tasks that emerges over time among learners and teachers in adult literacy classrooms. Lor [66] explores comprehension strategies in dyadic interactions among pairs of elder Hmong adults and a trusted family helper when filling out a health data form. Another aspiration is to develop HL measures that make multilinguality more visible in every day health navigation tasks, not merely focusing on competence tied to proficiency in the dominant language of healthcare (i.e., English in the United States) [138]. Finally, we invite serious reflection on why comparisons to L1-only speaking monolinguals (e.g., "native English speakers" in the United States) tend to be viewed as the benchmark of methodological rigor in HL studies. A research agenda on multilinguality in HL would invite new insights into HL competence within and across groups of "multilingual natives" [139], not in comparison to a monolingual norm.

Conclusion

We aimed to demonstrate that *new thinking* about language as a social determinant of health or as an indicator of competence in healthcare requires that we (both in applied linguistics and public health) interrogate *old thinking* about the nature of language and our conceptualizations of language users. To guide our exploration, we used the glasses of applied linguistics. We focused on six myths that are central to that interrogation. Most certainly, these are not the only trouble spots worth examining: for example, we did not raise questions about the historical under-representation of multilinguals in leadership roles in the applied linguistics or public health workforce, a trend that may skew our perception of who is championing the fight for linguistic equity in healthcare.

In view of the powerful links between language and health outcomes, we posit that there is a need to advance the *linguistics of healthcare* as a field of study in its own right. Within applied linguistics, the study of language and language-related issues in educational practice (including but not limited to schools and classrooms) is called *educational linguistics*. We would love to debate as to whether the forging of a subdiscipline we will refer to, for now, as *healthcare linguistics* might open up new channels of interchange, help to formalize provider training, and accelerate problem-solving toward linguistic equity in healthcare, as yet not fully recognized as a vital domain of professional knowledge and training.

Myth-busting work and the resulting need for changes at multiple levels (ideologically, in our regulatory policies around language access, within disciplines, and in daily practice) will require a tremendous investment of time, energy, and resources. That would be majorly unfair to lay at the feet of individual practitioners. We are thinking about organizations and individuals in power (e.g., funders, university researchers, and policymakers) where a leadership commitment to myth-busting and making multilinguality visible [138, 139] should help us imagine whether a "multilingual turn" in healthcare is realizable.

Finally, we appeal directly to practitioners who work in community-based classrooms and clinics: we hope this chapter inspires you to be myth-busters in their own right. Community-based practitioners shoulder some of the most emotionally demanding workloads responding to the needs of linguistically minoritized communities. Our sense of professional/personal accomplishment in these settings is often a function of how confident, entrusted, and efficacious we feel in our *own* capacity as communicators to the people we are trained to support [133]. Practitioners working on the front line with linguistically diverse communities know best the myriad of moment-to-moment adjustments we make in our communication practices to boost that sense of confidence, respect, and self-efficacy. We also know first-hand the pressures of wanting to make the best decision about how and what to communicate considering real constraints in time and resources. We trivialize this work if we see their communication efforts as ancillary to the work of healing, treating, and caring for people. In contrast, we would like to see language work, healthcare, and health equity not as separate from each other but as fundamentally interrelated. We hope this chapter sparked curiosity in the many relevant factors visible when exploring HL through the "glasses" of applied linguistics. Lastly, we hope it provides a working agenda for the creation of dissemination platforms and funding streams that bring greater visibility to the equity work taking place in our classrooms and clinics.

Highlights

- Applied linguistics perspectives are critical to our understanding of the complexities of language in healthcare and to the dismantling of health disparities for linguistically minoritized communities.
- Research and theories on social determinants of health and HL have shaped thinking about language as a mediator of health outcomes.
- There are myths about language and language use that need busting. With the expertise of applied linguists, we can improve our understanding of language, comprehension processes, multilinguality in healthcare, and healthcare environments.
- New thinking about healthcare linguistics can open up new channels of disciplinary interchange, help to formalize provider training, and accelerate problem-solving toward language equity in healthcare.

REFERENCES

1. Gee, J. (2015). *Social Linguistics and Literacies: Ideology in Discourses*. Routledge.
2. Auerbach, E. (ed.) (2002). *Community Partnerships*. Arlington, VA: Teachers of English to Speakers of Other Languages.
3. Santos, M.G., Showstack, R., Martínez, G. et al. (2022). *Health Disparities and the Applied Linguist*. Milton: Taylor & Francis Group.
4. Wallerstein, N., Duran, B., Oetzel, J.G., and Minkler, M. (2018). *Community-Based Participatory Research for Health: Advancing Social and Health Equity*. San Francisco: Jossey-Bass.
5. Quenzel, G., and Schaeffer, D. (2016) Health literacy–gesundheitskompetenz vulnerabler bevölkerungsgruppen. https://doi.org/10.13140/RG.2.1.2509.1604
6. World Health Organization (2017). *Beyond the Barriers: Framing Evidence on Health System Strengthening to Improve the Health of Migrants Experiencing Poverty and Social Exclusion*. Geneva: World Health Organization.
7. Ehlich, K., and München, L.-M.-U. (2007) *Recherche und Dokumentation hinsichtlich der Sprachbedarfe von Teilnehmenden an Integrationskursen DaZ*. München. Online: http://www.goethe.de/lhr/prj/daz/pro/InDaZ_Recherche.pdf.
8. Wrigley, H. (2007). Beyond the life boat: improving language, citizenship and training services for immigrants and refugees. In: *Toward Defining and Improving Quality in Adult Basic Education: Issues and Challenges* (ed. A. Belzer), 221–239. Routledge, New York: Erlbaum Publishing. Defin. Improv. Qual. Adult Basic Educ. Issues Chall.
9. Parrish, B. (2019). *Teaching Adult English Language Learners: A Practical Introduction*. Cambridge: Cambridge University Press.
10. Leong, M. and Santos, M. (2019). Taking our seat at the table: why the expertise of LESLLA educators is needed in the health literacy field. In: *Proceedings from the 9th annual Low Educated Second Language and Literacy Acquisition (LESLLA) Symposium 2017*, 53–68.
11. Harsch, S. (2022). Ein fremder, zweiter Blick auf Health Literacy–was uns die Zweitsprachen-Didaktik lehren kann. In: *Gesundheitskompetenz* (ed. K. Rathmann, K. Dadaczynski, O. Okan, and M. Messer). Berlin, Heidelberg: Springer. https://doi.org/10.1007/978-3-662-62800-3_124-1.
12. Andrulis, D.P. and Brach, C. (2007). Integrating literacy, culture, and language to improve health care quality for diverse populations. *Am. J. Health Behav.* 31 (Suppl 1): S122–S133.
13. Mohan, B.A. (1986). *Language and Content*. Reading, Mass: Addison-Wesley.
14. Wolf, J.A. (2018). Elevating the discourse on experience in healthcare's uncertain times. *Patient Exp. J.* 5 (3): 1–5.
15. Rudd, R. (2002). A maturing partnership. *Focus Basics Connect. Res. Pract.* 5 (C): 1–10.
16. Rubin, D. (2014). Applied linguistics as a resource for understanding and advancing health literacy. In: *The Routledge Handbook of Language and Health Communication* (ed. H. Hamilton and W.Y.S. Chou), 153–167. Routledge.
17. World Health Organization (1946). *Constitutions of the World Health Organization*. World Health Organization.
18. World Health Organization (1986). *Ottawa Charter for Health Promotion*. World Health Organization.
19. The US Department of Health and Human Services (n.d.). *Social Determinants of Health*. The US Department of Health and Human Services.
20. Giesecke, J. and Müters, S. (2009). Strukturelle und verhaltensbezogene Faktoren gesundheitlicher Ungleichheit: methodische Überlegungen zur Ermittlung der Erklärungsanteile. In: *Gesundheitliche Ungleichheit: Grundlagen, Probleme, Perspektiven* (ed. M. Richter and K. Hurrelmann), 353–366. Wiesbaden: VS Verlag für Sozialwissenschaften.
21. Tarlov, A.R. (1999). Public policy frameworks for improving population health. *Ann. N. Y. Acad. Sci.* 896: 281–293.

22. Marmot, M., Allen, J., Bell, R. et al. (2012). WHO European review of social determinants of health and the health divide. *The Lancet* 380 (9846): 1011–1029.
23. World Health Organization (2008) Closing the Gap in a Generation: Health Equity Through Action on the Social Determinants of Health - Final Report of the Commission on Social Determinants of Health.
24. González, H.M., Vega, W.A., and Tarraf, W. (2010). Health care quality perceptions among foreign-born Latinos and the importance of speaking the same language. *J. Am. Board Fam. Med. JABFM* 23 (6): 745–752.
25. Detz, A., Mangione, C.M., de Jaimes, F.N. et al. (2014). Language concordance, interpersonal care, and diabetes self-care in rural latino patients. *J. Gen. Intern. Med.* 29 (12): 1650–1656.
26. Jaramillo, J., Snyder, E., Dunlap, J.L. et al. (2016). The hispanic clinic for pediatric surgery: a model to improve parent–provider communication for Hispanic pediatric surgery patients. *J. Pediatr. Surg.* 51 (4): 670–674.
27. Cheng, E.M., Chen, A., and Cunningham, W. (2007). Primary language and receipt of recommended health care among Hispanics in the United States. *J. Gen. Intern. Med.* 22 (2): 283–288.
28. Jacobs, E.A., Karavolos, K., Rathouz, P.J. et al. (2005). Limited English proficiency and breast and cervical cancer screening in a multiethnic population. *Am. J. Public Health* 95 (8): 1410–1416.
29. Haviland, A.M., Elliott, M.N., Hambarsoomian, K., and Lurie, N. (2011). Immunization disparities by Hispanic ethnicity and language preference. *Arch. Intern. Med.* 171 (2): 158–165.
30. Hulme, P.A., Walker, S.N., Effle, K.J. et al. (2003). Health-promoting lifestyle behaviors of Spanish-speaking Hispanic adults. *J. Transcult. Nurs.* 14 (3): 244–254.
31. John-Baptiste, A., Naglie, G., Tomlinson, G. et al. (2004). The effect of English language proficiency on length of stay and in-hospital mortality. *J. Gen. Intern. Med.* 19 (3): 221–228.
32. Ratzan, S.C. and Parker, R.M. (2000). *Health Literacy*. US Department of Health and Human Services: National Institutes of Health.
33. World Health Organization. Regional Office for Europe (2018). *Report on the Health of Refugees and Migrants in the WHO European Region: No Public Health Without Refugee and Migrant Health*. Copenhagen: World Health Organization. Regional Office for Europe.
34. Schouten, B.C., Cox, A., Duran, G. et al. (2020). Mitigating language and cultural barriers in healthcare communication: toward a holistic approach. *Patient Educ. Couns.* 103 (12): 2604–2608.
35. Becerra, B.J., Arias, D., and Becerra, M.B. (2017). Low health literacy among immigrant hispanics. *J. Racial Ethn. Health Disparities* 4 (3): 480–483.
36. Berens, E.-M., Ganahl, K., Vogt, D., and Schaeffer, D. (2021). Health literacy in the domain of healthcare among older migrants in Germany (North Rhine-Westphalia). Findings from a cross-sectional survey. *Int. J. Migr. Health Soc. Care* 17 (1): 62–74.
37. Kickbusch, I., Pelikan, J.M., Apfel, F., and Tsouros, A. (2013). *Health Literacy*. Copenhagen: WHO Regional Office for Europe.
38. Scribner, S. and Cole, M. (1981). *The Psychology of Literacy*. Cambridge, MA: Harvard University Press.
39. Street, B.V. (1985). *Literacy in Theory and Practice*. New York: Cambridge University Press, Cambridge Cambridgeshire.
40. Baker-Bell, A. (2020). *Linguistic Justice: Black Language, Literacy, Identity, and Pedagogy*. New York: Routledge.
41. Charity, A.H. (2008). Linguists as agents for social change. *Lang. Linguist. Compass* 2 (5): 923–939.
42. Cioè-Peña, M. (2021). *(M)othering Labeled Children: Bilingualism and Disability in the Lives of Latinx Mothers*. Blue Ridge Summit, PA: Multilingual Matters.
43. Purcell-Gates, V. (ed.) (2007). *Cultural Practices of Literacy: Case Studies of Language, Literacy, Social Practice, and Power*. Mahwah, NJ: Lawrence Erlbaum Associates Publishers.
44. Purcell-Gates, V., Anderson, J., Gagne, M. et al. (2012). Measuring situated literacy activity: challenges and promises. *J. Lit. Res.* 44 (4): 396–425.
45. Raymond, C.W. (2014). Epistemic brokering in the interpreter-mediated

medical visit: negotiating "patient's side" and "doctor's side" knowledge. *Res. Lang. Soc. Interact.* 47 (4): 426–446.
46. Vieira, K. (2016). *American by Paper: How Documents Matter in Immigrant Literacy.* Minneapolis: University of Minnesota Press.
47. Weinstein, G. (1999). *Learners' Lives as Curriculum: Six Journeys to Immigrant Literacy.* McHenry, IL: Delta Systems.
48. Becerra, M.B., Becerra, B.J., Daus, G.P., and Martin, L.R. (2015). Determinants of low health literacy among Asian-American and Pacific islanders in California. *J. Racial Ethn. Health Disparities* 2 (2): 267–273.
49. Harris, L.M., Dreyer, B.P., Jimenez, J.J. et al. (2017). Liquid medication dosing errors by hispanic parents: role of health literacy and english proficiency. *Acad. Pediatr.* 17 (4): 403–410.
50. Lee, M., Lee, M.A., Ahn, H. et al. (2021). Health literacy and access to care in cancer screening among Korean Americans. *HLRP Health Lit. Res. Pract.* 5 (4): e310.
51. Masland, M.C., Kang, S.H., and Ma, Y. (2011). Association between limited English proficiency and understanding prescription labels among five ethnic groups in California. *Ethn. Health* 16 (2): 125–144.
52. Sarkar, M., Asti, L., Nacion, K.M., and Chisolm, D.J. (2016). The role of health literacy in predicting multiple healthcare outcomes among Hispanics in a nationally representative sample: a comparative analysis by English proficiency levels. *J. Immigr. Minor. Health* 18 (3): 608–615.
53. Sentell, T. and Braun, K.L. (2012). Low health literacy, limited English proficiency, and health status in Asians, Latinos, and other racial/ethnic groups in California. *J. Health Commun.* 17 (Suppl 3): 82–99.
54. Yeheskel, A. and Rawal, S. (2019). Exploring the "patient experience" of individuals with limited English proficiency: a scoping review. *J. Immigr. Minor. Health* 21 (4): 853–878.
55. Cuban, S. and Stromquist, N.P. (2009). It is difficult to be a woman with a dream of an education: challenging U.S. Adult Basic Education Policies to Support Women Immigrants' Self-Determination. *J. Crit. Educ. Policy Stud. JCEPS* 7 (2): 154–186.
56. Pettitt, N.M. and Tarone, E. (2015). Following Roba: what happens when a low-educated adult immigrant learns to read. *Writ. Syst. Res.* 7 (1): 20–38.
57. Wall, T. (2017). *L1 Literacy and Its Implications for Leslla Immigrant Women in Canada.* Theresa Wall, Hamline University.
58. Papen, U. (2009). Literacy, learning and health – a social practices view of health literacy. *Lit. Numeracy Stud.* 16/17 (2/1): 19–34.
59. Santos, M.G., Gorukanti, A.L., Jurkunas, L.M., and Handley, M.A. (2018). The health literacy of U.S. immigrant adolescents: a neglected research priority in a changing world. *Int. J. Environ. Res. Public. Health* 15 (10): 2108.
60. Harsch, S. (2022). *Health Literacy as a Situational, Social Practice in Context-Insights From Three Research Projects Among "Vulnerable Groups".* University of Education Freiburg.
61. Ortega, P. and Prada, J. (2020). Words matter: translanguaging in medical communication skills training. *Perspect. Med. Educ.* 9 (4): 251–255.
62. Ortega, P., Diamond, L., Alemán, M.A. et al. (2020). Medical Spanish standardization in U.S. medical schools: consensus statement from a multidisciplinary expert panel. *Acad. Med.* 95 (1): 22–31.
63. Altgeld, T. (2018) Bestandsaufnahme von Interventionen (Modelle guter Praxis) zur Gesundheitsförderung und Prävention bei Menschen mit Migrationshintergrund.
64. Nutbeam, D. (2000). Health literacy as a public health goal: a challenge for contemporary health education and communication strategies into the 21st century. *Health Promot. Int.* 15 (3): 259–267.
65. Brooks, E. (2022). Translanguaging health. *Appl. Linguist.* 43 (3): 517–537.
66. Lor, M., Schaeffer, N.C., Brown, R.L., and Bowers, B.J. (2020). Completing self-administered questionnaires: among older adults and their family helpers. *Field Methods* 32 (3): 253–273.
67. Santos, M.G., Mcclelland, J., and Handley, M. (2011). Language lessons on immigrant identity, food culture, and the search for home. *TESOL J.* 2 (2): 203–228.

68. Reder, S. (2013). Lifelong and life-wide adult literacy development. *Perspect. Lang. Lit.* 39 (2): 18–21.
69. Koch-Institus, R. (2020). *Gesundheitliche Lage der Frauen in Deutschland*. RKI: Gesundheitsberichterstattung Bundes Berl.
70. Jarvis, P. (2009). *The Routledge International Handbook of Lifelong Learning*. London: Routledge.
71. Hinkel, E. (2005). *Handbook of Research in Second Language Teaching and Learning*. Routledge.
72. Levy, S., Rasher, S., Carter, S. et al. (2008). Health literacy curriculum works for adult basic education students. *Focus Basics* 9 (B): 33–39.
73. Jacobson, E., Degener, S., and Purcell-Gates, V. (2003). *Creating authentic materials and activities for the adult literacy classroom: a handbook for practitioners*. National Center for the Study of Adult Learning and Literacy.
74. Wallerstein, N. and Auerbach, E. (2004). *Problem-Posing at Work: Popular Educator's Guide*. Grass Roots Press Edmonton.
75. Gibbons, P. (2002). *Scaffolding Language, Scaffolding Learning*. Portsmouth, NH: Heinemann.
76. Vygotskij, L.S. (2012). *Thought and Language*. Cambridge, MA, London, England: MIT Press.
77. Bandura, A. and Walters, R.H. (1977). *Social Learning Theory*. Englewood Cliffs Prentice Hall.
78. Kniffka, G. and Siebert-Ott, G. (2009). *Deutsch als Zweitsprache: Lehren und Lernen*. Paderborn München Wien Zürich: Schöningh.
79. Goethe-Institut (2016). *Rahmencurriculum für Integrationskurse Deutsch als Zweitsprache*. Munich, Germany: Goethe Institute.
80. Ramírez-Esparza, N., Harris, K., Hellermann, J. et al. (2012). Socio-interactive practices and personality in adult learners of English with little formal education. *Lang. Learn.* 62 (2): 541–570.
81. Barton, D., Hamilton, M., and Ivanič, R. (ed.) (2000). *Situated Literacies: Reading and Writing in Context*. New York: Routledge, London.
82. UNESCO (2022). *Literacy, Promoting the Power of Literacy for All*. UNESCO.
83. Reder, S. (2019). LESLLA learners in the United States: a portrait in Census Data, 1900-2015. *Lit. Educ. Second Lang. Learn. Adults* 102: 102–120.
84. Grotlüschen, A. and Buddeberg, K. (ed.) (2020). *LEO 2018: Leben mit geringer Literalität*. Bielefeld: wbv.
85. Bigelow, M. and Tarone, E. (2004). The role of literacy level in second language acquisition: doesn't who we study determine what we know? *TESOL Q.* 38 (4): 689–700.
86. Shapiro, S., Farrelly, R., and Curry, M.J. (ed.) (2018). *Educating Refugee-Background Students: Critical Issues and Dynamic Contexts*. Blue Ridge Summit, Bristol: Multilingual Matters.
87. Harsch, S. (2023). Promoting HL among LESLLA learners: empirical findings and practical implications. *LESLLA Symp. Proc.* 16 (1): 57–75.
88. Santos, M.G. (2021) Finding "low-literate populations" in U.S. health literacy research: a review of labels, descriptors, and measures. *Roundtable Presented at American Association of Applied Linguistics, Virtual* (20–23 March 2021).
89. Bruski, D.J. (2011) Do They Get the Picture?: Visual Literacy and Low-Literacy Adult ESL Learners. School of Education and Leadership Student Capstone Theses and Dissertations. Hamline University, Saint Paul, Minnesota.
90. Altherr Flores, J.A. (2021). The semiotics of writing: how adult L2 learners with emergent literacy make meaning in assessment texts through writing. *J. Second Lang. Writ.* 51: 100793.
91. Purcell-Gates, V., Degener, S.C., Jacobson, E., and Soler, M. (2002). Impact of authentic adult literacy instruction on adult literacy practices. *Read. Res. Q.* 37 (1): 70–92.
92. Martinez, G. (2008). Language-in-healthcare policy, interaction patterns, and unequal care on the U.S.-Mexico border. *Lang. Policy* 7 (4): 345–363.
93. Paris, D. and Alim, H.S. (2014). What are we seeking to sustain through culturally sustaining pedagogy? A loving critique forward. *Harv. Educ. Rev.* 84 (1): 85–100.
94. Egan, P. (2017) Teaching students with limited L1 literacy: a few strategies to get literacy off the page!

95. Phipps, A. and Sithole, T. (2021). *Hospitality Through Languages: Pain. Gist: Joy.*
96. Rudd, R.E. (2013). Needed action in health literacy. *J. Health Psychol.* 18 (8): 1004–1010.
97. World Health Organization (2022). *Geneva Charter for Well-Being.* World Health Organization.
98. Sørensen, K., Van den Broucke, S., Fullam, J. et al. (2012). Health literacy and public health: a systematic review and integration of definitions and models. *BMC Public Health* 12 (1): 80.
99. Dodson, S., Good, S., and Osborne, R. (2015). *Health Literacy Toolkit for Low- and Middle-Income Countries: a Series of Information Sheets to Empower Communities and Strengthen Health Systems.* New Delhi: World Health Organization, Regional Office for South-East Asia.
100. Knowles, M. (1973). *The Adult Learner: A Neglected Species.* Houston, TX: Gulf Publishing Company.
101. Wigglesworth, G. (2003). *The Kaleidoscope of Adult Second Language Learning: Learner, Teacher and Researcher Perspectives.* National Centre for English Language Teaching and Research, Macquarie University.
102. Vanpatten, B. and Cadierno, T. (1993). Input processing and second language acquisition: a role for instruction. *Mod. Lang. J.* 77 (1): 45–57.
103. Corder, S.P. (1967). The significance of Learner's Errors. *IRAL: Int. Rev. Appl. Linguistics Language Teaching* V (4): 161–170.
104. Pennington, M.C. (1996). When input becomes intake: tracing the sources of teachers'. In: *Teacher Learning in Language Teaching* (ed. D. Freeman and J.C. Richards). New York: Cambridge University Press.
105. Chi, D.-N. (2016). Intake in second language acquisition. *Hawaii Pac. Univ. TESOL Work. Pap. Ser.* 14: 76–89.
106. Swain, M. (2005). The output hypothesis - 1-Theory and research. In: *Handbook of Research in Second Language Teaching and Learning.* Routledge.
107. Lyster, R. and Ranta, L. (1997). Corrective feedback and learner uptake: negotiation of form in communicative classrooms. *Stud. Second Lang. Acquis.* 19 (1): 37–66.
108. Sheen, Y. (2004). Corrective feedback and learner uptake in communicative classrooms across instructional settings. *Lang. Teach. Res.* 8 (3): 263–300.
109. Echevarria, J., Vogt, M., and Short, D. (2008). *Making Content Comprehensible for English Learners: The SIOP Model.* Boston: Pearson Education, Inc.
110. Cazden, C., Cope, B., Fairclough, N. et al. (1996). A pedagogy of multiliteracies: designing social futures. *Harv. Educ. Rev.* 66 (1): 60–92.
111. Grosjean, F. (1989). Neurolinguists, beware! The bilingual is not two monolinguals in one person. *Brain Lang.* 36 (1): 3–15.
112. Dewaele, J.-M. (2008). The emotional weight of I love you in multilinguals' languages. *J. Pragmat.* 40 (10): 1753–1780.
113. Chamcharatsri, P.B. (2013). Emotionality and second language writers: expressing fear through narrative in Thai and in English. *L2 J.* 5 (1): 59–75.
114. Pavlenko, A. (2013). The affective turn in SLA: from 'affective factors' to 'language desire' and 'commodification of affect'. In: *The Affective Dimension in Second Language Acquisition*, vol. 3, 3–28. Multilingual Matters.
115. May, S. (2013). *The Multilingual Turn: Implications for SLA, TESOL, and Bilingual Education.* Routledge.
116. Alarcón, A., Di Paolo, A., Heyman, J., and Morales, M.C. (2018). Returns to Spanish–English bilingualism in the new information economy: the health and criminal justice sectors in the Texas border and dallas-tarrant counties. In: *The Bilingual Advantage*, 138–159. Bristol, Blue Ridge Summit: Multilingual Matters.
117. Martinez, G. and Schwartz, A. (2012). Elevating "low" language for high stakes: a case for critical, community-based learning in a medical Spanish for heritage learners program. *Herit. Lang. J.* 9 (2): 37–49.

118. Brega, A.G., Barnard, J., Mabachi, N.M. et al. (2015). *AHRQ Health Literacy Universal Precautions Toolkit*, 2ee. (Prepared by Colorado Health Outcomes Program, University of Colorado Anschutz Medical Campus under Contract No. HHSA290200710008, TO#10.) AHRQ Publication No. 15-0023-EF. Rockville, MD: Agency for Healthcare Research and Quality.

119. Kolpatzik, K. (2019). *Gesundheitskompetenz im Fokus*. KomPart Berl: Das Praxishandbuch.

120. Zarcadoolas, C. and Vaughon, W. (2014). If numbers could speak: numeracy and the digital revolution. In: *The Routledge Handbook of Language and Health Communication*. Routledge.

121. McNamara, D.S. and Magliano, J. (2009). Chapter 9 Toward a comprehensive model of comprehension. In: *Psychology of Learning and Motivation*, vol. 51, 297–384. Academic Press.

122. WHO (2021). *Health Promotion Glossary of Terms*. WHO.

123. Freire, P. (2020). Pedagogy of the Oppressed. In: *Toward a Sociology of Education*, 374–386. Routledge.

124. Schillinger, D., Duran, N.D., McNamara, D.S. et al. (2021). Precision communication: physicians' linguistic adaptation to patients' health literacy. *Sci. Adv.* 7 (51): eabj2836.

125. Walqui, A. (2006). Scaffolding instruction for English language learners: a conceptual framework. *Int. J. Biling. Educ. Biling.* 9 (2): 159–180.

126. Vozenilek, J. (2004). See one, do one, teach one: advanced technology in medical education. *Acad. Emerg. Med.* 11 (11): 1149–1154.

127. Mearns, T.L. (2012). Using CLIL to enhance pupils' experience of learning and raise attainment in German and health education: a teacher research project. *Lang. Learn. J.* 40 (2): 175–192.

128. Leisen, J. (2010). *Handbuch Sprachförderung im Fach: sprachsensibler Fachunterricht in der Praxis; Grundlagenwissen, Anregungen und Beispiele für die Unterstützung von sprachschwachen Lernern und Lernern mit Zuwanderungsgeschichte beim Sprechen, Lesen*. Varus: Schreiben und Üben im Fach.

129. Nutbeam, D., Levin-Zamir, D., and Rowlands, G. (2019). *Health Literacy in Context-Settings, Media, and Populations*. MDPI-Multidisciplinary Digital Publishing Institute.

130. Levin-Zamir, D., Leung, A.Y.M., Dodson, S., and Rowlands, G. (2017). Health literacy in selected populations: individuals, families, and communities from the international and cultural perspective. *Inf. Serv. Use* 37 (2): 131–151.

131. Menken, K. (2008). High-stakes tests as de facto language education policies. *Encycl. Lang. Educ.* 7: 401–413.

132. Shohamy, E. (1993). The power of tests: the impact of language tests on teaching and learning. NFLC occasional Papers.

133. Fillmore, L.W. and Snow, C.E. (2000). *What Teachers Need to Know About Language*. Washington, DC: Center for Applied Linguistics.

134. Pleasant, A. (2014). Advancing health literacy measurement: a pathway to better health and health system performance. *J. Health Commun.* 19 (12): 1481–1496.

135. Santos, M. and Landry, L. (2008). Partners in training: a cross-disciplinary approach to preparing adult literacy practitioners and health professionals. *Focus Basics* 9 (B): 21–25.

136. Showstack, R.E. (2021). Making sense of the interpreter role in a healthcare service-learning program. *Appl. Linguist.* 42 (1): 93–112.

137. Hohn, M.D. and Rivera, L. (2019). The impact and outcomes of integrating health literacy education into adult basic education programs in Boston. *HLRP Health Lit. Res. Pract.* 3 (3): S25–S32.

138. Ortega, L. (2019). SLA and the study of equitable multilingualism. *Mod. Lang. J.* 103: 23–38.

139. Ortega, L. (2010) The bilingual turn in SLA. *Plenary Delivered at the Annual Conference of the American Association of Applied Linguistics*, in Atlanta, GA (6–9 March 2010).

2 Sociolinguistics, Public Health, and Healthcare

DALIA MAGAÑA

Introduction

Communication is an essential aspect of quality healthcare. Language choices in healthcare contexts can impact how patients understand and react to health information and how they act on it. This includes micro-level language choices such as which variety and register (formal or informal) healthcare workers use. In multilingual and multicultural societies, it is vital that healthcare workers not only know patients' language but also make deliberate linguistic choices to support patient health. However, healthcare workers are not trained in this area and are usually neither sensitized to it nor equipped to handle it appropriately. This chapter uses sociolinguistic tools and concepts related to language and interaction to explain language-based disparities. It advances an argument regarding the value of local language in promoting healthcare equity. To contextualize the concepts introduced in the theoretical framework section, the proceeding sections will discuss issues at the intersection of Latinx identity in the United States, language, and health from a critical sociolinguistics perspective. This chapter will equip the reader to gain new insight into the languages in contact during healthcare interactions, the role of language in COVID-19 health communications, and issues around language access during clinical interactions. The final section offers practical implications for working against language prestige to promote local languages and create more equitable healthcare for minoritized language speakers.

Sociolinguistics as a theoretical framework in healthcare communication

Sociolinguistics

A recognized subdiscipline within linguistics since the 1930s, sociolinguistics is defined as "the study of language as a complex of resources, of their value distribution, right of ownership and effects" [1] (p. 28). People invest in language resources (e.g., learning standard English or Spanish) for a variety of reasons. For example, Medical Spanish students take such courses to support Spanish-speaking patients; these courses guide learners in developing formal and specialized language uses. The value distribution of language resources refers to how language varieties are distributed and the value placed on them as influenced by class, gender, age, and social status differences. Right of ownership (who has access to language resources) and effects (usefulness of language resources) point to social inequality as partially temporal and context-dependent while also structural and enduring. This perspective helps uncover why across societies, the language varieties of middle/upper-class and educated people are associated with standard, prestigious forms of speech; meanwhile, how working-class groups speak is considered nonstandard and often stigmatized in formal settings.

Sociolinguistics offers an understanding of how lack of access or control to prestige language varieties or literacy skills contributes to social inequalities among marginalized groups [2]. For instance, a patient in the United States without formal education and who does not speak English will face disadvantages in navigating the healthcare system and having access to information compared to a highly educated English speaker. Standard English speakers have advantages not only in the healthcare system but across a range of situations within and outside the United States. In this sense, the language resources of highly educated English speakers have "mobility."

Sociolinguistics of mobility

Sociolinguistics of mobility refers to language in motion in a changing society with stratified scales that are hierarchical and power-invested. This central concept views language as occurring in motion (not stagnant), meaning that both languages and their speakers change. New terms are added to language influenced by social changes, global emergencies, etc. (e.g., social media, pandemic, and migration). Migration results in languages in contact and language change. In this sense, people are mobile, promote multilingualism, and impact their linguistic resources. Sociolinguistics of mobility invites a more complex, dynamic, and multifaceted view of people and their languages' realities [1].

Language resources are not valued equally; they are stratified. Lower-scale language resources are fleeting, local, and situated in a specific context (e.g., a rural variety of Dominican Spanish). Higher-scale language resources are timeless, translocal (i.e., transcending geographical or political boundaries), and widespread (e.g., standard Spanish). To illustrate the concept of scales, we return to our example of Medical Spanish courses in the United States. Many of those use standard Spanish in addition to a specialized healthcare use of the language. Such courses typically do not focus on local uses of Spanish. In this sense, local varieties of Spanish would be placed on a lower scale than a translocal and widespread situation. An argument for prioritizing standard Spanish in educational settings is that a generalized context conveys practices beyond the local.

Sociolinguistics of mobility also offers a lens to explain how language norms can be transferred and transported from one context where it is spoken to another. Language varieties considered more prestigious (e.g., standard Spanish) are more mobile than those considered less prestigious (e.g., rural Dominican Spanish). Prestigious varieties are considered translocal and widespread, while low-prestige varieties are considered local and situated. Using this framework can shed light on language access and healthcare inequalities and point to recommendations for inclusivity. For instance, in practice, Medical Spanish students may realize that communicating effectively with local communities requires learning the varieties of the population they serve, even when it means going against standard language norms. This was the case for United States practitioners who volunteered in the Dominican Republic and faced challenges communicating with patients because some standard terms they used confused local patients [3]. These practitioners had to learn a rural Dominican variety of Spanish, adopt "Dominicanisms" in their speech and adapt medical intake forms to enhance communication and trust with the Dominican patients. This example illustrates the consequences of prioritizing higher-scale language varieties (e.g., miscommunication during initial interactions with rural Dominicans) and the need to value the local even when it means resisting standard language norms. Awareness of language varieties, their scales, prestige, and value is crucial as more people and languages come in contact with globalization and social diversification.

Translanguaging

Viewing language as characterized by mobility is timely as societies across the globe diversify due to globalization and migration. When people of different language and cultural backgrounds interact, they practice translanguaging, meaning when bilingual or multilingual speakers use their entire linguistic repertoire without regard to traditional language boundaries [4]. For instance, translanguaging among bilingual Spanish-English patients and health practitioners in the United States may entail using both English and Spanish to make sense of healthcare terms, enhance communication, and express solidarity (of living between two worlds). A translanguaging lens views speakers' linguistic repertoire holistically because it considers languaging (practicing language) a collection of linguistic features in the speakers' languages of equal value. As with sociolinguistics of mobility, translanguaging is seen as a fluid, flexible use of language and calls for avoiding "watchful adherence to the socially and politically defined boundaries of named (and usually national and state) languages" [5] (p. 283). Unfortunately, people who engage in translanguaging are often perceived as being language deficient, having language gaps, or having incomplete knowledge of their languages. Educational spaces in the United States often promote separating multilinguals' languages (e.g., speaking heritage languages at home and English at school). However, embracing translanguaging in schools not only leads to more successful learning but also serves to create inclusivity of learners' heritage and liberates them from strict language separation [5].

In multilingual contexts, which are widespread due to diversifying neighborhoods and ongoing globalization processes, translanguaging occurs since language tasks are collaborative and involve multilingual repertoires, often combining several languages and varieties [6]. Speakers draw on the language resources or communicative repertoires they have at their disposal when communicating with other language speakers. In multilingual interactions, people "very often pool their competencies and skills in particular languages when they have to accomplish demanding communication tasks" [1] (p. 7). They do this by serving as translators, providing other assistance, and pooling the language resources available to them.

Language is considered a resource in interpreted interactions in health communication studies where speakers draw on their communicative repertoires to mediate understanding. A study on antenatal consultations in a London hospital that serves a super-diverse population illustrates how speakers draw on their linguistic resources to negotiate patient information collaboratively [6]. The consultation involves an English-speaking midwife, a Portuguese-speaking patient, the patient's multilingual companion, and a professional Portuguese-to-English interpreter. During the consultation, the midwife asks in English whether the patient experiences blood clots, but the interpreter does not know the term for blood clots in Portuguese. The midwife uses another language repertoire to describe the condition in detail in plain English instead of using technical terms. With the patient's companion's help, the interpreter is able to convey this information to the patient and ask whether she has issues with her blood flow. Later the midwife asks whether the patient has had chickenpox, using a medicalized term, varicella, which the interpreter mistakenly interprets, given the Portuguese term for rabies. The patient's companion recognizes the problem and again collaborates with the healthcare practitioners, offering the correct translation. An excerpt of that interaction is provided below.

> Interpreter: chicken box, eh eh, chicken pox is . . .
> Midwife: in childhood
> Interpreter: *Quando tu era pequeno* [When you were small]
> (Turns to Patient companion) *o que era a palavra chickenpox erm é em Portuguées voceés é* [what was the word chicken pox uhm in Portuguese you all]
> Patient companion: chicken box
> Interpreter: yeah, *e´ chickenpox, aquele do* [yeah, chicken pox that one of the]
> Midwife: yes, little, skin spots
> Patient companion: aah, varicella
> Interpreter: rabies. rabies.
> Patient: okay okay

The study highlights the importance of collaborative translanguaging because it leads to correcting misunderstandings, enhancing communication, and overall improving patient care.

That study also shows how important it is for transnational patients to bring advocates to their consultation rooms. Besides helping to aid communication, as the patient's companion did in this case, a companion to a medical visit might offer emotional support and a sense of security to a transnational patient unfamiliar with complex and confusing healthcare systems such as those in the United Kingdom and the United States. The emotional support and protection that a companion provides contribute to the patient's reception of the information and the efficacy of the interaction in dealing with the health problem. For ethnic groups that value community orientation over individual orientation, such as Latinxs, bringing a family member or friend to the medical visit is typical, given the cultural value of *compañerismo* meaning, companionship, and togetherness [7]. Latinxs who value community orientation/collectivism may prefer to face health complications as shared experiences among family or friends rather than as a private/individual issue; bringing a companion to a consultation is part of inviting someone to share that health experience.

Sociolinguistics and COVID-19

Beyond case studies, research shows that attentiveness to sociolinguistics in healthcare communication, specifically in which language or language varieties are valued, can illuminate the causes of inequalities in healthcare and provide insights for moving toward equity. For example, English-centric communication has strongly exacerbated health disparities during the COVID-19 pandemic. The pandemic created the need for rapidly emerging neologisms (e.g., coronavirus, social distancing, quarantine, super-spreader, lockdown, and flattening the curve). This new scientific and medical language needed to be communicated to multilingual communities around the world [8]. Unfortunately, this crisis-based information does not reach all equally. For instance, inequitable access to COVID-19 information in Spanish intensified health disparities among Latinxs, who have been disproportionately affected by COVID-19. A study in Arkansas found that Spanish speakers "reported little awareness of public health messaging and low knowledge regarding SARS-CoV-2 transmission and disease characteristics. . .[they were] unaware of or unsure about how to access support services available in the local community, leading to confusion around prevention, testing, and services" [9] (p. 1809). These barriers were due to the lack of reliable information in Spanish, which complicated lowering virus transmission, and contributed to the crisis.

The literature has also pointed to lower vaccination rates among the Latinx community, partly due to communication and language-related issues. For example, Latinxs report more confusion about where to get vaccinated than Whites [10]. Many Latinxs are not getting the information they need. Even within the Latinx community, they face language-based disparities. A recent study surveyed the COVID-19-related knowledge and plans of Spanish monolingual Latinxs, English-proficient Latinxs, and English-proficient non-Latinxs [11]. They found that Spanish monolinguals were less likely to anticipate getting vaccinated, despite having higher cases of COVID-19 and more concerns about the virus than the other groups. Spanish monolinguals reported more concerns over vaccine side effects (62.6%) than English-proficient Latinxs (41.6%) and English-proficient non-Latinxs (41.2%). These differences between Spanish and English speakers (Latinxs and non-Latinxs) point to the need to improve services for language access.

Such cases suggest the adverse impacts of devaluing minoritized languages in emergency communication and the role of language repertoires in building trust with community members. The issues of overlooking minoritized languages go beyond disseminating accurate COVID-19 information and extend to the lack of creating relationships, which is crucial so that the audience can trust the information and feel comfortable acting on it [12]. Taking into account the role of culture in building relationships may be a crucial part of this process.

Sociolinguists have pointed out that members of some groups might be more receptive to the information if presented in culturally tailored ways; for instance, Mongolians may find comfort in traditional Mongolian fiddle stories, Chinese transnationals in Chinese social media, and other East Asian groups in classical Chinese poetry [2]. Other studies have found cross-cultural differences in receptiveness to metaphors across ethnic groups [13]. Definitions that include metaphors tend to have particular resonance for Spanish-speaking Latinxs, even in comparison to English-speaking Latinxs. Metaphors tend to boost recall and trust for this group as well. Awareness of such distinctions can support tailoring health information in linguistic and culturally specific-ways. The following section turns to the case of Latinxs in the United States to further explore the consequences of privileging English-centric communication and standard varieties of Spanish over local language.

Critical issues around latinx health and language

Latinxs and language in healthcare

To offer a specific example of how sociolinguistics, specifically the concepts of scales and mobility, intersects and affects people in one particular English-language dominant context, we turn to the situation of Latinxs in the United States. Understanding language scales or how our society values particular language or language varieties over minoritized or stigmatized varieties and viewing language and its speakers in terms of mobility can help uncover the dire consequences of privileging English in multilingual societies.

Latinxs are the largest racial/ethnic minority group in the United States, constituting approximately 57.5 million Americans and up to 18% of the population, with growing numbers [14]. About 72% of Latinxs over five years of age speak a language other than English at home, and 30% have limited English proficiency [15]. Nearly 20% have low educational attainment and live below the poverty line [16]. In California, the US state with the largest Latinx population (15.3 million), 41% of Latinxs 25 years or older have less than a high school education, which is five times greater than that of non-Latinxs [17]. Latinxs are sociolinguistically diverse. Some come to the United States as adults with a high level of education and speak prestigious varieties of Spanish and English; others are raised or born in the United States and have strong English language skills and a wide range of abilities in Spanish as a heritage language. Still, other groups speak an indigenous language along with Spanish or may not speak Spanish at all. The latter group, along with Spanish monolinguals, are among the most disadvantaged regarding language and healthcare access because US medical institutions are designed to privilege English speakers.

To explore the disadvantages that Spanish monolinguals face in accessing healthcare and risk communication, the following sections will discuss issues around interpreted interactions, patient experiences, and communicating risk. This section will also feature a clinical interaction where a doctor adjusts his language choices to offer patient-centered care and issues around promoting local language use.

Language access in healthcare

Poor access, bias, discrimination, and language and cultural barriers pose unique challenges to non-English speaking Latinxs in healthcare interactions with providers in the United States because there is a severe shortage of Latinx and Spanish-speaking providers [18–20]. Patients benefit when providers are culturally and linguistically competent [18, 21]. Language concordant providers promote confidence in asking questions and trust and lower the perception of discrimination [20, 22, 23]. Spanish-speaking patients report better consultation experiences and better health outcomes with Spanish-speaking providers [24]. Unfortunately, there is also a scarcity of language interpreters. Even when an English–Spanish interpreter is present, subtle nuances may be lost, and misinterpretation can occur [25, 26]. Another disadvantage that has been reported in language-discordant interactions is that patients tend to ask fewer questions and are less likely to have their questions answered when compared to patients in language-concordant consultations [27]. Further, interpreted consultations are not typically allotted more time than same language interactions despite the apparent need, and patients say their interactions with providers are very rushed [28]. More time between clinicians and language-minorized patients can help address some of these concerns by promoting opportunities to ask questions, clarify information, share concerns, and enhance patient-centered care.

Patient experiences

A sociolinguistics perspective in healthcare can raise critical awareness of languages and how the value society ascribes to them creates advantages for language majority speakers and disadvantages for minoritized groups. Language-minorized communities have identified the elevated status of English in the United States as a central issue in obtaining equitable care [26]. Spanish speakers report being disempowered during their consultations due to a lack of opportunities to speak and feeling profiled in medical encounters because they do not speak English [29–31]. Spanish-speaking Latinxs perceive that providers treat English-speaking patients better than minority language speakers; they report that medical personnel express frustration over their low English literacy levels and belittle them if they need extra support with tasks like completing paperwork [28]. For example, Amalia, a woman in her 60s living in rural California, reported that, *"Hay recepcionistas muy impacientes, más en contra de las personas que no hablan inglés. Como que lo ignoran a uno. Eso es muy duro."* [There are receptionists who are very impatient, more toward the people who don't speak English. It's like they ignore you. That's very hard.] These disadvantages also adversely affect general Latinx healthcare and distrust in providers and the healthcare system; for instance, how patients access or process complex medical paperwork affects their treatment and how they make sense of essential health information.

Risk communication in the digital age

Latinxs face a lack of access to science-based, accessible, trustworthy, and bilingual health information [32]. They also face a digital divide: Only 55% of low-income Latinx families have broadband at home, severely limiting access to COVID-19 bilingual information [33]. TV news is a prominent source of information for Latinxs, especially for immigrant Latinxs. About 89% of immigrant Latinxs get at least some of their news in Spanish [34]. Younger, United States-born Latinxs are turning to the internet for news consumption, but immigrant Latinxs, who tend to be older, prefer Spanish-language TV news sources. For these reasons, it is crucial that healthcare practitioners not assume their patients have digital access.

Language experts recommend that healthcare messages be patient-centered; evidence suggests that such communication boosts safe and effective practice of medicine [35]. This requires cultural and linguistic tailoring, drawing on knowledge from patients themselves [36, 37]. Patient-centered communication requires providers to be aware of the local linguistic practices that patients use and use plain language to de-jargonize specialized terms. This might mean, for instance, that local varieties of Spanish would be used, making locals feel represented (e.g., translanguaging, colloquialisms, regionalisms, refrains, and metaphors) and that speaks to their cultural values (community and family orientation, mutual trust and respect, etc.). This requires a move to the local and, in terms of sociolinguistics of mobility, "scaling down" and prioritizing the local. This recommendation aligns with the "plain language" approach to enhance health communication by replacing public health jargon with everyday words. A sociolinguistics lens complements the plain language approach. It sheds further light on why certain groups are excluded from access to health communication through the concepts of language scales and their associated value.

Clinical interactions

To contextualize this language use in a healthcare interaction, let us consider medical providers' move from a specific technical register to plain language, which would be translanguaging because the provider uses the linguistic codes at their disposal to enhance communication. For example, a study observed that a healthcare provider flattened epistemics to avoid possible face threats to the patient that technical and unfamiliar language might cause [6]. Similarly, an analysis of doctor-patient consultations observed that a Mexican doctor asked a rural Mexican woman about the delivery of her child when collecting clinical history using the colloquial phrase *"nacer por abajo"* (literally, to be born from down there) instead of mentioning vaginal delivery or a cesarean section [38]. This way, he avoided using taboo genital-related terms that might embarrass the patient or seem too direct in ways that violate the politeness norms of rural Mexican immigrants. This switch from a generalized term to a colloquial phrase would be considered a scale move to prioritize the local. In other cases, this same provider uses both English and Spanish when bilingual patients do, signaling to patients that he values translanguaging. Thus he creates an inviting space for patients to make meaning using their full linguistic repertoires without judgmental attitudes toward translanguaging practices.

Empowering the patient may also entail successively introducing medical terms (scaffolding). For instance, when another Mexican patient does not recognize the term *ataque de pánico* [panic attack], this doctor explains, *"Que siente que se le sale el corazón y empieza a sudar como si le fuera a dar un ataque y siente que se va a morir."* [You feel that your heart is going to burst, and you start sweating as if you were going to get a heart attack, and you feel that you're going to die.] [38]. As the example shows, the doctor replaces the terms with several phrases using plain language that illustrate the symptoms. The patient responds that she thinks she did indeed experience a panic attack.

Promoting local language

Accommodating the language varieties of patients is crucial in promoting inclusivity in healthcare. If rural Mexican Spanish is most common in southern Texas regions, that variety should be prioritized in healthcare messaging. However, their lower-scale status can breed resistance in those who formulate such messages. Similarly, Spanish language instruction in US schools tends to emphasize "standard" varieties and not, for example, the Spanish of working-class Mexicans or the Spanish spoken in the United States, which reflects significant English language influence. Educators may defend such resistance on the grounds of the diversity of Spanish speakers in the United States and the advantage of a language more widely spoken.

Textbooks support this view by elevating standard language use. In a thorough review of medical Spanish textbooks, a key finding was they lack discussion of practical issues that medical professionals encounter, including knowledge about people's social values and how people discuss health issues in colloquial or regional ways [39]. Medical

Spanish textbooks overlook regionalisms and colloquialisms, for instance, emphasizing the standard term for "health insurance" as *seguro médico* when many Spanish speakers in the United States use *aseguranza*. However, stigmatizing and silencing local varieties does real harm [40]. Interpreters, especially those not part of the communities they serve, internalize such stigma and may not use local varieties in clinical interactions. They miss a significant opportunity to make patients feel represented and valued in healthcare communication by including local language.

The media plays a role in normalizing how dominant groups discuss health. For instance, the *war* metaphor is common in COVID-19 news on Twitter, where the virus is portrayed as an invisible enemy, medication and vaccines as "weapons," and healthcare practitioners as "heroes" battling on the "front lines" [41]. Similarly, a study on TV news in Spanish in the United States showed that this war metaphor was prevalent, as in, "*Siguen luchando desde los hospitales y presentan obstáculos para ganarle la batalla a la pandemia.*" [They continue to **fight** from hospitals and face obstacles to **winning** the **battle** against the pandemic.] [42]. However, using the *war* metaphor in health messaging about diseases is dangerous because it negatively impacts prevention behavior in part because of the increased perceived difficulty through this framing [43] and stigmatizes individuals who die from the disease (e.g., "losing their battle to COVID-19" implies that dying is "defeat"). This war metaphor, which conveys violence, is imposed onto US Latinxs through the media without evidence of its effectiveness among this group. Studies on metaphor use in cancer discourse indicate that this war metaphor is not as prevalent among Latinas [44] or is problematic among black women who do not see themselves as "lone battlers" but rather deal with diseases more collectively [45].

A deliberate focus on inclusive linguistic varieties is essential because how language is used can be a way to build trust, which is vital when "communicating with vulnerable, marginalized, and underserved communities who regularly face systemic barriers and discrimination" [36].

Recommendations for health messaging, practice, education, and research

Practical recommendations for improving health messaging campaigns

Leading experts in Latinx healthcare have emphasized the crucial role of language and communication in reaching this population [37, 46, 47]. Professor of Medicine Alicia Fernández advises that healthcare providers must focus on improving communication to reach the Latinx community [46]. She calls for outreach from community health clinics and *promotoras* (translingual community health workers) because they have people who have cultural and linguistic competencies and experience educating those with low health literacy. She has suggested social marketing campaigns in Spanish (television, radio, billboards, and social media) for health information. This tailored outreach and collaboration with people and organizations Latinxs trust could make a significant difference. Focusing on language and sociolinguistics offers insights into the form and content such messages should have.

A study that included many Latinx and Black participants found that participants favor language that references people over companies or institutions [36]. For example, in healthcare messaging, participants indicated that they would trust "scientists, health and medical experts, and researchers" more than "science, health, and medical companies" (p. 99). Respondents also reported being more likely to get vaccinated for their families than for the nation or the economy. For some ethnic groups, this wording also aligns with their cultural values. For Latinxs, it speaks to their values of community orientation and *familismo* (meaning prioritizing the needs of a group over individual needs) and altruism (making burdensome sacrifices for family or others) [48]. These studies point to the need to tailor messages using local language varieties that are culturally informed, meaning tapping into the groups' cultural values.

Practical recommendation for improving interpretative encounters

The recommendations on healthcare messaging also apply to healthcare interactions. However, real-time communication complexities should be considered, including language/cultural barriers and power dynamics. Given the hierarchical roles of doctors and patients in healthcare interactions, empowering patients may entail minimizing interruptions, using informal language, lay terms, or colloquialisms, or engaging patients in small talk to create a more interpersonal relationship [38]. These measures may be essential with language-minoritized patients. Bilingual providers should use their total speech repertoire and engage in translanguaging practices to enhance communication with their patients, e.g., by switching to plain language to break down information or into a colloquial variety when asking about a stigmatized topic (e.g., drug use) or using other languages shared with patients to explain words.

Communicating with minoritized language speakers should be a collaborative effort to support patients who value a communal approach to healthcare and enhance communication. Spanish-speaking Latinxs prefer having someone they trust (like a family member or friend) to advocate for them in healthcare consultations, even when an interpreter is present. Several reasons for this include reported issues with remote interpreting (through voice or video call), such as incorrect interpretation and feeling dehumanized in having interpreting services through a device to call-in medical interpreters [49]. Having an advocate present mitigates some of these frustrations. In many US hospitals, only professional interpreters are allowed to interpret; it is prohibited to enable *ad-hoc* interpreters. However, research shows that professional interpreters can work with patients' advocates and patients to solve language barriers [6]. Early in the COVID-19 pandemic, many hospitals and clinics relied on remote interpreting, and patients were typically not allowed to bring anyone into the consultation room with them. For people whose culture calls for an individualistic orientation to healthcare, who are confident advocating for themselves, who trust the healthcare system, and who prefer independence and privacy, this did not pose a problem. But this restriction may create further barriers and stress for Latinxs, especially those who do not speak English and/or mistrust the healthcare system. Healthcare practitioners should actively encourage Spanish-speaking patients to bring someone into the consultation room with them and create space for using multiple repertoires and/or languages or translanguaging to enhance communication.

Educational recommendations for clinician and interpreter training

Given that provider time with patients is constrained, training providers and interpreters to make intentional language choices during patient interactions is crucial. As sociolinguistics of mobility informs us, language varieties can be stigmatized and create implicit biases. This stigma reflects class distinctions rather than intrinsic value, comprehensibility, or aesthetic features. Practitioners and interpreters must practice language acceptance, a concept that moves beyond language access [47]. Language access overlooks the relationship between language prestige associated with power, a crucial problem affecting language-minoritized groups in navigating the healthcare system. On the other hand, the concept of language acceptance can serve to train practitioners and interpreters to avoid marking inferiority or superiority distinctions between varieties. Acceptance entails sociolinguistic awareness of the varieties of Latinxs in the United States, a descriptive view and attitude about language varieties, and making strides to adapt the interaction to patients' language variety or displaying a willingness to learn. These steps require a critical reflection on language use, which can lead to more inclusive and welcoming healthcare experiences.

These sociolinguistic lessons could be a crucial addition to the clinical skills curriculum to support medical students in practicing medicine safely and effectively [35]. Ortega and Prada [35] emphasize patient-centered communication, a shift from focusing on technical language knowledge, as the principal goal for training medical students. The practical strategies they propose for including in medical language education work to center local, lower-scale language include the following approaches:

1. using supplemental resources that reflect local linguistic practices (adopting books or glossaries that incorporate such language or creating such resources),
2. partnering with students that have lived experience using local linguistic practices to serve as TAs or course consultants,
3. collaborating with community members as educators (community health workers, advocates, patients, and interpreters),
4. implementing service-learning opportunities for students to gain insight into language use in the local community,
5. integrating course activities that foment local language use (e.g., using ethnolinguistic material, and assigning ethnographic observations).

These recommendations align with a sociolinguistics approach by allowing students to reflect critically on the language varieties used in healthcare interactions. The suggestions are also crucial steps against the imposition of language prestige by promoting the local, lower-scaled varieties, which are recognized as vital in creating inclusivity in healthcare. Ortega and Prada suggest embracing translanguaging to encourage providers to expand their language repertoire and to view this as an ongoing learning experience, given language change. Strategies to enhance patient-centered communication skills in medical education are long-term learning experiences that should be adapted according to the communities served [35]. This movement requires multiple levels of stakeholder collaboration, such as the work of the National Association of Medical Spanish [50].

Increasing time allotted to minoritized patients

Minoritized language speakers should also be allotted more time with their health providers than other patients to account for time spent on interpretation and addressing low health literacy and barriers such as the digital divide. For instance, a patient with low health literacy, limited English language skills, and/or lack of access to the internet would need an oral explanation of their test results, which takes more time than referring them to an online portal. This step requires more time from the providers and interpreters. Greater time allotment would lessen patients' perception that providers are rude. Patients may perceive clinicians as rude because they may skip greetings or small talk, not make eye contact with patients, and take notes during the consultation [28]. For providers, these may be time-saving measures, but this behavior violates cultural values such as *personalismo* (friendliness and making an interpersonal connection before an institutional relationship). For these reasons, reducing time pressures on providers can enhance the quality of patient-centered care. This recommendation to increase time with language-minoritized patients is as much for health organizations as for providers.

Recommendations for research on the sociolinguistics of mobility in healthcare

More studies are needed to understand the different needs within diverse Latinx communities since Latinxs, like any language minority group, are not homogenous. Latinxs have different levels of privilege in terms of social access (income, education, immigration status, and insurance); some of this access is also language-based (health literacy, English language proficiency). These differences must be recognized to become attentive to those most vulnerable in healthcare. The first step is to critically reflect on which linguistic varieties should be prioritized, in which spaces, and for what purposes. A sociolinguistics of mobility perspective helps shed light on why a standard variety is valorized: because it is translocal and widespread. Healthcare communication (messaging and interpersonal interactions) might aim to reach the most people with a standard variety because Latinxs are diverse and speak numerous varieties of Spanish (Puerto Rican Spanish, Cuban Spanish, Salvadorean Spanish, and Mexican), English, Indigenous languages, and a mixture of multiple varieties, which beyond region also differ according to class, gender, and identity. A significant variation in these varieties is their colloquialisms. It is crucial to deliberately target the most vulnerable groups by uncovering knowledge around their colloquialisms, how they conceptualize health/illness, and how their language varieties and cultural understandings support more successful public health messaging. Equally urgent, we need a better understanding of which Latinx language groups are vulnerable to specific health issues; for instance, tobacco use and diet-release disease affect the English monolingual Latinx population at greater levels than Spanish monolinguals according to the acculturation paradox research [51–53].

Research questions that arise to help shed more light on these issues may include,

1. What is the role of language in the Latinx health paradox?
2. How do other Latinxs compare to each other regarding cultural constructs and communication issues?
3. How does Latinx culture impact gender differences in communication?

4. What is the role of translanguaging in medical consultations across Latinx groups?
5. What language choices (e.g., metaphors) most resonate with Latinxs and influence their perceptions of health and associated actions?

When considering Latinxs, it is also critical to consider non-Spanish speaking groups; for example, those who speak an indigenous language experience severe issues around language access. Indeed, a vital reflection of the local languages and varieties spoken in specific regions is essential in creating more inclusive and equitable healthcare for language minority groups.

Further language-based research focusing on medical discourse from a sociolinguistics perspective is needed. Such studies should consider patients' views and use a holistic approach that encompasses the context in which interactions occur and is systematic. Linguists who have studied healthcare discourse have pointed out barriers that only close attention to language can reveal and have provided potential solutions [54]. Future research to refine such solutions should be based on collaborations with stakeholders at various levels, including community healthcare advocates, medical education instructors, language instructors, public health scholars, interpreters, and medical providers. At the same time, to understand the healthcare experiences of minoritized language speakers in English-dominant countries and their suggestions for improvements, it is crucial to center their voices and engage them as partners in research [49]. Indeed, collaborations are vital in addressing issues in multilingual communication during a health crisis [2].

Conclusion

Research on language barriers from a critical sociolinguistics perspective is starting to gain attention and shed light on inequalities in healthcare, as well as point toward solutions for reaching underserved communities. This chapter has discussed concepts of translanguaging and sociolinguistics of mobility to discuss the role of local language varieties in healthcare. It has been proposed that further explicit understanding of translanguaging practices and training in creating spaces that invite those practices. It is critical to adopt a collaborative approach inviting translanguaging practices where all parties can draw on their linguistic resources and repertoires to mediate differences and enhance understanding [6].

Studies on language use and globalization in the context of COVID-19 shed light on which languages and language varieties are prioritized, who has access to this information, and who is left behind. Language plays an important role, among other factors, contributing to disparities in healthcare. For instance, when health messaging does not reach everyone, it contributes to higher levels of COVID-19 transmission and lower COVID-19 vaccination rates among Spanish speakers. The Latinx community is diverse, and there are evident differences within the group according to their language proficiency, nation of origin, socioeconomic differences, etc. For these reasons, it is crucial that healthcare practitioners have knowledge about local language use to target communities in culturally tailored ways. Unfortunately, problematic attitudes against local varieties of Spanish in the United States pervade our society. Sociolinguistics of mobility helps shed light on these attitudes. In health messaging, a "standard" variety of Spanish, sometimes even peninsular Spanish, is prioritized over the local. While the stated objective is to target a larger audience through language that is "translocal," this inevitably stigmatizes local varieties and those who speak them. It can impede communication with those who do not understand the "standard" variety and consistently interferes with the comfort of those who are more comfortable speaking other varieties. Including local knowledge and language varieties in healthcare, communication is vital if patients are to feel seen, heard, and understood.

Healthcare systems need to be deliberate about reaching low-income communities; otherwise, inequalities will continue. Critical language awareness about the role of sociolinguistics and translanguaging in healthcare communication can offer insights into solutions for reaching communities in deliberate ways. A sociolinguistics perspective in improving healthcare interactions aligns with general health communication but contributes by uncovering an understanding of the root of the problem around language prestige and power. Sociolinguistics of mobility sheds light on why certain languages or language varieties are disparaged and excluded from formal spaces like classrooms and training materials. It reinforces why a deliberate focus on the local is needed to resist the powerful forces upholding the superiority of languages and language varieties.

A sociolinguistics approach emphasizes that healthcare practitioner training should be oriented towards expanding their repertoire of various ways to communicate so that interventions can be linguistically and culturally adequate. Indeed, improving communication between minoritized patients and their medical providers is a way to strengthen relationships between them, build trust, and thus improve public health for marginalized groups in the United States whose healthcare needs are inadequately met.

Highlights

- This chapter introduces sociolinguistic concepts to shed new light on the role of language in healthcare.
- Deliberate attention to language is essential in bridging gaps that affect non-English speakers in healthcare.
- A sociolinguistics approach emphasizes that healthcare practitioner training should be oriented toward expanding their repertoire of various ways to communicate so that interventions can be linguistically and culturally adequate.
- Healthcare systems should actively encourage language-minoritized patients to bring someone into the consultation room and invite using multiple repertoires and/or languages to enhance communication.
- Local language should not be overlooked in healthcare interactions and communications because it aids in reaching language minoritized groups and promotes health equity.

REFERENCES

1. Blommaert, J. (2010). *The Sociolinguistics of Globalization*. Cambridge University Press.
2. Piller, I., Zhang, J., and Li, J. (2020). Linguistic diversity in a time of crisis: language challenges of the COVID-19 pandemic. *Multilingua* 39 (5): 503–515.
3. Bloom-Pojar, R. (2018). Translanguaging outside the academy: negotiating rhetoric

and healthcare in the Spanish Caribbean. In: *Conference on College Composition and Communication*. National Council of Teachers of English.
4. García, O. and Wei, L. (2014). *Translanguaging: Language, Bilingualism and Education*. London: Palgrave Pivot.
5. Otheguy, R., García, O., and Reid, W. (2015). Clarifying translanguaging and deconstructing named languages: a perspective from linguistics. *Appl. Linguist. Rev.* 6 (3): 281–307.
6. Brooks, E. (2022). Translanguaging Health. *Appl. Linguist.* 43 (3): 517–537.
7. Albarran, C.R., Heilemann, M.V., and Koniak-Griffin, D. (2014). Promotoras as facilitators of change: Latinas' perspectives after participating in a lifestyle behaviour intervention program. *J. Adv. Nurs.* 70 (10): 2303–2313.
8. Dong, J. (2021). Language and globalization revisited: life from the periphery in COVID-19. *Int. J. Sociol. Lang.* 2021 (267–268): 105–110.
9. Center, K.E., Da Silva, J., Hernandez, A.L. et al. (2020). Multidisciplinary community-based investigation of a COVID-19 outbreak among Marshallese and Hispanic/Latino communities—Benton and Washington Counties, Arkansas, March–June 2020. *Morb. Mortal. Wkly. Rep.* 69 (48): 1807.
10. Hamel, L., Kirzinger, A., Lopes, L. et al. (2021). *KFF COVID-19 Vaccine Monitor: January 2021*. San Francisco, CA: Kaiser Family Foundation.
11. Himmelstein, J., Himmelstein, D.U., Woolhandler, S. et al. (2022). COVID-19-related care for Hispanic elderly adults with limited English proficiency. *Ann. Intern. Med.* 175 (1): 143–145.
12. Li, Y., Rao, G., Zhang, J., and Li, J. (2020). Conceptualizing national emergency language competence. *Multilingua* 39 (5): 617–623.
13. Ondish, P., Cohen, D., Lucas, K.W., and Vandello, J. (2019). The resonance of metaphor: evidence for Latino preferences for metaphor and analogy. *Pers. Soc. Psychol. Bull.* 45 (11): 1531–1548.
14. Vespa, J., Armstrong, D.M., and Medina, L. (2018). *Demographic turning points for the United States: Population projections for 2020 to 2060*. Washington, DC: US Department of Commerce, Economics and Statistics Administration, US Census Bureau. https://www.census.gov/library/publications/2020/demo/p25-1144.html (accessed 10 November 2021).
15. Office of Minority Health (2021). *Profile: Hispanic/Latino Americans*. Washington, DC. https://minorityhealth.hhs.gov/omh/browse.aspx?lvl=3&lvlid=64#:~:text=According%20to%20the%202019%20U.S.,the%20largest%20at%2061.4%20percent (accessed 10 November 2021).
16. Fontenot, K., Semega, J., and Kollar, M. (2018). *Income and poverty in the United States: 2017*. Washington, DC: US Government Printing Office. https://www.census.gov/library/publications/2018/demo/p60-263.html (accessed 7 October 2021).
17. California Senate Office of Research (CSOR). *A Statistical Picture of Latinos in California: 2017 update*. 2017. https://latinocaucus.legislature.ca.gov/sites/latinocaucus.legislature.ca.gov/files/forms/Statistical%20Picture%20of%20Latinos%20in%20California%20-%202017%20Update.pdf (accessed 22 September 2021).
18. Bustamante A, Felix Beltran L. *Latino Physician Shortage in California: The Patient Perspective*. 2019. https://latino.ucla.edu/wp-content/uploads/2019/08/The_Patient_Perspective-UCLA-LPPI-Final.pdf (accessed 22 September 2021).
19. Martínez LE, Solis G, Gomez V, Mendez-Vargas J, Diaz SFM, Hayes-Bautista DE. *California's Language Concordance Mismatch: An Analysis of Language Proficient Physicians and Limited English Proficient Individuals Who Speak Spanish, Tagalog, Thai, Lao or Vietnamese*. 2019. https://latino.ucla.edu/wp-content/uploads/2019/03/LPPI_Californias_Language_Concordance_Mismatch_2019.pdf (accessed 11 October 2021).
20. Steinberg, E.M., Valenzuela-Araujo, D., Zickafoose, J.S. et al. (2016). The "battle" of managing language barriers in health care. *Clin. Pediatr.* 55 (14): 1318–1327.
21. Kanter, M.H., Abrams, K.M., Carrasco, M.R. et al. (2009). Patient-physician

language concordance: a strategy for meeting the needs of Spanish-speaking patients in primary care. *Perm. J.* 13 (4): 79.
22. Detz, A., Mangione, C.M., de Jaimes, F.N. et al. (2014). Language concordance, interpersonal care, and diabetes self-care in rural Latino patients. *J. Gen. Intern. Med.* 29 (12): 1650–1656.
23. Valdez, C.R., Dvorscek, M.J., Budge, S.L., and Esmond, S. (2011). Provider perspectives about Latino patients: determinants of care and implications for treatment. *Counsel. Psychol.* 39 (4): 497–526.
24. Fernandez, A., Schillinger, D., Warton, E.M. et al. (2011). Language barriers, physician-patient language concordance, and glycemic control among insured Latinos with diabetes: the Diabetes Study of Northern California (DISTANCE). *J. Gen. Intern. Med.* 26 (2): 170–176.
25. Elderkin-Thompson, V., Silver, R.C., and Waitzkin, H. (2001). When nurses double as interpreters: a study of Spanish-speaking patients in a US primary care setting. *Soc. Sci. Med.* 52 (9): 1343–1358.
26. Martinez, G. (2008). Language-in-healthcare policy, interaction patterns, and unequal care on the US-Mexico border. *Lang. Policy* 7 (4): 345–363.
27. Davidson, B. (2000). The interpreter as institutional gatekeeper: the social-linguistic role of interpreters in Spanish-English medical discourse. *J. Socioling.* 4 (3): 379–405.
28. Magaña, D. (2020). Local voices on health care communication issues and insights on Latino cultural constructs. *Hisp. J. Behav. Sci.* 42 (3): 300–323.
29. Barr, D.A. and Wanat, S.F. (2005). Listening to patients: cultural and linguistic barriers to health care access. *Fam. Med.* 37 (3): 199–204.
30. Cheng, H.L., Lopez, A., Rislin, J.L. et al. (2018). Latino/Hispanic community adults' healthcare experience in a New Mexico borderland region. *J. Health Disparities Res. Pract.* 11 (4): 5.
31. Martínez, G. (2010). Language and power in healthcare: towards a theory of language barriers among linguistic minorities in the United States. In: *Readings in Language Studies: Language and Power*, vol. 2, 59–74.
32. American Public Health Association. *AHPA Leader Calls for Greater Access to COVID-19 Resources for Hispanics*. 2020. https://www.apha.org/news-and-media/news-releases/apha-news-releases/2020/hispanics-and-covid-19 (accessed 18 April 2021).
33. Latino Community Foundation. *Love Not Fear Fund (COVID-19 Response)*. 2021. https://latinocf.org/covid/ (accessed 20 April 2021)
34. Flores, A. and Lopez, M.H. (2018). *Among US Latinos, the Internet Now Rivals Television as a Source for News*, 11. Pew Research Center.
35. Ortega, P. and Prada, J. (2020). Words matter: translanguaging in medical communication skills training. *Perspect. Med. Educ.* 9: 251–255.
36. Miller, M.R. (2021). Language choice about COVID-19 vaccines can save lives. *J. Commun. Healthc.* 23: 1–3.
37. Ortega, P., Martínez, G., and Diamond, L. (2020). Language and health equity during COVID-19: lessons and opportunities. *J. Health Care Poor Underserved* 31 (4): 1530–1535.
38. Magaña, D. (2021). *Building Confianza: Empowering Latinos/as Through Transcultural Health Care Communication*. The Ohio State University Press.
39. Hardin, K. (2012). Targeting oral and cultural proficiency for medical personnel: an examination of current medical Spanish textbooks. *Hispania* 1: 698–713.
40. Martínez, G. and Schwartz, A. (2012). Elevating "low" language for high stakes: a case for critical, community-based learning in a medical Spanish for heritage learners program. *Herit. Lang. J.* 9 (2): 175–187.
41. Wicke, P. and Bolognesi, M.M. (2020). Framing COVID-19: how we conceptualize and discuss the pandemic on Twitter. *PloS One* 15 (9): e0240010.
42. Magaña, D., Durazo, A., Ramos, L., and Matlock, T. Conveying COVID-19 information in TV news: an analysis of metaphors in English and Spanish. *J. Commun. Healthc.*.
43. Hauser, D.J. and Schwarz, N. (2020). The war on prevention II: battle metaphors undermine cancer treatment

and prevention and do not increase vigilance. *Health Commun.* 35 (13): 1698–1704.

44. Magaña, D. (2020). Praying to win this battle: cancer metaphors in Latina and Spanish Women's narratives. *Health Commun.* 35 (5): 649–657.

45. Mathews, H.F. (2000). Negotiating cultural consensus in a breast cancer self-help group. *Med. Anthropol. Q.* 14 (3): 394–413.

46. Fernandez, A. (2021). *We need to get more Latinx people vaccinated. Here's how*, 11. AAMC. www.aamc.org/news-insights/we-need-get-more-latinx-people-vaccinated-heres-how (accessed 7 September 2021.

47. Martínez, G.A. (2020). *Spanish in Health Care: Policy, Practice and Pedagogy in Latino Health*. Routledge.

48. Manzo, R.D., Brazil-Cruz, L., Flores, Y.G., and Rivera-Lopez, H. (2020). *Cultura y corazón: A decolonial methodology for community engaged research*. University of Arizona Press.

49. Martínez, G.A., Showstack, R.E., Magaña, D. et al. (2021). Pursuing testimonial justice: language access through patient-centered outcomes research with Spanish speakers. *Appl. Linguist.* 42 (6): 1110–1124.

50. Ortega, P., Diamond, L., Alemán, M.A. et al. (2020). Medical Spanish standardization in US medical schools: consensus statement from a multidisciplinary expert panel. *Acad. Med.* 95 (1): 22–31.

51. Ramírez, A.S., Wilson, M.D., and Miller, L.M. (2022). Segmented assimilation as a mechanism to explain the dietary acculturation paradox. *Appetite* 169: 105820.

52. Ramírez, A.S. and Carmona, K.A. (2018). Beyond fatalism: information overload as a mechanism to understand health disparities. *Soc. Sci. Med.* 219: 11–18.

53. Ramírez, A.S., Golash-Boza, T., Unger, J.B., and Baezconde-Garbanati, L. (2018). Questioning the dietary acculturation paradox: a mixed-methods study of the relationship between food and ethnic identity in a group of Mexican-American women. *J. Acad. Nutr. Diet.* 118 (3): 431–439.

54. Santos, M.G., Showstack, R., Martínez, G. et al. (2022). *Health Disparities and the Applied Linguist*. Taylor & Francis.

3 A Critical Overview of Illness Narratives: Sociolinguistic, Literary, and Graphic Perspectives

ROXANA DELBENE

Introduction

In his essay "Two Models of Thought," Jerome Bruner [1] proposed that narrative is a mode of thought, an apprehension of reality, and a mode of communication fundamental to the human cognitive makeup. Bruner distinguished between the logico-scientific mode, based on the need to either confirm or reject hypotheses through their testing against empirical data, and the narrative mode of knowledge. The latter is concerned with making sense of experiences from a subjective perspective rather than finding objective truths. The emphasis of the narrative mode lies in the unique way in which classic human dramas are emploted. Illness, conceptualized as an interruption [2] or as a biographical disruption [3] that threatens physical, emotional, social, and even spiritual losses, is an occasion for narrative in all forms. As Hyden and Brockmeier [4, p. 4], put it, "it appears that people who are ill tend to weave the threads of their illnesses and their presumed origins and therapeutic trajectories together with their personal life stories and identity constructions."

The valorization of narrative as a form of knowledge and its consequent use in the social sciences and medicine has received the name of the "narrative turn." This umbrella term focuses on the study of narratives in different disciplines such as the humanities, the social sciences, medicine, and law. Czarniawska [5] notes that the impulse toward the study of and emphasis on narrative originated in the humanities with hermeneutic studies of religious texts. In the second part of the twentieth century, the narrative turn will offer a new lens to the practice of medicine and to the patient's voice.

In the 1980s, illness narratives as first-person accounts of illness experiences became a publishing phenomenon in the United States and the United Kingdom [6, 7]. Literature and medicine slowly began to be studied in American universities as part of the humanistic

---

The Handbook of Language in Public Health and Healthcare, First Edition.
Edited by Pilar Ortega, Glenn Martínez, Maichou Lor, and A. Susana Ramírez.
© 2024 John Wiley & Sons, Inc. Published 2024 by John Wiley & Sons, Inc.

formation of medical students, and it can be speculated that this might have paved the way for the current teaching of illness narratives [8]. Since then, scholarly literature on illness narratives has dedicated great attention to examining these narratives also known as "pathographies" [11] resulting in an association of illness narratives with pathographies. I argue, though, that the term illness narrative is polysemic and transcends the study of pathographies. The term, illness narratives, refers, on the one hand, to narrative co-constructions [9, 10] in face-to-face interactions between patients and healthcare professionals, caregivers, or family members; and on the other, it refers to memoirs or "pathographies" [11] achieved by means of introspection, as narrative reconstruction [12, 13] and, ultimately, it refers also to graphic novels or "graphic pathographies" [14].

In this chapter, I provide a critical overview of the different modes of expression of illness narratives (oral, written, and graphic) from the viewpoints of sociolinguistics, literary studies, and graphic medicine. I use a communicative and genre-oriented approach [15] that sees the different modes of expression of illness narratives as a matter of communicative specialization depending on the speech situation, audience, and communicative intention. This view sees the communicative affordances of each genre as equally effective. Readers particularly interested in a practice-oriented approach to graphic medicine are encouraged to read Chapter 24 of this volume.

The linguistic and narrative turns in the genesis of illness narratives

With the emergence of the field of medical humanities in the 1970s [8] and in recent decades, the fields of autobiographical studies [16], narrative medicine [17, 18], and the health humanities [19], the term illness narrative has been predominantly associated with written memoirs as "pathographies." The term pathography appeared in Hawkins's pioneering book *Reconstructing Illness*, originally published in 1993. Hawkins states, "a pathography is an extended narrative situating the illness experience within the author's life and the meaning of that life" [11, p. 13]. Hawkins's work delimited the boundaries of pathographies to "written narratives and only to narratives [written] by an ill person or by someone who is very close to that person" [11, p. viii]. Like Hawkins, medical sociologist Arthur Frank [12] focused his study on literary, autobiographical, illness narratives as he agreed with Hawkins' characterization of illness narratives as written works. Frank [12, p. 249] states, "Hawkins correctly places pathographies as second-order formulations of illness. Because they are literary constructions, pathographies reformulate illness experiences; publication is the final stage in the process of formulation." Thus, the pioneered studies of Hawkins and Frank placed the study of illness narratives within the field of literature. In his book *Recovering Bodies*, Couser [20] acknowledges that personal narratives of sickness and disability have taken forms other than autobiographical accounts, including self-portraiture as in the paintings of Frida Kahlo; however, he also delimits the term illness narrative to refer to written autobiographical episodes. Couser states, "Illness narrative refers to writing about the episode of one's illness, whereas full-life narrative refers to a comprehensive account of one's life, including illness" [20, p. 6]. Thus, the genre of illness narratives has become almost synonymous with the written form, that is, pathographies, as memoirs about illness experiences [6, 11, 13, 20, 21]. However, oral accounts of illness that a person may tell family members or may deliver in consultations with healthcare providers are also named illness narratives [22].

As initially appeared in Kleinman [22], the term illness narrative referred to the patient's account to his or her doctor, as interactively co-constructed between the two of them, or to others, such as family members and researchers [23–26]. Since the 2000s, the old genre of comics has been reborn, drawing on medical and health content as graphic pathographies [14]. These graphic novels combine texts and images, and they are flourishing in the field of graphic medicine [27]. Thus, graphic pathographies add to the diversity of modes of expression in illness narratives. I will start with an overview of the oral and written versions of illness narratives, followed by graphic pathographies or graphic novels.

Oral and written versions of illness narratives

As noted earlier, the term illness narrative appeared in the influential book titled *Illness Narratives: Suffering, Healing, and the Human Condition* by psychiatrist and medical anthropologist, Arthur Kleinman [22]. The book has had a lasting impact on medicine, the social sciences, and the humanities because it shifted the focus of attention from the physician's voice to the patient's [28]. In describing illness narratives, Kleinman [22, p. 49] states,

> Patients order their experience of illness – what it means to them and to significant others – as personal narratives. The illness narrative is a story the patient tells, and significant others retell, to give coherence to the distinctive events and long-term course of suffering. The plot lines, core metaphors, and rhetorical devices that structure the illness narrative are drawn from cultural and personal models for arranging experiences in meaningful ways and for effectively communicating those meanings. Over the long course of chronic disorder, these model *texts shape and even create experience*. The personal narrative does not merely reflect illness experience, but rather it *contributes to the experience of symptoms and suffering.* (emphasis added)

This definition contains several conceptual aspects that I would like to unpack. First, although the oral form of illness narratives is not explicitly stated, Kleinman seems to see the person's illness narrative as an oral account that they may share with others (including their physician). However, Kleinman's definition of illness narratives has been applied indistinctively to either oral or written accounts, including authors who write on their experiences as patients, as Gygax and Locher observe [29]. Second, Kleinman points out that persons' illness narratives may be used to find meaning and convey their explanatory model of illness, which is simultaneously entrenched in cultural belief systems. And third, in his definition, Kleinman points out how the linguistic and structural forms of the patient's narrative inform the experience of illness while the experience of illness may reinforce and even change those belief systems altogether.

Kleinman's observation that the patient's narrative contributes to the experience of symptoms and suffering foregrounds the reciprocal interconnection between language, culture, and experience; that is, how illness may inform our plots and, also, how the plots we create about illness inform our experience of illness in either hopeful or pessimistic ways. Kleinman's position can be placed in dialogue with sociolinguists and discourse analysts who share consensus regarding the interconnections of language and the lifeworld. For instance, sociolinguist Barbara Johnstone asserts, "Discourse both reflects and creates human beings' 'worldviews'" [30], p. 35. Similarly, psychiatrist Howard Brody, in his book *Stories of Sickness*, notes, "The way we experience the world influences the language we use and the stories we tell, but just as important, the ways we use language and tell stories influence the way we experience the world" [31], p. 24. Another important aspect of Kleinman's [22] conceptualization of illness narratives is his emphasis on the interactional aspect of the face-to-face clinical encounter. Kleinman [22, p. 52] states,

> Even before the physician identifies an elusive illness into a precise disease, the very ways of auditing the illness account influence the giving of the account and its interpretation. Patients are usually aware of the demands of different settings ... and how these [demands] help cast the story in a certain form. ... The way they [physicians] nod their head, fidget, or look at the patient influences how the patient tells the illness story.

Kleinman's statement acknowledges the influence of the context, as cocreated in the clinical encounter between patient and doctor, as a specific conversational genre with its specific "demands" or rather with its idiosyncratic conversational constraints. The quotation pays great attention to the fact that meaning in interactions is negotiated and co-constructed. Kleinman's observation about the clinical encounter as an interactional achievement has been supported by studies in sociolinguistics at the time of the publication of *Illness Narratives* [22]. For instance, sociolinguists such as Duranti [10] and Goodwin [32] initially observed that the interlocutor can influence and shape the trajectory and outcome of the conversation. The form and content of verbal exchanges, like storytelling, are continuously reshaped by the co-participants through their ability to create certain alignments, which suggest or impose certain interpretations. Goodwin also commented on how an unsympathetic or uncooperative audience can deeply affect the performance of any speech act, as professional stage actors who repeat the same lines at every performance can tell [32].

Another influential study [23] analyzed two doctor-and-patient encounters. Mishler's study shows the impact that the conversational trajectory has in these encounters, as shaped by the interaction between the participants. Through analysis of discourse strategies, Mishler demonstrated how one interaction was favorable and the other unfavorable to enable or prevent each patient, respectively, from articulating their stories [23]. Mishler concluded that the difference in the quality of these interactions could not have been solely attributed to the patients' storytelling abilities but rather to the different interactive practices between patient and doctor, that shaped the online coproduction of their encounters [23]. Thus, Kleinman's [22] observation about the cultural and linguistic interactive aspects of illness narratives reflects the knowledge developed in sociolinguistic studies, concerned with interactive encounters. However, this interactive aspect in the co-construction of narratives that Kleinman observed, has received less attention in the literature on illness narratives. A possible reason is that Kleinman's most observed contribution lies in his emphasis on the illness narrative as the patient's explanatory model and the patient's subjective experience of suffering in contrast to the biomedical perspective of disease. Because this has been a major contribution, it has then received most of the attention.

Kleinman's notion of illness narrative emerged in the context of Engel's [33] biopsychosocial model, as Kleinman himself referred to Engel's research. Within Engel's biopsychosocial model, the physician's professional role is not only limited to curing but is also expected to facilitate the individual's healing process. Thus, this view created the necessary basis for the significance of the patient's narrative, not only because of its clinical relevance but also because of the need to consider the patient's account. As Hyden [28, p. 52] acutely observes, "This [contribution] makes it possible to study the patient's illness experience and illness world as a social reality apart from the conception and definition of illness as formulated by biomedicine." Another study considering a historical review of the evolution of the genre of illness narratives encompassing linguistic and literary perspectives is the publication of Hydén and Mishler [34], from which I draw in this chapter.

In their "Language and Medicine" article, Hydén and Mishler [34] reviewed the evolution from what they called the "linguistic turn" to the "narrative turn" in the study of patients' narratives in the 1970s and 1980s. The linguistic turn focused its concern on the forms and functions of language in medical practice and training and produced many publications on doctor–patient interactions that analyzed the verbal characteristics and linguistic organization of the medical consultation, including the patient's story. A classic study of the linguistic turn is the work of Byrne and Long [35], which examines the different speech events involved in clinical consultation. Hydén and Mishler characterized these initial studies as "speaking to patients" [34, p. 174]. These studies aimed to examine how well physicians communicated with their patients to achieve their clinical tasks. However, as observed by Hydén [28], the publication of Kleinman's book would shift the research interests by changing the perception of the patient's narrative as an object of biomedicine, useful for diagnostic purposes, to an appreciation of the patient as a subject whose experience needs to be acknowledged.

A second group of studies on doctor–patient interactions that emerged in the 1980s drew on sociolinguistics and conversation analysis methodologies. Within the frame of sociolinguistics, these studies were categorized as "speaking with patients" [34, p. 175]. Speaking with patients' studies approached clinical encounters as "speech events," [36] susceptible to being shaped by the listener in contact with their context of situation, thus considering sociocultural and socioeconomic variables [37, 38]. Other studies in this category adopted the frame of conversation analysis. These studies focused on how participants socially organize means of interaction, including membership and the sequential organization of the turn-taking between physicians and patients [39]. Their contributions illuminated significant aspects of the asymmetry between doctors and patients in interactions that required immediate attention in order to improve patients' satisfaction.

The third category of studies described by Hydén and Mishler is "speaking about patients" [34, p. 181]. This category leads us to a shift toward the conceptualization of illness narratives as seen from the perspective of the narrative turn. The influential trend among studies [11, 20, 40] identified in this category, "speaking about patients," emerged simultaneously during the studies described earlier as "speaking with patients," as part of the linguistic turn. But given that the narrative turn cannot be reduced to written texts, I suggest that a better description of the category "speaking about patients" in Hydén's and Mishler's [34] description would be to say that this one is a highly literary and literacy-oriented category within the narrative turn. A characteristic of this literary and literacy-oriented category is that influential authors, who conducted research on narrative and illness or narrative and medicine, are scholars trained in literature studies. Kathryn Hunter's [40] book *Doctor's Stories* is one of these influential studies. Hunter argued that despite the scientific basis, narrative is pervasive in medicine. Hunter claims that the narrative structure of medicine can be seen from the narratological ways in which doctors construct their diagnoses, the way in which physicians make chronological sense of their patients' stories, to the different storytelling events (e.g., case presentations, case conferences, medical charts, and others) that organize the medical day, and beyond [40, p. 5].

> The patient's account of illness is the first account but not the only one. The physician's own discourse about illness takes the form of a story. The space between the patient's first words to the physician and the physician's closing recommendations to the patient is filled with medicine's narratives . . . Medical stories are a well-established way of sorting through and tackling problems of diagnosis and treatment.

The view of patients' illness narratives, as elaborated by Hunter [40], Charon [41], Hawkins [11], and Frank [13], highlighted a link between medicine and narrative, as it is summarized in the following quote from Hunter [41, p. 8]:

> The patients are the texts to be examined and studied and understood by the physician. Sometimes, they can be read like the text of a newspaper story or a piece of straightforwardly expository prose. In other instances, the "interesting" cases, patients' stories resemble novels or poems, those more complicated works that do not always readily yield an easy paraphrase at their meaning.

As shown in this quote, the narrative link is emphasized in the sense that the patient is meant to be "read" as a written text and the patient is even compared with a written text. If a less complex text unfolds, the patient is compared with a newspaper story; and if a more complex one unfolds, the patient is compared with a poem or a novel. Thus, literacy and literature are emphasized.

Literacy, as a technology [42], has enjoyed a privileged position in Western culture and it has contributed to the development of consciousness along with the articulation of personal experiences, as in the case of memoirs [43]. Thus, I suggest that the emphasis on seeing the patient as a written text and the association of medicine with literature [17, 44] could be explained, in part, by this privileged position that literacy and literature have enjoyed in our culture leading to an explosion of autobiographical works since the 1980s [6]. For this reason, I prefer to call this approach "the literary/literature approach" rather than the narrative approach as other authors in the study of illness narratives do [45].

A critique about the methodological absence of oral illness narratives in the influential works of Frank and Hawkins comes from Hydén and Mishler [34, p. 183]:

> The exclusive reliance on written texts . . . limits the generalizability of their analyses. The study of written narratives cannot give us access to important features in the production and structuring of illness narratives that reflect the social contexts of storytelling – identifying the setting as medical or nonmedical, establishing the relations of other participants to the patient and understanding the contributions of these other participants to the story.

The focus on autobiographical memoirs as illness narratives is also noted by writing studies researcher, Debra Journet [46]. She observes that a shift through the 1980s and 1990s began to take place at that time when composition research started to emphasize social contexts and personal histories. This thematic shift in composition research gave rise not only to different discursive formats but it contributed to "foreground narrative's capacity to render the complexities of individual and social experience" [46, p. 14].

The time of publishing boom of illness narratives was identified in the United States with the emergence of the AIDS pandemic in the 1980s and 1990s [6]. Such an explosion of illness narratives is in stark contrast to the absence of narratives associated with the 1918 flu pandemic [6]. Although the HIV/AIDS epidemic waned thanks to the advances in antiretroviral treatment in the mid-1990s, writing about illness and disability continued to grow, and it became a motive of research in the social sciences and humanities. Illness narratives as pathographies were seen as a means of reclaiming patients' voices from the biomedical constraints as acts of resistance to the medical establishment [26]. For instance, in the prologue of her book *Bite Me*, Ally Hilfiger, a person living with Lyme disease, claims that she wrote her memoir not because her story was unusual, but because she wanted to give voice to others: "No, my story is not unusual, but I believe it needs to be told if only to give others a voice" [47], p. xvii. Polly Murray, a pioneered advocate against Lyme disease and a survivor, was living in Lyme, Connecticut, when she got infected in the early 1970s. At the time, the infection with Lyme had not been properly identified, thus, her symptoms were not believed to be physically based. Her memoir, *The Widening Circle*, was written to remind physicians that the patient's experience, knowledge of their own body, and environment need to be listened to and considered [48], p. xi.

> The purpose of my book is to tell the story of a disease from the viewpoint of the patient, and to emphasize that what patients tell their doctors can be important in the diagnostic procedure. The doctor who enters the examining room to see a patient is armed with knowledge ... The patient is armed with a different type of knowledge – that of experiencing the disease or living within the disease. When these two perspectives are brought into balance, good medical caretaking ensures.

Illness narratives are seen as a means of reclaiming the self [13] from the voice of biomedicine and as means of restoring the patient's voice [26] by increasing self-awareness and connection with others. The act of disclosure is seen as a therapeutic agent [49]. "The act of converting emotions and images into words changes the way a person organizes and thinks about stress and crisis," assert Smyth and Pennebaker [49, p. 79]. In terms of reading, illness narratives may offer a reparative reading, a term coined by feminist scholar Eve K. Sedgwick [50], as an alternative position to the "hermeneutics of suspicion" that has dominated literary criticism [6, p. 3]. In this case, reparative reading means the ability to find solace and companionship in reading about others' experiences with illness. Reparative reading also claims the value of narratives to inspire compassion vicariously, and, consequently, to serve as a source of moral education [51].

With the development of writing studies in recent years, several studies in the humanities and the social sciences [52–56] have documented the healing power of writing as an act of gaining control over reality and as a means of organizing and understanding oneself. Many writers of memoirs are often heard saying that writing saved their lives, or that they write to live. For instance, in her article, "Writing for our lives," physician Kate

Scannell [56, p. 781] (an infectious disease doctor) tells us about the therapeutic meaning that writing her memoir during the early years of the AIDS epidemic had for her:

> I first discovered the urgency to write during my clinical work with AIDS patients in the early epidemic years. During that time, I looked to traditional narratives about physicians' lives but found little that resonated with my personal and professional experience of working with young patients who would all die. Writing my memoir about that time became an exercise in staying alive – to my patients' stories, to their felt experiences of life near death, to my evolving identity as a doctor, to the changing cultural norms contextualizing medical practice.

In recent years, the field of narrative medicine, founded by physician and literary scholar Rita Charon and her colleagues at Columbia University [17, 18], has emphasized the need for healthcare professionals to develop narrative skills or "narrative competence" understood as "the ability to acknowledge, absorb, interpret, and act on the stories and plights of others" [44, p. 1897]. In its pedagogical approach, narrative medicine has turned to the use of literature and literacy skills such as reflective writing and close reading as signature methods. Reflective writing, a practice that usually takes place after the close reading of a text, is seen as a form of knowledge and self-knowledge that promotes the perception and representation of narrative acts. The actual activity of writing endows reflections with shape and form, which brings reflection into awareness and existence [17].

Charon et al. [18, p. 165] claims that "close reading develops the capacity for attentive listening," given that the same level of alertness and attentiveness to the written word that is required from the reader will be transferred to the listener who undergoes this training. It can be said that Charon has amplified Hunter's [40] comparison of the patient to a (literary) text by equating the act of reading a narrative text with the act of listening to patients' narratives in consultations. As Charon et al. [18, p. 168] states, "these skills of the attentive reader are then transferrable to the skills of the attentive listener." A critique of this formulation, which also favors written texts, is that Charon's conceptualization of the reader as a listener seems to be devoid of the contextual and interactional aspects that influence the coproduction of narratives in face-to-face interactions, as reviewed earlier. Narrative medicine has not yet addressed how the components of oral communication, as observed by Hymes [36] (e.g., purpose, setting, emotional tone, participants, message, rules of interaction, and cultural norms of interpretation), and its units of analysis (i.e., communicative situation, event, and act) involved in face-to-face encounters including the clinical encounter, are transferred from close reading into attentive listening. In the next section, I elaborate on the emergence of graphic novels and their contributions to the study of illness narratives.

Graphic pathographies/graphic novels

In their article, "Graphic medicine: use of comics in medical education and patient care," Michael Green and Kimberly Myers [14, p. 574] define graphic pathographies as "a distinctive sub-genre or graphic stories – illness narratives in graphic form [that] has emerged to fill a niche for patients and doctors." As clearly stated in their definition, these authors conceptualize illness narratives as graphic novels.

The genre of comics combining image and text is not a new medium; its first golden age can be traced to the 1930s and 1940s [57]. However, despite their popularity, comics were not legitimized by the high culture; as in the past, other genres in literature or painting were initially rejected (e.g., the novel itself versus poetry). Renowned author of comic books Will Eisner [58, p. 26] explains this rejection, "Since comics are easily read, their reputation for usefulness has been associated with people of low literacy. . . . Little wonder that encouragement and acceptance of this medium by the education establishment was for a long time less than enthusiastic." But this ill perception of comics started to change in the 1990s thanks in part to what Eisner [58, p. 30] identified as "the beginning of the new literacy" in which a younger generation brought up with television, computers, and video games has been trained to process visual information on several levels at once, as a habitual activity. Thus, reading in its purely textual/ print sense has lost its exclusivity as a means of communication, Eisner notes.

The name "graphic novel" emerged strategically in the early 2000s to refer to the revival of the comic as a serious and respectable genre that not only can depict superheroes but can also address serious, taboo topics, such as illness and disability. Thus, the renaming was a way to draw the attention of the literary critics to grant these texts the same cultural recognition as traditional literary texts [57]. Around 2006, Ian Williams, a medical doctor living in England, coined the term "graphic medicine" for his new website, in which he started cataloging all comic books related to medical content. As a result of his website, several authors of graphic novels who had previously met online, gathered in London in 2010 for the first conference on graphic medicine organized by Williams. This event formally marked the beginning of graphic medicine not only as embracing graphic pathographies as an artistic form but also as a movement [27, p. 2]: "A movement for change that challenges the dominant methods of scholarship in healthcare, offering a more inclusive perspective of medicine, illness, disability, caregiving, and being cared for," as the voice of Susan Squier says through her iconic avatar (the chicken) in the *Graphic Medicine Manifesto* [27].

The successful emergence of graphic pathographies has contributed to the fact that some authors begin to consider graphic novels as the "comics' passports to recognition as a form of literature" [59, p. 21]. Eisner [58, p. 33] also defended this medium as literature because, as he argues, in comics "images are employed as a language" thanks to recognizable, conventionalized relationships between the iconography and the logographic. Whether graphic novels are considered literature, there is no doubt that they are an artistic expression in which meaning is conveyed at the intersection of image and text with a specific purpose. As Williams [59, p. 21] claims, graphic novels can effectively relate the patient experience and, indeed, the experience of the caregiver or healthcare provider. Also, comics might have a part to play in discussing difficult, complex, or ambiguous subject matters. The benefits of using graphic pathographies in medical education and patient care have been documented. The following is a summary of some of the benefits of graphic novels presented in the literature:

Enhance literacy and access to health information. Graphic novels are seen as a medium particularly appropriate for educating patients because of the linguistic challenges experienced by diverse populations. The process of reading verbal text alone involves word-to-word conversion, but comics accelerate the reading process because it involves word-to-image conversion. Thanks to graphic conventions, readers can easily understand the relationship between logography and iconography [58, p. 32]. Sarah McNicol's [60] experimental study about the potential of educational comics reports positive benefits in terms of access to health literacy. One of these benefits, as expressed in semi-structured interviews with her participants, is that readers find in comics an opportunity not only to learn more about their own conditions but also to educate others about their conditions, especially to family members. The general information presented in the comic may speak on behalf of the patient, especially when patients do not wish to disclose or explain their personal symptoms in detail to others. Although most of the participants in McNicol's study found comics easy to understand and to be relatable, some participants expressed their concerns about the negative impact of some images on their mood as well as the confusion they experienced in trying to integrate both codes of interpretation [60]. This is an important observation given that most studies tend to report universal acceptance of comics as intuitively easy to understand [14, 58, 59].

Regarding the claim concerning the easy readership of graphic novels, it can be counterargued that this may depend on the author's communicative intention, the content, style, and the targeted audience, among other possible factors. Considering these factors, some comics might be easier to read than other types of texts. Nevertheless, to read comics or graphic novels effectively, readers not only need to decode and combine the meaning of the images and verbal texts, but they also need to make inferences about "the context of situation" [36] and the cultural context, especially when the meaning is not made graphically explicit, but it is exophoric. This is a type of challenge that any teacher using comics with students could confirm.

Observational skills. Because authors in graphic medicine argue that in comics, images can carry as much information as verbal texts, the claim is that reading graphic novels may help increase observational and interpretative skills that parallel those needed for diagnostic reasoning in clinical medicine [61, 62]. As a sequential art [58] in which images and texts are arranged in a certain order to tell a story, reading comics demands attention to detail to grasp the process of meaning-making. For instance, details may vary from one panel to another to convey a sense of temporality or duration and several layers of information may be overlapped in a panel or divided into one single panel. Thus, authors claim that the observational skills deployed to read comics may parallel those used for diagnostic reasoning by observing the progressive development of clinical signs in a patient. However, scholars working in the field of memoirs and literature and medicine have also made similar claims about the use of literature for the education of healthcare professionals [17, 18, 63–65].

Empathy. Graphic pathographies serve as a direct confirmation to those who have lived through a similar illness experience that they are not alone; like them, other people have experienced something similar and survived to tell and draw the tale [59, p. 25].

Representational mediacy. Comics offer the advantage of a safe space where readers are not frightened by the immediate resonance of a video documenting trauma. Because graphic novels portray iconic avatars in lieu of the authors or protagonists, it is believed that they can reduce emphatic concerns for the subject, in contrast to videos or films that feature real people. The reader can still feel and understand a character's suffering, but "at something of a distance and without the conditioned response of lens-based media," asserts Williams [59, p. 26]. However, the view that comics may offer a mediated form of representation was not always shared. In the 1950s, comics were seen as a potential source of maladjustment and violence in children, as criticized in publications by psychiatrist Fredric Wertham as cited in Saji's and Venkatesan's book [66].

Literalization of metaphors. Metaphors used in texts in prose as part of figurative language (e.g., comparing depression with a black dog) must be imagined by the reader in order to be understood. Graphic novel scholars [66] claim that by virtue of the visual representation (i.e., a black dog is illustrated as a metaphor that represents depression) [67], the process of literalization may help patients visualize the intricacies of their internal minds. However, reading literature is also claimed to have therapeutic value [68] by theory of mind [69], in part, because of the benefits for readers to develop their imagination and visualization skills.

In sum, scholars in the graphic medicine field tend to point out the communicative advantages and efficiency of comics versus illness narratives in prose, with the intention, perhaps, to reclaim the values of graphic novels as a genre. For instance, Williams [59] claims that comics seem to allow more leeway in terms of meaning than illness narratives in prose. Similarly, Green and Myers [14] analyze selected panels from Marchetto's [70] graphic novel *Cancer Vixen* to illustrate the advantageous, communicative effectiveness of graphic novels over illness narratives in prose. The dreaded moment before the eventuality of cancer that fills Marchetto with angst while she is trying to listen to her doctor's explanation, is portrayed in three graphic levels within one panel (i.e., upper and lower green bubbles representing the narrator's and the protagonist's voice respectively, a white bubble representing the doctor's voice, and the picture of the scene representing Marchetto and her mother looking at the doctor with bulging eyes expressing terror). The syntax between these three levels of representation indicates the discrepancy in Marchetto's mind between what the doctor says and her understanding of his words. Thus, the doctor's explanation of the diagnostic procedure is cut off, as represented by scribbles punctuated only by the few, but significant, words that she can retain ("cancer," "lumpectomy," "may not be invasive," "lymph nodes"). Aware of her inability to listen to her doctor (or understand him), the lower green bubble containing the protagonist's voice states, "the last doctor's visit without a tape recorder." Green and Myers assert that this type of graphic expression, as it has been described, "accomplishes something that is almost impossible to do with pure text: the representation of a conversation along with the hidden, unspoken meaning behind the words" [14, p. 575].

Although Williams recognizes that writers of illness narratives have a range of rhetorical and communicative devices available, he also claims that the number of possible strategies in comics is multiplied [59, p. 25]. Whereas language may fail to describe bodily sensations or complex emotional states, he argues that the plurality of graphic resources (e.g., panels, borders, layouts, lettering, chiaroscuro, and others) can compensate for the faults of linguistic expression. Notwithstanding, Williams's [59], and Green's and Myers' [14] claims can be disputed.

Rhetorical and even typographic strategies used by authors of pathographies or illness narratives in prose have access to an equal variety of devices that can convey similar topics and concerns, emotions, and communicative purposes although the experience of reading these types of texts would be different for each case. Some of these rhetorical devices are lexical choices, repetitions, enumerations, similes and metaphors, direct speech, reported speech, free indirect speech, use of ellipses, internal monologue, and italics, among other possible devices. Not to mention the array of speech resources available to speakers to tell stories, such as tone of voice, pitch, intonation, emphasis, repetitions, comparisons, contextual and pragmatic cues, among others. Because each genre is highly specialized in its form of expression and artistic representation, I argue here that their effectiveness may depend on external variables to the texts, such as audience, speech situation or context of communication, and communicative intention [71]. Drawing on semiotician Gunther Kress, I suggest that using different genres – with their respective, specialized artistic conventions – renders specialized communicative works that not only attract diverse audiences but also have different receptions and communicative purposes [71]. I cannot compare here, in detail, the communicative competencies of the three genres (oral, written, and graphic), but I suggest that the claim of exclusive communicative resources of graphic novels would need further examination. The success of communication, observes Kress, depends on its purpose and to whom – that is, to what audience – the message is directed [71]. Rather, the communicative intention informs the mode of communication (e.g., speech, writing, image, or both). One single mode of communication cannot fully carry all the meaning. Each mode (i.e., speaking or writing, or graphic) may be assessed to be better suited depending on the specialized tasks that are intended to achieve, that is, "the tasks which are best done with that mode" as Kress asserts [71, p. 20]. This means that graphic novels convey meaning in a specialized way – as well as illness narratives in print or oral do the same – according to the affordances of their genres. In this manner, the claim is how different genres communicate in specialized ways, serving different communicative purposes, and impacting readers differently. For instance, not all readers may need to communicate by means of the same genre and not all readers may be prepared to absorb the nuances of all genres in the same manner and benefit equally from them. Comparative studies of different genres of illness narratives, considering linguistic, semiotic, and literary perspectives would be needed to explore the communicative affordances of each genre in interdisciplinary ways.

Conclusion

Although illness narratives are overwhelmingly seen as beneficial for the reasons explained earlier, some scholars have argued about the limits of narratives. Angela Woods [72] challenges the claim that narrative articulation is essential to create a sense of self, as this has been one of the major claims formulated by the narrative turn in the social sciences and humanities. Woods points out that the universalization of narrative as the only means to the construction of self and to provide authentic insight into someone's subjectivity is not an ethical imperative for achieving true or full personhood for everybody. This position, she observes, neglects those who cannot employ narrative competence and those whose preferences are not narratively oriented. A more compromising perspective is offered by Hilde Lindemann Nelson [73], who addresses the pros and cons of a narrative approach to ethics. Nelson observes that in contrast to abstract ethical principles, narratives allow revising moral understandings, considering the contexts and the particularities of the characters in which the plots are formed. Yet narratives cannot exhaust the work of moral justification, and neither do ethical principles.

Although the publication of illness narratives has been a social phenomenon in North America and England, this movement is no longer circumscribed to the English language. In Spain and Latin America, pathographies and graphic pathographies are growing to consider Spanish as an influential language in the United States. The graphic medicine website (www.graphicmedicine.org) has begun to catalog graphic novels in Spanish and other languages. Scholarly publications, such as the work of Inés González Cabeza [74] from the University of León, offer an analysis of the most acclaimed graphic novels in Spain. An important observation about some distinctions between the illness narrative movement in North America and Latin America is attributed to the tradition of "testimony," which is considered the dominant narrative form in Latin America [75, 76]. Testimonial narratives tend to denounce and resist the status quo and are written with political intentions. The use of the first person in testimonial narratives is, however, a collective "I" that juxtaposes the personal voice with the voices of the community in one single voice. Chávez [77] observes that "pathographies of struggle," as represented in Castro's and Mondragón's memoir *Una Caricia de Dios* [78], mix the subjective with the collective. The elements of the pathography, concerned with the cognitive and emotional needs of the subject to process personal experiences, tend to overlap with the collective and social concerns of the testimonial narrative in Latin America.

In conclusion, this chapter critically overviewed the different expressive modes of illness narratives (the oral, written, and graphic) with a communicative focus on the specialized affordances of each genre. It has called attention to the polysemy of the term "illness narratives," although frequently associated with pathographies and therefore with literacy and literature. Also, it has been argued that a communicative perspective considering the context of situation, the audience, and the communicative purpose is necessary to appreciate the communicative efficiency of each illness narrative genre and how they complement each other.

Key highlights

- Illness narratives became typically associated with "pathographies." However, the term, illness narratives, is polysemic and refers, on the one hand, to narrative co-constructions in face-to-face interactions between patients and healthcare professionals, caregivers, or family members; and on the other, it refers to memoirs or pathographies achieved by means of introspection as narrative reconstruction and, ultimately, it refers also to "graphic novels" or graphic pathographies.
- Each illness narrative genre conveys meaning in a specialized way. One single mode of communication cannot fully carry all the meaning. The effectiveness of each genre may depend on variables that transcend the rhetorical devices of each genre, such as audience, context or speech situation, and communicative intention. The communicative affordances of each genre of illness narratives (oral, written, or graphic) may be better assessed by looking at the specialized communicative tasks that each genre is intended to achieve, that is, the tasks which are best done with that mode.
- The claim concerning the communicative advantages and efficiency of graphic pathographies or graphic novels over other illness narratives in prose would need further examination considering the special affordances of each genre.
- Comparative studies of different genres of illness narratives addressing linguistic, semiotic, and literary perspectives are needed to explore the communicative affordances of each genre in interdisciplinary ways.
- Although the publication of illness narratives has been a social phenomenon in North America and England, this movement is no longer circumscribed to the English language. Further studies examining illness narratives and testimonial narratives in Latin America are encouraged.

REFERENCES

1. Bruner, J. (1986). *Actual Minds, Possible Worlds*. Cambridge, MA: Harvard University Press.
2. Frank, A. (1992). What kind of phoenix? Illness and self-knowledge. *Second Opinion* 18 (2): 31–41.
3. Bury, M. (1982). Chronic illness as biographical disruption. *Sociol. Health Illness* 4 (2): 166–182.
4. Hyden, L.C. and Brockmeier, J. (2008). *Health, Illness and Culture: Broken Narratives*. London: Routledge.
5. Czarniawska, B. (2004). *Narratives in Social Science Research*. London: SAGE Publications, Inc.
6. Jurecic, A. (2012). *Illness as Narrative*. Pittsburgh: University of Pittsburgh Press.
7. Rak, J. (2004). Are memoirs autobiography? A consideration of genre and public identity. *Genre Forms Discourse Culture* 37 (3–4): 483–504.
8. Cole, T.R., Carlin, N., and Carson, R.A. (2015). *Medical Humanities: An Introduction*. New York: Cambridge University Press.
9. Schegloff, E.A. (1997). Narrative analysis thirty years later. Oral versions of personal experience: three decades of narrative analysis. Special issue. *J. Narrative Life Hist.* 97–106.
10. Duranti, A. (1986). The audience as co-author: an introduction. *Text* 6 (3): 239–247.
11. Hawkins Hunsaker, A. (1999). *Reconstructing Illness: Studies in Pathography*. West Lafayette, IN: Purdue University Press.
12. Frank, A. (1993). Reconstructing illness: studies in pathography. *Literature Med.* 12 (2): 248–252.
13. Frank, A. (1995). *The Wounded Storyteller*. Chicago: The University of Chicago Press.
14. Green, M. and Myers, K.R. (2010). Graphic medicine: use of comics in medical education and patient care. *BMJ* 340: 574–577.
15. Kress, G. (2003). *Literacy in the New Age*. London: Routledge.
16. Smith, S. and Watson, J. (2010). *Reading Autobiography: A Guide for Interpreting Life Narratives*. Minneapolis: University of Minnesota Press.
17. Charon, R. (2006). *Narrative Medicine: Honoring the Stories of Illness*. Oxford: Oxford University Press.
18. Charon, R., DasGupta, S., Herman, N. et al. (2017). *The Principles and Practices of Narrative Medicine*. New York, NY: Oxford University Press.
19. Crawford, P., Brian, B., Baker, C. et al. (2015). *Health Humanities*. New York: Palgrave MacMillan.
20. Couser, G.T. (1997). *Recovering Bodies: Illness, Disability, and Life Writing*. Madison: University of Wisconsin Press.
21. Couser, G.T. (2012). *Memoir: An Introduction*. New York: Oxford University Press.
22. Kleinman, A. (1988). *The Illness Narratives: Suffering, Healing, and the Human Condition*. New York: Basic Books.
23. Mishler, E. (1997). The interactional construction of narratives in medical and life-history interviews. In: *The Construction of Professional Discourse* (ed. B. Gunnarsson, P. Linell, and B. Nordberg), 223–245. UK: Longman Limited.
24. Shapiro, J. (1993). The use of narrative in the doctor-patient encounter. *Family Syst. Med.* 11 (1): 47–53.
25. Riessman, C.K. (1990). Strategic uses of narrative in the presentation of self and illness: a research note. *Soc. Sci. Med.* 30 (11): 1195–1200.
26. Sakalys, J.A. (2003). Restoring the patient's voice: the therapeutics of illness narratives. *J. Holistic Nurs.* 21 (3): 228–241.
27. Czerwiec, M., Williams, I., Squier, S.M. et al. (2015). *Graphic Medicine Manifesto*. University Park, PA: The Pennsylvania State University Press.
28. Hyden, L.C. (1997). Illness and narrative. *Sociol. Health Illness* 19 (1): 48–69.
29. Gygax, F. and Locher, M.A. (2015). Introduction to narrative matters in medical contexts across disciplines. In: *Narrative Matters in Medical Contexts across Disciplines* (ed. F. Gygax and M.A. Locher), 13–14. John Benjamins Publishing Company.

30. Johnstone, B. (2018). *Discourse Analysis*. Hoboken, NJ: John Wiley & Sons, Inc.
31. Brody, H. (2003). *Stories of Sickness*, seconde. New York: Oxford University Press.
32. Goodwin, C. (1986). Audience diversity, participation, and interpretation. *Text* 6 (3): 283–316.
33. Engel, G. (1977). The need for a new medical model: a challenge for biomedicine. *Science* 196 (4286): 129–135.
34. Hydén, L.C. and Mishler, E. (1999). Literature and medicine. *Annu. Rev. Appl. Ling.* 19: 147–192.
35. Byrne, P. and Long, B. (1976). *Doctors Talking to Patients: A Study of the Verbal Behaviors of Doctors in the Consultation*. Her Majesty's Stationery Office.
36. Hymes, D. (1972). Models of the interaction of language and social life. In: *Directions in Sociolinguistics: Ethnography of Communication* (ed. J. Gumperz and D. Hymes), 35–71. New York: Holt, Rinehart & Winston.
37. Fisher, S. (1983). *A Dundas Todd. The Social Organization of Doctor-Patient Communication*. Washington, DC: Center for Applied Linguistics.
38. Mishler, E. (1984). *The Discourse of Medicine: Dialects of Medical Interviews*. Norwood, NJ: Ablex.
39. Frankel, R.M. (1990). Talking in interviews: a dispreference for patient-initiated questions in physician-patient encounters. In: *Interaction Competence* (ed. G. Sathas), 231–260. Washington, DC: International Institute for Ethnomethodology and Conversation Analysis. University Press of America.
40. Hunter, M.K. (1991). *Doctors' Stories: The Narrative Structure of Medical Knowledge*. Princeton, NJ: Princeton University Press.
41. Charon, R. (1989). Doctor-patient/reader-writer: learning to find the text. *Soundings Interdiscip. J.* 72 (1): 137–152.
42. Ong, W. (1982). *Orality and Literacy: The Technologizing of the Word*. London: Methuen & Co. Ltd.
43. Gusdorf, G. (1980). Conditions and limits of autobiography. In: *Autobiography: Essays Theoretical and Critical* (ed. J. Olney), 28–49. Princeton, NJ: Princeton University Press.
44. Charon, R. (2001). Narrative medicine: a model for empathy, reflection, profession, and trust. *JAMA* 286: 1897–1902.
45. Whitehead, A. (2014). The medical humanities: a literary perspective. In: *Medicine, Health and the Arts: Approaches to the Medical Humanities* (ed. V. Bates, A. Bleakley, and S. Goodman), 107–128. London: Routledge.
46. Journet, D. (2012). Narrative turns in writing studies research. In: *Writing Studies Research in Practice: Methods and Methodologies* (ed. L. Nickoson and M.P. Sheridan), 13–24. Southern Illinois Press.
47. Hilfiger, A. (2017). *Bite Me: How Lyme Disease Stole My Childhood, Made Me Crazy and Almost Killed Me*. New York: Hachette Book Group.
48. Murray, P. (1996). *The Widening Circle: A Lyme Disease Pioneer Tells Her Story*. New York: St. Martin's Press.
49. Smyth, J. and Pennebaker, J. (1999). Sharing one's story: translating emotional experiences into words as a coping tool. In: *Coping: The Psychology of What Works* (ed. C.R. Snyder), 70–89. New York: Oxford University Press.
50. Sedgwick, E.K. (2003). *Touching Feeling: Affect, Pedagogy, Performativity*. London, UK: Duke University Press.
51. Nussbaum, M.C. (1997). *Cultivating Humanity: A Classical Defense of Reform in Liberal Education*. Cambridge, MA: Harvard University Press.
52. De Salvo, L.A. (2000). *Writing as a Way of Healing: How Telling Our Stories Transformed Our Lives*. Boston: Beacon.
53. Pennebaker, J.W. (1997). Writing about emotional experiences. *Psychol. Sci.* 8 (3): 161–166.
54. Pennebaker, J.W. (2000). Telling stories: the health benefits of narrative. *Literature Med.* 19 (1): 3–18.
55. Pennebaker, J.W. and Smyth, J.M. (2016). *Opening Up by Writing It Down: How Expressive Writing Improvs Health and Eases Emotional Pain*, thirde. New York: Guildford Publications, Inc.
56. Scannell, K. (2002). Writing for our lives: physicians' narratives and medical practice. *Ann. Int. Med.* 137 (9): 779.

57. Kan, K. (2010). *Graphic Novels and Comic Books*. New York: H.W. Wilson Co.
58. Eisner, W. (1996). *Graphic Storytelling and Visual Narrative*. Paramus, NJ: Poorhouse Press.
59. Williams, I.C. (2012). Graphic medicine: comics as medical narrative. *Med. Humanit.* 38: 21–27.
60. McNicol, S. (2016). The potential of educational comics as a health information medium. *Health Inform. Lib. J.* 34: 20–31.
61. Dolev, J., Friedlaender, L., and Braverman, I. (2001). Use of fine art to enhance visual diagnostic skills. *JAMA* 286: 1020–1021.
62. Naghshineh, S., Hafler, J., Miller, A. et al. (2008). Formal art observation training improves medical students' visual diagnostic skills. *J. Gen. Intern. Med.* 23: 991–997.
63. Trautmann, J. (1978). The wonders of literature in medical education. In: *The Role of the Humanities in Medical Education* (ed. D.J. Self), 32–44. Norfolk: Eastern Virginia Medical School.
64. Hudson, J.A. (2013). Why teach literature and medicine? Answers from three decades. *J. Med. Humanit.* 35: 415–428.
65. Hunter, M.K. (2015). Narrative, literature, and the clinical exercise of practical reason. In: *Humanitas: Readings in the Development of the Medical Humanities* (ed. B. Dolan), 187–207. San Francisco, CA: University of California Press.
66. Saji, S. and Venkatesan, S. (2022). *Metaphors of Mental Illness in Graphic Medicine*. New York: Routledge.
67. Johnstone, M. (2006). *Living with a Black Dog: His Name Is Depression*. Kansas City, MO: Andrews McMeel.
68. Aubry, T. (2011). *Reading as Therapy: What Contemporary Fiction Does for Middle-Class Americans*. Iowa City: The University of Iowa.
69. Kidd, D.C. and Castano, E. (2013). Reading literary fiction improves theory of mind. *Science* 342: 377–380.
70. Marchetto, M.A. (2006). *Cancer Vixen: A True Story*. New York: Alfred A. Knop.
71. Kress, G. (2003). *Literacy in the New Age*. London: Routledge.
72. Woods, A. The limits of narrative: provocations for the medical humanities. *Med. Humanit.* 37: 73–78.
73. Nelson, H.L. (1997). *Stories and Their Limits: Narrative Approaches to Bioethics*. New York: Routledge.
74. Cabeza IG. La patografía gráfica en España: Un género emergente más allá de Arrugas. In: *La escritura y su órbita: Nuevos horizontes de la crítica literaria Hispánica*. Ana Abello Verano, Arciello Daniel, Fernández Martínez Sergio (eds.). Spain: University of León; 2018. p. 293–305.
75. Beverley, J. (1987). Anatomía del testimonio. *Rev. Crít. Latinoamericana.* 13 (25): 7–16.
76. Beverley, J. (1991). Through all things modern: second thoughts on testimonio. *Boundary 2* 18 (2): 1–21.
77. Chávez, W.V. Cuando el paciente se vuelve biógrafo. Las narrativas de enfermedades en una Caricia de Dios. *Dialogía* 10: 237–258.
78. Castro, R.B. and Mondragón, G.F. (2012). *Una Caricia de Dios*. Paulinos, México: Editorial Alba.

4 Anthropological Linguistics, Health, and Healthcare

MILENA A. MELO, CARLA PEZZIA, WILLIAM J. ROBERTSON, AND K. JILL FLEURIET

Introduction

Linguistic borders and boundaries permeate health and healthcare practices, often reinforcing inequalities [1]. In this chapter, we consider how linguistic bordering practices shape healthcare access and experiences in three vulnerable populations. Each case study is grounded in ethnographic methodologies, especially participant observation; structured and semi-structured interviews; and collection of cultural texts. We use our disciplinary approach of inductive analysis. Inductive approaches allow us to enter the field with disciplinary knowledge of what we expect to encounter but leave open the possibilities to generate new theories based on the lived experiences of participants. Herein, our analysis focuses on communicative acts and other linguistic practices that influence health outcomes for undocumented immigrant patients with end-stage renal disease (ESRD) in the south Texas borderlands; indigenous Maya in the Guatemalan highlands, and LGBTQI+ patients at an anal cancer research clinic in Chicago.

Theoretical framework

We frame these case studies within bordering theory [2, 3], performativity [4], and Latourian translation and purification [5]. We apply bordering theory to consider how linguistic practices can exclude (border) or include (deborder) people from historically oppressed communities in the production of health and wellbeing. Bordering theory contributes to our understanding of the potential of communicative practices in and around health/care to produce both illness and health, especially in vulnerable populations marked by marginalized identities.

Broadly, borderlands research advances the study of health, language, and boundary-making in three principal ways: (1) the emphasis on how borders are often material,

---

The Handbook of Language in Public Health and Healthcare, First Edition.
Edited by Pilar Ortega, Glenn Martínez, Maichou Lor, and A. Susana Ramírez.
© 2024 John Wiley & Sons, Inc. Published 2024 by John Wiley & Sons, Inc.

metaphorical, and textual as well as inherently unstable [6, 7], (2) how borderlands as third spaces can produce new social formations that challenge hegemonic thinking [8, 9], and (3) how borders can be transcended through cooperative action [2, 9].

Communicative and other linguistic practices can border, deborder, or reborder social identities [2, 3, 6, 7, 10, 11]. One mechanism by which linguistic practices can border or deborder identities that impact health is performativity [4], or the constant reenactment of identity through embodied communicative acts. Because identity must be continuously fashioned and refashioned, each act has the potential for change and challenge [4]. Our ethnographic attention to the quotidian communicative and other linguistic practices in health/care documents how these moments can enact [12] new social formations and values or reinscribe old ones, such as racism, sexism, heteronormativity, and classism [13]. In our case studies, we address how people use linguistic practices to navigate identity binaries that shape health and healthcare: noncitizen/citizen, nonwhite/white, straight/queer, transgender/cisgender, indigenous/nonindigenous, patient/doctor, living/dying and human/animal.

Our theoretical substrate is Latour's contention that a hallmark of our modern world is the belief that binaries structure our world while our daily practices regularly elide those binaries [5]. While Latour emphasized ontological binaries, his work has applications with common social boundaries, including race, gender, citizenship, sexuality, and indigeneity, which are slippery in practice but conceptually rigid. In Latourian terms, *purification* is the process of maintaining binaries, and *translation* is the suite of practices that blur them. One cannot exist without the other [5]. Recent work in communicative practices across epistemologies of different medical systems [14] emphasizes the generative potential of translation and purification [5, 15], or boundary crossing and boundary maintenance, respectively. For our purposes, communicative practices surveil and police boundary zones of identity (purification), while at the same time, they can cross boundaries (translation). We consider how translation and purification practices around normative binaries of identity can shape health/care experiences for marginalized populations.

Bordering theory within a Latourian frame highlights the role of performative, communicative practices in healthcare settings in the reinscription, rejection, or creation of boundaries between people, objects, and bodily conditions that shape health and healthcare experiences. Latour argues that translation can produce hybrids and new social formations; borderlands theorists point toward the friction (e.g., [8, 16]), flows (e.g., [17]), and partnerships [2] of people and goods that create new social formations to challenge existing hierarchies and boundaries of identity. Below, we integrate both theoretical strands to show that communicative practices such as labeling, metaphor, storytelling, and boundary-making can generate and convey meaning within and across social and illness categories. We highlight power asymmetries embedded in such linguistic practices and the semiotic process of translation itself [15].

Case studies

The boundary of life and death: Constructing deservingness in the United States–Mexico borderlands

Rodrigo can barely walk as he stumbles into the hospital emergency room. It is 6:30 a.m., 30 minutes before the shift change that will usher in a new rotation of emergency room doctors and nurses. Rodrigo hopes that this time he will be found worthy – deserving of the emergency dialysis treatment he so desperately needs in order to be able to breathe easy again and finally get some sleep. Just yesterday, he was sent away from the emergency room without treatment because his potassium was at 5.8, a fraction shy from the threshold of a "true emergency." This time he hopes for a different outcome – for the physician to read his results and determine they fit the linguistic bounds of the Emergency Medicaid criteria, granting him access to dialysis treatment to cleanse his blood of toxins and excess fluid and keep him alive.

I (Melo) utilize experiences of undocumented patients with ESRD as an extreme case study to illustrate how communicative practices that reinforce borders of citizenship and healthcare inclusion in the United States push people toward the border between life and death. I draw from over two years of ethnographic fieldwork in the Rio Grande Valley (RGV) in south Texas. The region is known for its alarmingly high rates of Type II diabetes (30.7%) [18], obesity, and a largely low-income and immigrant population. As a native of the RGV and formerly undocumented immigrant, I focus my work on the relationship of citizenship, health, and healthcare.

Deservingness, exclusionary violence, and belonging

In the United States, access to healthcare is not a human right. Everyone must prove their "deservingness" of healthcare, whether through ability to obtain health insurance, qualify for aid in the form of federal, state, or local funding, like Medicare or individual county indigent healthcare programs, or self-pay for treatment. Undocumented immigrants do not qualify for most federal and state funding options because of their "non-citizen" status. Undocumented immigrants without means to pay out-of-pocket must rely on hospital emergency departments that follow the Emergency Medical Treatment and Active Labor Act (EMTALA) regulations. EMTALA obligates the treatment and stabilization of all patients who seek care at emergency departments irrespective of ability to pay or citizenship status. However, there are criteria for cases to be marked as emergencies. The policy language of EMTALA and emergency Medicaid reinforces notions of deservingness, determining healthcare inclusion only when the patient is determined to be in a life-or-death state [19].

Labeling people as noncitizens and therefore undeserving of care is a moral claim [20] that dramatically impacts health [21]. Juridico-political criteria draw a line between citizen and noncitizen as well as immigrant and non-immigrant. Categorized as "other," noncitizen patients must prove themselves worthy based on limiting criteria for emergency care. Even when qualifying for emergency care, noncitizen patients can be turned away. Some healthcare institutions take this exclusion even further through actions that make them feel threatened and unwelcome. In the 1990s, one of the largest hospitals of the RGV had their security guards dressed in green uniforms to resemble those of United States Border Patrol agents to deter and instill fear into undocumented immigrant patients. Uniforms were yet another communicative practice and performance, rebordering the exclusion of undocumented immigrants in the hospital. In the geopolitical borderlands where identities can easily blur, the uniforms also were a means of Latourian purification [5] to reinforce binaries of belonging. Recognizing such acts of "exclusionary violence" [22] lets us question boundaries of citizen/noncitizen, deserving/ undeserving, life/death, standard care/substandard care, and inclusion/exclusion.

Fieldwork setting and methods

My data included 42 semi-structured interviews with healthcare professionals (primary care doctors, social workers, dieticians, hospital administrators, nurses, financial directors, dialysis technicians, nephrologists, radiologists, bio-technicians, and dialysis facility administrators); 100 semi-structured interviews with low-income Mexican immigrant dialysis patients (50 undocumented; 50 documented); and participant observation. I followed eight dialysis patients (four undocumented; four documented) for six months to observe and document their daily lives and impacts of ESRD. I drove dialysis patients to hospital emergency departments; attended family barbecues and birthday parties, doctor's appointments; ran errands with them; and had casual conversations with patients and their families around kitchen tables, living rooms, or in backyards trying to enjoy the evening breeze on hot Texas days.

Bordering access and inclusion/exclusion

In the United States, citizens and lawful permanent residents with enough working credits who are diagnosed with ESRD are given the medical standard of treatment: thrice weekly dialysis treatment in private outpatient facilities, scheduled and guaranteed at the same time and place. All others must go through emergency care, where treatment is not guaranteed. For example, Diego was a 56-year-old naturalized United States citizen from Matamoros, Tamaulipas, Mexico. He was diagnosed with Type II diabetes and hypertension at 26 years old. Coming from a family of diabetics, Diego had a basic understanding of Type II diabetes and he regularly sought treatment. When his kidneys began failing, his primary care doctor referred him to a nephrologist who prepared Diego for a possible future of dialysis. When Diego was 55 years old, after almost three decades of living with diabetes, he began dialysis. He was referred to an outpatient dialysis center, where the social worker helped him process his Medicare claim to qualify for standard dialysis care – three treatments a week in this same outpatient facility. Once his paperwork based on citizenship, work history, and kidney failure was processed, Diego was granted Medicare and assigned a regular shift at the dialysis center. Subsequently, Diego reported to the same center every Monday, Wednesday, and Friday at 10:00 a.m. for his four-hour-long dialysis session. He was never turned away from treatment, regardless of his potassium level.

Patients like Diego at outpatient facilities do not have their potassium levels checked before each treatment but rather are monitored monthly, along with protein, phosphorus, and several other analyses. These analyses are checked regularly to modify the patient's diet, dialysis filter type and machine speed, and medications. Registering a "normal" potassium level does not mean that they no longer need treatment or that they can go several days without it, but that the treatment and patient's efforts are working to replace the kidneys. Their biological integrity remains unquestioned, but closely supervised to detect any threats.

Undocumented patients, however, must prove their deservingness and need of treatment for every dialysis session. The boundary that determines whether they will receive treatment is based in their biology: potassium levels. Undocumented immigrants throughout most of the United States only receive emergency dialysis through hospitals when their condition has been deemed as question of "life and death state," another boundary dictated by Medicaid criteria and determined by hospital healthcare professionals. Emergency Medicaid is granted when "absence of immediate medical attention could reasonably be expected to result in – (a) placing the patient's health in serious jeopardy" [23]. As a result, most undocumented immigrants receive dialysis once or twice a week when the emergency physician determines that they are "sick enough" to need dialysis according to signs of physical distress and potassium levels.

Such elevated potassium levels place patients at risk of cardiac arrest. In these instances, healthcare professionals must justify inclusion or exclusion in determining a course of treatment relying on the language of exclusionary healthcare policies that deem undocumented patients as "undeserving" or unworthy of care if they do not fit qualifying criteria [20].

A peculiar kind of Latourian translation and purification occurs in which treatment is justified based on their emergency state and not by citizenship. Undocumented immigrants must prove and construct their "deservingness" each time. Their health must deteriorate to the blurred state between life and death. Communicative practices in the clinics then attempt to re-establish boundaries by labeling undocumented patients as "regulars," "frequent flyers," or "freebies," terminology that denotes these patients are taking advantage of the system. They must be "other," and difference is reinscribed. By enforcing Emergency Medicaid criteria, the healthcare system does not allow them to die, but only to maintain a "bare life" [24]. Hospital emergency departments become "zones of abandonment" [25] where undocumented patients succumb to hovering between life and death.

If an undocumented patient's potassium comes back normal, they are sent home with only two options: return when the potassium level is higher, although they may be in incredible pain, discomfort, and have possible serious complications such as pneumonia or stroke, or do something to raise it themselves. However, potassium is not the only factor or side effect affecting patient comfort and quality of life. Other symptoms such as being incredibly swollen and full of excess toxins, struggling to breathe, and having dangerously high amounts levels checked irregularly, such as phosphorus, can also have detrimental effects on the physical status of patients.

Rodrigo, the 51-year-old undocumented Mexican immigrant on dialysis for the last 12 years, was denied dialysis when his potassium did not meet hospital criteria. He suffered severe consequences because of insufficient dialysis. As we sat around the kitchen table, snacking on some crackers and drinking a fresh Mexican Joya soda, which Rodrigo's sister brought from Mexico that morning, we discussed his experiences being rejected.

MM Have you ever been denied dialysis?
Rodrigo Ah, yes, but they denied it because I did not have the potassium and when I don't have potassium they tell me 'You are good, come another day or when you get sick.' That's what they say.
MM How many times has this happened?
Rodrigo Many times, yes, many times.
MM Those times that they sent you back home, did you still feel that you needed it?
Rodrigo Yes, because it was the potassium. I don't have potassium but, like I told you, it's not just the potassiumIt's the potassium, it's the water and the toxins. . .If I don't have potassium but I do have toxins they are going to build up, so I needed it but they say "You know what? Sign here [discharge papers]" and they send me home.
MM Did you have any consequences as a result of not receiving dialysis regularly, like pneumonia or a heart attack?
Rodrigo Three times. In the last 12 years, I've had three, one stroke and two heart attacks.

Rodrigo was continuously evaluated solely based on potassium. Potassium minimums are perhaps the most obvious of hospital policies that anchor communicative practices that restrict access to care and force many patients to become "at risk" in order to receive treatment to stay alive. Exclusionary policy language, biological measurements, and uniforms worn by security personnel – each a communicative practice, enact biopolitical exclusion. Bodies become boundaries. In her work with undocumented immigrants in France and the French "illness clause" that grants citizenship to the chronically ill [26], Ticktin argues:

> The citizens produced by the joining of humanitarian ethics and politics have inequality literally inscribed on their bodies. They are forever marked and interpellated as sick, as already handicapped – they can never realize equality. . . Immigrants are stripped of their legal personas when identified solely as suffering bodies, and, as such, they cannot be protected by law; they are rendered politically irrelevant (44).

For undocumented immigrants in the United States, the humanitarian ethics that relegate care to emergency departments when patients are on the verge of death due to immigration politics cause detrimental physical and emotional scars on their bodies. Just as Ticktin argues that inequality is inscribed on the body, exclusion becomes embodied, physically and emotionally for undocumented dialysis patients. Borders are literally inscribed upon their bodies. Biopolitical exclusion pushes undocumented immigrants closer each week to the border between life and death.

The boundary between humans and animals: Indigeneity and alcoholism in Guatemala

> Marco, an indigenous Maya man in his 50's, was reserved and spoke in hushed tones as he told me about his life-long struggles with alcoholism. But then his anger was palpable as he recounted the death of someone he knew who also suffered from alcoholism:

> "The life in the street is of dogs. And the alcoholic on various occasions has been seen to die like an animal. One time we saw a drunk that was run over by a truck and he was drunk and he died like a dog."

> For Marco, there is also an embodied correlation to this metaphor of the alcoholic individual as animal as he recalled instances during his most severe binges where he sifted through trash for food, "like a dog."

> The comparison of alcoholic individuals to dogs was a common one. Rosa's husband was an indigenous Maya man in his 40s. After he spent a month at a drug and alcohol rehabilitation center, she felt like he had returned even more abusive than before. She told me how, when she turned to his family for help, "his brothers said he is a dog, just let him die they said."

Marco and Rosa's stories illustrate how discursive practices can dehumanize indigenous and alcoholic individuals and legitimize substandard healthcare for alcoholism. In this case study, I (Pezzia) present evidence illustrating how historical public discourse persists in national and local discourse by both indigenous and nonindigenous Guatemalans that drunkenness is innate to indigeneity. I argue that prevailing metaphors among community members construct human–nonhuman boundaries that equate subhumanism (dogs) to indigenous alcoholic populations, as well as criminal (vagrants) –noncriminal binaries. The Latourian translation [5] of the human-nonhuman border of alcoholic indigenous people by healthcare professionals and community leaders directly affects individual care and community interventions.

Concept-metaphor and borderwork

For my analysis, I draw upon two bodies of literature. The first is based in Moore's concept-metaphor that generates ambiguity around a concept while producing a "tension between universal claims and specific historical contexts" [27]. Concept-metaphors are often examined and scrutinized for the ways in which they impact society [2]. For this case study, I consider "indigeneity" to be a concept-metaphor that informs understandings of alcoholism among the Guatemalan Maya throughout history, and arguably transcends sociopolitical borders as similar understandings are applied to other indigenous peoples across the globe. Beyond the concept-metaphor, linguistic metaphors further delineate and divide notions of indigeneity.

The second is literature on bordering or borderwork (or boundary work). Borderwork, for the purposes of this case study, refers to the ways in which non-state actors ("ordinary people") create, shape, and erase borders [28], physical and social. This type of borderwork can sometimes serve to create ideological boundaries that socially determine "good"/"bad" behaviors [29]. These boundaries, in turn, reinforce social distinctions that allow for one group to flourish and another to be disenfranchised, with limited access to healthcare for example.

Methods and setting

Data are derived from observations, textual data, and 105 semi-structured interviews with people in recovery (n = 35), community members (n = 23), and healthcare providers (n = 17) from August 2010 to November 2011 in the Western Highland community of Panajachel, Guatemala. Panajachel is a primary tourist destination with a population of local, national, and foreign-born residents, approximately 70% of whom are indigenous Maya [30]. For my linguistic analysis, I focused on the experiential value of words and metaphors [31]. I compared interview and observational analyses to newspaper articles from *Nuestro Diario* and *Prensa Libre* and state-sponsored pamphlets on alcoholism to measure how these texts interacted with each other.

Alcoholism and indigeneity

Contemporary understandings of indigeneity have been shaped by historical processes and continue to reflect the ways in which indigenous peoples are treated by the state. Alcoholism and indigeneity in Guatemala became one and the same thing through public discourse [32]. Prior to colonialism, excessive alcohol consumption was not common among the ancient Maya [32]). Both distilling practices introduced by Europeans and state-enforced labor laws had a major influence on increasing alcohol consumption by the Maya [32]). By the nineteenth and early twentieth centuries, Guatemalan politicians and scholars associated alcoholism as a defining component of indigenous culture and leading cause of death. Contemporary Maya were portrayed as inferior to their ancestors, marked by ignorance, poverty, ill-health, and drunkenness. They were regularly referred to as "beasts" and subhuman by social and political elites of the time [32].

My discursive analysis suggests this conflation continues to occur in contemporary Guatemala. First, state-sponsored pamphlets on alcoholism only included images of indigenous people or people of ambiguous ethnicity. Second, in my interviews, everyone agreed outright that alcoholism affected people regardless of race/ethnicity, social, or economic status. However, a linguistic distinction suggested that alcohol-related problems are naturalized as part of indigenous culture. Interviewees who self-identified as Maya would state, "*we* have a problem with alcohol," while Ladinos and foreign-born residents claimed, "*they* have a problem with alcohol." Drinking alcohol was considered problematic for specific individuals in the Ladino and foreign population, whereas it was classified as an issue for the entirety of the indigenous Maya population, highlighting indigenous–nonindigenous divides. Similarly, interviewed health professionals would state that they saw patients of various ethnic and cultural backgrounds, yet emphasis was continuously placed on linkages between alcoholism and indigenous culture.

According to the physicians interviewed, alcoholic individuals were not interested in therapeutic care but rather in medical solutions to allow them to continue drinking. This assumption has consequences for the health of the indigenous alcoholic patient. Medical advice on the benefits of quitting drinking was rarely discussed as part of standard of care for alcoholic individuals. Furthermore, alcoholic indigenous individuals were more likely to provide examples of substandard care when presenting to various care facilities. For example, Gustavo reported medical professionals at the general hospital saw him as nothing more than male and indigenous and, thus, alcoholic. He presented to the hospital several times complaining about headaches, stomach pains, and "nervios" (a common condition that typically gets a referral to the psychiatrist). However, he was never referred to the psychiatrist, and his overarching physical ailments were reduced to an alcoholic-induced gastritis. He felt like the doctors did not listen to him because of their assumptions about his alcohol use based on his indigeneity. With my intervention, he was finally able to see the psychiatrist who diagnosed Gustavo with generalized anxiety disorder, which may have been a contributing factor to both his alcoholism and his gastrointestinal problems.

Borderwork through linguistic metaphor

The human–nonhuman border is further reflected through the metaphor describing indigenous alcoholic individuals "like a dog." Dogs are multivalent symbols for the alcoholic individual with both figurative and nonfigurative discursive representations. The first articulation of the alcoholic individual in relation to dogs comes in the form of the legend of "El Cadejo." The most common version throughout Guatemala is of a large black dog-like creature who guides drunk men home. This version usually has just one black Cadejo, but more recently a story with two different colored Cadejos has emerged, where the black Cadejo now kills drunken individuals and a different white Cadejo watches over them when passed out in the street.

There is little available literature documenting the reasons for the changes in the story. The two Cadejo versions along with the shift of the black Cadejo to a malevolent spirit brings forth certain racial implications providing another articulation of alcoholism and indigeneity. The black Cadejo, who is considered by some to have indigenous roots, transitions from the protector to the bringer of death. The white Cadejo can be interpreted as the Europeanized Ladino savior who protects the "drunk Indian." The literary connection between dogs and alcoholic individuals has transitioned into a more direct equation of alcoholic individuals to dogs. Both recovering alcoholic individuals and nondrinking community members consistently referred to alcoholic individuals as dogs, as noted in Marco and Rosa's stories above. Notably, Rodrigo compares the alcoholic individual to a dog ("like"), while Rosa's family equates the two ("is"). This linguistic distinction underlies people's attitudes toward the alcoholic "nonhuman" individual and impacts treatments.

Present-day discussions on how to address alcoholism directly reflect previous public discourse intertwining alcoholism, indigeneity, and criminality. Newspaper articles and local security commissions regularly suggest reinstating the Vagrancy Law, an early twentieth century law that disproportionately affected indigenous men and was eventually deemed a human rights violation. The law would make alcohol consumption during working hours a criminal offense resulting in jail time or fines. Newspaper article writers further associate criminality with alcoholism by regularly portraying a direct connection between alcohol consumption and violence, albeit not limited to indigenous men. In various articles, drinking alcohol was stated as the activity a murder victim was involved in immediately prior to their death or, in one case, directly responsible for the person's death. In contrast, interviewees often mentioned alcohol consumption prior to experiences of intimate partner violence.

The portrayal of the criminal and violent character of alcohol drinkers encourages community-level distrust and resentment. A healthcare provider I interviewed blamed both alcohol and drug addicts for the high murder rate in the country:

> So every time an alcoholic or a drug addict needs to maintain their addiction, how are they going to do it? If they do not have a source of income? Stealing, and if they steal, well, probably next comes the delinquency. And a lot of times, it is not just theft, but crime, homicides-

Here we see a discursive progression within the connections between the alcoholic individual and criminality. In the first examples regarding new laws and regulations on drinking, the act of drinking in and of itself was considered criminal, not necessarily the alcoholic individual. The next examples showed an association between alcohol consumption and a criminal life, suggesting that perhaps the alcoholic individual might be a criminal. This last example from the healthcare provider directly identifies an alcoholic individual as a criminal. An alcoholic individual steals, commits crimes, and kills people just to maintain his addiction.

This conceptualization of alcoholics as criminals is not lost on the alcoholic individual. Marco tried to get a job as a guidance counselor for children, assuming his experiences would help provide an example for the kids to avoid the mistakes of his past. However, the hiring manager told Marco, "You do not have moral character." Importantly, Marco was recently diagnosed with bipolar disorder that, according to the psychiatrist who diagnosed him, may have been a contributing factor to his alcoholism throughout his life. Yet he is still viewed by community members as a moral failure. These reinforced moral understandings of alcoholism contribute to the struggle of those in recovery developing a new sober identity and looking to dissociate from negative associations and detrimental behaviors of the alcoholic criminal and subhuman identity.

The conflation of alcoholism and indigeneity affects identity and experience, and the translation of these borders [5] by physicians directly affects the care they provide. First, assumptions that indigenous alcoholic patients do not seek medical care for their alcohol use reflect what is sometimes referred to by hospital physicians in the United States as "the culture of alcoholism" [33]. Furthermore, physicians regularly do not address comorbid mental health conditions that may be a contributing factor to someone's alcoholism, like in the case of Gustavo's anxiety and Marco's bipolar disorder. At the population level, the continued conflation of alcoholism and indigeneity further limits proper targeting for potential interventions. Indeed, data reported elsewhere suggest that nonindigenous populations, at least in Panajachel, may be more likely to suffer from alcoholism [34]. By targeting indigenous populations for alcoholism interventions (legal or otherwise), a significant percentage of the alcoholic population remains untreated, thus maintaining high degrees of alcohol-related health problems within these populations.

Bordering sex/gender and sexuality: Anal cancer prevention

"How detailed do you want this history to be?" Brad asked.

After several months and witnessing hundreds of procedures, the day I had been anticipating since before going into the field had arrived: I was to undergo an anal cancer prevention examination. Brad, a Physician's Assistant at the Anal Dysplasia Clinic-MidWest, was required to do several of these procedures as part of his certification. I took this as an opportunity to add some autoethnographic depth to my fieldwork experience.

"Whatever you need to know. Just ask me what you'd ask any patient," I responded.

Brad began with a series of questions aimed at gathering information about my health and medical histories to estimate my risk for developing anal cancer. As he asked each question, he marked boxes and typed notes in my electronic medical record. He inquired about my age, history of same-sex encounters, HIV status, whether or not I smoked, and if I had a history of anogenital warts.

"So, out of the five risk factors, you're only positive for one. . .and a half. Kind of. With the former smoking."

After his declaration of my minimal risk level, he moved on to social history.

"Marital status?"

"Single," I replied.

"Sexual preference for men, women, or both?"

"Men."

"When you play, do you prefer top –"

"Is that how you ask it?" I interrupted, intrigued by his turn of phrase as I had not noticed it before. "'When you play'?"

"I think so! I think the other providers say that," he said.

"Vers," I replied, knowing he was asking me to pick a category from a set of gay sexual categories top, bottom, and versatile, which refer to people's preferences during sexual activities.

He checked a box in the medical chart and continued asking questions about things like substance use and condom use. When we completed the medical history, I returned to my desk to wait for the exam to begin, nervously anticipating the fraught experience of an anal cancer prevention procedure.

In this case study, I (Robertson) draw on ethnographic fieldwork at an anal cancer prevention clinic in Chicago, United States, to explore how communicative practices, clinical environments, and their associated objects work to border sex/gender and sexuality. These bordering practices both reinforce and challenge sex/gender and sexual norms and categories while also destigmatizing and rehumanizing queer and trans people and their health interests, otherwise routinely ignored and often actively stigmatized in other biomedical environments.

Boundary objects, biomedicalization, and sex/gender and sexuality

Within Science and Technology Studies (STS), processes of bordering, debordering, and rebordering have alternatively been referred to as *boundary work* [35]. This term denotes the ideologically informed practices of scientists attempting to delimit science from non-science and, more recently, the "processes by which people continuously draw, maintain, and dissolve boundaries" [36]. Some scholars [37] describe boundary work as the ongoing interplay between symbolic boundaries and social boundaries, where symbolic boundaries are conceptual distinctions used to create/dissolve social boundaries that separate people into different groups with varying social statuses. A useful concept for understanding how people in different social worlds work to bridge boundaries is *boundary objects* [38]. In current articulations, "object" refers to "something people act toward and with" [39] that derives its materiality from actions rather than as "a thing." Boundary objects, then, are adaptable objects with both loosely structured general forms and specific local forms that aid in the collaborative practices of de/rebordering.

Herein, I argue that boundary objects in the clinic can work to de/reborder broader social categories of sex/gender and sexuality within and beyond medical environments. Discursive clinical interactions among patients and providers are everyday sources of de/rebordering sex/gender and sexual norms and normativities. Deviations from these normativities – in this case, queer and trans subjectivities – are often pathologized and biomedicalized [40], treated as risk factors deserving of biomedical surveillance and technological intervention. Through these processes, queer and trans people are more easily stigmatized within medical environments and society more generally. Only within the last few years have some mainstream biomedical environments begun to incorporate more positively affirming language and practices aimed at improving care for trans and queer patients.

Fieldwork setting and methods

Over the course of 12 months in 2018 and 2019, I conducted ethnographic fieldwork at Anal Dysplasia Clinic-MidWest (ADC), owned and operated by Dr. Gary Bucher (not anonymized per Dr. Bucher). Clinicians specialize in the procedure high-resolution anoscopy, an invasive procedure used to detect cancerous lesions and anal dysplasia caused by human papillomavirus (HPV), the same virus that causes cervical cancer as well as cancers in the genitals, throat, and mouth. I spent most time working as a medical and clinical trial research assistant, assisting clinicians during procedures, processing specimens in the lab, data entry, consenting patients into an ongoing clinical trial, conducting patient retention calls, and helping to keep exam rooms clean and stocked. In addition to participant observation during these kinds of duties, I conducted interviews with clinic staff and patients.

Queer and trans people, especially those living with HIV, experience disproportionately high rates of anal dysplasia and anal cancer. In the general population, the incidence rate of anal cancer is about 2 per 100,000 [41]; among the LGBTQ+ population, incidence rates among LGBTQ+ people vary based on methodology, HIV status, and geographic location, but are estimated to be anywhere between 18 and 173 per 100,000 [42]. Accordingly, most ADC patients and staff during my fieldwork were members of the LGBTQ+ community. The overrepresentation of trans and queer people at ADC – and the taboo status of the body part and diseases the clinic focuses on – led to the development of medical discourses and care practices specifically aimed at de-stigmatizing sexual and bodily health concerns otherwise frequently ignored.

Boundary objects and bordering gender and sexuality

At ADC, queer and trans subjectivities were treated as defaults – a radically different clinical orientation than mainstream medical environments where trans and queer patients have to decide whether or not to disclose their identities and risk being treated poorly. While ADC's bordering processes often worked to reborder normative ideas of sex/gender and sexuality, they also simultaneously debordered clinical spaces as exclusionary of trans and queer needs, effectively de-stigmatizing and re-humanizing queer and trans patients. I focus on two boundary objects engaged in these processes: the patient intake form and electronic medical record (EMR).

Like any clinic, new patients at ADC are required to fill out paperwork. The first form collects basic identity and demographic information (see Figure 4.1). Of particular interest is the "Gender Identity" section, situated near the top reflecting its primacy in medical conceptualizations of patients. Gender identity is (re)bordered as a binary: male and female. Importantly, these two categories are meant to be selected by cisgender (non-transgender) patients. Trans patients are expected to select the "transgender" box and follow with either "male to female" or "female to male." Leaving the terms "male" and "female" unmarked while including a "transgender" category enacts a rebordering of a cisgender/transgender binary.

Within these two categories, the form further presumes patients will identify as *either* male *or* female. No options are offered for nonbinary people. While possible to read the form's gender categorization in other ways (e.g., as providing three gender identity options ([cisgender] male, [cisgender] female, and transgender), the "male to female" and "female to male" categories reborder "transgender" as always already occurring within a binary male/female gender system. Someone is considered transgender not because they do not identify with the gender they were assigned at birth, but because they have moved from one gender category to its "opposite." Whether that movement is social, medical, or legal is unreadable through the form. In practice, these categories were usually marked by people who had begun or completed medical transitioning, usually through the use of hormones and/or surgeries. In my experience processing intake forms, trans people regularly marked the assumed cisgender categories *as well as* the transgender categories. Trans women, for example, would regularly mark "female" then "transgender," but sometimes leave the "male to female" box blank. These moments can be interpreted as practices of de-bordering gender, aimed at dissolving the assumed cisgender default of "male" and "female" gender identity boxes with this boundary object.

Another remarkable bordering activity this boundary object enables is "ethnicity" and "race," which reborder biopolitical categories of race and ethnicity derived from the United States Census. These categories were sometimes confusing to patients. I regularly encountered Hispanic and Latino patients who did not want to select any racial category because they did not identify as white, black, or American Indian, but as Latino

Bucher Medical Services, S.C. - PATIENT REGISTRATION FORM

Please complete the following confidential information:

How did you hear about the ANCHOR study?

Patient's Name: _____, _____, _____
 Last   First   MI

Gender Identity: Male ☐ Female ☐ Transgender ☐ Male to Female ☐
                                                  Female to Male ☐

Patient's Date of Birth: _____ Age: _____ Patient SS#: _____

Preferred Language: ☐ English   ☐ Spanish   ☐ Other

Ethnicity: ☐ Hispanic or Latino   ☐ NOT Hispanic or Latino

Race: ☐ American Indian or Alaska Native   ☐ Asian   ☐ White
         ☐ Black or African American   ☐ Native Hawaiian or Other Pacific Islander

---

Address: _____
 Street   City   State   Zip

Please provide a phone number where we could leave detailed messages at: (___) ___-____

Employer: _____

E-mail: _____

Married ☐   Single ☐   Divorced ☐   Significant Other ☐

ALTERNATE CONTACTS (if we can't reach you at your number)

Name	Relationship	Phone	Email
Name	Relationship	Phone	Email

The name of my Insurance Company is: _____

Patient Signature: _____   Date: _____

Figure 4.1 ADC patient intake form.

or Hispanic. They expressed discomfort with such a limited set of racial categories and often debordered these categories by refusing to select a racial category. Additionally, the boxes for relationship status – married, single, divorced, significant other, effectively reborder (hetero)normative relationship categories and kin structures. There are, for example, no options for polyamorous relationships, friendships, or other forms of queer relatedness that do not presume significant relationships as only monogamous and romantic.

After new patients complete the paperwork, a clinician conducts a thorough medical and social history, documenting each response in the EMR. The medical history is fairly standard, but the social history includes some questions uncommon in mainstream medical settings. The most obvious of these relate to sexual behaviors. They first ask, "is your sexual preference for men, women, or both?" The answer is combined with the patient's gender identity to mark a "sexual orientation" box in the EMR. The available categories within the EMR, however, are not sexual orientation categories. They do not use lay categories such as "gay," "lesbian," or "bisexual," or categories commonly used by insurance providers like "homosexual" and "heterosexual." Instead, the EMR includes risk-based categories like "men who have sex with men" (MSM) or "women who have sex with men" (WSM), which originate from public health.

If a male-identified patient replies saying he has sex with men or both men and women, the provider then asks of their sexual preference, "do you prefer top, bottom, vers [versatile], vers top, or vers bottom?" Unlike the sexual orientation option, these categories are based on popular lay sexual identity categories (especially among gay men) meant to indicate whether a person prefers to penetrate, be penetrated, or do both during anal sexual intercourse. The clinician documents the patient's response in the EMR using these lay categories, effectively rebordering them generally as medically relevant risk categories and simultaneously biomedicalizing sexual identities and practices as risk categories specifically relevant for the screening and diagnosis of anal dysplasia and cancers. Those who bottom are considered to have a higher risk for developing HPV-related anal disease and anal cancer compared to those who are exclusively top. In practice, the clinicians examine patients the same way regardless of their answers to this question. However, such biomedicalized risk categories can shape the kinds of behavior changes and frequency of follow-up visits the provider recommends to the patient.

De/rebordering gender and sexuality in an anal dysplasia clinic

The intake form and EMR are boundary objects because these conceptual categories of sex/gender and sexuality are both loosely structured common categories and have specific local meanings. Asking a queer male patient if he is a top, bottom, or vers draws on common categories that both clinician and patient understand, but the answer to this question is translated [5] to work in specifically clinical ways that may or may not reflect the patient's experiences or conceptualizations of their bodies and/or identities. All along, these boundary objects and their associated discursive practices de/reborder gender and sexual categories.

Despite the biomedicalization, the inclusion of queer and trans categories nonetheless does important work to destigmatize queer and trans subjectivities and health needs. During my fieldwork, trans and queer patients regularly praised the clinic and its staff for creating an inclusive, affirming environment, centering their concerns and needs, and making them want to come back despite the procedure's fraught nature. Notwithstanding problematic categories such as "male to female" and "female to male" on the intake form, clinicians expressed support and affirmation rather than judgment and condemnation for trans and queer sexual subjectivities. ADC's boundary objects may have worked to reborder heteronormative and cisnormative ideas of sex/gender and sexuality, but clinicians' everyday communicative work debordered the clinic as queer/trans-exclusionary space and rebordered it as welcoming and even celebratory.

Discussion

Our chapter has analyzed health and healthcare linguistic practices through the lens of borderlands theory and border practices by "talking about the social processes that define (border), reinforce (reborder), or challenge (deborder) them" [2]. Utilizing bordering theory, performativity, Latourian translation, and purification, our three case studies demonstrate how communicative practices shape health and healthcare experiences for vulnerable populations. In Melo's case study, undocumented immigrants are judged by their biology through communicative practices including blood labs and emergency Medicaid criteria in order to be deemed worthy of treatment. Pezzia's case study analyzes experiential word values and metaphors that dehumanize indigenous and alcoholic individuals. Robertson's case study examines the patient intake form and the EMR to showcase how boundary objects can both reinforce and challenge sex/gender and sexual norms. While each varies in how language shapes identities and healthcare access, all three case study subjects are seen as "at risk" and in need of "biomedical surveillance" and intervention because of their indigeneity, sexuality, or citizenship.

Recommendations for research, education, and practice

Our chapter seeks to make novel contributions to the field of linguistics and healthcare by applying borderlands and bordering theory to communicative and discursive practices. Borderlands, whether biopolitical, linguistic, or metaphorical, are places of emergence. Bordering theory focuses analysis on the ways in which we draw, erase, or revise lines of difference. While the cultural competency framework – ubiquitous in medical education and training today – calls for medical professionals to recognize and respect cultural differences, our recommendations are instead based on the concept of cultural humility. More than mere appreciation or "listing of traits" that too often gets glossed as racial/ethnic difference [43], cultural humility is a critically reflexive approach based on recognizing power imbalances in clinical interactions. It requires practitioners to be humble and open to learning from and with patients *and* demands the development of "mutually beneficial and non-paternalistic clinical and advocacy partnerships with communities" [44]. Through ethnography, we find spaces in healthcare where translation happens; these are spaces where we can intervene to do the work of debordering to improve health outcomes for populations marked by inequality. Our recommendations are grounded in the recognition of medicine as a sociocultural endeavor thoroughly entangled with political and economic institutions.

Conclusion

Each of our case studies demonstrates that who and how you are defined by the healthcare system through communicative practices matters when it comes to determining if, what, where, and when you will receive care and treatment. Boundaries of inclusion-exclusion can become hazy through performance and Latourian translation whether in an anal cancer research clinic in Chicago, an emergency department in south Texas, or a public health clinic in highland Guatemala. Approaches from linguistic anthropology and cultural anthropology demonstrate how communicative and other linguistic practices border, deborder and reborder identities, in health and healthcare. Linguistic barriers can be reimagined as they are remade and challenged in everyday life.

Highlights

- Include a quality-of-life measure in emergency care criteria for chronically ill patients that could help identify additional clinical and nonclinical resources.
- Standardize a brief intervention for all patients who drink with stigmatized conditions to minimize provider bias on patient racial/ethnic identity.
- Reconsider how medical categories are deployed in research and practice to make clinical materials like intake forms affirming of patients' identities.

REFERENCES

1. Piller, I. (2016). *Linguistic Diversity and Social Justice: An Introduction to Applied*. New York, NY: Oxford University Press.
2. Fleuriet, K. (2021). *Rhetoric and Reality on the U.S.-Mexico Border: Place, Politics, Home*. New York, NY: Palgrave Macmillan.
3. DeChaine, D. (2012). *Border Rhetorics: Citizenship and Identity on the US-Mexico Border*. Tuscaloosa, AL: University of Alabama Press.
4. Butler, J. (1990). *Gender Trouble*. New York, NY: Routledge.
5. Latour, B. (1993). *We Have Never Been Modern*. Cambridge, MA: Harvard University Press.
6. Agnew, J. (2008). Borders on the mind: re-framing border thinking. *Ethics Global Polit.* 1 (4): 175–191.
7. Heyman, J., Slack, J., and Guerra, E. (2018). Bordering a "crisis": Central American asylum seekers and the reproduction of dominant enforcement practices. *J. Southwest.* 60 (4): 754–786.
8. Anzaldua, G. (2012). *Borderlands/La Frontera: The New Mestiza*, 4 ee. San Francisco, CA: Aunt Lute Books.
9. Licona, A. (2012). *Zines in Third Space: Radical Cooperation and Borderlands Rhetoric*. New York, NY: SUNY Press.
10. Nevins, J. (2010). *Operation Gatekeeper and Beyond: The Way on "Illegals" and the Remaking of the U.S.-Mexico Boundary*. New York, NY: Routledge.
11. Ono, K. and Sloop, J. (2002). *Shifting Borders: Rhetoric, Immigration, and California's 187 Proposition*. Philadelphia, PA: Temple University Press.
12. Mol, A. (2002). *The Body Multiple: Ontology in Medical Practice*. Durham, NC: Duke University Press.
13. Hill, J. (2008). *The Everyday Language of White Racism*. Malden, MA: Wiley-Blackwell.
14. Lang, C. (2018). Translation and purification: Ayurvedic psychiatry, allopathic psychiatry, spirits and occult

violence in Kerala, South India. *Anthropol. Med.* 25 (2): 141–161.
15. Gal, S. (2015). Politics of translation. *Annu. Rev. Anthropol.* 44: 225–240.
16. Tsing, A. (2005). *Friction: An Ethnography of Global Connection*. Princeton, NJ: Princeton University Press.
17. Richardson, C. and Pisani, M. (2017). *Batos, Bolillos, Pochos, and Pelados: Class and Culture on the South Texas Border, Revised Edition*. Austin, TX: University of Texas Press.
18. Millard, A., Graham, M., Mier, N. et al. (2017). Diabetes screening and prevention in a high-risk, medically isolated border community. *Front. Public Health* 5 (135): 1–8. https://www.frontiersin.org/articles/10.3389/fpubh.2017.00135/full.
19. Melo MA. Stratified access: seeking dialysis care in the borderlands. In Castaneda JMaH. *Unequal Coverage: The Experience of Health Care Reform in the United States*. New York: New York University Press; 2017.
20. Black, S. (2018). The ethics and aesthetics of care. *Annu. Rev. Anthropol.* 47: 79–95.
21. Willen, S. (2011). Do "illegal" Im/migrants have a right to health? Engaging ethical theory as social practice at a Tel Aviv Open Clinic. *Med. Anthropol. Q.* 25 (3): 303–330.
22. Willen, S. (2021). On exclusionary violence and its subcutaneous consequences: a commentary. *Cult. Med. Psychiatry* 45: 65–73.
23. Campbell, G.A., Sanoff, S., and Rosner, M.H. (2010). Care of the undocumented immigrant in the United States with ESRD. *Am. J. Kidney Dis.* 55 (1): 181–191.
24. Agamben, G. (1998). *Homo Sacer: Sovereign Power and Bare Life*. Stanford University Press.
25. Vita, B.J. (2005). *Life in a Zone of Social Abandonment*. University of California Press.
26. Ticktin, M. (2006). Where ethics and politics meet: the violence of humanitarianism in France. *Am. Ethnol.* 33 (1): 33–49.
27. Moore, H. (2004). Global anxieties: concept-metaphors and pre-theoretical commitments in anthropology. *Anthropol. Theory* 4 (1): 71–88.
28. Rumford, C. (2012). Towards a multiperspectival study of borders. *Geopolitics* 17 (4): 887–902.
29. Sibley, D. (2002). *Geographies of Exclusion: Society and Difference in the West*. New York: Routledge.
30. (INE) INE. *Censos Nacionales XI de Población y VI de Habitación*; 2002.
31. Fairclough, N. (1989). *Language and Power*. London: Longman.
32. Garrard-Burnett, V. (2000). Indians are drunks and drunks are Indians: alcohol and indigenismo in Guatemala, 1890–1940. *Bull. Latin Am. Res.* 19: 341–356.
33. Pezzia, C., Pugh, J., Lanham, H., and Leykum, L. (2018). Psychiatric consultation requests by inpatient medical teams: an observational study. *BMC Health Serv. Res.* 18 (1): 1–9.
34. Pezzia, C. (2013). *The Sober Self: Discourse and Identity of Recovering Alcoholics in the Western Highlands of Guatemala*: PhD Dissertation. San Antonio: The University of Texas at San Antonio.
35. Gieryn, T. (1983). Boundary-work and the demarcation of science from non-science: strains and interests in professional ideologies of scientists. *Am. Sociol. Rev.* 48 (6): 781–795.
36. Meier, N. (2015). Collaboration in healthcare through boundary work and boundary objects. *Qual. Sociol. Rev.* XI (3): 60–82.
37. Lamont, M. and Molńar, V. (2002). The study of boundaries in the social sciences. *Annu. Rev. Sociol.* 28: 167–195.
38. Star, S. and JR G. (1989). Institutional Ecology, 'translations' and boundary objects: amateurs and professionals in Berkley's Museum of Bertebrate Zoology, 1907–39. *Soc. Stud. Sci.* 19 (3): 387–420.
39. Star, S. (2010). This is not a boundary object: reflections on the origin of a concept. *Sci. Technol. Human Val.* 35 (5): 601–617.
40. Clarke, A., Shim, J., Mamo, L. et al. (2003). Biomedicalization: technoscientific transformations of health, illness, and U.S. biomedicine. *Am. Sociol Rev.* 68 (2): 161–194.
41. National Cancer Institute. *National Cancer Institute*; 2022. https://seer.cancer.gov/statfacts/html/anus.html (accessed 2022).
42. Palefsky, J., Lee, J., Jay, N. et al. (2022). Treatment of anal high-grade squamous intraepithelial lesions to prevent anal cancer. *N. Engl. J. Med.* 386 (24): 2273–2282.

43. Jenks, A. (2011). From "lists of traits" to "open-mindedness": emerging issues in cultural competence education. *Cult. Med. Psychiatry* 35: 209–235.
44. Tervalon, M. and Murray-García, J. (1998). Cultural humility versus cultural competence: a critical distinction in defining physician training outcomes in multicultural education. *J. Health Care Poor Underserved.* 9 (2): 117–125.

5 Applied Linguistics, Public Health, and Healthcare

HOLLY E. JACOBSON

Introduction

This chapter provides a critical overview of applied linguistic empirical research in two of the most critical arenas in healthcare: patient–provider interaction and health literacy (HL). It surveys the themes and sites, methodologies, and types of authentic data used in exploring language in healthcare. Many recent definitions of applied linguistics include reference to investigations that are driven by real-world problems ("linguistics applied") [1, 2]: this chapter focuses in particular on research which is consistent with that perspective. It provides an overview of studies that set out to understand the crucial role of language, both spoken and written, in healthcare access and patient health outcomes. This chapter does not specifically explore language acquisition and teaching (traditionally falling under the umbrella of applied linguistics). Elsewhere in this volume (Chapter 1), Harsch and Santos propose practical and conceptual responses to some of the complexities and problems linked to language proficiency and language acquisition: they provide practical insights for innovative reforms in the healthcare system derived primarily from research on adult education, language acquisition, and teaching. The representative applied research described here was conducted with the aim of identifying linguistic barriers to the quality of healthcare: it deals with the complexities of provider–patient interaction; the impact of HL; the approaches and materials used in patient education; and the "problems" that emerge in the sociocultural and structural environments in which these issues are embedded.

Applied linguists began to seek answers to questions related to real-world language problems in healthcare contexts by looking at provider–patient discourse through different theoretical lenses and using a variety of tools and approaches, primarily qualitative. The linguistic literature on interaction in healthcare settings during the past several decades has primarily focused on the asymmetry of the medical encounter; specifically: the unequal nature of medical discourse [3]; power relations, [4–6]; issues of gender and socioeconomic status in doctor–patient interaction [7–9]; and the impact of specific medical conditions on interaction [10]. Much of the research examines the miscommunication that occurs in healthcare interactions, potentially impacting patient healthcare outcomes [11–14]. A limited amount of quantitative research has explored larger databases (often referred to as corpora) of recordings of provider–patient consultations, as well as clinical print materials (see section on HL and written documents below). Applied linguistic research has tended to be interdisciplinary, involving collaborations among healthcare providers, public health researchers, and experts in communication studies, among others [15]. In recent years, applied linguists have also begun to explore many of the problems and conundrums that have long been attributed to HL. Studies have evaluated instruments used to assess HL and probed the development and implementation of patient education materials using "plain language" protocols and translation. Both public health and applied linguistic research have contributed to the debunking of previous beliefs about HL by revealing practices and structures within the healthcare system that impact the communicative process as much as, or more than HL (for practical approaches to these issues see the chapter by Harcsch and Santos in this volume). However, literacy and factors inherent in the overall healthcare system have proven difficult to tease apart, and much more research is needed to understand the complex relationship that exists among the many variables.

The first section of this chapter focuses on studies that have been conducted on provider–patient interaction during the past several decades. Early research is discussed, followed by an overview of approaches informed by linguistic theory. In the second section, we turn to research in HL, starting with a historical overview, followed by discussion of incursions by applied linguists. The last section provides recommendations for future research directions in applied linguistics and health and discusses the importance of dissemination of findings.

Provider–patient interaction

Historical context

Since the 1950s one of the most common major themes in language research in healthcare has been doctor–patient interaction. Early studies (driven primarily by experts in health communication, public health, and medicine) focused on the ways doctors and patients use language throughout the multiple phases of medical encounters, and were both descriptive and experimental, deriving primarily from traditions in communications research. The work of Balint [16], for example, was seminal in that it drew attention to the patient's linguistic contributions and the importance of focused listening by the provider. Byrne and Long [17] explored physicians' language contributions during different phases of the medical consultation, and described a continuum of provider language styles, from provider-centered to patient-centered. Sudnow's [18] seminal research analyzed the utterances of hospital emergency staff reporting the death of patients to each other and to the deceased's relatives. His analysis showed that whether or not staff decided to revive patients depended on the social value they believed the patients to have: such perceptions were reflected in the lexicon and phrasing used to report or announce the death of patients (this was followed 22 years later by an insightful qualitative study by Timmermans [19] suggesting that, despite the current legal initiatives to support resuscitative efforts, social inequality in death and dying still exists). The findings of these and other pioneering communications researchers led to subsequent "non-linguistic" language research which emerged within the fields of communication, public health, psychology, and other fields. These studies explored doctor–patient interaction in terms of distinct communication features and dimensions, including culture; the doctor–patient relationship (particularly shared decision-making and language concordance); disease characteristics; communicative "behaviors"; patient outcomes (measured as patient satisfaction, patient compliance, and recall and understanding of information); and long-term health status of patients. A particularly productive area of research in medical communication in the past several decades involves coding systems referred to as interaction analysis systems [20]. These coding schemes make it possible to analyze large numbers of doctor–patient interactions more efficiently than when implementing detailed linguistic analysis because the analysis is done using audio data, and transcription is not required [21]. For example, the Roter Interaction Analysis System (RIAS) which is perhaps the most widely known, has high interrater reliability, and has provided clinically meaningful data in a number of studies [22]. However, the RIAS system has received criticism for not being sufficiently fine-tuned. According to Sanvik et al. [22], RIAS analyzes the verbal dialogue of medical consultations by categorizing utterances into poorly delimited task-focused and socioemotional categories and lacks the nuance that linguistic approaches can provide. In contrast, the linguistic methodological approaches that have subsequently been implemented in provider–patient interaction allow for a more nuanced "turn-by-turn" analysis with greater focus on how the interaction systematically unfolds between speakers. Although the data analyses involved are much more tedious, they provide researchers with a more comprehensive perspective of the complexities of discourse in medical consultations. Two of the predominant approaches are referred to as Conversation Analysis (CA) and Interactional Sociolinguistics (IS) and are discussed in detail below.

Applied linguistic methodological approaches and concepts in provider–patient interaction

Applied Conversation Analysis

One of the applied linguistic approaches that has contributed most, in terms of sheer numbers of studies, to our understanding of communication in healthcare settings, especially the clinical setting, is Conversation Analysis (CA). The goal of CA is to "provide empirically grounded explication of the social organization of naturally occurring action and interaction" [23]. CA explores both informal, every day and institutional conversations with a focus on turn-taking, organization of sequences, conversational repair, and epistemics (how participants orient to shared knowledge) [24]. CA involves detailed analyses of both linguistic and paralinguistic (eye gaze, breaths, gasps, silences, facial expressions, gestures) features of authentic audio-recorded or video-recorded data, and involves the use of extremely detailed transcription of talk. Conversation analysis involves Jeffersonian transcriptions [25, 26] or adaptations thereof depending on the particular objectives and questions posed by the researcher. When video recordings are used (which are not always possible due to ethical considerations in sensitive medical encounters) visual body activity, positioning, and other paralinguistic cues can be included in the transcription and subsequent analyses [27]. The goal of CA in healthcare contexts is to identify recurrent patterns of interaction [28] and to explore how and why they occur and their impact on the overall objectives of the encounter (both provider objectives and patient objectives) [27, 29].

Because CA focuses on the organizational structure and participants' orientation to that structure and to each other, issues such as power, gender, and other demographic and sociocultural variables do not form part of the analysis unless they are explicitly represented or referred to in the conversational data. For this reason, applied CA has proven to be particularly powerful in analyzing healthcare communication: it allows for a microscopic, granular focus on the "give and take" between patients and healthcare professionals allowing for precise identification of points of miscommunication: CA analysts are able to pinpoint exactly where conversational derailing occurs. Because of its strength in identifying problematic discourse, applied CA analyses have focused specifically on persistent communication problems in medical consultations. Collaborative work between healthcare providers and linguists is iterative: Heritage [27] recommends identifying problems in interaction through consultation with healthcare providers and patients a priori, preferably with the participation of collaborators on an interdisciplinary team. CA analyses illuminate conversational features and strategies that are directly linked to these problems. The data also bring to light other points in the interaction that contribute to miscommunication that both patients and providers were unaware of (these issues "emerge" from the data). A few examples of the problems inherent in provider–patient interaction that have been explored through CA in healthcare contexts are: Why do doctors overprescribe antibiotics? [30, 31] Why do patients feel unable to address all of their concerns during medial consultations, and what strategies can be used to resolve this [29]? At what point in communication between receptionist and patient do problems in triaging occur, causing much-needed healthcare to be postponed [32]? At what phases in the medical consultation do physicians exert control over the interaction in a medical encounter, and how does this impact the patient [33]?

In a survey of the past 30 years of medical CA literature, Gill and Roberts [34] identified three "streams" of applied CA research in medical settings, based on the social identity of participants, the interactional settings, and the activities accomplished during the encounters in those settings. These streams include (1) physician–patient interaction in primary care and secondary care where the activities include evaluation, diagnosis of illness, and treatment recommendations; (2) interactions among patients and other categories of medical providers besides physicians, where the activities include assessment, screenings, and treatment provisions; and (3) interaction among medical professionals, where the activities include discussion of diagnoses, professional training, and administrative issues. Gill and Roberts provide a comprehensive overview of these streams, with detailed descriptions of representative research. Their overview reveals the enormous impact that applied CA has had thus far not only in understanding interaction in healthcare, but also in the application of findings within the medical professions. However, it also illuminates the enormous gap that exists in the application of conversational analytic methods in the area of intercultural communication, which will be discussed in the following subsections.

Conversation Analysis and intercultural communication in healthcare

Candlin and Candlin [35] point to this gap in the literature and contend that applied CA research has had minimal influence on intercultural communication in healthcare, including interpreter-mediated interaction. Indeed, a search of the literature reveals that few CA researchers have focused on interactions involving more than one language. One outstanding recent example, however, of how applied CA research can be implemented in multilingual settings is that of Jansson, Wadensjö and Plejert [36]: the investigators examined complaint making in older people in multilingual care encounters using CA methodology embedded in an overall ethnographic study. The analysis focuses on the challenges faced by home healthcare workers in responding to patient complaints given their need to provide emotional support to the patient, and illuminates the importance of understanding how interaction is negotiated among patients and providers with different L1. There is an urgent need for applied research in similar language-discordant contexts. The contexts that would most benefit from the micro-analysis offered by CA approaches, according to Roberts [37], include (1) "frontstage" intercultural communication, especially interaction between healthcare providers and patients who speak different L1 and involving a language mediator or interpreter; and (2) "backstage" interaction or interaction among healthcare providers themselves; and (3) interaction involving providers who are second language speakers of English (in the United States).

Conversation Analysis and interpreting in healthcare contexts

Although there has been a proliferation of research on healthcare interpreting in the past several decades, the nature of the focus and linguistic analyses being conducted have remained fairly static, focusing primarily on the interpreter role and how it manifests in the interaction. In the early 1990s, this interest in the interpreter role emerged in part with the work of Wadensjö [38]. She focused on community interpreting from an interactional perspective, using conversation analytic approaches. Her seminal research suggests that the interpreter's role is anything but neutral and invisible and led to further exploration of the interpreter's role by other investigators [39–42]. As stated by Jacobson [41, p. 570], "Interpreting, far from occurring in a neutral, noninvolved manner, requires an active, direct interlocutor who is constantly shifting roles, aligning herself with primary interlocutors, and managing the flow of conversation. The interpreter creates and takes turns, manages overlap, and initiates talk..." According to Jacobson, in her exploratory analysis of data on mediated interaction among student interpreters, interpreters manage (or mismanage) the flow of conversation between providers and patients, leading to miscommunication. She calls for further applied linguistic research, including CA analyses, to determine how interpreters orient to turn-taking and other conversational tasks in interpreted healthcare contexts. This remains a much-needed area of investigation with potential for informing interpreter and provider training and education.

Applied conversation analysis has been criticized because it does not consider the broader workings of power on the level of institutions, societies, and cultures. CA studies tend to be less sensitive to the ways particular encounters are embedded within wider arrangements of medical work, institutional systems and policies that may have a profound effect on participants even when they do not explicitly orient toward them [43]. Nevertheless, CA has proven to be an extremely useful and productive tool in understanding the "online" interaction between practitioners and patients at a more "micro-linguistic" level. The macro-level issues have been tackled using other approaches, such as IS.

Interactional Sociolinguistics

Interactional Sociolinguistics (IS) is a discourse analytic approach that has a strong tradition in applied research in the workplace and healthcare settings in particular. IS evolved from the early sociolinguistic work of Goffman [44], Gumperz [45, 46], and Tannen [47]. IS developed through contributions from linguistics, sociology, and anthropology and involves analyses both at the micro level, similar to conversation analysis (which it draws on, including the transcription conventions of CA), and the macro levels of situational context and sociocultural context [48, 49]. IS researchers concern themselves primarily with how language is used to signal and maintain social relationships among interactants. It allows for both fine-grained micro-linguistic and discourse-level analyses while also illuminating the role of both context, culture, and social structures (macro analyses). From the perspective of IS, interaction involves "inferences": that is, interlocutors infer what other speakers intend to convey and are constantly self-monitoring their own contributions to the discourse. The focus is on shared interpretations, rather than just meaning or semantics. The aim of IS analyses is to "show how individuals participating in such exchanges use talk to achieve their communicative goals in real-life situations by concentrating on both the verbal processes and the taken-for-granted background assumptions that underlie the negotiation of interpretations" [50, p. 63]. These background assumptions can include interpretive frame (definition of the situation), repertoire of signaling devices, sociocultural knowledge, and expectations. From an IS perspective, assumptions drive the norms of interaction, and vary not only crosslinguistically, but also across language varieties, institutions, professions, and genres [51]. IS is characterized by an analytical focus on the role of signaling devices and assumptions-as-meaning: roles, power, and identity are dynamically negotiated and constructed through talk. Signaling devices include prosody, intonation, loudness, stress, phrasing, shifts, tempo, pausing and hesitation, latching, overlapping, and even code-switching, which Gumperz [46] refers to as "contextualization cues." Because interlocutors do not always share the same repertoire of assumptions and cues, they constitute key sites for misinterpretation, leading to miscommunication [52].

Like CA, IS involves the collection of video-recorded, authentic data and involves sequential, detailed analysis. IS researchers identify points where the communication derailed or miscommunications occurred, creating significant asymmetry and serious repercussions for the patient [53]. IS differs from CA in that it investigates *both* interactional patterns and interpretive processes of interaction: IS analyses combine the conversational data and factors external to the data to understand how meaning is negotiated.

IS studies have shed light on our understanding of many different aspects of health communication. Some examples include: inequalities in medical discourse [54, 55]; co-construction of asymmetrical power relations [4, 5]; impact of medical conditions on the flow and shape of the consultation [10]; assessment of health risk [33]; and exploration of features of interaction between health professionals and patients which lead to success in promoting preventive behavior [56].

Interactional Sociolinguistics and intercultural communication in healthcare

IS has also contributed to research on intercultural communication in healthcare contexts, including interaction mediated by an interpreter, but to a much lesser extent. A review of some of the most recent collections on communication in health (cf Hamilton and Chou [51] and Demjén [57]) shows that intercultural communication and interpreting studies seem to have been included as an afterthought. Considering the enormous communicative challenges represented by the changing demographics in the United States and throughout the world, and the continued significance of language as a social determinant of health disparities, more intensive and extensive applied research on interactional intercultural communication, especially where the mediation of an interpreter is required, is urgently needed.

There are, however, a handful of studies that serve as examples of the types of analysis that can illuminate the urgent issues that exist at the intersection of health disparities, language, and interaction and point in the direction of future exploration. Vickers's [58] study on "transnational" medical consultations involving Spanish-speaking patients uses IS and CA analytic approaches. Her findings reveal contextualization cues in medical interactions which play a crucial role in the development of power asymmetries "in which English is hegemonically dominant and interpretive frames are contested" [58, p. 570]. Additional work has been conducted by Vickers et al. [59] on language-concordant interaction in which a medical professional uses L2 Spanish to communicate with a Spanish-dominant patient. This study, focusing on stance and identity, shows how language used by the English-dominant healthcare professionals establishes English as normative and Spanish as marked. Another study by Vickers et al. [60] sheds light on the use of Spanish to English codeswitching by medical professionals as a means of controlling the ongoing discourse, leading to power asymmetries. These findings point to the need for further quantitative, qualitative, and mixed-methods research that explores discrete conversational practices using interactional approaches in healthcare contexts. Such studies have the potential to reveal interactional impact on health outcomes, including understanding patient experiences of illness and diagnosis; "compliance" with treatment regimens; and success in continuity of care. It is essential that the results of such interactional studies be interpreted in light of systemic and sociocultural factors to fill the research void identified by Feuerheum et al. "on the relationship between linguistic differences and health disparities, which remain largely under-theorized and under-researched" [61, p. 128].

This section has provided an overview of the methodologies that have been implemented by applied linguists to explore spoken-language interaction between providers and patients. Another strand of research, HL, involves the analysis of both spoken and written documents, and constitutes a broad area of research covering several decades. The history and methodologies of HL are discussed in the next section.

Health literacy

Historical context

HL has been a focus of research on language in healthcare settings and in public health primarily since the 1990s [62]. HL scholarship has a long and problematic history: early investigations on "low HL" attempted to establish correlations of this poorly defined construct with poor patient outcomes in a number of healthcare contexts, primarily clinical, using a variety of measurement tools. These investigations provided evidence of a link between individual low HL levels and poor patient processing of information which, in turn, serves as an obstacle to healthcare access and patient compliance, resulting in poor health outcomes. However, the overwhelming majority of early studies involved individual testing in clinics using instruments based on narrow definitions of literacy. Throughout the early literature and even more currently, HL has been presented as a patient condition that medical professionals must "treat" or "work around" [63], and has failed to consider the myriad of factors contributing to poor patient outcomes, such as those related to the healthcare system in which provider–patient clinical encounters are embedded, and other linguistic, social and cultural issues linked to poor outcomes. Because of this, public health approaches to HL began to move away from the clinical view to take a broader, more sociocultural and community perspective [64]. Applied linguists have taken an interest in this turn in the research and have illuminated the role of language proficiency and multilingualism [65], which add layers of complexity to understanding HL and impact on healthcare access (also see Harsch and Santos, this volume). A few applied linguistic studies have also contributed to understanding how people make sense of and use medical and media texts, such as health promotion pamphlets, patient education materials, and pharmaceutical advertisements by conducting macro and micro-analyses of the linguistics of these texts, and through recall and other comprehension protocols with readers (see below in HL and Written Documents). For more on media analyses, see Part "Mass Communication and Health: Theory, Research, and Application with and for Linguistically Diverse Populations" in this volume.

Defining and operationalizing HL

HL is one of the areas at the intersection of language and health that has seen the fewest incursions by applied linguists. The concept of "health literacy" emerged as a significant issue in the national dialogue in the 90s. In 2000, the improvement of HL was identified as one of the objectives of Healthy People 2010 by the United States Department of Health and Human Services, leading to the Institute of Medicine designating HL as a "national priority" in 2004 [66]. HL has always been plagued by conceptual and measurement conundrums. There have been many proposed definitions for HL in the past nearly two decades since 2004, although there is of yet no general consensus on how to define or operationalize the concept. Perhaps the most commonly disseminated definition in the literature has been that used by both DHHS and IOS in early reports: "the capacity of individuals to obtain, process, and understand basic health information and services needed to make appropriate health decisions" [67]. Since 2004, a number of federal initiatives have been established to address HL, including the Affordable Care Act of 2010; the Department of Health and Human Services' National Action Plan to Improve HL; and the Plain Writing Act of 2010 [68]. The many different definitions proposed for HL have led to generalized confusion surrounding exactly what it is, the purpose of measuring it, and which measurement tools to use in research and clinical practice. Despite this confusion, or perhaps because of it, the NIH provided extensive support for "a wide array of prevention-focused HL research," funding 192 studies between 2004 and 2017. According to Villani and Trivedi's evaluation of NIH-funded HL research [67], 88% of these grants focused on the HL of patients and only 2.1% "evaluated the health literacy skills of providers," and a mere 1.0% addressed the health care system. Linguistic research does not figure prominently in any of this research.

A myriad of instruments for measuring HL have been developed and utilized in both clinical practice and research. According to Pleasant et al. [69], more than 100 instruments had been developed to test HL skills at the time of publication. In 2014, Haun et al. [68] conducted a descriptive review of 51 measurement tools, developed between 1999 and 2013, to include the conceptual dimensions the instruments purport to assess, the test parameters of each of the tools, in addition to their psychometric properties. The authors' system of evaluation of the tools was derived from the taxonomy of HL skills developed by Sørensen et al. [70]: their evaluation focused particularly on the components of *literacy* (defined as a reading skill); *interaction*; *comprehension*; and *numeracy*. According to Haun et al., the tools included in their exhaustive review vary greatly in terms of the dimensions they measure and their level of psychometric rigor. Most of the tools are performance-based and are administered in person, requiring pen and paper. Haun et al. conclude that "the field still lacks in a single rigorously validated HL measure that addresses the full range of dimensions which represent this complex construct" [68, p. 327]. Their systematic evaluation of these HL instruments points to the need for the development of metrics that meet the needs of diverse populations and derive from the many components or dimensions represented in conceptual models of HL, such as that of Sørensen et al. And yet, it merits pointing out that taxonomies of components of HL have proven to be elusive and difficult to develop [71]. The process of developing the taxonomy of Sørensen et al. serves to illustrate this point. Their team conducted a content analysis of HL definitions and conceptual frameworks through an exhaustive review of the HL literature (in English) that existed in 2012. However, out of 170 publications, only 19 defined HL explicitly, and a mere 12 provided conceptual frameworks for the construct. These conceptual frameworks varied depending on whether the research was clinically focused or utilized a broader public health approach (see Pleasant and Kuruvilla [63] and Nutbeam [72]). From these limited definitions and frameworks, a conceptual model was developed which included a taxonomy of 12 different literacy "skills." The work of Sørensen et al. served to illuminate the need for consensus in defining HL and in establishing measurable core competencies, constructs, and systems that promote healthcare access. However, the existing taxonomies of competencies remain as vague and obscure and difficult to measure as the literature they are derived from, and the consensus on a definition of HL, called for by Bauer [73] in 2010, McCormack et al. [74] in 2011, and again by Pleasant et al. [69] in 2016, has never been reached.

The literature to date suggests that the persistent focus on "health literacy" constitutes an unfortunate attempt to repackage the many different facets of healthcare, including communication, face-to-face interaction, cognition, culture, education, the healthcare infrastructure and system, and sociocultural variables, among many others. The question remains whether a consensus can be reached on "the definition" of HL with discrete, measurable components. The search for such a consensus may be severely limiting our quest to answer a myriad of research questions (see the next section) and the funding to do so. Until the need for quantitative and qualitative research to examine healthcare access, dissemination of health information, and the healthcare system is recognized both by the academy and at the community level, and informed by the many disciplines that can contribute, including applied linguistics, changes and solutions may not be forthcoming.

Applied linguistics methodological approaches and concepts in health literacy

Health literacy and multilingualism

Directly related to HL, and presenting further complexities, is critical examination of the role of multilingualism, and language proficiency in understanding how non-native English-speaking patients engage with health information (in the United States). In their chapter on developing health and risk messages, Santos et al. [75, p. 1] point out that "While the negative effects of limited proficiency in English have been widely documented in risk messaging and health communication research, the processes by which LEP patients actually come to understand risk messages, seeking out health information from different social networks and resources in different languages, remain poorly researched and understood." Applied linguistic research into HL among diverse language communities, including speakers of minoritized languages, has been limited and is urgently needed. An exhaustive review conducted by Nguyen et al. [76] in 2015 considered the problem of validity in the use of HL instruments with ethnic minorities who speak languages other than English. Their review of 37 non-English measures of HL revealed that they were not sufficiently explicit in the ethnic, linguistic, and cultural makeup of their validation samples. The same was true of 72 English language measures: in the studies utilizing these HL measures with speakers of minoritized languages or English-as-a-second language, language obviously becomes a confounding factor, as discussed also by Jacobson et al. [65]. Nguyen et al. state "The ethno-linguistic and cultural diversity of a given population will influence the extent to which this may pose a problem for any particular project" [76, p. 1501].

There have been few actionable proposals for resolving issues linked to the concept of HL and the intersection with bilingualism and multilingualism, whether at the individual, interactional, or systemic level. A number of researchers, including Santos et al. [75], Soto Mas and Jacobson [77]; Soto Mas et al. [78]; Soto Mas et al. [79], have explored multilingualism and HL by integrating HL modules into English as a Second Language (ESL) classes as a means of promoting HL and proficiency in English. A review conducted by Chen et al. [80] indicates that these types of interventions in ESL classes constitute an effective approach to Improving "limited-English-proficient" students' HL. Harsch and Santos (this volume) also discuss HL among L2 learners of English and multilinguals in this volume and offer viable options for confronting these issues.

Health literacy and written documents

Plain language

Another focal point for applied linguistic research within the realm of HL, healthcare access, and public health is the analysis of the written documents that patients engage with as they navigate the healthcare system. There is a plethora of documents in healthcare contexts that have been developed according to the principles of "plain language," presenting an opportunity for quantitative studies of large databases or corpora as well as mixed-methods research to better understand the use and impact of these materials. The plain language movement grew in parallel with the HL movement: It emerged in the 1970s as a means of simplifying the writing of legal documents [81] and was eventually presented as a way to deal with the challenges of producing comprehensible education materials for patients with low HL, in addition to other documents, such as informed consent documents and patient discharge instructions [82, 83]. In 2010, President Obama signed the "Plain Writing Act" which requires that all public documents written by the federal government be written in plain language. Eventually, the use of plain language was incorporated into guidelines for the National Standards for Culturally and Linguistically Appropriate Services (CLAS standards) in Health and Health Care [84].

The plain language guidelines developed by federal agencies focus on surface-level linguistic features, in particular on short words, short sentences, the use of the active voice, and a number of other prescriptive rules developed to simplify documents provided to the public to make them more accessible [85]. The rules were designed as a means of meeting the criteria for "appropriate" readability levels determined by archaic readability formulae. However, no empirical research to date has provided clear evidence demonstrating that plain language improves the comprehensibility of health-related print materials. Zarcadoolas [64] contends that "surface level language simplification as it is generally practiced in health promotion and communication, is not ideal for communicating complex information effectively." She developed a novel approach to health message development that involves nuanced textual and pragmatic features that are essential to reading comprehension. Her approach, "health literacy load analysis," involves "conducting a structural and functional analysis of any given text" to determine how demanding it will be for the patient to read [86, p. 339]. This analytic approach was used to analyze consumer messaging about overweight and obesity, and the findings led to the development of health materials on the prevention of obesity and overweight for dissemination to the public. Zarcadoolas's research is an example of how in-depth, multi-feature, and multi-componential linguistics combined with sociocultural analyses can lead to enhanced practices in developing comprehensible messages and other oral and written texts. Further research is called for that explores other text types: these include communication campaign materials; patient education brochures provided in hard copy to patients in clinics and hospitals (or available online); pharmaceutical labels and instructions, and documents such as informed consent forms, patient intake and discharge forms, instructions for advanced directives, research questionnaires and surveys, and other written artifacts that providers and patients engage with as they negotiate healthcare encounters and the healthcare system. There are many gaps in our understanding of these documents, including how they are developed; how and when they are used in healthcare encounters and presented to patients; how comprehensible they are to the end user; and the level of impact they have on patient understanding of diagnosis; treatment; medication and treatment compliance, health decisions, and overall health outcomes. There is also a scarcity of research that looks at similar materials developed in other languages, usually through a process of translation, and provided to patients who speak (and read) languages other than English as L1 or who are multilingual.

Minoritized languages and written health documents
In the past several decades, a minimal amount of research in applied linguistics has explored these written health materials developed for speakers of minoritized languages. Development of these materials (whether print or digital) continues to be conducted through a process of translation and what is commonly referred to as "back translation," (a highly controversial method used to determine the quality and accuracy of translations) [87]. There have been a handful of studies exploring non-English health materials that have been informed by applied linguists and translation studies. Jacobson [88] conducted a multi-faceted, mixed-methods study that involved the comparative analysis of a corpus of health brochures from the United States translated from English into Spanish and a corpus of health brochures developed originally in Spanish from Mexico. Her linguistic analyses of the texts involved what she referred to as a mixed-methods, micro-linguistic analysis grounded in Speech Act Theory. This analysis provided evidence for markedly different linguistic realizations of the persuasive interactional goals in the two text types, translated and non-translated. She also conducted a

multifeature–multidimensional factor analysis adapted from the methods proposed by Biber [89–91] to compare the patterning and co-occurrence of linguistic features serving informational and persuasive functions across the two corpora. She attributed the qualitative and quantitative differences revealed in the analyses to the different sociocultural contexts in which the documents were developed and used. Her study also implemented pre-test and post-test and recall protocols with Spanish-speaking adults to compare the translated and non-translated texts. Her multi-level research revealed stark differences between the two text types and impact on the reader. It provided evidence to support developing and field-testing health materials among and for the communities who will be using them, and avoiding translations altogether.

In a recent mixed-methods study also involving both text analysis and participant testing, Ratajczak [92] explored the comprehensibility of health-related documents based on a limited number of linguistic features, including average word frequency, average word length; passive voice forms, cohesive markers, gerunds, frequency of occurrence of superordinate words, combined with scores of readability indices. He collected demographic data (age, education, English proficiency, HL level) from native English and native Polish, L2 speakers of English in the United Kingdom, and administered a reading comprehension test to these participants. His goals, as reflected in the research questions, were threefold: (1) to determine how reader attributes predict comprehension of written health-related information; (2) to determine how textual features predict the comprehensibility of written health-related information; and (3) to determine whether reader attributes and textual characteristics interact in predicting the comprehension of health-related information. Two intriguing findings of his study, and relevant to current thinking on HL and plain language, are (1) plain language adaptations for different users did not impact comprehension, and (2) differences between individual attributes are more important than differences in the texts themselves. He concludes that "the lack of supporting evidence for the effects of text features indicates that the most effective way to improve comprehension of health-related texts is likely to be offered by interventions focusing on individuals rather than on texts" (p. 288) providing further evidence to support work such as that of Zarcadoolas, [64, 86] and her contention that "plain language" does not provide a ready answer to problems linked to HL (see also Harsch and Santos, discussion of plain language, linguistic simplification and empowerment in Chapter 1). Another study conducted by Villareal [93] involved a lengthy linguistic analysis of translated (English to Spanish) texts on pediatric cancer diagnosis and treatment. Villareal used Halliday's Systemic Functional Linguistics framework to explore the Interpersonal, Ideational, and Textual Meta functions. Her findings shed light on translation problems, particularly those related to differences in culture and ideologies.

The studies conducted by these scholars demonstrate the importance of digging deep both qualitatively and quantitatively to illuminate how written health materials in languages other than English in the United States are developed, and their impact on the communities who use them.

Recommendations

The intent of this chapter has been to discuss the incursion of applied linguistics into areas of public health and healthcare by focusing on key areas of linguistic research. It has sought to elucidate the prominent research trends at the intersection of language and health during the past several decades and to point to the many pressing questions that remain to be addressed through rigorous empirical research. Methodological diversity is essential to this challenge: conversation analysis; IS; discourse analysis; first and second language acquisition studies; language teaching; bilingualism and multiculturalism; text and genre analysis; interpreting and translation studies, and other linguistic fields all offer powerful quantitative and qualitative analytical tools and approaches and theoretical frameworks that have the potential to shed further light on how language impacts health.

Future research

This chapter has brought up a list of salient (but by no means exhaustive) topics in healthcare and public health that call for an applied linguistic perspective:

First, there is much-unexplored research territory in the area of linguistic and cultural discordant provider–patient interaction. Richly descriptive qualitative "micro-analyses" at the conversational level are needed, as well as approaches that "zoom out" and focus on systemic and sociocultural factors and variables that directly influence what happens at the conversational, face-to-face level. Quantitative analyses of larger corpora of healthcare encounters will inform these more qualitative and critical approaches. Medical encounters involving interpreters have been notably neglected in the literature: the educational approaches for interpreters and providers who collaborate with them in providing healthcare need reforming. However, curricula revision must derive from the findings of rigorous empirical research that goes beyond what has been done on the "interpreter role" to date, and by expanding our perception of what HL is and what it involves. As discussed above in relation to Villani and Trivedi's [67] evaluation of NIH-funded HL studies, linguistic research was not represented in any of this research. If "the ability to obtain, process and understand basic health information and services" is core to HL, then provider–patient interaction mediated by an interpreter should be central to the research agenda in pursuit of improving HL. It merits reiterating that the decades-long mission to arrive at consensus on a "definition" of HL may be severely limiting our quest to answer some of the most pressing questions, as well as the funding to do so.

This leads to a second area of applied linguistic collaboration that of HL instruments. The implementation of applied linguistic methodologies has the potential to inform many of the challenges that have emerged in the development and use of these tools. There are a number of questions to address regarding confounding variables in their administration and in interpretation of the results. For example, referring back to Nguyen et al.'s review [76], Jacobson et al. [65], and Santos et al. [84], linguistic and cultural diversity needs to be taken into account when developing HL tools and when interpreting their results. There are many questions still unanswered about "how to measure health literacy within... richly layered social and linguistic contexts" [15, p. 59] including taking into account the bilingual status of the communities of participants.

Third, regarding efforts to improve HL in multilingual communities, experts in English-as-a-Second-Language have already been active in conducting innovative adult education interventions. These have involved the integration of health components into ESL classes as a means of improving HL, with some degree of success. As suggested by Feuerherm et al. [15] building partnerships with public health, nursing, and other healthcare entities is essential to continued collaborations of this sort.

Finally, healthcare information disseminated in print and digitally should constitute a key focal point for applied linguistic research. A few exhaustive linguistic analyses have been conducted to explore plain language and translated documents and their impact on comprehensibility. There is a need for further research that builds on these studies, and for additional innovative analytic approaches to be proposed and implemented.

Dissemination of findings

However, it is not enough to conduct the research: applied linguists must also be involved in the dissemination of research findings to assure their "uptake" by professionals in the health field. Roberts and Sarangi [94] bring this problem to our attention in their discussion of discourse analytic research in medical consultancies. Applied linguists conduct research, in part, because they are working to invoke change. However, finding ways to transition from findings to practice is a continual challenge, as demonstrated by other researchers in this volume. Making findings practically relevant can be done in a number of ways. One involves conducting further research in order to demonstrate the impact of findings on defined outcomes. Heritage and Robinson [95], for example, demonstrate the approach of conducting an intervention protocol using findings from CA research on provider–patient consultations. The aim of the example interventions they describe is "research fully focused on the relationship between interactional practices and medically relevant outcomes" (p. 212). Community and institutional partnerships such as those established by the ESL researchers mentioned in this chapter, are key to making all parties, including health practitioners and patients, feel vested in the ultimate goal of creating impact. Developing clear research questions from the beginning is essential, and if these can be co-authored with collaborators from the health disciplines who are working "on the front lines," then the subsequent uptake of the findings in health contexts will be much easier [96].

Dissemination and uptake of the findings of research in applied linguistics remains a challenge and will require innovative approaches, multidisciplinary collaboration, and effective planning and design of projects. Dissemination and implementation cannot be an afterthought.

With the continued growing diversity of the United States population and the discouraging trends in health disparities, continued involvement of applied linguists in the endeavors discussed in this chapter is essential. Findings derived from both applied linguistic research alone and multidisciplinary collaborations involving applied linguists have the potential of impacting public health policy and informing best practices in health communication, leading to future reduction in health disparities.

Highlights

- Applied linguistic methodological approaches, such as conversation analysis and IS, have illuminated provider–patient interaction by allowing for a more nuanced "turn-by-turn" analysis with greater focus on how the interaction systematically unfolds between speakers.
- Applied linguists have confronted the challenges of HL and multilingualism by integrating HL modules into ESL classes as a means of promoting HL and

proficiency in English. These types of interventions in ESL classes constitute an effective approach to improving "limited English proficient" students' HL.
- Applied linguistic research demonstrates the importance of digging deep both qualitatively and quantitatively to illuminate how written health materials in languages other than English in the United States are developed and their impact on the communities who use them.

REFERENCES

1. Brumfit, C.J. (1995). Teacher professionalism and research. In: *Principle and Practice in Applied Linguistics* (ed. G. Cook and B. Seidhofer), 27–41. Oxford: Oxford University Press.
2. Simpson, J. (2011). *The Routledge Handbook of Applied Linguistics*. Abingdon: Routledge.
3. Heller, M.S. and Freeman, S.H. (1987). *Medical Discourse (Ser. Text, v. 7-1)*. Mouton de Gruyter.
4. Ainsworth-Vaughn, N. (1998). *Claiming Power in Doctor–Patient Talk*. Oxford: Oxford University Press.
5. Wodak, R. (1997). Discourse-sociolinguistics and the study of doctor–patient interaction. In: *The Construction of Professional Discourse* (ed. B.L. Gunnarsson, P. Linell, and B. Nordberg), 173–2000. London: Longman.
6. Ten Have, P. (1995). Medical ethnomethodology: an overview. *Hum. Stud.* 18 (2–3): 245–261. Available from: https://libproxy.unm.edu/login?url=https://www.proquest.com/scholarly-journals/medical-ethnomethodology-overview/docview/61412768/se-2?accountid=14613.
7. Fisher, S. (1995). *Nursing Wounds: Nurse Practitioners/Doctors/Women Patients and the Negotiation of Meaning*. New Brunswick, NJ: Rutgers University Press.
8. West, C. (1984). *Routine Complications: Troubles in Talk Between Doctors and Patients*. Bloomington, IN: Indiana University Press.
9. Todd, A.D. (1984). The prescription of contraception: negotiations between doctors and patients. *Discourse Process.* 7 (2): 171–200.
10. Hamilton, H.E. (2004). Symptoms and signs in particular: the influence of the medical concern on the shape of physician-patient talk. *Commun. Med.* 1 (1): 59–70.
11. Cicourel, A. (1983). Hearing is not believing: language and the structure of belief in medical communication. In: *The Social Organisation of Doctor–Patient Communication* (ed. S. Fisher and A.D. Todd), 221–239. Washington, DC: Bloomsbury Academic.
12. Atkinson, P. (1995). *Medical Talk and Medical Work: The Liturgy of the Clinic*. London: Sage.
13. Tannen, D. and Wallet, C. (1986). Medical professions and parents: a linguistic analysis of communication across contexts. *Lang. Soc.* 15: 295–312.
14. Silverman, D. (1996). *Medical Talk and Medical Work: The Liturgy of the Clinic*, Sociology of Health and Illness, vol. Vol. 18, 277–278. London: Sage.
15. Feuerherm, E., Showstack, R., Santos, M.G. et al. (2021). Language as a social determinant of health: partnerships for health equity. In: *Extending Applied Linguistics for Social Impact: Cross-Disciplinary Collaborations in Diverse Spaces of Public Inquiry* (ed. L. Miller and D. Warriner), 125–148. Bloomsbury Academic.
16. Balint, M. (1957). *The Doctor, His Patient, and the Illness*. New York: International Universities Press.
17. Byrne, P. and Long, B. (1976). *Doctors Talking to Patients: A Study of the Verbal Behaviours of Doctors in the Consultation*. London: HMSO.
18. Sudnow, D. (1967). *Passing on: The Social Organization of Dying*. Englewood Cliffs, NJ: Prentice-Hall.

19. Timmermans, S. (1998). Social death as self-fulfilling prophecy: David Sudnow's passing on revisited. *Sociol. Q.* 39 (3): 453–472.
20. Ong, L.M.L., de Haes, J.C.J.M., Hoos, A.M., and Lammes, F.B. (1995). Doctor-patient communication: a review of the literature. *Soc. Sci. Med.* 40 (7): 903–918.
21. Roter, D. and Larson, S. (2002). The Roter interaction analysis system (RIAS): utility and flexibility for analysis of medical interactions. *Patient Educ. Couns.* 46 (4): 243–251.
22. Sandvik, M., Eide, H., Lind, M. et al. (2002). Analyzing medical dialogues: strength and weakness of Roter's interaction analysis system (RIAS). *Patient Educ. Couns.* 46 (4): 235–241.
23. Pomerantz, A. and Fehr, B. (2009). Conversation analysis: an approach to the analysis of social interaction. In: *Discourse Studies: A Multidisciplinary Introduction* (ed. T. Van Dijk), 165–190. London: Sage.
24. ten Have, P. (2007). *Doing Conversation Analysis: A Practical Guide*, 2e. London: Sage.
25. Kasper, G. and Wagner, J. (2014). Conversation analysis in applied linguistics. *Annu. Rev. Appl. Linguist.* 34: 171–212.
26. Edwards, J.A. and Lampert, M.D. (1993). *Talking Data: Transcription and Coding in Discourse Research*. Hillsdale, NJ: Lawrence Erlbaum Associates.
27. Heritage, J. (2011). Conversation analysis: practices and methods. In: *Qualitative Research*, 3e (ed. D. Silverman), 209–228. Sage Available from: http://books.google.com/books?hl=en&lr=&id=77wHtzvtYM0C&oi=fnd&pg=PA208&dq=Conversation+Analysis:+Practices+and+Methods&ots=iFzIJInOrs&sig=ppNu0BKFPQ7fzUjql9Uir6kOaH4.
28. Halkowski, T. and Gill, V. (2010). Conversation analysis and ethnomethodology: the centrality of interaction. In: *The Sage Handbook of Qualitative Methods in Health Research* (ed. I. Bourgeault, R. Dingwall, and R. de Vries), 212–228. London: Sage Publications.
29. Heritage, J. and Robinson, J.D. (2011). 'Some' versus 'any' medical issues: encouraging patients to reveal their unmet concerns. In: *Applied Conversation Analysis* (ed. C. Antaki), 15–31. Palgrave Macmillan UK.
30. Stivers, T. (2021). Managing patient pressure to prescribe antibiotics in the clinic. *Pediatr. Drugs* 23: 437–443. https://doi.org/10.1007/s40272-021-00466-y.
31. Stivers, T. and Timmermans, S. (2020). Medical authority under siege: how clinicians transform patient resistance into acceptance. *J. Health Soc. Behav.* 61 (1): 60–78.
32. Sikveland, R. and Stokoe, E. (2020). Effective triaging in general practice receptions: a conversation analytic study. In: *Applying Linguistics in Illness and Healthcare Contexts* (ed. Z. Demjén), 271–294. London: Bloomsbury Academic.
33. Rodney, H.J. (2013). *Health and Risk Communication: An Applied Linguistic Perspective*. Routledge.
34. Gill, V. and Roberts, F. (2012). Conversation analysis in medicine. In: *The Handbook of Conversation Analysis* (ed. J. Sidnell and T. Stivers), 575–592. Blackwell-Wiley.
35. Candlin, C.N. and Candlin, S. (2003). 8. Health care communication: a problematic site for applied linguistics research. *Annu. Rev. Appl. Linguist.* 23: 134–154.
36. Jansson, G., Wadensjö, C., and Plejert, C. (2017). Managing complaints in multilingual care encounters. *Multilingua* 36 (3): 313–345.
37. Roberts, C. (2008). Intercultural communication in healthcare settings. In: *Handbook of Intercultural Communication* (ed. H. Kotthoff and H. Spencer-Oatey), 243–262. De Gruyter Mouton.
38. Wadensjö, C. (2014). *Interpreting as Interaction*. Routledge.
39. Davidson, B. (2000). The interpreter as institutional gatekeeper: the social-linguistic role of interpreters in Spanish-English medical discourse. *J. Socioling.* 4 (3): 379–405.
40. Davidson, B. (2001). Questions in cross-linguistic medical encounters: the role of the hospital interpreter. *Anthropol. Q.* 74: 170–178.
41. Jacobson, H.E. (2009). Moving beyond words in assessing mediated interaction:

measuring interactional competence in healthcare settings. In: *Testing and Assessment in Translation and Interpreting*, American Translators Association Scholarly Monograph Series XIV, 1–10 (ed. C. Angelelli and H. Jacobson), 49–70. Amsterdam: John Benjamins Publishing Co.
42. Raymond, C.W. (2014). Conveying information in the interpreter-mediated medical visit: the case of epistemic brokering. *Patient Educ. Couns.* 97 (1): 38–46.
43. Pappas, G. (1990). Some implications for the study of the doctor-patient interaction: power, structure, and agency in the works of Howard Waitzkin and Arthur Kleinman. *Soc. Sci. Med.* 30 (2): 199–204.
44. Schegloff, E.A. (1988). Goffman and the analysis of conversation. In: *Erving Goffman: Exploring the Interaction Other* (ed. P. Drew and A. Wootton), 89–135. Polity Press.
45. Gordon, C. (2010). Gumperz and interactional sociolinguistics. In: *The SAGE Handbook of Sociolinguistics* (ed. R. Wodak, B. Johnstone, and P.E. Kerswill), 67–84. Sage Publications.
46. Rampton, B. (2019). Interactional sociolinguistics. In: *The Routledge Handbook of Linguistic Ethnography* (ed. K. Tusting), 13–27. Routledge.
47. Scollon, R. and Scollon, S.W. (2001). *Intercultural Communication*, 2e. SocioLinguistics.
48. Gordon, C. and Kraut, J. (2017). Interactional sociolinguistics. In: *The Routledge Handbook of Language in the Workplace* (ed. B. Vine), 3–14. Routledge.
49. Toomaneejinda, A. and Saengboon, S. (2022). Interactional sociolinguistics: the theoretical framework and methodological approach to ELF interaction research. *Learn. J. Lang. Educ. Acquis. Res. Netw.* 15 (1): 156–179.
50. Gumperz, J.J. and Cook-Gumperz, J. (2012). Interactional sociolinguistics: perspectives on intercultural communication. In: *The Handbook of Intercultural Discourse and Communication* (ed. C.B. Paulston, S.F. Kiesling, and E.S. Rangel), 63–76. John Wiley.
51. Hamilton, H.E. and Chou, W.Y.S. (2014). *The Routledge Handbook of Language and Health Communication*. Routledge.
52. Pickering, L. (2009). Intonation as a pragmatic resource in ELF interaction. *Intercult. Pragmat.* 6 (2): 235–255.
53. Vickers, C.H., Goble, R., and Lindfelt, C. (2013). Narrative co-construction in the medical consultation: how agency and control affect the diagnosis. *Commun. Med.* 9 (2): 159–171.
54. Vickers, C.H., Zychowicz, S., and Morones, J.R. (2010). Living with pain: narrating an ideological position toward healthcare. *Commun. Med.* 7: 85–92.
55. Goble, R. and Vickers, C.H. (2015). "Shift" 'n "control": the computer as a third interactant in Spanish-language medical consultations. *Commun. Med.* 12 (2–3): 171–185.
56. Chimbwete-Phiri, R. and Schnurr, S. (2020). Improving HIV/AIDS consultations in Malawi: how interactional sociolinguistics can contribute. In: *Applying Linguistics in Illness and Healthcare Contexts* (ed. Z. Demjén), 131–158. Bloomsbury Academic.
57. Demjén, Z. (2016). *Applying Linguistics in Illness and Healthcare Contexts*. Bloomsbury Academic.
58. Vickers, C. and Goble, R. (2011). Well, now, okey dokey: English discourse markers in Spanish-language medical consultations. *Can. Mod. Lang. Rev.* 67 (4).
59. Vickers, C.H., Deckert, S.K., and Goble, R. (2014). Constructing language normativity through the animation of stance in Spanish-language Medical consultations. *Health Commun.* 29 (7): https://doi.org/10.1353/cml.2011.0025.
60. Vickers, C.H., Goble, R., and Deckert, S.K. (2015). Third party interaction in the medical context: code-switching and control. *J. Pragmat.* 84: 154–171.
61. Feuerherm, E.M., Showstack, R.E., Santos, M.G. et al. (2021). Language as a social determinant of health: partnerships for health equity. In: *Extending Applied Linguistics for Social Impact* (ed. D.S. Warriner and E.R. Miller), 125–148. Bloomsbury Publishing.
62. Cutilli, C.C. and Bennett, I.M. (2009). Understanding the health literacy of America. *Orthop. Nurs.* 28 (1): 27–32.
63. Pleasant, A. and Kuruvilla, S. (2008). A tale of two health literacies: public health and

clinical approaches to health literacy. *Health Promot. Int.* 23 (2): 152–159.
64. Zarcadoolas, C. (2011). The simplicity complex: exploring simplified health messages in a complex world. *Health Promot. Int.* 26 (3): 338–350.
65. Jacobson, H.E., Hund, L., and Soto, M.F. (2016). Predictors of English health literacy among U.S. Hispanic immigrants: the importance of language, bilingualism and sociolinguistic environment. *Lit. Numer. Stud.* 24 (1): 43–64.
66. Institute of Medicine (US) Committee on Health Literacy (2004). *Health Literacy: A Prescription to End Confusion* (ed. L. Nielsen-Bohlman, A.M. Panzer, and D.A. Kindig). Washington (DC): National Academies Press (US).
67. Villani, J. and Trivedi, N. (2020). Health literacy research funded by the NIH for disease prevention. *Heal. Lit. Res. Pract.* 4 (4): e212–e223.
68. Haun, J.N., Valerio, M.A., McCormack, L.A. et al. (2014). Health literacy measurement: an inventory and descriptive summary of 51 instruments. *J. Health Commun.* 19: 302–333.
69. Pleasant, A., Rudd, R.E., O'Leary, C. et al. (2016). *Considerations for a New Definition of Health Literacy*. Washington, DC: National Academy of Medicine.
70. Sørensen, K., Van Den Broucke, S., Fullam, J. et al. (2012). Health literacy and public health: a systematic review and integration of definitions and models. *BMC Public Health* 12: 80.
71. Jørgensen, M.B. and Larsen, A.K. (2022). Occupational health literacy: healthy decisions at work. In: *International Handbook of Health Literacy* (ed. O. Okan, U. Bauer, D. Levin-zamir, et al.), 347–358. Policy Press.
72. Nutbeam, D. (2008). The evolving concept of health literacy. *Soc. Sci. Med.* 67 (12): 2072–2078.
73. Baur, C. (2010). New directions in research on public health and health literacy. *J. Health Commun.* 15 (SUPPL. 2): 42–50.
74. McCormack, L.A., Rush, S.R., Kandula, N.R., and Paasche-Orlow, M.K. (2011). Health literacy research: looking forward. *J. Health Commun.* 16 (SUPPL. 3): 5–8.
75. Santos, M.G., Handley, M.A., Omark, K., and Schillinger, D. (2014). ESL participation as a mechanism for advancing health literacy in immigrant communities. *J. Health Commun.* 19: 89–105.
76. Nguyen, T.H., Park, H., Han, H.R. et al. (2015). State of the science of health literacy measures: validity implications for minority populations. *Patient Educ. Couns.* 98 (12): 1492–1512.
77. Soto Mas, F. and Jacobson, H.E. (2019). Advancing health literacy among Hispanic immigrants: the intersection between education and health. *Health Promot. Pract.* 20 (2): 251–257.
78. Soto Mas, F., Schmitt, C.L., Jacobson, H.E., and Myers, O.B. (2018). A cardiovascular health intervention for Spanish speakers: the health literacy and ESL curriculum. *J. Community Health* 43 (4): 717–724.
79. Soto Mas, F., Mein, E., Fuentes, B. et al. (2013). Integrating health literacy and ESL: an interdisciplinary curriculum for Hispanic immigrants. *Health Promot. Pract.* 14 (2): 263–273.
80. Chen, X., Goodson, P., and Acosta, S. (2015). Blending health literacy with an English as a second language curriculum: a systematic literature review. *J. Health Commun.* 20 (d): 101–111.
81. Rubin, D.L. and Floyd, D.H. (1992). A functional approach to writing for trial court judges. *J. Teach. Writ.* 11 (2): 187–202.
82. Davis, T.C., Holcombe, R.F., Berkel, H.J. et al. (1998). Informed consent for clinical trials: a comparative study of standard versus simplified forms. *J. Natl. Cancer Inst.* 90 (9): 668–674.
83. Williams, D.M., Counselman, F.L., and Caggiano, C.D. (1996). Emergency department discharge instructions and patient literacy: a problem of disparity. *Am. J. Emerg. Med.* 14 (1): 19–22.
84. Santos, M.G., Jacobson, H.E., and Manneh, S. (2017). Limited English proficiency as a consideration when designing health and risk messages. *Oxford Res. Encycl. Commun.* (August): 1–30.
85. Federal plain language guidelines. [Internet]. [cited 2022 Oct 1]. Available

from: https://www.plainlanguage.gov/guidelines.
86. Zarcadoolas, C., Sealy, Y., Levy, J. et al. (2011). Health literacy at work to address overweight and obesity in adults: the development of the obesity action kit. *J. Commun Healthc.* 4 (2): 88–101.
87. Behr, D. (2017). Assessing the use of back translation: the shortcomings of back translation as a quality testing method. *Int. J. Soc. Res. Methodol.* 20 (6): 573–584.
88. Jacobson, H.E. (2002). *Translation of the Health Brochure and Impact on the Target Reader: A Contrastive Analysis of the Structural and Pragmatic Features of Texts Translated into Spanish Versus Texts Written Originally in Spanish*. Tucson, AZ: The University of Arizona Available from: https://repository.arizona.edu/handle/10150/280112.
89. Friginal, E. (2013). Twenty-five years of Biber's multi-dimensional analysis: introduction to the special issue and an interview with Douglas Biber. *Corpora* 8: 137–152.
90. Charles, M. (2015). Corpus-based research in applied linguistics: studies in honor of Doug Biber. *System* 53: 164–165. https://doi.org/10.1016/j.system.2015.07.009.
91. Biber, D. (2019). Text-linguistic approaches to register variation. *Reg. Stud.* 1 (1): 42–75.
92. Ratajezak, M. (2020). *The Effects of Individual Differences and Linguistic Features on Reading Comprehension of Health-Related Texts* Michael Ratajczak Doctoral Thesis Submitted in Fulfilment of the Requirements for the Degree of Doctor of Philosophy in Linguistics April 2020 L. Lancaster University.
93. Villareal, A. (2017). Constructing meaning: a systemic functional review of translated health texts and community narratives. *Fac. Dep. Hisp. Stud. Univ. Houst.* 53 (9): 1689–1699. Available from: https://search.proquest.com/docview/2206580420?accountid=43860.
94. Roberts, C. and Sarangi, S. (2003). Uptake of discourse research in interprofessional settings: reporting from medical consultancy. *Appl. Linguist.* 24 (3): 338–359+421.
95. Heritage, J. and Robinson, J.D. (2011). "Some" versus "any" medical issues: encouraging patients to reveal their unmet concerns. In: *Applied Conversation Analysis: Intervention and Change in Institutional Talk* (ed. C. Antaki), 15–16. London: Palgrave Macmillan UK.
96. Tomlinson, J. (2020). Epilogue. In: *Applying Linguistics in Illness and Healthcare Contexts* (ed. Z. Demjen), 372–378. London: Bloomsbury Academic.

Part II   Language Interpretation and Translation in Public Health and Healthcare

Introduction to Part II

Maichou Lor

Over the past five decades, the number of international migrations has increased globally. Between 1970 and 2020, the number of people living in a country other than their country of birth tripled from 94 million to 281 million [1]. Approximately two-thirds of all international migrants live in high-income countries [2], such as Australia, Switzerland, and the United States, while the top ten countries with the highest number of emigrants in 2020 were India, Mexico, Russia, China, Syria, Bangladesh, Pakistan, Ukraine, the Philippines, and Afghanistan [3]. Given the increase in global migration, there is growing diversity among migrants in terms of language, literacy, and cultural background. Additionally, the proportion of individuals who have limited ability to speak, write, and read English is likely to increase as emigrants migrate to high-income countries where English is likely to be the primary language.

Research shows that people with limited English proficiency are more likely to have low health literacy compared to those who are English proficient [4–6]. Inadequate health literacy and limited English proficiency are associated with poor healthcare access and outcomes [7–9]. Both limited English proficiency and low health literacy pose significant structural barriers to healthcare communication [10–13], placing linguistically diverse populations at risk of experiencing health disparities.

Effective health communication is critical for all aspects of health and well-being, including disease prevention, health promotion, and quality of life [14], yet when

---

The Handbook of Language in Public Health and Healthcare, First Edition.
Edited by Pilar Ortega, Glenn Martínez, Maichou Lor, and A. Susana Ramírez.
© 2024 John Wiley & Sons, Inc. Published 2024 by John Wiley & Sons, Inc.

patients and health professionals do not share the same language (i.e., language discordance), communication is likely to be compromised. The consequences of language discordance are well documented and significant, including reduced patient access to healthcare [15]; poorer diagnostic and therapeutic outcomes [16]; longer hospital stays [17, 18]; lower use of primary prevention services, such as Pap smears and mammograms [19]; poorer understanding of discharge instructions [20]; and lower patient satisfaction [21]. These outcomes highlight the need for linguistically diverse populations to access language services to address health and reduce healthcare disparities.

Research and practice efforts have been made across different countries to address language discordance between patients and clinicians in healthcare settings. These efforts have focused on studying and implementing interpreter services, healthcare translation, plain language, and health literacy to promote effective communication (see glossary for definitions). The research in these areas has expanded in the past five decades, yet has varied in focus between countries. Therefore, in this section of the volume, we present the latest evidence for the benefits and proper use of strategies to facilitate communication with linguistically diverse populations in language-discordant scenarios. Specifically, by collating literature from different disciplines and theories, the chapters provide detailed information and a discussion about the research on interpreter services, healthcare translation, plain language, and health literacy in public health and healthcare. At the end of each chapter, there is a summary of recommendations for policy, practice, and research.

Chapter 6 provides an overview of the key issues that contribute to language-discordant situations in healthcare settings, using the United States as a case exemplar. This chapter also focuses on how recent policy changes are moving the healthcare industry toward improving health outcomes for people with non-English language preferences.

Chapter 7 focuses on spoken language interpreting in a medical context. This chapter reports on the function and impacts of medical interpreters in healthcare settings, including the historical development of interpreter roles, and the continuum of roles interpreters interactively negotiate and construct as they manage their tasks, identities, and relationships in interpreter-mediated interactions. Moreover, the authors present a summary of different interpreter types (i.e., professional interpreters and dual role bilingual medical professionals [i.e., are not specifically trained as interpreters], and non-professional interpreters) – using the Model of Bilingual Health Communication – and report the latest findings on the impact of each interpreter type.

Chapter 8 reports on the written translation of health-related texts for linguistically diverse patients across the healthcare spectrum. The author reports on the different text genres translated, summarizes the challenges of text translation, and provides good practices and recommendations.

Chapter 9 focuses on health literacy and plain language by providing an overview of the critical issues and topics. This chapter highlights the prevalence, historical development, and theoretical framework of health literacy followed globally by focusing on the United States' initiatives to address health literacy and plain language as an exemplar.

REFERENCES

1. McAuliffe, M. and Triandafyllidou, A. (ed.) (2021). *World Migration Report 2022*. Geneva: International Organization for Migration. https://worldmigrationreport.iom.int/wmr-2022-interactive/ (accessed 22 March 2023).
2. Department of Economic and Social Affairs (2021). International migration 2020 highlights. United Nations. https://www.un.org/development/desa/pd/sites/www.un.org.development.desa.pd/files/international_migration_2020_highlights_ten_key_messages.pdf (accessed 22 March 2023).
3. World Population Review (2022). Immigration by country 2022. https://worldpopulationreview.com/country-rankings/immigration-by-country (accessed 22 March 2023).
4. Kindig D.A., Panzer A.M., Nielsen-Bohlman L. (Eds.). *Health Literacy: A Prescription to End Confusion*. 2002. National Academies of Press. https://www.nap.edu/catalog/10883/health-literacy-a-prescription-to-end-confusion (accessed 22 March 2023).
5. Leyva, M., Sharif, I., and Ozuah, P.O. (2004). Health literacy among Spanish-speaking Latino parents with limited English proficiency. *Ambul. Pediatr.* 5 (1): 56–59.
6. Sentell, T. and Braun, K. (2012). Low health literacy, limited English proficiency, and health status in Asians, Latinos, and other racial/ethnic groups in California. *J. Health Commun.* 17 (3): 82–99.
7. Sentell, T. and Braun, K.L. (2012). Low health literacy, limited English proficiency, and health status in Asians, Latinos, and other racial/ethnic groups in California. *J. Health Commun.* 17 (sup3): 82–99.
8. Leyva, M., Sharif, I., and Ozuah, P.O. (2005). Health literacy among Spanish-speaking Latino parents with limited English proficiency. *Ambul. Pediatr.* 5 (1): 56–59.
9. Sentell, T., Braun, K.L., Davis, J., and Davis, T. (2013). Colorectal cancer screening: low health literacy and limited English proficiency among Asians and Whites in California. *J. Health Commun.* 18 (sup1): 242–255.
10. McKee, M.M. and Paasche-Orlow, M.K. (2012). Health literacy and the disenfranchised: yhe importance of collaboration between limited English proficiency and health literacy researchers. *J. Health Communn.* 17 (sup3): 7–12.
11. Bernhardt, J.M. (2004). Communication at the core of effective public health. *Am. J. Public Health* 94: 2051–2053.
12. Fernandez, A., Schillinger, D., Grumbach, K. et al. (2004). Physician language ability and cultural competence. *J. Gen. Internal Med.* 19 (2): 167–174.
13. Graham, E.A., Jacobs, T.A., Kwan-Gett, T.S., and Cover, J. (2008). Health services utilization by low-income limited English proficient adults. *J. Immigr. Minor. Health* 10 (3): 207–217.
14. Paasche-Orlow, M.K. and Wolf, M.S. (2007). The causal pathways linking health literacy to health outcomes. *Am. J. Health Behav.* 31 (1): S19–S26.
15. Gulati, R.K. and Hur, K. (2022). Association between limited English proficiency and healthcare access and utilization in California. *J. Immigr. Minor. Health*. 24 (1): 95–101.
16. Herbert, B.M., Johnson, A.E., Paasche-Orlow, M.K. et al. (2021). Disparities in reporting a history of cardiovascular disease among adults with limited English proficiency and angina. *JAMA Netw. Open* 4 (12): 1–11.
17. Levas, M.N., Cowden, J.D., and Dowd, M.D. (2011). Effects of the limited English proficiency of parents on hospital length of stay and home health care referral for their home health care–eligible children with infections. *Arch. Pediatr. Adolesc. Med.* 165 (9): 831–836.
18. Patel, A.T., Lee, B.R., Donegan, R. et al. (2020). Length of stay for patients with limited English proficiency in pediatric urgent care. *Clin. Pediatr.* 59 (4-5): 421–428.
19. Jacobs, E.A., Karavolos, K., Rathouz, P.J. et al. (2005). Limited English proficiency and breast and cervical cancer screening in a multiethnic population. *Am. J. Public Health* 95 (8): 1410–1416.

20. Choe, A.Y., Thomson, J.E., Unaka, N.I. et al. (2021). Disparity in nurse discharge communication for hospitalized families based on English proficiency. *Hosp. Pediatr.* 11 (3): 245–253.

21. Al, S.H., Almutair, A.G., Al, M.S. et al. (2020). Implications of language barriers for healthcare: a systematic review. *Oman Med. J.* 35 (2): e122.

6 Recognizing and Addressing Language Discordance

ALLISON SQUIRES

Introduction

Imagine you need medical care. You walk into a primary care office, an emergency department, or find yourself suddenly hospitalized.

Then you do not understand a word being spoken around you. It is clear people are trying to communicate with you using hand gestures and pointing to places on their bodies, and you partially understand what they are asking. Complicating the situation further, there is no one with you for this health visit or sudden hospitalization. The uncertainty and the fear are becoming overwhelming because you just do not understand what is happening. The risk for harm to yourself is great because you cannot communicate with the people around you; yet, there is nothing you can do about it.

On a daily basis, millions of people have this experience of "language discordance" or "language barriers." They may be tourists, traveling for work, immigrants, or refugees – with hearing abilities or not. Language discordance occurs when two people cannot communicate with each other in the same language [1]. During a healthcare encounter, language discordance presents a very real threat to the safety of the person seeking health services. For example, in primary care, patients who anticipate that their healthcare provider does not speak their preferred language will often delay seeking preventive services which results in more acute illnesses later on and increases their risk for hospitalization [2–4]. During a hospitalization, language discordance results in patients experiencing higher risk for complications related to their treatment or the handling of their care [5, 6]. They are also less likely to receive home healthcare services, and, when they do, providing those services requires more time on the part of the agency and the provider [7, 8].

All these challenges related to language discordance can be bridged by qualified human interpreters or healthcare professionals who speak the same language as the person seeking care. Health and system outcomes improve with interpreter use across all age groups but rarely achieve equivalent rates when language discordance is not an issue [9]. Computer technology has not quite reached the point where automated translation software (e.g., Google translate) can be used to safely communicate across

---

The Handbook of Language in Public Health and Healthcare, First Edition.
Edited by Pilar Ortega, Glenn Martínez, Maichou Lor, and A. Susana Ramírez.
© 2024 John Wiley & Sons, Inc. Published 2024 by John Wiley & Sons, Inc.

languages during a healthcare encounter [10]. As such, healthcare professionals and organizations are still required to mitigate the effects of a language-discordant encounter.

This chapter will provide a general overview of the key issues related to addressing language discordance during a healthcare encounter and how it becomes a source of structural inequities in health outcomes. It begins with an overview of the historical and legal aspects of addressing language discordance during a healthcare encounter. The succeeding sections will further review the gaps in the research literature and associated measurement challenges. The chapter concludes with several recommendations for research, education, policy, and clinical practice.

Conceptual definitions

Working to address language discordance requires operating under a common set of definitions. Refer to Squires and Youdelman (2019) for common terms used in relation to address language in healthcare [10]. These terms could be considered variables or coding terms for research purposes. It is important to remember, however, that the terms listed may have different conceptual meanings based on the context where they are used and the linguistic diversity found in a country [11, 12].

Historical overview

Global migration patterns since the early twentieth century have contributed to the current and growing demand for language access services in healthcare in many countries around the world. While war, conflict, and economic stressors have always driven human migration, people's ability to travel around the globe has facilitated it. Countries that previously had small minorities of their populations not speaking the official or dominant language of a country now find themselves with more linguistic diversity than ever before. There is also a greater sensitivity to the impact of language diversity and language discordance on individual persons, even in countries where the population may speak multiple languages.

Combined, these factors have increased demand for language access services in many countries around the world. To illustrate how policies have shifted over time in response to changing demands and an improved evidence-based around the consequences of language discordance on health, the policy responses of the United States are highlighted as a case example.

Case example: Language access policies and laws in the United States

Language access in the United States was codified as a civil right in the 1964 Civil Rights Act. The law states that every person has the legal right to have an interpreter present during any encounter where they do not speak the language [1]. In 2011, Executive Order 13166 strengthened the initial Civil Rights Act and required all federal agencies to provide "meaningful access" to language services. Meaningful access means that the services provided demonstrate a level of quality that can ensure clear and safe communication means for all persons regardless of the languages they speak. Organizations are held accountable through fines and other penalties if they fail to provide adequate access to language services [10]. These services must also be provided if organizations would like to receive federal funding to support their operations.

To regulate these practices, multiple actors are involved. The Joint Commission – the United States hospital accreditor – has identified that documenting a person's preferred language – e.g., the language in which they *prefer to communicate with healthcare providers and related personnel* – in the healthcare record (paper or electronic) as a standard and best practice for delivering quality healthcare [13]. Documenting a person's language preference also meets the requirements of the Office of Minority Health's National Standards for Culturally and Linguistically Appropriate Services (CLAS), the Centers for Medicare and Medicaid Services Meaningful Use criteria, and the Institute of Medicine's Race, Ethnicity, and Language Data: Standardization for Healthcare Quality Improvement report. Failure to document preferred language accurately is a violation of the person's civil rights [10]. Over time, as persons with limited English proficiency (LEP) exercised their civil rights and increasingly sued healthcare and other organizations for failing to provide language-appropriate care [14], more layers of accountability have emerged for healthcare organizations and providers.

In addition to the far-reaching changes to access to health insurance, the 2010 Affordable Care Act (ACA) also strengthened language access requirements in healthcare. Implemented in 2016, Section 1557 of the ACA requires every healthcare organization receiving federal funding to provide no-cost language access services implemented by qualified interpreters[1] [10]. These services, including written materials, also had to be provided in the top 15 languages in the healthcare organizations local market service area [10]. For example, if the organization does not regularly serve Vietnamese speakers, they should have access to Vietnamese interpreting services by video or phone but may not need to employ or contract with interpreters who speak the language nor provide translations of common documents. It also stipulates that computer-based interpretation modalities, e.g., where someone speaks into a smartphone and it provides a text translation, are not considered a legal substitute for interpreter services.

Another new component for language access services brought by Section 1557 was a formal assessment of language competence for healthcare providers who indicated they spoke another language. Research has found that providers' self-assessment of their language skills can differ significantly from their actual language competence [15, 16]. It has also shown that providers who speak other languages than English are often overburdened with additional interpreting tasks compared to monolingual ones [7, 17–22]. Healthcare providers, however, often have little to no training or preparation for working with interpreters [17, 23–27]. Thus, the intent of the formal assessment of language competence of the legislation was to reduce the risks associated with providers, who thought they were fluent in another language; yet, there is no minimum level of competency required in the language nor the healthcare vocabulary (known as medical language proficiency) to communicate safely and effectively during a healthcare encounter in the legislation [21]. It is also designed to encourage the appropriate use of interpreters whenever possible. Simply speaking a standard few sentences in another language is not sufficient for safe communication during a healthcare encounter. Healthcare organizations were also encouraged to designate qualified speakers on their identification badges so they could be more easily identified as assigned to work with patients who spoke the language. Table 6.1 provides an outline of activities organizations need to take to adequately address Section 1557.

Table 6.1 Recommendations for Healthcare Organizations When Implementing the United States Affordable Care Act's Section 1557.

Governance

- Conduct a needs assessment to identify target linguistic groups in your practice area.
- Develop a language access plan that ensures the needs of patients with non-English language preference are addressed and relevant policies and procedures are developed and implemented.
- Ensure meaningful participation of consumers from linguistically diverse communities (and their advocates) in governance, advisory, and oversight committees of healthcare facilities.
- Create a health inequities committee or other formal mechanisms to identify and address language and cultural needs in marketplace governance.
- Develop procedures to reassess and update the language access plan yearly.
- Designate a staff member who directly reports to the organization's director or Chief (C)-suite executives to coordinate and oversee language services.

Provision of Healthcare Services Involving Interpretation

- Utilize methods of identifying patients with non-English language preference in advance and schedule language services.
- Ensure all people providing services in a non-English language are competent. This should include language proficiency (including relevant healthcare terminology) and training. Certification for healthcare interpreters is also available.
- Prohibit individuals who have not demonstrated sufficient language proficiency and the knowledge, skills, and abilities required of interpreters or translators from interpreting or translating in an "ad hoc" manner.

Notices and Information for Consumers

- Translate documents, notices, and wayfinding signs into the most common languages in your state.
- Include taglines in the top 15 languages in your state or healthcare service area on all significant patient documents to inform consumers with non-English language preference about the availability of written translations, oral language services, and in-person assistance.

Website

- Include taglines or a language portal on the homepage of the marketplace website with information in the top 15 languages in your state or healthcare service area to inform patients with non-English language preference about the availability of written translations, oral language services, and in-person assistance.
- Consider translating the website in whole or in part for frequently encountered languages.
- Provide a prominent link from the homepage of the website to a directory of in-person and consumer assistance programs that allow patients to request language services or make an appointment with a bilingual/bicultural provider.

- Provide training on assessing language needs, securing interpreter services, and working with interpreters for all of the entity's staff.
- Develop formal mechanisms to collect feedback from consumers with non-English language preference and solicit input from navigator and consumer assistance programs to help identify and address problems.
- Collect and publicly report institutional data, including the numbers of interactions with consumers with non-English language preference, languages spoken, and the use of language services.

Telephonic and Answering Systems
- Ensure any voicemail system or answering system has information readily available for consumers with non-English language preference. This could include having competent, bilingual consumer service representatives in frequently encountered languages and providing access to competent oral interpreters at all times.
- Provide training to call center representatives on responding appropriately to callers with non-English language preference, how to access bilingual staff or interpreters, and procedures for referring consumers to in-person enrollment assistance and consumer assistance programs.
- If using an automated telephone system, include voice prompts in multiple languages that provide access to bilingual representatives or interpreter services or have direct telephone lines for in-language assistance.
- Collect and publicly report call center data, including the number of calls by consumers with non-English language preference, languages spoken, and the use of language services.

Outreach and Education
- Develop culturally appropriate outreach and education plans that are tailored to populations with non-English language preference, particularly those experiencing health disparities.
- Engage trusted messengers and community-based organizations that work with populations with non-English language preference in developing and implementing outreach plans.

Source: Adapted from Squires & Youdleman [10].

This case example from the United States highlights one way a centralized national strategy to reduce inequities in health outcomes associated with language barriers. The goal is to reduce the common sources of structural inequities found in healthcare delivery that fail to account for the linguistic diversity of the population. Given that most health systems have similar ways of organizing care delivery, these structural inequities are likely to be quite common across countries.

Critical issues related to addressing language discordance

To reduce the aforementioned disparities in health outcomes for people with language preferences that differ from the dominant language, there are several key issues that are related to research, practice, and workforce preparation that require more attention from funders, practitioners, educators, and policymakers. Few studies, for example, have captured the patient perspective of how language concordance improves the care experience. Most studies focus on the clinician or interpreter perspectives. This section provides an overview of several of these issues.

The labor market of healthcare interpreters

Interpreters in healthcare, including the languages they are qualified to interpret in, are poorly tracked as a distinct labor group in most countries. Economic data are inconsistently tracked for this worker cadre, if noted at all in national labor statistics. Wages for healthcare interpreters vary extensively. Paradoxically, languages in high demand do not always translate into higher wages. Practice context is also important as local, regional, state, provincial, and other regulatory elements may influence wages. For example, if insurance reimburses for interpreter services, having a reliable interpreter workforce in healthcare is easier to sustain. When there is no insurance reimbursement, services are outsourced at higher rates and interpreter wages will depend on the contracted rates between the healthcare organization and the external interpreter services.

Healthcare interpreters and their regulation and training

In most countries, the healthcare interpreting industry – e.g., those who provide telephone and video interpreting services to healthcare organizations – is not regulated by a minimum set of language competence standards for employing interpreters. In the majority of circumstances, a healthcare interpreter needs to have a high school education or equivalent number of years of schooling along with training to work as an interpreter. When hiring interpreters to work in healthcare settings, the credentials and resume evaluation falls on the agency hiring the interpreter. Interpreters are hired to work in healthcare in one of two ways: (a) as contractors employed by an agency or (b) as a direct employee of the facility when the demand for a specific language is sufficiently high that it is less expensive to hire someone full time than to contract them through an agency. The hiring agent has legal responsibility for the performance of the interpreter. The quality of interpreter performance depends on feedback received during annual performance reviews if hired by a healthcare organization. If the interpreter is employed by an agency, performance evaluation is based on feedback received from the healthcare organizations where the interpreter has provided services. Performance concerns about interpreters hired by agencies, however, are often not communicated by healthcare providers because reporting mechanisms are not often convenient.

Many countries around the world are grappling with similar challenges associated with healthcare interpreter regulation and training. The United States presents an interesting case study in terms of healthcare interpreters' regulation and training. First, there are no national standards for training healthcare interpreters nor are they licensed [28]. There is also no minimum level of education to become a healthcare interpreter. Nonetheless, with regard to healthcare interpreter training, the National Council for Interpreting in Healthcare (NCIHC), the national professional organization for interpreters working in healthcare, and the Certification Commission for Healthcare Interpreters (CCHI), the organization that administers the certification exam, both recommend that individuals undergoing healthcare interpreting training receive no less than 40 hours of formal training that includes in-person interpreting practice. The preference of these groups, however, is that interpreters seeking to work in healthcare settings undergo no less than 100 hours of formal training. They have yet to make a policy statement about industry regulation. Nonetheless, there is a nascent national movement in the United States toward educational standardization for healthcare interpreters. The challenge at present, however, is that the lack of standardization in educational preparation of healthcare interpreters can pose risks to patient safety.

Poor quality interpretation poses threats to patient safety

Even though many healthcare organizations now require interpreters to have a healthcare interpreting credential, this requirement is inconsistently implemented. Inconsistent language access services implementation in addition to the quality of interpreting experienced by patients and healthcare professionals in language-discordant situations may be contributing to health and healthcare outcome disparities for linguistically diverse communities.

Two decades of research have captured how language discordance and poor-quality interpretation affect patient safety across healthcare settings. The greatest risks come from using ad hoc interpreters – defined as those with no formal training in medical interpretation. These individuals lack the vocabulary needed to perform interpretation accurately and of good quality [29–33]. Beyond the risk for errors in care due to this lack of vocabulary, poor-quality interpretation can lead to higher risks for adverse events experienced by hospitalized persons with non-English language preference, longer lengths of stay due to communication issues, and higher risks for 30-day readmission to the hospital [34–36]. Incorrect patient education could also occur when interpretation is of poor quality and thus increase threats to safety.

A lack of data about language capacity in health professions

The United States and most countries do not consistently track the language skills and proficiency levels of healthcare professionals and the interpreters with whom they work. Most often, employers track these data based on self-report and it may or may not include a formal assessment. Organizational-level statistics are also not publicly available, so it is difficult to know exactly how many healthcare professionals speak other languages. Without this data, policymakers cannot determine where to direct resources for capacity building. Moreover, without the data, educators cannot develop ways to recruit more individuals with needed language skills into the health professions nor can educational institutions justify investing in developing curricula that can build language capacity among existing students.

To understand the scope and deficits in language capacity among healthcare professionals, capturing data about this skill in the workforce is essential. The easiest point to capture these data is during professional or occupational license or credentialing, either initial or during renewals. Sample questions that could be asked on the licensure or credentialing application are:

- Do you speak another language?
    - If yes, which language: [Select from a list of all languages or the 15 most common spoken locally]
    - Please rate yourself on how well you:
        - Speak: Not at all; not very well; well; very well
        - Read: Not at all; not very well; well; very well
        - Understand: Not at all; not very well; well; very well
        - Write: Not at all; not very well; well; very well
- Did you grow up speaking a language other than English [or the country's dominant language] at home? [Yes, No]

Licensure or credentialing bodies could also ask candidates who answer "Yes" if they would like to have a formal language skills assessment. The results of their assessment could be included in their licensure documents. That would also make recruitment of healthcare professionals with language skills easier for employers.

Documentation of language-related data in the electronic health record

Documentation of a person's preferred language in the medical record is poor although some organizations are making improvements. Researchers, practitioners, and policymakers thought that the use of electronic health records would improve the capture of these data, but that has yet to prove true [37–40]. The two most common issues are (a) the complete absence of language preference information or (b) the "dominant" language is documented as the preference even if the person only speaks a few sentences of the locally dominant language. Because the documentation of a patient's preferred language is generally of such poor quality, it is difficult to conduct patient outcomes analyses with sample sizes that are large enough to be sufficiently powered for the complex statistical analyses required to capture the extent of health outcome disparities in linguistically diverse populations [41–43]. These gaps also mean that healthcare organizations are likely underestimating demands for language access services due to incomplete data.

Documentation of interpreter use in the electronic health record depends entirely on the healthcare organization making it easy for providers to do so [37–40]. Interpreters should also be able to document their encounters in the patient's record. Implementation of these practices in the system requires those working with the documentation system and the information technology department coming together to determine how to facilitate documentation. Said features, however, are inconsistently implemented at present but have potential to improve over time.

Language access services implementation as a source of structural inequities in healthcare: The need for a common set of measures

Sources of structural inequities in healthcare are systems and processes built into the delivery of healthcare that contribute to inequitable health outcomes once controlling for other potential confounders [44–47]. The dearth of implementation research about language access services means there is not a common set of quality measures to gauge their impact on addressing structural inequities nor how much can be attributed to them. Consensus on a common set of structural measures that can reliably and validly evaluate language access services implementation by the multiple actors involved is needed.

Researchers lack training in cross-language research methods

Language differences across human subjects can pose significant threats to the rigor of research studies [48]. Yet, most researchers do not receive training on addressing language discordance when they are learning how to design studies involving populations with nondominant language preferences. The threats to rigor are also different for qualitative and quantitative studies [48]. The following paragraphs highlight the key language-related methodological threats to rigor in research studies.

In qualitative research, the first threat to rigor centers on who will conduct the interpreting and translation activities. It is common for qualitative studies to not describe how interpreters were used in the study [49–51]. Failure to describe their roles means the quality of the qualitative data and subsequent analysis could pose a threat to the rigor of the research. Researchers may also rely on untrained graduate students to conduct interpreting and translation in research [48, 51, 52]. Even if the student is a native speaker, the principal investigator still needs to provide training to the student on best practices for interpreting and translation to address the threat to rigor. As described above, interpretation and translation are highly skilled activities that require formal training to be done well and with quality. When designing research studies, consulting with local interpretation service providers or subject matter experts will help ensure quality training. Since there is usually insufficient word count in peer-reviewed publications to describe how interpreters were trained, a brief descriptor of the identity of the interpreter's qualifications will help evaluate a study's rigor and the potential threat to rigor that translation/interpretation may have posed.

The second threat to rigor is the timing of interpreting and translation activities [51]. Will data collection occur in the same language of the participant or will an interpreter be used? How many team members are genuinely proficient in the study's language(s) if they differ from that of the principal investigator? Will data analysis occur in the participant's language or the researcher's? These are key study implementation considerations when implementing research. The timing of translation matters, therefore, when conducting a research study and should be explicitly detailed in research publications involving its use.

For quantitative studies, threats to the rigor of research can occur at several points in the research process. These include the translation of the instrument, the data collection process, and analysis of data.

First, survey instrument translation is not simply a matter of forward and backward translation; it requires a much more rigorous process to ensure a reliable and valid translation [48, 52]. Content validation, cognitive interviewing, and psychometric analyses of translated instruments ensure the best quality translations of survey instruments.

A second threat to research rigor comes from existing translations of survey instruments. Many have rarely had reliability and validity studies completed and also have poor quality translations, making them inadequate measures for the targeted populations. Researchers often assume that if an instrument's translation was published in a journal, it was an official translation, yet that may not be the case. For many instruments, evaluating the translation prior to including it in a study would be a useful step. This is also important for languages where there are country level variations or dialects that may substantively alter the meaning of words, e.g., Spanish, Arabic, and Russian.

When collecting survey data, ideally it occurs with a reliable and valid translation of the instrument. Nonetheless, for some languages, there are no written versions or the researcher may be working with populations with limited literacy in their language. In this case, it may require live interpretation as part of the data collection process. Researchers should work with the interpreters to determine a standardized interpretation process when collecting data to ensure the conceptual, content, semantic, and technical meanings of the words in the instrument are translated as closely as possible. The research team should also ensure that the words in the instrument have a conceptual equivalent in the language. In health research, for some diseases or conditions – mental health is a good example – there may not be words for the condition itself but the symptoms of it may translate. This is why a standardized translation plan for data collection is necessary.

Finally, some survey instruments contain open-ended questions at the end. Participants will respond in their preferred language. For studies involving a data collector, the research team needs to decide if they will either (a) write down an interpreted version of the participants' answers or (b) capture the response in the participants' language. The latter approach will present limitations for data quality that researchers will need to consider for their analytic plan and report in the limitations sections of their studies. The team should also plan in advance if data will be analyzed in the language of the participants or when translation will occur. These details should be made explicit in the methods section of the paper.

These exemplars highlight only a few issues that could arise when conducting research in healthcare when an interpreter is needed. They are highlighted to reinforce the importance of good quality interpretation and translation practices when creating the evidence-based that clinicians use to guide their work. A poor-quality evidence-based does not help to address outcome inequities in linguistically diverse groups. Overall, for the conduct of research involving translation and/or interpretation of languages, rigor is most easily evaluated through transparent reporting of how the translation process was managed as part of the methods.

Recommendations for research, education, practice, and policy

From each of the issues identified above, the following steps are recommended to address identified gaps in research, health professions education, and practice.

Research

- Increase the number of studies documenting the impact of language concordance, language discordance, and language-appropriate care on patient outcomes.
  - Improved data capture in electronic health records will make these studies easier to complete.

- Increase the diversity of languages studied when examining patient outcomes.
  - Most studies in the United States are of Spanish speakers and those of Mexican heritage. People who speak other languages, especially non-European ones, are understudied in general and are not well-represented in the research literature. These gaps in the evidence leave some groups under-represented and contribute to health outcome inequities.
- Capture the experiences of patients seeking healthcare in their preferred language.

Education

- Increase the number of people entering healthcare professions who are proficient in multiple languages.
- Invest in medical language education and assessment for health professionals in training who wish to improve and evaluate their skills in languages beyond the dominant language.
- Integrate working with interpreters into health professions education. Simulation-based education approaches are optimal for creating "real world" scenarios.
  - See Latimer et al. for an example of how to integrate interpreters into simulation-based education [27]. Simulation does not need to be high-fidelity to be effective.

Practice

- Conduct documentation quality checks of electronic health records to ensure that language preferences are being consistently recorded as well as healthcare interpreter use.
- Interpreters should be able to document their work with patients in the health record, including the electronic one.
- Consistently document a person's language preference in the healthcare record.
- Provide healthcare professionals with training in working effectively with professional interpreters and avoidance of ad hoc interpreter use.
- Use interpreters appropriately during healthcare encounters and document their use in the electronic health record.

Policy

- Collect data regarding self-reported language skills on occupational licensure or credentialing materials for health professionals.
- If formal language assessments were completed by the healthcare professional or interpreter, include those on licensure or credentialing documentation.

Conclusion

Language access is a structural factor in the delivery of healthcare. When healthcare organizations fail to provide adequate language access services, they create a source of structural inequities that contribute to health outcome inequities among those who do not speak the dominant language of a country. Said implementation failures become costly for everyone involved, but the greatest burden of the costs rests with the individual.

The structural factors in care delivery identified in this chapter can be common across countries. It is important to be mindful of the international variations in these variables, however, because resources to bridge language differences, cultural sensitivity to their significance, and the human resources capacity to maximize language access will vary widely. By addressing the structural challenges to providing language-appropriate healthcare services, clinicians, educators, and institutions can take meaningful steps to improving health equity for linguistically diverse populations.

Highlights

- Global migration patterns contribute to the growing demand for language access services in healthcare, resulting in policy change around the world.
- In the United States, ACA Section 1577 is an example of centralized national strategies that aim to reduce inequities in health outcomes associated with language discordance.
- There are several critical issues that must be considered to properly address language discordance. These issues include the varied labor market, mixed regulation and training for healthcare interpreters, inadequate documentation of language-related data in electronic health records, and lack of researcher training in crosslinguistic research methods.
- Language access service implementation is a source of structural inequities in healthcare; to resolve existing inequities, common sets of measures for evaluation need to be established.

NOTE

1 Qualified interpreters in healthcare have had specialized training in medical vocabulary and understanding care delivery. While training is not standardized in the United States, the National Council for Interpreting in Healthcare recommends that healthcare interpreters need a minimum of 40 hours of specialized training. Certification as a healthcare interpreter remains voluntary at the time of this printing.

REFERENCES

1. *Commonly Asked Questions.* http://LEP.gov, https://www.lep.gov/commonly-asked-questions (accessed 13 January 2022).
2. Rocque, R. and Leanza, Y. (2015). A systematic review of patients' experiences in communicating with primary care physicians: intercultural encounters and a balance between vulnerability and integrity. *PloS One* 10: e0139577.
3. Oh, H., Trinh, M.P., Vang, C. et al. (2020). Addressing barriers to primary care access for latinos in the U.S.: an agent-based model. *J. Soc. Soc. Work Res.* 11: 2334–2315.
4. Yu, M., Kelley, A.T., Morgan, A.U. et al. (2020). Challenges for adult undocumented immigrants in accessing primary care: a qualitative study of health care workers in Los Angeles County. *Health Equity* 4: 366–374.

5. Rawal, S., Srighanthan, J., Vasantharoopan, A. et al. (2019). Association between limited English proficiency and revisits and readmissions after hospitalization for patients with acute and chronic conditions in Toronto, Ontario, Canada. *JAMA* 322: 1605.
6. Anderson, T.S., Karliner, L.S., and Lin, G.A. (2020). Association of primary language and hospitalization for ambulatory care sensitive conditions. *Med. Care* 58: 45–51.
7. Narayan, M.C. and Scafide, K.N. (2017). Systematic review of racial/ethnic outcome disparities in home health care. *J. Transcult. Nurs.* 28: 598–607.
8. Squires, A., Ma, C., Miner, S. et al. (2022). Assessing the influence of patient language preference on 30 day hospital readmission risk from home health care: a retrospective analysis. *Int. J. Nurs. Stud.* 125: 104093.
9. Flores, G. (2005). The impact of medical interpreter services on the quality of health care: a systematic review. *Med. Care Res. Rev.* 62: 255–299.
10. Squires, A. and Youdelman, M. (2019). Section 1557 of the affordable care act: strengthening language access rights for patients with limited English proficiency. *J. Nurs. Regul.* 10: 65–67.
11. Hsieh, E. (2018). Reconceptulizing language discordance: meanings and experiences of language barriers in the U.S. and Taiwan. *J. Immigr. Minor. Health* 20: 1–4.
12. Terui, S. (2017). Conceptualizing the pathways and processes between language barriers and health disparities: review, synthesis, and extension. *J. Immigr. Minor. Health* 19: 215–224.
13. Medical Record—Preferred Language. Hospital and Hospital Clinics. Record of Care Treatment and Services RC. The Joint Commission, https://www.jointcommission.org/standards/standard-faqs/hospital-and-hospital-clinics/record-of-care-treatment-and-services-rc/000001373 (accessed 16 January 2022).
14. CyraCom International, Inc. *The First Section 1557 Language Access Lawsuit Has Arrived*. https://blog.cyracom.com/ciiblog/the-first-section-1557-language-access-lawsuit-has-arrived (2022), (accessed 13 January 2022).
15. Diamond, L., Chung, S., Ferguson, W. et al. (2014). Relationship between self-assessed and tested non-English-language proficiency among primary care providers. *Med. Care* 52: 435–438.
16. Diamond, L.C., Schenker, Y., Curry, L. et al. (2009). Getting by: underuse of interpreters by resident physicians. *J. Gen. Intern. Med.* 24: 256–262.
17. Jacobs, E.A., Diamond, L.C., and Stevak, L. (2010). The importance of teaching clinicians when and how to work with interpreters. *Patient Educ. Couns.* 78: 149–153.
18. Gerchow, L., Burka, L.R., Miner, S. et al. (2021). Language barriers between nurses and patients: a scoping review. *Patient Educ. Couns.* 104: 534–553.
19. Kirby, J.B., Berdahl, T.A., and Torres Stone, R.A. (2021). Perceptions of patient-provider communication across the six largest Asian subgroups in the USA. *J. Gen. Intern. Med.* 36: 888–893.
20. Dilworth, T.J., Mott, D., and Young, H. (2009). Pharmacists' communication with Spanish-speaking patients: a review of the literature to establish an agenda for future research. *Res. Social Adm. Pharm.* 5: 108–120.
21. Hull, M. (2016). Medical language proficiency: a discussion of interprofessional language competencies and potential for patient risk. *Int. J. Nurs. Stud.* 54: 158–172.
22. Chang, H., Hutchinson, C., and Gullick, J. (2021). Pulled away: the experience of bilingual nurses as ad hoc interpreters in the emergency department. *Ethn. Health* 26: 1045–1064.
23. Hsieh, E. (2015). Not just "getting by": factors influencing providers' choice of interpreters. *J. Gen. Intern. Med.* 30: 75–82.
24. Hsieh, E. (2006). Understanding medical interpreters: reconceptualizing bilingual health communication. *Health Commun.* 20: 177–186.
25. Hsieh, E. and Kramer, E.M. (2012). Medical interpreters as tools: dangers and challenges in the utilitarian approach to interpreters' roles and functions. *Patient Educ. Couns.* 89: 158–162.

26. Hsieh, E. (2010). Provider-interpreter collaboration in bilingual health care: competitions of control over interpreter-mediated interactions. *Patient Educ. Couns.* 78: 154–159.
27. Latimer, B., Robertiello, G., and Squires, A. (2019). Integrating health care interpreters into simulation education. *Clin. Simul. Nurs.* 32: 20–26.
28. NCIHC. *National Council on Interpreting in Health Care – Language Access Resources*, https://www.ncihc.org/home (2022), (accessed 13 January 2022).
29. Kwok, M.M.K., Chan, R.K., Hansen, C. et al. (2021). Access to translator (AT&T) project: interpreter on wheels during the COVID-19 pandemic. *BMJ Open Qual.* 10: 1062. https://doi.org/10.1136/bmjoq-2020-001062. PMID: 33547156.
30. Boylen, S., Cherian, S., Gill, F.J. et al. (2020). Impact of professional interpreters on outcomes for hospitalized children from migrant and refugee families with limited English proficiency: a systematic review. *JBI Evid. Synth.* 18: 1360–1388. https://doi.org/10.11124/JBISRIR-D-19-00300. PMID: 32813387.
31. Nápoles, A.M., Santoyo-Olsson, J., Karliner, L.S. et al. (2015). Inaccurate language interpretation and its clinical significance in the medical encounters of Spanish-speaking Latinos. *Med. Care* 53 (11): 940–947. https://doi.org/10.1097/MLR.0000000000000422. PMCID: PMC4610127.
32. VanderWielen, L.M., Enurah, A.S., Rho, H.Y. et al. (2014). Medical interpreters: improvements to address access, equity, and quality of care for limited-English-proficient patients. *Acad. Med.* 89 (10): 1324–1327. http://content.wkhealth.com/linkback/openurl?sid=WKPTLP:landingpage&an=00001888-201410000-00011. PMID: 25054413.
33. Nápoles, A.M., Santoyo-Olsson, J., Karliner, L.S. et al. (2010). Clinician ratings of interpreter mediated visits in underserved primary care settings with ad hoc, in-person professional, and video conferencing modes. *J. Health Care Poor Underserved* 21 (1): 301–317. https://doi.org/10.1353/hpu.0.0269. PMCID: PMC3576468.
34. van Rosse, F., de Bruijne, M., Suurmond, J. et al. (2016). Language barriers and patient safety risks in hospital care. A mixed methods study. *Int. J. Nurs. Stud.* 54: 45–53.
35. Taira, B.R., Kim, K., and Mody, N. (2019). Hospital and health system–level interventions to improve care for limited English proficiency patients: A systematic review. *Jt. Comm. J. Qual. Patient Saf.* 45: 446–458.
36. Betancourt, J.R., Renfrew, M.R., Green, A.R. et al. (2012). *Improving Patient Safety Systems for Patients with Limited English Proficiency: A Guide for Hospitals*. Rockville, MD: Agency for Healthcare Research and Quality.
37. Rodriguez, J.A., Fossa, A., Mishuris, R., and Herrick, B. (2021). Bridging the language gap in patient portals: an evaluation of google translate. *J. Gen. Intern. Med.* 36 (2): 567–569. https://doi.org/10.1007/s11606-020-05719-z. PMCID: PMC7878638.
38. Lyles, C.R., Fruchterman, J., Youdelman, M., and Schillinger, D. (2017). Legal, practical, and ethical considerations for making online patient portals accessible for all. *Am. J. Public Health* 107 (10): 1608–1611. https://doi.org/10.2105/AJPH.2017.303933. PMCID: PMC5607665.
39. Ochoa, A., Kitayama, K., Uijtdehaage, S. et al. (2017). Patient and provider perspectives on the potential value and use of a bilingual online patient portal in a Spanish-speaking safety-net population. *J. Am. Med. Inform. Assoc.* 24: 1160–1164. https://doi.org/10.1093/jamia/ocx040. PMID: 28460130.
40. Casillas A, Abhat A, Vassar SD, Huang DYC, Mahajan AP, Simmons S, Lyles C, Portz J, Moreno G, Brown AF. Not speaking the same language-lower portal use for limited English proficient patients in the Los Angeles safety net. *J. Health Care Poor Underserved*. 2021;32:2055–2070. doi:https://doi.org/10.1353/hpu.2021.0182 https://muse.jhu.edu/article/837336
41. Peterson, P.N., Campagna, E.J., Maravi, M. et al. (2012). Acculturation and outcomes among patients with heart failure. *Circ. Heart Fail.* 5: 160–166.

42. Meuter, R.F.I., Gallois, C., Segalowitz, N.S. et al. (2015). Overcoming language barriers in healthcare: a protocol for investigating safe and effective communication when patients or clinicians use a second language. *BMC Health Serv. Res.* 15: 371.
43. Aspinall, P.J. (2007). Language ability: a neglected dimension in the profiling of populations and health service users. *Health Educ. J.* 66: 90–106.
44. Essex, R., Markowski, M., and Miller, D. Structural injustice and dismantling racism in health and healthcare. *Nurs. Inq.* 29: e12441. Epub ahead of print 2021. DOI: https://doi.org/10.1111/NIN.12441.
45. Liu, S.Y., Fiorentini, C., Bailey, Z. et al. (2019). Structural racism and severe maternal morbidity in New York state. *Clin. Med. Insights Womens Health* 12: https://doi.org/10.1177/1179562X19854778.
46. Gee, G.C. and Hicken, M.T. (2021). Commentary-structural racism: the rules and relations of inequity. *Ethn. Dis.* 31: 293–300.
47. Bailey, Z.D., Krieger, N., Agénor, M. et al. (2017). Structural racism and health inequities in the USA: evidence and interventions. *Lancet* 389: 1453–1463.
48. Squires, A., Sadarangani, T., and Jones, S. (2020). Strategies for overcoming language barriers in research. *J. Adv. Nurs.* 76: 706–714.
49. Squires, A. (2009). Methodological challenges in cross-language qualitative research: a research review. *Int. J. Nurs. Stud.* 46 (2): 277–287. http://www.pubmedcentral.nih.gov/articlerender.fcgi?artid=2784094&tool=pmcentrez&rendertype=abstract. PMID: 18789799.
50. Croot, E.J., Lees, J., Grant, G. et al. (2011). Evaluating standards in cross-language research: a critique of Squires' criteria. *Int. J. Nurs. Stud.* 48 (8): 1002–1011. http://linkinghub.elsevier.com/retrieve/pii/S0020748911001830.
51. Squires, A. (2008). Language barriers and qualitative nursing research: methodological considerations. *Int. Nurs. Rev.* 55 (3): 265–273. http://www.pubmedcentral.nih.gov/articlerender.fcgi?artid=2697452&tool=pmcentrez&rendertype=abstract. PMID: 19522941.
52. Maneesriwongul, W. and Dixon, J.K. (2004). Instrument translation process: a methods review. *J. Adv. Nurs.* 48: 175–186.

7 The Role of Healthcare Interpreters

ELAINE HSIEH

Introduction

Whereas translators transfer information of written texts from one language to another, interpreters relay verbal messages between different interlocutors who do not share the same language. As such, interpreters' roles and functions in interpersonal, dynamic interactions have been studied extensively in the last 40 years [1], facilitating the paradigm shift from a blind preference for the interpreter-as-conduit model in healthcare settings to the recognition of interpreters as active participants in provider-patient interactions [2]. In this chapter, I use providers to refer to all healthcare clinicians, including physicians, nurses, therapists, and other health professionals who interact with patients directly.

The conduit model (i.e., interpreters as passive conduits who transfer information from one language to another) has been influential in shaping the early development of healthcare interpreting, conceptualizing interpreters as invisible linguistic machines that transfer information from one language to another. Interpreters are trained to adopt a neutral, faithful, and non-interfering presence in medical encounters. Various professional standards also view interpreter-as-conduit as the default role, reflecting institutional efforts to minimize interpreters' control and influence over medical encounters [3]. However, due to the differences in provider-patient health literacy, communicative norms, and illness ideologies, a conduit role can reinforce the power hierarchy, social injustice, and miscommunication in cross-cultural healthcare [3, 4].

Many researchers and interpreters, thus, have argued that a conduit-only model is unrealistic and impractical in healthcare settings [2]. By noting a continuum of roles enacted by healthcare interpreters in practice, from the passive conduit role to active advocacy roles, researchers found that interpreters strategically shift between various levels of visibilities to ensure the quality of care and to facilitate other speakers' identity performances, communicative competence, and communicative goals [5, 6].

In this chapter, I will first explore how interpreter roles are conceptualized and investigated in the literature, exploring the functions and impacts of such role performances. By recognizing the strengths and limitations of various typologies of interpreter roles, I will then examine an alternative approach to conceptualizing different types of

---

The Handbook of Language in Public Health and Healthcare, First Edition.
Edited by Pilar Ortega, Glenn Martínez, Maichou Lor, and A. Susana Ramírez.
© 2024 John Wiley & Sons, Inc. Published 2024 by John Wiley & Sons, Inc.

interpreters. Using the typology of interpreter types proposed by the Model of Bilingual Health Communication (BHC) model [3], I will examine how interpreters' professionalism and social positioning in healthcare settings can shape the process, outcome, and quality of cross-cultural care [7].

Historical development and moving beyond interpreter roles

Early typologies of interpreter roles are often proposed by researchers and training programs in a top-down manner [8]. For example, the Cross Cultural Health Care Program (CCHCP), one of the first and leading training programs for healthcare interpreters, proposed four interpreter roles [9]. A *conduit* is the default role and involves rendering in one language literally what has been said in the other without any additions, omissions, editing, or polishing. A *clarifier* is a role interpreters assume when they adjust speakers' register, interject their explanations, describe terms that have no linguistic equivalent, or check for understanding when necessary. A *cultural broker* provides a necessary cultural framework for understanding the message being interpreted. An *advocate* works on behalf of the patient outside the bounds of an interpreted interview, ensuring the patients' quality of care in addition to quality of communication. The CCHCP training program suggests, "the 'appropriate' role for the interpreter is the least invasive role that will assure effective communication and care" [10]. However, in practice, interpreters do not always actively move between these roles due to various concerns and institutional constraints [11].

Starting from the early 2000s, researchers increasingly abandoned a top-down approach and relied on empirical data (e.g., interviews and surveys with providers, patients, and interpreters) to explore interpreter roles [5]. Some researchers focused on elaborating the complexities of a specific role (e.g., mediator and co-diagnostician) [12, 13]. Others aimed to present comprehensive typologies of interpreter roles [6, 14, 15]. While some roles (e.g., conduit and cultural broker) are primarily enacted during the medical encounters, others (e.g., patient advocate and system agent) may be adopted both inside and outside of medical appointments. Some of the roles (e.g., institutional gatekeeper and co-diagnostician) also appear to adopt organizational goals in monitoring resource utilization and institutional ethics. Based on a meta-ethnographic analysis of 61 studies on interpreter roles, Brisset and colleagues concluded that all interpreter roles fit into a continuum in which "interpreters oscillate between the Lifeworld and the System" (see Table 7.1) [5].

Although there appear to be some overlapping roles (e.g., voice box, black box, linguistic agent, and conduit) across various studies, each typology represents a unique perspective in conceptualizing healthcare interpreters' roles and functions. For example, Leanza created a typology grounded in *interpreters' management of cultural differences* between the patient and the provider [16]. An interpreter who adopts the *system agent* role is likely to ignore cultural differences between the provider and the patient by actively overlooking the patients' cultural needs and working in favor of providers' cultural expectations. An interpreter who acts as an *integration agent* would actively locate resources to facilitate migrants to make sense of and negotiate meanings as well as an "in-between" way of behaving. On the other hand, Hsieh's typology was based on interpreters' self-perceived roles by identifying the *communicative goals and strategies* that are associated with specific role performances [11]. For example, when adopting the role

Table 7.1 Typologies of Interpreter Roles in Lifeworld-System Continuum.

Kaufert (1984/1999)	Language interpreter	Informant			
		Culture broker			
			Advocate		
Drennan & Swartz (2002)	Language specialist	Institutional therapist			
		Culture specialist			
			Patient advocate		
Hatton & Webb (1993)	Voice box	Collaborator			
			Excluder		
Davidson (2001)		Covert co-diagnostician			
		Institutional gatekeeper			
Miller (2005)	Black box	Therapy conduit			
Leanza (2005)	Linguistic agent	System agent		Lifeworld agent	Integration agent
Hsieh (2008)	Conduit	Professional	Manager	Advocate	
		← System		Lifeworld →	

Source: Brisset et al. [5]/With permission of Elsevier.

of *conduit*, an interpreter's goals include transferring complete information and reinforcing the provider-patient relationship. When assuming the role of *manager*, an interpreter's goals are to conserve medical resources, regulate appropriate and ethical performances (of others), and manage the optimal exchange of information. In short, despite similar roles identified, different typologies highlight distinctive perspectives and approaches to the understanding of interpreter roles and their management of interactional dynamics.

The investigation of interpreter roles has provided valuable momentum to the theoretical development of interpreter-mediated medical encounters. Based on Goffman's work, role as a theoretical concept allows researchers to examine how by assuming certain roles, individuals can define and control the contexts, the interactional frame, and the performances of others [17, 18]. In other words, interpreter roles highlight the issues of *contexts* and *others*. By conceptualizing interpreter performances as role performances, researchers can expand the scope of analysis to "the dynamics of interpreter-mediated interactions" [19] and the "different interrelated relational issues" associated with roles [5]. With role, there are specific expectations, perceptions, and actions that are implied (in the normative model), which is what allows the participants (i.e., providers, patients, and interpreters) to perform in the frame. From this perspective, understanding interpreter performances through interpreter roles allow researchers to discuss these aspects of a frame (e.g., the coordination of tasks, identities, and relationships), examine how interpreters use their roles to define contexts and impose control over others' performances [20]. By strategically constructing their relationships with others, interpreters not only define the communicative contexts but also shape the appropriate behaviors and role performances for others.

More importantly, role allows researchers to examine *other participants'* performance. This is because all participants in medical encounters are involved in the negotiation of role performance and interactional frame. As such, an interpreter may face specific pressure due to the roles projected and frames constructed by other speakers (e.g., two providers arguing about patient diagnosis in front of a patient while assuming that the interpreter would not relay their arguments to the patient projects) [21–23]. In addition, role is not static. As such, providers, patients, and interpreters often challenge each other's role performances and negotiate to achieve a mutually agreeable frame [17, 20, 21, 24, 25]. By conceptualizing interpreter performances as roles, interpreters are viewed as performers, and roles are dynamically and emergently co-constructed between the participants of the frame/event. The success of healthcare delivery is dependent on all participants' ability to identify and negotiate their goals and expectations [3].

In summary, as researchers have examined interpreters' role performances, their scope of analysis has expanded significantly as communicative contexts and other speakers' performances come into play. Rather than viewing the interpreter as the central *and* only person who is responsible for the quality of interpreter-mediated interactions, this new theoretical expansion recognizes all participants can actively influence the content and process of communication. A successful interpreter-mediated medical encounter is a collaborative achievement among all participants.

Finally, as studies identifying interpreters' roles proliferated, the literature is now saturated with typologies of interpreter roles. The efforts to develop a unified, comprehensive list of interpreter roles are likely to be unfruitful, if not impractical. This is because depending on the researchers' specific conceptual framework, theoretical perspectives, and clinical contexts, interpreter roles can entail and/or highlight different aspects of their unique functions. More importantly, interpreters' role performances are strategic actions that aim to address dynamic interactional challenges that emerge in cross-cultural, provider-patient interactions. As a result, interpreter roles do not conform to a restricted or prescribed list of role performances but are creative solutions that tackle contextual, situational challenges in a particular provider-patient interaction. Thus, recent research trends have shifted away from identifying interpreters' roles or generating new typologies. Increasingly, researchers have argued that we should explore other contextual variables that may be essential in guiding healthcare providers and anticipating interpreters' performances in interpreter-mediated medical encounters.

The Model of Bilingual Health Communication and the diversity of healthcare interpreters

The BHC model is a communicative model that explains how interpersonal dynamics can shape the process and content of interpreter-mediated interactions in cross-cultural care [3]. The BHC model views interpreter-mediated interactions as a socially constructed, goal-driven communicative activity that requires multi-party coordination on the meanings and processes of healthcare delivery. In addition, by recognizing that experiences of language barriers are contextually situated [26], the BHC model argues that healthcare providers and researchers must consider the distinctive impacts and relationships when working with different types of interpreters in healthcare settings.

Because there is a wide range of interpreters, with varying levels of language proficiency, clinical expertise, and cultural/patient familiarity, in healthcare settings, the BHC model argues that the quality of care is best protected when providers can effectively work with different types of interpreters, understand their strengths and limitations, and monitor the effectiveness and appropriateness of interpreter-mediated

Table 7.2 Comparisons Between Different Types of Interpreters.

	Type	Availability	Professionalism	Comfort to Patient	Interpreting Quality
Professionals interpreters	In-person interpreters	Varied	High	Moderate-high	High
	Technology-based Interpreters	High	Moderate-high	Moderate-high	Moderate-high
Bilingual medical professionals	Bilingual providers	Low	N/a	Moderate-high	Varied
	Bilingual medical staff	Varied	Low-moderate	Low-moderate	Varied
Nonprofessional interpreters	Chance interpreters	Moderate	Low	Low	Low
	Family interpreters	Moderate-high	Low	Moderate-high	Varied

Source: Hsieh [3]/Taylor & Francis.

interactions. The BHC model proposed three major categories of interpreters (i.e., professional interpreters, bilingual medical professionals, and nonprofessional interpreters), each with unique subgroups. In the following section, I will provide a synthesized summary of these interpreters, including their unique characteristics and corresponding impacts on healthcare delivery. Table 7.2 represents the typology of interpreters under the BHC Model.

Professional interpreters

Several recent reviews have concluded that professional interpreters can significantly improve a patient's quality of care [27]. In particular, professional interpreters can significantly improve provider-patient communication, resource utilization, patient satisfaction, and health outcomes. Professional interpreters include a wide variety of interpreters with varying levels of training. Although common training programs (e.g., CCHCP) typically are limited to 40 hours, a study found that interpreters with at least 100 hours of training are significantly less likely to commit interpreting errors than those with fewer than 100 hours of training [28]. Although there are several national organizations promoting national certification programs and/or examinations in the United States, none has been recognized as the official federal standard [29].

There are two types of professional interpreters in healthcare settings: (a) in-person interpreters and (b) technology-based interpreters. Several studies have found that *in-person professional interpreters* are reported as the preferred choice for patients, providers, and interpreters [30–33]. In-person interpreters, however, can include both hospital interpreters and contract interpreters. *Hospital interpreters* are paid professionals/employees within the health organization who provide interpreting services in healthcare settings and may work in shifts to provide 24-hour services. Because hospital interpreters are members of healthcare institutions, they have the benefit of developing long-term working relationships and effective collaborations with providers. In addition, depending on institutional policies, hospital interpreters may be able to coordinate with other colleagues so that each is responsible for specific clinics, allowing them to develop specialty-specific medical expertise over time. Hospital interpreters also provide telephone interpreting in situations that involve short, simple interactions or medical emergencies [34].

In contrast, *contract interpreters* are professional interpreters hired through interpreting agencies as needed and are often paid hourly wages. They often provide interpreting services to different healthcare facilities. Because they are outside of the organizational structure of the healthcare facilities, they often do not have institutional badges/outfits and can be viewed as outsiders by providers of the healthcare institutions. Although hospital interpreters and contract interpreters may appear to share similar tasks, their work environment and provider-interpreter relationship can be drastically different, which may also have a significant impact on their interpreting strategies [5, 24]. From this perspective, as future studies examine the practice of in-person interpreters, it may be useful to explore whether the types of employment may impact in-person interpreters' behaviors and practices.

The second type of professional interpreters is *technology-based interpreters*, which can include telephone, video-based, or web/app-based interpreters. Australia was the first country to introduce telephone interpreting services in 1973 [35], while the first telephone interpreting services in the United States were offered in 1981 [36]. Video remote interpreting (VRI) has been embraced by the deaf and mute communities for sign language interpreting. VRI also allows both the interpreter and other speakers to assess others' nonverbal communication, providing a comparable experience to in-person interpreting. VRI can be delivered through a wide range of mediums, including dedicated mobile stations, tablet computers (e.g., iPad), or personal smartphones [37]. While the literature on technology-based interpreting has often focused on its cost-effectiveness in relation to patient satisfaction, few studies have examined its impact on the quality of care or health outcomes.

There are several unique characteristics of these technology-based interpreters that may have an impact on the quality of interpreting. First, they often are employed by interpreting agencies, working from their home offices in remote locations [38]. Second, in order to maintain competitiveness, many interpreting agencies have set up call centers in foreign countries to reduce costs and to supplement the interpreter shortage in the United States [36]. Third, interpreting agencies may have better control over the quality of interpreting services as they can maintain quality control by requiring regular web-based training as well as monitoring their performances through recorded interpretation.

While these characteristics may appear straightforward, they have significant implications that providers may not consider when working with technology-based interpreters. For example, because the industry trend has been to establish offshore call centers, technology-based interpreters may not only work in a time zone significantly different from that of the providers but also be unfamiliar with the norms and practices of healthcare settings in the United States. Also, because technology-based interpreters often work for a wide range of clients (e.g., banks, police, airports, and hospitals) with subpar wages, they have minimal incentives to develop advanced skills for healthcare interpreting. In addition, these interpreters are unlikely to develop long-term relationships with providers or patients as they are randomly assigned to different tasks as needed. This also means that, unlike in-person interpreters, these interpreters are unlikely to have any background knowledge about provider-patient relationships/interactions based on prior interactions nor access to patient records through the institutional database. In short, while technology-based interpreters are often considered and touted as professional interpreters, their unique characteristics suggest that they may have very different interpreting styles than in-person interpreters.

Finally, in recent years, healthcare providers have increasingly relied on translation technologies (e.g., Google translate), often combined with voice capabilities, when interacting with patients with whom they are language-discordant. It is important to note that these technologies should not be understood as replacements that are interchangeable with professional interpreters because they are not specifically designed for healthcare delivery and often entail high rates of significant errors [39]. Nevertheless, some researchers have argued that such technologies can improve significantly over time and serve as low-cost, convenient solutions that may be suitable for highly routinized, standardized tasks (e.g., discharge instructions) [40, 41].

Bilingual medical professionals

Due to cost concerns, many healthcare facilities purposefully recruit bilingual providers and staff members to work with their language-discordant patients. These individuals are dual-role interpreters as their primary job responsibilities usually do not involve interpreting. It is important to note that bilingual medical professionals often are not hired or recognized as interpreters. Nevertheless, many bilingual providers and staff members have noted that they often are asked to serve as an interpreter for their colleagues [42]. It is also important not to confound them with other types of interpreters (e.g., chance interpreters) because their medical training and institutional status give them distinctive influences and authority in interpreter-mediated medical encounters. In the United States, Section 1557 of the Affordable Care Act of 2010 (Section 1557 of the ACA) requires the use of qualified interpreters, when reasonable, for communication with language-discordant patients [43]. As such, health organizations are encouraged to develop training programs and certifications to assess whether bilingual medical professionals are qualified to serve as interpreters in specific contexts. There are no current federal or state standards for such assessments [43, 44].

The BHC model proposes that bilingual medical professionals include: (a) *bilingual providers* who work with patients directly and (b) *bilingual medical employees* who are clinic-based medical professionals interpreting for their colleagues. Bilingual medical professionals are a unique category of interpreters due to their medical expertise, in-clinic availability, and institutional roles in healthcare settings.

Because of their medical expertise and ability to communicate with patients directly, *bilingual providers* are often viewed as the gold standard for working with language-discordant patients. Bilingual providers' level of proficiency in their patients' native language can vary significantly. In several comparative studies about interpreting modalities in healthcare settings, bilingual attending providers are treated as one of the conditions [45–48]. The presumption is that if patients can communicate with the provider directly, they should have the best quality of care and health outcomes, similar to that of language-concordant pairs. Several studies have found that patients who had bilingual physicians received similar care when compared to language-concordant provider-patient interactions [49, 50]. A review concluded that bilingual providers could significantly improve patients' quality of care, satisfaction, and outcomes [51].

In the United States, medical students and residents often learn medical Spanish as a way to facilitate care for patients with Spanish language preference. A 10-week medical Spanish course for pediatric emergency physicians was associated with decreased interpreter utilization and increased patient family's satisfaction [52].

However, not all findings of bilingual providers are positive. While a true bilingual provider can be extraordinarily valuable, it is important to recognize that being able to speak a second language does not necessarily mean that a provider has the language skills to interact with patients across different clinical contexts (e.g., patient education, discharge instructions, and informed consent). Providers often overlook the threat posed by bilingual providers' limited language proficiency due to the benefits of bilingual providers' medical expertise and in-clinic availability [24]. In fact, physicians and nurses with limited Spanish proficiency regularly communicated with patients directly even when interpreters were readily available [42]. In addition, providers' self-reports of their linguistic skills do not always reflect their true ability [53, 54]. A short-term class on medical Spanish, while valuable, is unlikely to replace the need for professional interpreters. In fact, researchers found that emergency physicians with medical Spanish training make minor errors in 50% of their consultations and major errors (e.g., misunderstanding duration of symptoms and misunderstanding of vocabulary) in 14% of their consultations [55]. In other words, medical Spanish may give providers false confidence that they are able to communicate directly with their patients, resulting in problematic assessments about the quality of care [56, 57].

This may also help address some intriguing findings in the literature, in which bilingual providers are not always perceived to be the most desirable form of communication for language-discordant patients. For example, one study found that patients are more satisfied with family interpreters (85.1%) and in-person professional interpreters (92.4%) than bilingual providers (75%) [58]. In Grossman's study [46], patients in the bilingual-provider cohort were less satisfied with their language service than those in the in-person and telephonic cohorts. While bilingual providers may be satisfied with their information needs for diagnostic purposes, they may not be able to communicate with the patients effectively about patients' illness-related concerns [59]. A patient may not feel comfortable asking for professional interpreters even when they recognize that the bilingual provider does not have sufficient skills to communicate with them directly due to concerns about rapport with or threat to face, authority, or identity for the provider [60].

From this perspective, it is essential for researchers, practitioners, and healthcare institutions to develop a meaningful assessment of and clear institutional guidelines for providers' language proficiency. This is especially important when various studies continue to demonstrate that physicians and nurses who self-report have low language proficiency frequently rely on their limited language skills when delivering care. In addition, future studies should expand beyond the investigation of patient satisfaction and examine the specific processes and impacts bilingual providers, especially those who use their non-native language skills for care delivery, have on patients' quality of care and health outcomes [61, 62].

The second category of bilingual medical professionals, *bilingual medical employees*, are any medical professionals who serve as an interpreter in healthcare settings, including bilingual physicians, nurses, and residents. A bilingual medical employee is both a bilingual provider and a bilingual medical employee. If a bilingual medical employee works with language-discordant patients directly, they are functioning as bilingual providers; in contrast, if they provide interpreting services to their colleagues, they should be understood as bilingual medical employees. They often offer higher availability and convenience than professional interpreters because they are readily available within the clinic. Several studies have found that bilingual staff is one of the most frequently used types of interpreters, often second only to family interpreters [63–66]. Bilingual medical employees share similar challenges with bilingual providers. For example, one study found one in five dual-role staff interpreters do not have adequate language skills to serve as interpreters [67]. Although many hospitals encourage bilingual staff members to be registered in their language banks, individual facilities often have different testing and training requirements.

Bilingual medical employees face additional challenges when serving as dual-role interpreters [68]. First, they may not assume a neutral role in medical encounters as their primary responsibilities often align with the physician and/or the healthcare team. For example, bilingual nurses' interpretation is more likely to align with providers' preferences and clinical expectations rather than with patients' needs [69, 70]. This can be particularly problematic because providers often have strong, implicit trust for bilingual medical employees due to their medical expertise [24], failing to recognize that their institutional role and hierarchy may prompt them to be biased, resulting in compromised care. For example, because these interpreters are locally based, they may feel pressured to provide interpreting services, even when they feel uncomfortable or inadequate for the task at hand [71]. Thus, to ensure the quality of care, providers need to be aware of these interpersonal dilemmas and provide opportunities for bilingual medical employees to refuse assignments for tasks that they are not prepared for or qualified to take on.

Second, because they are bilingual medical professionals, rather than trained interpreters, there appear to be higher variations in their interpreting styles. Researchers have argued that the complexity of language used and the interpersonal dynamics in medical encounters may contribute to the variations in the interpreting quality for these dual-role interpreters [70, 72]. For example, because providers are likely to assume that the bilingual medical employees are familiar with the medical knowledge and procedure, they may not recognize that complex questions (e.g., "Does she know what the diagnosis is?") or serial questions (e.g., "Would she describe this pain as a sharp, dull, or burning pain? Can she describe it at all?") may present challenges for bilingual medical employees. (Nonprofessional interpreters are likely to face similar challenges as well.) This also highlights the importance of providers' role in ensuring the quality of interpreter-mediated interactions.

Finally, despite the popularity of using bilingual medical employees as a solution to the shortage/inconvenience of professional interpreters, many studies have noted that dual-role interpreters, including bilingual nurses and social workers, face significant challenges in balancing their workload with the interpreting responsibilities [68, 73, 74]. For example, one study found that bilingual resident physicians (i.e., medical school graduates with a medical degree who are taking part in a postgraduate training program) estimated that they spent a mean of 2.3 hours per week interpreting for other residents although hospital interpreters were readily available [42]. This can pose a significant challenge to bilingual providers' workload. If organizations recruit bilingual medical employees and clinic staff with the intention of having them serve as stationed interpreters for a specific clinic, it is essential to develop organizational policies to address the allocation and expectations of their responsibilities and workload [68]. By doing so, other providers would feel more comfortable requesting their assistance and thus decrease the likelihood of avoiding or minimizing communication with patients who have non-English language preference. Finally, in addition to increased workload, researchers have raised concerns about how these dual-role interpreters' medical background and clinic status may shape the provider-patient communication and quality of care [22, 62, 70].

Nonprofessional interpreters

Nonprofessional interpreters, also known as ad hoc, untrained, or informal interpreters, include a wide variety of interpreters, usually referring to any individual who does not have formal training in interpreting in healthcare settings. This can include any individual who does not have training in either interpreting or medical expertise, such as receptionists and janitors. It is important to note that nonprofessionals are often the norm, rather than the exception, in interpreter-mediated medical encounters even in places where there are legislations mandating language access to language-discordant patients [65, 75–77]. One study found that 86% of physicians reported using family interpreters within the 12 months prior to the survey, compared to 71% for bilingual staff, 41% for in-person interpreters, and 21% for telephone interpreters [78]. A national survey in the United States found that when facing language barriers, 77% of residents reported using professional interpreters; in contrast, 84% reported using adult family interpreters, and 22% (including 37% of pediatric and emergency medicine residents) reported using children [79]. Section 1557 of the ACA has provided additional guidelines and conditions for the use of nonprofessional interpreters [43].

Greenhalgh et al. [80] argued, "Interpreting by family members (and other ad hoc contacts) is probably the most widespread and also the most under-researched of all the models in use in United Kingdom health care." This is likely to be true in any other country as well. The few comparative studies between professional and nonprofessional interpreters have suggested conflicting findings. For example, Flores et al. [81] found that although there are no significant differences in frequencies of interpreting errors (e.g., omission, substitution, addition, editorialization, and false fluency) committed by nonprofessional versus professional interpreters, the percentage of nonprofessional interpreters' errors that have potential clinical consequences is significantly higher than that of professional interpreters' (77% versus 55%, $p < 0.001$). A recent study by Flores et al. [28] found that a significantly lower portion of interpreting errors have potential clinical consequences (18%), while the nonprofessional interpreters' errors are still more likely to have potential clinical consequences than that of professional interpreters' (22% versus 12%, $p < 0.01$). In contrast, Butow et al. [82] found that although professional interpreters are less likely to produce nonequivalent speech than family interpreters ($p = 0.02$), they have a higher (but statistically nonsignificant) proportion of negative alterations than family interpreters (26% versus 21%; $p = 0.2$). Pham and colleagues found that 55% of professional interpreters' interpretation involves some form of alterations, among which 93% have negative impacts [83]. Part of the challenges in this line of research is that researchers still differ in how they define interpreting errors and/or measure clinical impacts. In short, there have been some mixed findings about whether professional interpreters and family interpreters differ in the frequencies and types of interpreter alterations and the corresponding positive/negative consequences.

It is important to note that providers' use of nonprofessional interpreters does not appear to be a random decision or a choice of convenience. The BHC model proposed that providers' choice of interpreters are shaped by: (a) time constraint, (b) alliances of care, (c) therapeutic objectives, and (d) organizational-level considerations (see Table 7.3) [3, 84]. These findings are also supported by other studies [78, 85]. Diamond et al. [86] found that providers with different levels of language proficiency differ in their strategies in communicating with patients; in addition, their choice also reflected their consideration for the task at hand. For example, although 100% of physicians

Table 7.3 Factors Shaping Providers' Choice of interpreters.

Factors	Corresponding dimensions	Sample narratives
Time constraints	Disruption to providers' schedule and priorities	I would use [professional interpreter] SO MUCH MORE OFTEN if they were just right there where I could just say, "Hey, can you come here? I need to ask you something real quick," instead of having to call and wait 25 min for them to get up here. (Nora[NUR])
	Increased responsibilities and competing demands	It is [an] unfair burden to carry on a regular patient load and then having to interpret for every family that needs it. [...The bilingual staff/provider who should be] making medical decisions or parting medical therapy [is] now tied up doing interpretation. (Eric[EM])
Alliances of care	Management of patient empowerment and patient receptiveness / Facilitation of provider agenda	[When disclosing poor prognosis,] I want somebody [who] stands in there WITH me. [...] I just couldn't use a telephone [interpreter]. (Cecil[ONC]) PROFESSIONAL interpreter is supposed to be working for ME, as a go-between with the patient. Whereas the family member, may be working for themselves, or may be xworking for the patient, or who knows what. They are not THERE FOR ME. (Gloria[OB/GYN])
Therapeutic objectives	Clinical complexity	I would trust (bilingual nurses much more than professional interpreters). Because they have more medical experience so they would know better how to explain exact procedures and diagnosis. (Eli[EM])
	Clinical urgency	If somebody is critically ill, we will get whatever information we can whether that'll be a family member that speaks very little English, or even a younger child [...] I have a few phrases of Spanish [...] we will utilize what we can till we get an interpreter. (Ed[EM])
	Patient privacy	[When working with family interpreters,] the obvious concern would be confidentiality issues. If the patient will not be forthcoming with the interpreter, then I cannot really ask [sensitive topics] I need to ask through a family interpreter. (Michael[MH])
Organizational-level considerations	Resource limitations	I agree that professional interpreters are our preference, but unfortunately, financially, it's nearly impossible to do that. (Gloria[OB/GYN])
	Ethical guidelines	You don't have to worry about somebody saying back later, "You never told me that. I was translating and you never said that." So, yeah, it's an extra level of protection to have a hospital hired [interpreter] as opposed to the family. The level of malpractice protection. (Cara[ONC])

Source: Hsieh [84]/Springer Nature.

with high Spanish proficiency would communicate to a patient directly to update them about clinical conditions, only 15% of physicians with low Spanish proficiency would do so. However, when it comes to discussing end-of-life issues, 33% of physicians with high Spanish proficiency and 90% with low Spanish proficiency would use a professional interpreter. In other words, providers' use of interpreters is a calculated decision [87].

In the category of nonprofessional interpreters, the BHC model proposed two subcategories of interpreters: (a) chance interpreters, and (b) family interpreters. Although traditionally, these two subgroups of interpreters have been viewed as one, recent studies have highlighted the importance of viewing them as two separate groups. After all, a bilingual bystander in the emergency department who happens to serve as an interpreter would have very different communicative styles than a bilingual daughter who is also the primary caretaker for an elderly parent.

Chance interpreters are untrained individuals who provide interpreting services by chance (e.g., bilingual bystanders). For example, in an emergency department, providers may ask a bilingual janitor or even call a local ethnic restaurant in hopes of finding a person to help with the interpreting task [88, 89]. Researchers have raised concerns about misinterpretation, patient privacy, and litigation risks as chance interpreters have minimal training in medical knowledge and interpreting skills [90, 91]. Many studies have demonstrated that chance interpreters often are prone to problematic interpreting styles and patient outcomes [47, 92].

Family interpreters are patients' family members or friends who also serve as interpreters in healthcare settings. Family interpreter is a unique category of healthcare interpreters due to their relationship with and knowledge of the patient outside of the clinical contexts. Although providers do share concerns about using family interpreters, including bilingual children [93, 94], family interpreters continue to be one of the most common types of interpreters in healthcare settings. Recently, Section 1557 of the ACA has prohibited the use of bilingual children as interpreters except in emergencies and significantly limited the use of family interpreters [43]. Although this is consistent with Western biomedical ideology, it is important to note that several prominent researchers have noted that when bilingual children serve as healthcare interpreters for their parents, both the parents and bilingual children work together as a team and become empowered in facing life adversities – for both the immediate medical encounters and the long-term individual and communal resilience as a whole[95, 96]. Researchers also have argued that respecting patients' preferences, cultural expectations, and larger decision-making contexts for family interpreters may be more appropriate in certain situations than imposing the Western biomedical ideology of and preference for professional interpreters [97, 98].

Recent studies have highlighted that family interpreters and professional interpreters differ in systematic ways. For example, family interpreters do not separate their other social roles (e.g., caregiver and family member) when acting as an interpreter, prompting them to adopt advocacy roles to facilitate understanding and ensure quality care [90, 99, 100]. They actively engage in provider-patient interactions, controlling the process and content of communication. Compared to professional interpreters, family interpreters are also more likely to initiate talk on their own behalf, promoting their own agenda [82, 101]. In addition, providers appear to interact with family interpreters differently than with professional interpreters, relying on them to report symptoms that the patient does not mention, provide interpreting services after the visit, and establish relationships with the whole family [94].

While there are concerns about the quality of interpreting from family interpreters, several studies have provided important findings. For example, although family interpreters have a significantly higher rate of nonequivalent interpretations than professional interpreters, the nonequivalent interpretations appear to be mostly inconsequential [82]. After comparing interpreting strategies between family interpreters and professional interpreters, Leanza et al. [101] concluded, "Adult family interpreters might be considered, at a linguistic level, as reliable as trained interpreters." Because family interpreters are not professionally trained, it is unlikely that they would share the same ethics and/or interpreting strategies as professional interpreters. Nevertheless, the family interpreters' understanding of their roles often entails "a sense of linguistic advocacy between speakers of minority languages and a society that struggles to accommodate the linguistic needs of its members" [102], which is likely to shape their communicative strategies as interpreters. In short, when conceptualizing and examining family interpreters, researchers should not use professional interpreters as the gold standard, hoping that the "best" family interpreters would act the same. They would not because they are not the same. Family interpreters know a lot more background information about the patient, share a stronger trust and bond with the patient, and can be a great ally for the provider to derive an accurate diagnosis and shared decision-making. The challenges for researchers and healthcare providers are to identify the specific processes and functions family interpreters can serve in a medical encounter and develop meaningful and ethical boundaries for collaboration.

Conclusion

The literature on bilingual health communication made significant progress in the last few decades. By conceptualizing interpreter performances as role performances, researchers began to recognize interpreters as active participants in the healthcare team, collaborating with other participants to achieve quality and equality of care [3]. Rather than focusing on the use of professional interpreters, researchers and practitioners have emphasized that quality of care is best protected when healthcare providers can effectively and appropriately work with different types of interpreters in healthcare settings, including bilingual medical professionals and nonprofessional interpreters. In addition, by recognizing the complexity of language concordance and the impact of different types of interpreters in provider-patient interactions, researchers have urged for more investigations of the corresponding impact to the content and process of provider-patient communication, quality of care, and patient outcomes (e.g., behavioral and health outcomes).

The literature indicates that at times, the presence of an interpreter may allow a language-discordant patient to do *better* than a language-concordant patient [103, 104]. This suggests that interpreters must function at a level that is more than simply transferring information from one language to another; otherwise, the best interpreters could do is to allow patients to have the same outcomes and quality of care as monolingual others. However, researchers know little about how such processes can be accomplished.

Our understanding and conceptualization of interpreters should move beyond ideological claims. By detailing the unique characteristics and impacts of different types of interpreters, my goal is to highlight and clarify some of the conflicting findings in the literature. Different types of interpreters have their unique strengths and weaknesses. They are not interchangeable.

Providers were inherently aware of these differences, resulting in calculated choices for different types of interpreters depending on the task at hand [86, 87]. However, it is unclear whether these choices were appropriate as we still know little about how different types of interpreters influence the processes, content, and outcomes of interpreter-mediated medical encounters. From this perspective, the important question to ask is: In what ways do different types of interpreters shape the processes, content, and outcomes of interpreter-mediated medical encounters? The goal of identifying the unique communicative patterns is not to demonstrate whether one type of interpreter is categorically better than others. This approach ignores the reality of healthcare delivery. Effective and meaningful utilization of interpreters cannot be completely dependent on a single type of interpreter because each type of interpreter has distinctive strengths and weaknesses. In other words, identifying when and how to best utilize each type of interpreter to achieve optimal care would allow researchers and practitioners to develop meaningful guidelines for best practices for language-discordant patients.

By recognizing that the different types of interpreters entail distinctive interpersonal dynamics, institutional relationships, and social responsibilities (beyond the immediate medical encounters), researchers can further explore how providers' and patients' expectations and behaviors may differ in response to the unique characteristics of the interpreters. This approach highlights providers' and patients' agency, preferences, and needs in the communicative process, emphasizing the collaborative and coordinated nature of interpreter-mediated provider-patient interactions.

Highlights

- Rather than viewing the interpreter as the central and only person who is responsible for the quality of interpreter-mediated interactions, researchers and practitioners increasingly argue that all participants can actively influence the content and process of communication.
- The BHC model views interpreter-mediated interactions as a socially constructed, goal-driven communicative activity that requires multi-party coordination on the meanings and processes of healthcare delivery.
- Different types of interpreters entail distinctive interpersonal dynamics, institutional relationships, and social responsibilities (beyond the immediate medical encounters) that can enhance or compromise patients' equality and quality of care.
- Effective and meaningful utilization of interpreters in healthcare settings cannot be completely dependent on a single type of interpreter because each type of interpreter has distinctive strengths and weaknesses.
- Further research and institutional guidelines are necessary to identify when and how to utilize different types of interpreters effectively and appropriately to achieve optimal care.

REFERENCES

1. Sleptsova, M., Hofer, G., Morina, N., and Langewitz, W. (2014). The role of the health care interpreter in a clinical setting—A narrative review. *J. Community Health Nurs.* 31 (3): 167–184.
2. Loach, B.L. (2019). A time to speak and a time to keep silent: Professional ethics, conscience, and the medical interpreter. *Ethics, Med. Public Health* 11: 52–59.
3. Hsieh, E. (2016). *Bilingual Health Communication: Working With Interpreters in Cross-Cultural Care*. New York, NY: Routledge.
4. Hsieh, E. (2013). Health literacy and patient empowerment: The role of medical interpreters in bilingual health communication. In: *Reducing Health Disparities: Communication Intervention* (ed. M.J. Dutta and G.L. Kreps), 41–66. New York, NY: Peter Lang.
5. Brisset, C., Leanza, Y., and Laforest, K. (2013). Working with interpreters in health care: A systematic review and meta-ethnography of qualitative studies. *Patient Educ. Couns.* 91 (2): 131–140.
6. de Cotret, F.R., Brisset, C., and Leanza, Y. (2021). A typology of healthcare interpreter positionings: When "neutral" means "proactive". *Interpreting* 23 (1): 103–126.
7. Hsieh, E. and Kramer, E.M. (2021). *Rethinking Culture in Health Communication: Social Interactions as Intercultural Encounters*. Wiley.
8. Dysart-Gale, D. (2005). Communication models, professionalization, and the work of medical interpreters. *Health Commun.* 17 (1): 91–103.
9. Roat, C.E. (1996). *Bridging the Gap: A Basic Training for Medical Interpreters*. Seattle, WA: Cross Cultural Health Care Program.
10. Roat, C.E., Putsch, R.W. III, and Lucero, C. (1997). *Bridging the Gap Over the Phone: A Basic Training for Telephone Interpreters Serving Medical Settings*. Seattle, WA: Cross Cultural Health Care Program.
11. Hsieh, E. (2008). "I am not a robot!" Interpreters' views of their roles in health care settings. *Qual. Health Res.* 18 (10): 1367–1383.

12. Hsieh, E. (2009). Bilingual health communication: Medical interpreters' construction of a mediator role. In: *Communicating to Manage Health and Illness* (ed. D.E. Brashers and D.J. Goldsmith), 135–160. New York, NY: Routledge.
13. Hsieh, E. (2007). Interpreters as co-diagnosticians: Overlapping roles and services between providers and interpreters. *Soc. Sci. Med.* 64 (4): 924–937.
14. Kilian, S., Swartz, L., Hunt, X. et al. (2020). When roles within interpreter-mediated psychiatric consultations speak louder than words. *Transcult. Psychiatry* 1363461520933768. https://doi.org/10.1177/1363461520933768.
15. Suarez, N.R.E., Urtecho, M., Jubran, S. et al. (2021). The roles of medical interpreters in intensive care unit communication: A qualitative study. *Patient Educ. Couns.* 104 (5): 1100–1108.
16. Leanza, Y. (2005). Roles of community interpreters in pediatrics as seen by interpreters, physicians and researchers. *Interpreting* 7 (2): 167–192.
17. Goffman, E. (1959). *The Presentation of Self in Everyday Life*. Garden City, NY: Doubleday.
18. Goffman, E. (1974). *Frame Analysis: An Essay on the Organization of Experience*. Cambridge, MA: Harvard University Press.
19. Wadensjö, C. (1998). *Interpreting as Interaction*. London: Longman.
20. Hsieh, E. (2010). Provider-interpreter collaboration in bilingual health care: Competitions of control over interpreter-mediated interactions. *Patient Educ. Couns.* 78 (2): 154–159.
21. Hsieh, E. (2006). Conflicts in how interpreters manage their roles in provider-patient interactions. *Soc. Sci. Med.* 62 (3): 721–730.
22. Aranda, C.Á., Gutiérrez, R.L., and Li, S. (2020). Towards a collaborative structure of interpreter-mediated medical consultations: Complementing functions between healthcare interpreters and providers. *Soc. Sci. Med.* 269: 113529.
23. Martínez-Gómez, A. (2020). Who defines role?: Negotiation and collaboration between non-professional interpreters and primary participants in prison settings. *Transl. Interpreting Stud.* 15 (1): 108–131.
24. Hsieh, E., Ju, H., and Kong, H. (2010). Dimensions of trust: The tensions and challenges in provider-interpreter trust. *Qual. Health Res.* 20 (2): 170–181.
25. Hsieh, E. and Kramer, E.M. (2012). Medical interpreters as tools: Dangers and challenges in the utilitarian approach to interpreters' roles and functions. *Patient Educ. Couns.* 89 (1): 158–162.
26. Hsieh, E. (2018). Reconceptualizing language discordance: Meanings and experiences of language barriers in the U.S. and Taiwan. *J. Immigr. Minor. Health* 20 (1): 1–4.
27. Karliner, L.S., Jacobs, E.A., Chen, A.H., and Mutha, S. (2007). Do professional interpreters improve clinical care for patients with limited English proficiency? A systematic review of the literature. *Health Serv. Res.* 42 (2): 727–754.
28. Flores, G., Abreu, M., Barone, C.P. et al. (2012). Errors of medical interpretation and their potential clinical consequences: A comparison of professional versus ad hoc versus no interpreters. *Ann. Emerg. Med.* 60 (5): 545–553.
29. International Medical Interpreters Association. *National Certificaiton*. http://www.imiaweb.org/advocacy/nationalcertificatereport.asp (accessed 10 December 2021).
30. Bagchi, A.D., Dale, S., Verbitsky-Savitz, N. et al. (2011). Examining effectiveness of medical interpreters in emergency departments for Spanish-speaking patients with limited English proficiency: Results of a randomized controlled trial. *Ann. Emerg. Med.* 57 (3): 248–256.
31. Nápoles, A.M., Santoyo-Olsson, J., Karliner, L.S. et al. (2010). Clinician ratings of interpreter mediated visits in underserved primary care settings with ad hoc, in-person professional, and video conferencing modes. *J. Health Care Poor Underserved* 21 (1): 301–317.
32. Locatis, C., Williamson, D., Gould-Kabler, C. et al. (2010). Comparing in-person, video, and telephonic medical interpretation. *J. Gen. Intern. Med.* 25 (4): 345–350.

33. Jungner, J.G., Tiselius, E., Blomgren, K. et al. (2019). Language barriers and the use of professional interpreters: A national multisite cross-sectional survey in pediatric oncology care. *Acta Oncol.* 58 (7): 1015–1020.
34. Angelelli, C.V. (2004). *Medical Interpreting and Cross-Cultural Communication*. Cambridge: Cambridge University Press.
35. Mikkelson, H. (2003). Telephone interpreting: Boon or bane? In: *Speaking in Tongues: Language Across Contexts and Users* (ed. L.P. González), 251–269. Valencia: Universitat de València.
36. Kelly, N. (2007). *Telephone Interpreting: A Comprehensive Guide to the Profession*. Victoria, BC: Trafford.
37. Ji, X., Chow, E., Abdelhamid, K. et al. (2021). Utility of mobile technology in medical interpretation: A literature review of current practices. *Patient Educ. Couns.* 104 (9): 2137–2145.
38. Phillips, C. (2013). Remote telephone interpretation in medical consultations with refugees: Meta-communications about care, survival and selfhood. *J. Refug. Stud.* 26 (4): 505–523.
39. Kreger, V., Aintablian, H., Diamond, L., and Taira, R.B. (2019). Google Translate as a tool for emergency department discharge instructions? Not so fast! *Ann. Emerg. Med.* 74 (4): S5–S6.
40. Khoong, E.C., Steinbrook, E., Brown, C., and Fernandez, A. (2019). Assessing the use of Google Translate for Spanish and Chinese translations of emergency department discharge instructions. *JAMA Intern. Med.* 179 (4): 580–582.
41. Birkenbeuel, J., Joyce, H., Sahyouni, R. et al. (2021). Google Translate in healthcare: Preliminary evaluation of transcription, translation and speech synthesis accuracy. *BMJ Innov.* 7 (2): 422–429.
42. O'Leary, S.C.B., Federico, S., and Hampers, L.C. (2003). The truth about language barriers: One residency program's experience. *Pediatrics* 111 (5 Pt 1): e569–e573.
43. Squires, A. and Youdelman, M. (2019). Section 1557 of the Affordable Care Act: Strengthening language access rights for patients with limited English proficiency. *J. Nurs. Regul.* 10 (1): 65–67.
44. Kasten MJ, Berman AC, Ebright AB, Mitchell JD, Quirindongo-Cedeno O. Interpreters in health care: A concise review for clinicians. *Am. J. Med.* 2020.133(4):424-8.e2. https://doi.org/10.1016/j.amjmed.2019.12.008.
45. Grover, A., Deakyne, S., Bajaj, L., and Roosevelt, G.E. (2012). Comparison of throughput times for limited English proficiency patient visits in the emergency department between different interpreter modalities. *J. Immigr. Minor. Health* 14 (4): 602–607.
46. Crossman, K.L., Wiener, E., Roosevelt, G. et al. (2010). Interpreters: Telephonic, in-person interpretation and bilingual providers. *Pediatrics* 125 (3): e631–e638.
47. Lee, L.J., Batal, H.A., Maselli, J.H., and Kutner, J.S. (2002). Effect of Spanish interpretation method on patient satisfaction in an urban walk-in clinic. *J. Gen. Intern. Med.* 17 (8): 641–645.
48. Diamond, L., Izquierdo, K., Canfield, D. et al. (2019). A systematic review of the impact of patient–physician non-English language concordance on quality of care and outcomes. *J. Gen. Intern. Med.* 34 (8): 1591–1606.
49. Eamranond, P.P., Davis, R.B., Phillips, R.S., and Wee, C.C. (2009). Patient-physician language concordance and lifestyle counseling among Spanish-speaking patients. *J. Immigr. Minor. Health* 11 (6): 494–498.
50. Hampers, L.C. and McNulty, J.E. (2002). Professional interpreters and bilingual physicians in a pediatric emergency department: Effect on resource utilization. *Arch. Pediatr. Adolesc. Med.* 156 (11): 1108–1113.
51. Flores, G. (2005). The impact of medical interpreter services on the quality of health care: A systematic review. *Med. Care Res. Rev.* 62 (3): 255–299.
52. Mazor, S.S., Hampers, L.C., Chande, V.T., and Krug, S.E. (2002). Teaching Spanish to pediatric emergency physicians: Effects on patient satisfaction. *Arch. Pediatr. Adolesc. Med.* 156 (7): 693–695.

53. Lion, K.C., Thompson, D.A., Cowden, J.D. et al. (2013). Clinical Spanish use and language proficiency testing among pediatric residents. *Acad. Med.* 88 (10): 1478–1484.
54. Diamond, L.C., Luft, H.S., Chung, S., and Jacobs, E.A. (2012). "Does this doctor speak my language?" Improving the characterization of physician non-English language skills. *Health Serv. Res.* 47 (1, Pt 2): 556–569.
55. Prince, D. and Nelson, M. (1995). Teaching Spanish to emergency medicine residents. *Acad. Emerg. Med.* 2 (1): 32–37.
56. Diamond, L.C. and Jacobs, E.A. (2010). Let's not contribute to disparities: The best methods for teaching clinicians how to overcome language barriers to health care. *J. Gen. Intern. Med.* 25 (Suppl. 2): S189–S193.
57. Ortega, P., Avila, S., and Park, Y.S. (2022). Patient-reported quality of communication skills in the clinical workplace for clinicians learning medical Spanish. *Cureus* 14 (2): 1–12.
58. Kuo, D. and Fagan, M.J. (1999). Satisfaction with methods of Spanish interpretation in an ambulatory care clinic. *J. Gen. Intern. Med.* 14 (9): 547–550.
59. Diamond, L.C. and Reuland, D.S. (2009). Describing physician language fluency: Deconstructing medical Spanish. *JAMA* 301 (4): 426–428.
60. Fryer, C.E., Mackintosh, S.F., Stanley, M.J., and Crichton, J. (2013). 'I understand all the major things': How older people with limited English proficiency decide their need for a professional interpreter during health care after stroke. *Ethn. Health* 18 (6): 610–625.
61. Fernandez, A., Schillinger, D., Warton, E.M. et al. (2011). Language barriers, physician-patient language concordance, and glycemic control among insured Latinos with diabetes: The Diabetes Study of Northern California (DISTANCE). *J. Gen. Intern. Med.* 26 (2): 170–176.
62. Gerchow, L., Burka, L.R., Miner, S., and Squires, A. (2021). Language barriers between nurses and patients: A scoping review. *Patient Educ. Couns.* 104 (3): 534–553.
63. Kuo, D.Z., O'Connor, K.G., Flores, G., and Minkovitz, C.S. (2007). Pediatricians' use of language services for families with limited English proficiency. *Pediatrics* 119 (4): e920–e927.
64. Bischoff, A. and Hudelson, P. (2010). Communicating with foreign language-speaking patients: Is access to professional interpreters enough? *J. Travel Med.* 17 (1): 15–20.
65. Ginde, A.A., Sullivan, A.F., Corel, B. et al. (2010). Reevaluation of the effect of mandatory interpreter legislation on use of professional interpreters for ED patients with language barriers. *Patient Educ. Couns.* 81 (2): 204–206.
66. Gill, P.S., Beavan, J., Calvert, M., and Freemantle, N. (2011). The unmet need for interpreting provision in UK primary care. *PloS One* 6 (6): 1–6.
67. Moreno, M.R., Otero-Sabogal, R., and Newman, J. (2007). Assessing dual-role staff-interpreter linguistic competency in an integrated healthcare system. *J. Gen. Intern. Med.* 22 (Suppl 2): S331–S335.
68. Chang, H., Hutchinson, C., and Gullick, J. (2021). Pulled away: The experience of bilingual nurses as ad hoc interpreters in the emergency department. *Ethn. Health* 26 (7): 1045–1064.
69. Elderkin-Thompson, V., Silver, R.C., and Waitzkin, H. (2001). When nurses double as interpreters: A study of Spanish-speaking patients in a US primary care setting. *Soc. Sci. Med.* 52 (9): 1343–1358.
70. Mueller, M.-R., Roussos, S., Hill, L. et al. (2011). Medical interpreting by bilingual staff whose primary role is not interpreting: Contingencies influencing communication for dual-role interpreters. In: *Access to Care and Factors That Impact Access, Patients as Partners in Care and Changing Roles of Health Providers*, vol. 29 (ed. J.J. Kronenfeld), 77–91. Bingley: Emerald.
71. Yang, C.-F. and Gray, B. (2008). Bilingual medical students as interpreters—what are the benefits and risks? *N. Z. Med. J.* 121 (1282): 15–28.
72. Ebden, P., Bhatt, A., Carey, O., and Harrison, B. (1988). The bilingual medical consultation. *Lancet* 331 (8581): 347.

73. Engstrom, D.W., Piedra, L.M., and Min, J.W. (2009). Bilingual social workers: Language and service complexities. *Adm. Soc. Work* 33 (2): 167–185.
74. Squires, A., Miner, S., Liang, E. et al. (2019). How language barriers influence provider workload for home health care professionals: A secondary analysis of interview data. *Int. J. Nurs. Stud.* 99: 103394–1033401. https://doi.org/10.1016/j.ijnurstu.2019.103394.
75. Schenker, Y., Pérez-Stable, E.J., Nickleach, D., and Karliner, L.S. (2011). Patterns of interpreter use for hospitalized patients with limited English proficiency. *J. Gen. Intern. Med.* 26 (7): 712–717.
76. Papic, O., Malak, Z., and Rosenberg, E. (2012). Survey of family physicians' perspectives on management of immigrant patients: Attitudes, barriers, strategies, and training needs. *Patient Educ. Couns.* 86 (2): 205–209.
77. Gray, B., Hilder, J., and Donaldson, H. (2011). Why do we not use trained interpreters for all patients with limited English proficiency? Is there a place for using family members? *Aust. J. Prim. Health* 17 (3): 240–249.
78. Rose, D.E., Tisnado, D.M., Malin, J.L. et al. (2010). Use of interpreters by physicians treating limited English proficient women with breast cancer: Results from the provider survey of the Los Angeles Women's Health Study. *Health Serv. Res.* 45 (1): 172–194.
79. Lee, K.C., Winickoff, J.P., Kim, M.K. et al. (2006). Resident physicians' use of professional and nonprofessional interpreters: A national survey. *JAMA* 296 (9): 1050–1053.
80. Greenhalgh, T., Robb, N., and Scambler, G. (2006). Communicative and strategic action in interpreted consultations in primary health care: A Habermasian perspective. *Soc. Sci. Med.* 63 (5): 1170–1187.
81. Flores, G., Laws, M.B., Mayo, S.J. et al. (2003). Errors in medical interpretation and their potential clinical consequences in pediatric encounters. *Pediatrics* 111 (1): 6–14.
82. Butow, P.N., Goldstein, D., Bell, M.L. et al. (2011). Interpretation in consultations with immigrant patients with cancer: How accurate is it? *J. Clin. Oncol.* 29 (20): 2801–2807.
83. Pham, K., Thornton, J.D., Engelberg, R.A. et al. (2008). Alterations during medical interpretation of ICU family conferences that interfere with or enhance communication. *Chest* 134 (1): 109–116.
84. Hsieh, E. (2015). Not just "getting by": Factors influencing providers' choice of interpreters. *J. Gen. Intern. Med.* 30 (1): 75–82.
85. Bischoff, A. and Hudelson, P. (2010). Access to healthcare interpreter services: Where are we and where do we need to go? *Int. J. Environ.* 7 (7): 2838–2844.
86. Diamond, L.C., Tuot, D., and Karliner, L. (2012). The use of Spanish language skills by physicians and nurses: Policy implications for teaching and testing. *J. Gen. Intern. Med.* 27 (1): 117–123.
87. Diamond, L.C., Schenker, Y., Curry, L. et al. (2009). Getting by: Underuse of interpreters by resident physicians. *J. Gen. Intern. Med.* 24 (2): 256–262.
88. Weaver, C. and Sklar, D. (1980). Diagnostic dilemmas and cultural diversity in emergency rooms. *West. J. Med.* 133 (4): 356–366.
89. Pöchhacker, F. (2007). Giving access—or not: A developing-country perspective on healthcare interpreting. In: *Interpreting Studies and Beyond* (ed. F. Pöchhacker, A.-L. Jakobson, and I.M. Mees), 121–137. Frederiksberg: Samfundslitteratur.
90. Meeuwesen, L., Twilt, S., ten Thije, J.D., and Harmsen, H. (2010). "Ne diyor?" (What does she say?): Informal interpreting in general practice. *Patient Educ. Couns.* 81 (2): 198–203.
91. MacFarlane, A., Dzebisova, Z., Karapish, D. et al. (2009). Arranging and negotiating the use of informal interpreters in general practice consultations: Experiences of refugees and asylum seekers in the west of Ireland. *Soc. Sci. Med.* 69 (2): 210–214.
92. Meeuwesen, L. (2012). Language barriers in migrant health care: A blind spot. *Patient Educ. Couns.* 86 (2): 135–136.

93. Cohen, S., Moran-Ellis, J., and Smaje, C. (1999). Children as informal interpreters in GP consultations: Pragmatics and ideology. *Sociol. Health Illn.* 21 (2): 163–186.
94. Rosenberg, E., Leanza, Y., and Seller, R. (2007). Doctor-patient communication in primary care with an interpreter: Physician perceptions of professional and family interpreters. *Patient Educ. Couns.* 67 (3): 286–292.
95. Guntzviller, L.M., Jensen, J.D., and Carreno, L.M. (2017). Latino children's ability to interpret in health settings: A parent–child dyadic perspective on child health literacy. *Commun. Monogr.* 84 (2): 143–163.
96. Kam, J.A., Basinger, E.D., and Guntzviller, L.M. (2017). Communal coping among Spanish-speaking mother–child dyads engaging in language brokering: A latent class analysis. *Commun. Res.* 44 (5): 743–769.
97. Ho, A. (2008). Using family members as interpreters in the clinical setting. *J. Clin. Ethics* 19 (3): 223–233.
98. Pollock, S. (2020). More than words can say: Why health and social care policy makers should reconsider their position on informal interpreters. *Crit. Soc. Policy* 41 (1): 128–147.
99. Rosenberg, E., Seller, R., and Leanza, Y. (2008). Through interpreters' eyes: Comparing roles of professional and family interpreters. *Patient Educ. Couns.* 70 (1): 87–93.
100. Valdés, G. (2003). *Expanding Definitions of Giftedness: The Case of Young Interpreters From Immigrant Communities*. Mahwah, NJ: Erlbaum.
101. Leanza, Y., Boivin, I., and Rosenberg, E. (2010). Interruptions and resistance: A comparison of medical consultations with family and trained interpreters. *Soc. Sci. Med.* 70 (12): 1888–1895.
102. Angelelli, C.V. (2010). A professional ideology in the making: Bilingual youngsters interpreting for their communities and the notion of (no) choice. *Transl. Interpreting Stud.* 5 (1): 94–108.
103. Andrulis, D., Goodman, N., and Pryor, C. (2022). *What a Difference an Interpreter Can Make: Health Care Experiences of Uninsured With Limited English Proficiency*. Boston, MA: Access Project. https://www.migrationpolicy.org/sites/default/files/language_portal/interpreter.report_0.pdf (accessed 11 November 2022).
104. Bernstein, J., Bernstein, E., Dave, A. et al. (2002). Trained medical interpreters in the emergency department: Effects on services, subsequent charges, and follow-up. *J. Immigr. Health* 4 (4): 171–176.

8 Healthcare Translation for Patients

WIOLETA KARWACKA

Introduction

Healthcare translation is a factor that contributes to improving access to health services. The problems in accessing healthcare intersect with language preferences and health literacy. Existing structural barriers to effective health communication in nondominant languages pose considerable difficulties in obtaining quality healthcare or may even prevent patients from seeking medical help [1–6]. Moreover, structural barriers to language-appropriate care may lead to sociodemographic exclusion and consequently insufficient participation of linguistically diverse groups in clinical trials, which in turn may lead to inaccurate conclusions related to risk factors, disease prevalence, or treatment response in various ethnocultural groups [7]. Medical translation and interpreting help bridge communication gaps and secure access to healthcare information for marginalized/minoritized groups, migrants, or patients with limited language or health proficiency. Patients who are deaf or hard of hearing should be provided with sign language interpreting; patients with visual impairment need access to intralingual transcription into Braille. Intralingual translation and using plain language to produce lay-friendly, easy-to-read materials is a channel through which patients with limited health literacy access health-related information.

This chapter discusses overcoming language discordance between patients and providers through the translation of health-related texts for linguistically diverse patients across the healthcare spectrum. This is referred to as "healthcare translation" in this chapter, which is a narrower category than "medical translation," which generally refers to translating any text pertaining to medicine. Text genres translated for patients include factsheets, patient information leaflets, informed consent forms (ICFs), brochures, and other forms, which may include discharge instructions for patients. They need to be translated in a way ensuring their usability by the patients, i.e., adapted to recipients' needs and edited in a clear and comprehensible manner. This chapter also discusses common practices in healthcare translation and relevant recommendations. It addresses problems specific to translation, understood as written translation, i.e., "the rendering

---

The Handbook of Language in Public Health and Healthcare, First Edition.
Edited by Pilar Ortega, Glenn Martínez, Maichou Lor, and A. Susana Ramírez.
© 2024 John Wiley & Sons, Inc. Published 2024 by John Wiley & Sons, Inc.

of a written text in one language in a comparable written text in another language" [8]. Interpreting, i.e., "the oral rendering of spoken or signed communication from one language into another" [8], is discussed in Chapter 7. Finally, this chapter addresses intralingual translation, i.e., adapting and simplifying texts for patients within the same language.

Background and theoretical framework: Communication with patients through medical text genres

Theoretical framework

Translation studies is a multidisciplinary field diverse in terms of approaches and methodologies, but it is probably safe to say that all or nearly all the branches of the field seem to share an interest in the relationship between the source and the target text (i.e., the original and its translation). There is certainly a diversity of approaches observed in research into healthcare translation, reflecting the diversity of approaches across the whole field of translation studies. There are prescriptive approaches, indicating how a text should be translated and descriptive ones, which focus on tracing norms, conventions, or strategies employed by translators [9–11]. In terms of the focus of research, product-oriented studies concentrate on the target texts, while process-oriented research strives to gain insight into the translation project and translatorial activity itself as a cognitive, cultural, or social process [9–11]. The main directions of healthcare translation studies include qualifications and translator training, history of medical translation, terminology, lay-friendliness, and genre shift [12, 13]. It is important to note that systematic research into medical and – for that matter – healthcare translation is a fairly young branch of translation studies as it started developing at the turn of the twenty-first century [12–14]. Early research into medical and healthcare translation was predominantly prescriptive with a strong tendency to assess specialized terminological equivalence, while more recent approaches tend to be descriptive and are open to a range of problems, concepts, text types, communicative situations, contexts, and participants [13].

Within the process-oriented research into healthcare translation, there are propositions of models for healthcare translation, which describe how the source text is (descriptive) or should be (prescriptive) handled, what steps are taken to commission a translator, verify the translation and prepare the final target text [15–18]. The purpose of those models seems to be to ensure adequate quality and usability of such documents. The full range of translation quality assessment methods is quite broad and includes intuitive assessment (based on experience or anecdotal judgment), error analysis, corpus-based evaluation, scale-based methods, mixed-methods scoring (using scales and error analysis), item-based assessment and comparative judgment [18, 19]. There is also diversity in approaches to quality assessment: experiential approaches lean toward intuitive assessment, while textual or pragmatic approaches may use raters and scale-based or mixed-method scoring [18–20]. In terms of quality assurance tools used in healthcare translation, one of the prevalent features of number of proposed models is back-translation of various documents or instruments in a multistep process [18, 21, 22], a tool proposed in the 1970s [23], which is used in a model that involves translating the source text (ST) into the target language (TL) (forward translation, sometimes two parallel forward translations are prepared), then blind translation of the target text (blind, meaning performed by another translator who did not have access to the ST) "back" into the source language. The versions are then compared to detect inaccuracies or omissions, verified, reconciled, and proofread – various organizations follow this general outline, but the steps or project phases may slightly differ [16, 24]. Such an equivalence-based approach, however, is problematic for more than one reason. First, the back-translation method can detect omissions or certain changes in denotative meaning, but it is not a reliable or suitable tool for detecting poorly constructed sentences or register problems [22], while those areas can affect the readability and comprehensibility of materials for patients. Second, it seems to be based on an outdated premise that perfect equivalence is always possible between source and target – a view that has been vastly debated and criticized in the field of translation studies [9, 23, 25, 26]. Traditionally, equivalence was understood as the goal and condition of translation as every translation was expected to strive for equivalence. Equivalence is, however, a problematic concept, as it is not uniform and various translation researchers use different criteria to categorize it [10, 11, 26–30]. The very notion of equivalence is controversial because it defines a category that is too narrow and does not account for the function or the purpose of translation, which is why the assessment of equivalence as part of the evaluation of translations is replaced for instance with the determination of how comprehensible the translation is for the recipient (i.e., the determination of readability) [30]. Equivalence determines only one possible type of relationship between the source and the target text [9]. More recent approaches are sensitive to tensions between accuracy and adequacy of language in the target texts, norms, and conventions, the role of translation and translator, the power relations, the purpose and function of translation and target texts, their genres and registers within which they operate [9, 30].

The approaches to the healthcare translation process which are function-oriented and based on genre features and text purpose are more sensitive to the problematic areas in the translation of health information for patients, such as comprehensibility issues resulting from using too specialized language or omitting information, which are common healthcare translation problems [31]. The shift from equivalence-based models to more functional approaches is parallel to the tendencies observed in the field of translation studies as a whole. The models which are not limited to verifying accuracy and adequate use of terminology but also assess the functional fit and genre-specific features of texts are worth considering in order to achieve better usability of translated healthcare documents [18]. An ideal or universal design of a translation process does not exist – various models utilizing various translation quality assessments have been shown to have issues regarding their validity, reliability, or practicality [19]. Additionally, there are inconsistencies between theoretical models and practical approaches [20, 32]. In order for a healthcare translation model to produce satisfying results, it needs to account for specific qualifications and skills of healthcare translators, and the purpose and function of texts that are translated [16]. An adequately trained translator is proficient in the source and TL and is familiar with various registers, knows a range of translation strategies or procedures and uses them at the lexical, syntactic, and pragmatic level, knows healthcare terminology and text type features, and has background knowledge about the subject matter of the text as well as the source and target cultures [16, 33–35].

Healthcare text genres

Written healthcare communication is mediated through text genres (i.e., classes of texts which have a conventional text structure) [36] and a set of other formal features, such as text organization, length, level of specialization, level of formality and also a "communicative activity" whereby a specific goal is achieved; for instance, the readers are convinced to comply with the recommendations included in the text or to accept that the conclusions reached by authors are adequate [37]. Examples of text genres encountered in healthcare settings include informed consent forms or fact sheets. Text genres may have different rhetorical purposes in the context of healthcare: there are instructional, expository, and argumentative genres. The goal intended to be achieved through instructional genres is to give instructions, like those included in patient information leaflets containing drug dosing directions. Expository texts present information; for instance, patient information in the first part of an ICF or a fact sheet is intended as such informative texts for patients. The purpose of argumentative text genres is to convince; for example, a poster in a health campaign is designed to convince patients to follow particular treatment, prevention, or other guidelines [37]. Text genres have a range of functions: preventing disease, educating patients, helping in carrying out treatment, and communicating discoveries to nonscientific readers [37, 38]. Some genres are designed to overcome barriers and bridge communication gaps within the same language – between laypersons and researchers or patients and healthcare professionals, e.g., fact sheets for patients (FSP), package information leaflets (PIL), and popularizing articles [37]. They are also among frequently translated healthcare documents to meet the requirements specified in legal acts regulating clinical trials and drug marketing and ensure access to healthcare information to migrants and refugees. They are widely used by various healthcare institutions, organizations, and professionals for patient education and health promotion to promote prevention, treatment, and compliance [39].

Fact sheets for patients

Fact sheets for patients (FSPs) are also called patient (information) brochures or patient (information) leaflets contain information on a disease, and their aim is to educate patients, help them prevent a disease or its progress, or manage it once it develops. The information comes from reliable sources, such as medical association reports or guidelines, peer-reviewed research papers, etc. FSPs tend to be written by health professionals, but their language should be comprehensible for laypersons. FSPs are usually relatively concise – they contain only the most relevant information about a particular disease, such as the symptoms, causes, treatment methods, and recommendations (e.g., diet). The information is organized under headings that follow a hierarchic order – starting with the most basic information [37].

Package information leaflet

A package information leaflet (PIL) contains information and instructions which ensure safe and effective drug application by a patient, such as the name and indications of the product, information a patient should know before taking a product, instructions for use, side effects, storage instructions, etc. The contents of the document are regulated by the European Union law [40]. While it is usually the case for most genres to evolve gradually, as a result of changing social and cultural conventions, some genres are subject to abrupt changes resulting from regulations in force [36]. PIL is an excellent example of such a case. It is a mandatory European document submitted as part of the registration documentation in English. It is then translated into all European Union official languages. It is worth noticing that there are specific differences between PILs in different languages; for instance, English PILs tend to be more scientifically oriented, while the translated Dutch PILs are more lay-friendly [41]. In the United States, Medication Guides (MG), Patient Package Inserts (PPI), and Patient Instructions for Use (PIFU) fulfill the same function as the European PIL. The Australian equivalent of the document is called Consumer Medicine Information.

The European Medicines Agency regulates the structure and contents of a patient information leaflet, and its template is part of the Quality Review of Documents (QRD template) [24, 36, 42]. It provides information on the number and sequence of headings, indicates the necessary information a PIL should contain and even insists on particular wording in some sections. In the United States, Medication Guides also follow a mandatory template. The readability of MG, PPI and PIFU is regulated in the United States Food and Drug Administration documents [24]. In Australia, Consumer Medicine Information leaflets accompany all prescription and pharmacist-only medicines and follow an official template [36]. In Europe, PILs are developed based on a document entitled Summary of Product Characteristics (SmPCs), which is a detailed and specialized description of drug properties addressed to medical professionals. It provides information on pharmacodynamic and pharmacokinetic properties of a drug, preclinical safety data, list of excipients, incompatibilities, shelf life and special precautions for storage, and special precautions for disposal [38, 42].

The templates for PILs and SmPCs follow a similar order, but SmPCs are much more detailed and specialized – this phenomenon is referred to as structural simplification [37, 38, 42]. Simplifying the leaflets, which are addressed to lay audiences, is crucial because simplification ensures better comprehension, which means that a patient who reads a PIL should be able to find, read, understand, and retain the information in the texts in all European languages [41, 43]. Consequently, structural simplification contributes to increasing comprehension and improving accessibility to crucial health-related information, which is vital for the safe and effective application of medicines, while reducing patients' uncertainty about the therapy they are receiving [38, 41, 43]. To that end, popularization strategies are applied, including explicitation of scientific terms, determinologization, i.e., replacing specialized terms (notably, including those of Latin and Greek origin) with lay words [41]. This chapter uses the European PILs as an example because their development process always involves translation into 23 languages (altogether 24 language versions including the source English document) and the readability requirements are equally applicable to source and target PILs.

Informed consent form

Informed consent form (ICF) or informed consent document (ICD) is a mandatory document in which patients confirm they agree to specific medical procedures, including experimental ones. Under the Declaration of Helsinki, patients and clinical trial participants can only be treated or enrolled in a clinical trial if they are informed of the risks related to the treatment and procedures and express their consent. The ICF is a form that confirms that the patient or candidate participant has received sufficient explanation and also ushers the informed consent process. It contains relevant information on the procedure and/or the nature of the experiment, risks and/or discomforts, benefits, alternative course of treatment, etc. Ideally, it is read out and discussed with a healthcare provider/researcher overseeing the course of treatment or involved in the experimental project. The form and the process of obtaining consent are subject to diligent review to ensure that the ICF is available in the patient's or candidate participant's preferred language to ensure that the information is presented clearly, accurately, and in an unbiased way. Such lay friendliness of the ICF allows for better patient or candidate participant comprehension, which is conducive to ensuring that the consent is in fact informed. However, as the sections below indicate, they only partly fulfill this task.

Other healthcare text genres

Of course, there are other texts translated into healthcare contexts, such as medication labels or healthcare-related websites, which need to be localized (i.e., not only translated but also adapted to the conventions of the target community [44]), and made accessible to linguistically diverse patients. They can serve the purposes of patient-centered care provided they are prepared and translated in a lay-friendly and comprehensible manner.

Impacted populations

Understanding the challenges of healthcare translation involves understanding the needs of the recipients of translation, translated texts, and their purpose. In general, the recipients of healthcare-related documents include medical professionals and patients, and the latter are the focus of this chapter. "Patients" are a very diverse group in terms of literacy, health literacy, and disability status, all of which may affect the usability of documents translated for them. What is more, the reasons why patients need translation are also diverse. Texts are translated as part of pharmaceutical registration and marketing processes. For instance, a product information leaflet included in the drug packaging is translated into the languages where the drug will be sold for regulatory and business-related reasons, but its primary purpose is to ensure safe and effective use. Healthcare information is also translated to accommodate the needs of migrant and refugee populations in the context of health services.

It is important to note that there are, in fact, two major migration trajectories – the first one involves asylum-seeking and the second one is migration for occupational reasons; asylum-seeking refugees may have very little knowledge of how the healthcare system (in the country they reach or where they eventually reside) works, while occupational migrants may be more knowledgeable in that respect since they have time to prepare and get information online even prior to relocating to a given country or get some support from the local migrant community originally from their own country [45]. Consequently, if there is available information translated for migrants on how a healthcare system in a given country operates, they can have better access and actually utilize a range of possibilities that the system offers.

It is estimated that more than 70 million people worldwide have been "forcibly displaced from their homes as a result of persecution, conflict, violence, or human rights violations" [2, 3]. That number includes persons with refugee status and asylum seekers [4]. They resettled in countries where official languages, cultural norms, and administrative structures are different from those in their countries of origin. Thus, groups of refugees may show limited language proficiency or health literacy, both of which are associated with poorer health status [3]. In this respect, individuals with limitations in the dominant language face barriers in accessing healthcare [5, 6], and these barriers contribute to health disparities between migrants and populations proficient in the dominant language [4, 46]. Language discordance and the resulting communication problems are among the most common challenges refugees have to overcome when attempting to access and use health services in their country of resettlement [4]. Patients with limited language proficiency, including recently arrived immigrants, are reported to have poorer access to healthcare [46, 47]. Moreover, language discordance contributes to poorer patient assessment, misdiagnosis, and/or delayed treatment on the part of service providers and on the part of patients – lack of confidence in the received health services, insufficient understanding of their condition, and recommended medication [48]. Other problem areas include access to preventive services, such as screening for cancer and mental health services [46].

Refugee women are particularly affected in terms of accessing healthcare due to several factors, including especially language discordance and unfamiliar healthcare systems [4, 46, 49, 50]. Refugee women have relatively lower foreign language proficiency than men [4]. There is a share of illiterate women among refugees, and they are reported to face the most significant challenges in accessing healthcare [49]. It is also worthy to note that reproductive and health behavior are also mediated through literacy skills, which means that literacy may affect access to information or care in those areas [51]. Healthcare translation can help improve access to reproductive healthcare.

Translating healthcare information for migrant and refugee populations means addressing language discordance, which in turn can help overcome inequalities [45]. Achieving language concordance between patients and providers is reported to be beneficial in terms of more efficient reporting and a smoother referral process if patients require specialized consultations [52]. Migrants and refugees may need language assistance and cultural and social support, which means that (healthcare) translators are often expected to act as community guides and social and cultural mediators [53]. Ideally, written translation is complimented with access to adequately trained interpreters and staff who can effectively communicate in the patients' language. Quality translation and interpreting by skilled and professional translators may help bridge communication gaps provided that mediation is person-centered, informative, and sensitive to cultural differences, for instance, in communicating healthcare needs [4]. Quality translation is usually associated with an accurate and adequate rendition of the original message in the TL. However, in the context of healthcare translation, the usability of translated healthcare information materials needs to be considered. It involves offering translation in the preferred language and in the preferred format to ensure comprehensibility (easily understood texts), readability (easily read contents and form in terms of finding or processing information in the text), and lay-friendliness (information that is relevant, easily understood and retained by nonspecialists).

Challenges of healthcare translation

Ensuring translation in healthcare settings is critical – as signaled in the section above, if translation is not available to linguistically diverse patients, they are limited in their access to healthcare services or healthcare information, they face delays in the diagnosis or referral processes, they are likely to be confused about their treatment regimen and fail to adhere to relevant instructions, which makes them vulnerable to further health risks [36, 46–48].

The types of errors encountered in healthcare translation to an extent reflect the problems seen across all specialized translation, and they include lexical mismatches, such as using an incorrect term or an incorrect collocation, or those resulting from so-called false friends between languages (i.e., words in which may appear similar but have different meanings), changes in pragmatic meaning, including those related to register shifts or, finally, syntactic problems such as those resulting from source language patterning (i.e., copying the structure of the original sentence); see for example, Refs. [34, 54, 55]. There are also cultural differences generating lack of direct equivalents (for instance, for names of institutions, food ingredients, or home remedies for ailments) and posing additional translation challenges. The problem is the potential gravity of such errors, considering the fact that they may affect the accuracy and usability of healthcare documents and thus impact clinical outcomes. The main translation problems traced particularly in healthcare translation include: (a) shifts in register, especially the use of more specialized (i.e., less lay-friendly) language, (b) omissions that affect the clarity of the message, comprehension of the text, and (c) changes of the denotative meaning conveyed through a text, including terminology [17, 31, 55]. Shifts in register and omissions may be due to an asymmetrical relation between the senders of translated healthcare documents and their target readers [13]. Sometimes this lack of symmetry consists in the fact that the source text is written by an expert who does not use lay-friendly language or sometimes a translator fails to convey a lay-friendly message from the source and produces a more specialized material which requires some expert background knowledge [13, 34].

The challenges in healthcare translation are related to adapting texts to the specific communicative and socio-cultural needs of the target recipients (i.e., patients across the care spectrum), including, for instance, persons with low health literacy (who need lay-friendly texts), persons who have recently migrated to a country (and may not be familiar with the socio-cultural specificity of the country including its healthcare structure, names of common medicines, as well as social practices, customs, etc. and need texts which will be transparent and comprehensible in those respects), persons with disabilities (blindness and severe vision impairment exclude the use of written forms, so health information should be communicated through other media and formats, such as audio recordings or Braille transcriptions). Problem areas in this respect are related to usability affected by poor comprehensibility, accessibility, readability, or lay-friendliness.

Adapting translations to the needs of patients is paramount to the usability of healthcare information texts – if the purpose of a text is to inform patients, it needs to be translated in a comprehensible, readable, and lay-friendly manner. Texts for patients are frequently written and/or translated by medical professionals, who tend to produce texts that patients find difficult to understand because they are not adapted to patients' command of specialized terminology and level of health literacy [35]. Apparently, when texts for patients are translated by trained translators, they are more comprehensible than those produced by healthcare professionals [34, 35]. Although meeting the communication needs of lay recipients is such a challenge, the skills necessary to perform such tasks are rarely incorporated in medical translator training programs [35]. The difficulty in securing a skilled translator for a task is even more accentuated in the case of less-commonly encountered languages, whereby interpreters (individuals who are trained in mediating oral communication across languages) provide written translation of documents that are not prepared in advance. Moreover, such requests are made irrespective of text length or its complexity and lack of consistent guidance on those matters or adequate training – performing interpreting tasks requires a different skillset and thus different preparation than written translation tasks [8].

Another issue that seems particularly problematic in the translation for asylum seekers and refugees is the lack of terminological equivalents between source and TL, which hinders communication [4, 56]. Terminological lacunae (i.e., lack of equivalents) may result from the differences in healthcare systems (e.g., job titles or names of institutions) or cultural differences (e.g., the terminology related to sexual health or Sexual Orientation and Gender Identity rights; see Ref. [57]).

In terms of genre-specific problems, several issues need to be addressed by translators and providers who face the challenges related to translating texts for patients, which can be observed in the case of PILs and ICFs and extrapolated to other healthcare genres. Quite contrary to expectations and guidelines, patients still struggle with PILs, documents translated into all European languages, which are not regarded as reader-friendly [33, 41, 43]. They have been shown to be counterintuitive [36]. According to studies on PILs on various subjects, leaflets generally require relatively high reading skills – higher than the actual level of skills in target populations. The major problems affecting readability and usability are specialized content, writing style, or organization [39, 58]. Studies conducted in three continents show that patient information does not always meet patients' needs as they cannot find, understand or retain relevant information contained in leaflets, thus not feeling motivated to adhere to instructions [36]. PILs are not sufficiently user-friendly in terms of linguistic complexity, design, and layout [39, 43, 59]. The prominent features affecting the usability of PILs include the wording used to present risks, which in fact leads to the overestimation of the risks and side-effects by patients; there is insufficient emphasis on the benefit information; what is more the information about interactions, contraindications, dosage instructions, and side effects is too complex, creating comprehension problems to the patient with lower literacy. The fonts used are too small, and the lines are too dense. As a result, patients may skip entire sections, including important information vital to patient adherence and safe and effective use of medicines [43, 59]. The language used in current PILs to convey risk information provokes anxiety in readers, who consequently alter their prescribed regimen without consulting a physician [59]. Contrary to the primary purpose of PILs, i.e., "to inform patients about application and risks of the prescribed medication in a clear, understandable and readily readable way," reading PILs is reported to be associated with worse adherence to treatment instructions [59]. Consequently, the primary purpose of PILs (i.e., to ensure safe and effective drug application) is not fulfilled. Instead, entire populations of patients are at health risk resulting from refraining from applying a drug or applying it in a manner that is not compliant with instructions.

Similar, though not identical, readability-related issues are relevant to ICFs: studies on ICFs indicate candidates for participation in clinical trials do not understand and retain the information contained in the forms they sign and/or do not read these documents carefully [60, 61]. It means that the forms do not meet their communicative needs. That, in turn, affects enrollment rates, patient compliance with the regimen in the research protocol and leads to patient dissatisfaction [60]. It becomes an even greater issue for ethnic or racial minority participants. Although the inclusion of participants of a range of ethnic backgrounds in clinical research is paramount to the generalizability of research findings, removing disparities in the provision of healthcare and improving the accuracy of ethnicity-specific subgroup analyses, racial and ethnic minorities remain underrepresented in clinical research [61, 62]. Therefore, the process of obtaining informed consent should be improved with regard to recruiting minorities who have so far been underrepresented in clinical trials [61]. What stakeholders need to take into consideration is the fact that cultural and contextual factors affect informed decision-making for participants who identified with a racially/ethnically minoritized group. Contextual factors identified include lack of trust resulting from mistreatment endured in the past, misinformation about the informed consent as such, and, finally, low comprehensibility of the text of the form [61]. That is why, also in the case of ICFs used for ethnically or racially minoritized groups, it is important to ensure translation and/or use plain language, summaries, and images [61].

Good practices and recommendations

Removing barriers and improving access to language-appropriate healthcare can be achieved by offering language assistance services such as translation to patients and adequate training in cultural competence to providers [47]. Bridging communications gaps requires translating written materials into appropriate languages with all necessary adaptations performed by culturally and linguistically competent professionals who can identify those gaps [62]. This can contribute to providing the quality written translation of documents used in patient encounters [8]. According to the Guidance Memorandum on Persons with Limited English Proficiency, language assistance should involve ensuring that written materials and especially vital documents and forms are translated into the languages regularly encountered by the population [8, 63]. It is essential that patients receive the documents translated into their preferred language. In order to ensure the best usability of such documents, providers should be sensitive to the fact that some patients communicate orally better in their mother tongue but prefer reading in the language of their schooling [8]. Patients who do not read should be offered adequate language assistance – audio or video recordings are suggested as alternatives to written translation, also to be considered when a translation is needed to a language that does not have a commonly used written form (for instance, Navajo or Hmong) [8].

To provide patients with non-dominant language preference with full access to health information or instructions, relevant texts should be translated in advance rather than sight-translated by an interpreter as the latter is more ephemeral and less likely to contribute to clear communication and complete comprehension [8]. While simple instructions can be sight-translated, educational materials and documents containing background information are not suitable for sight translation and need to be translated in writing [8]. Moreover, healthcare materials should be translated by adequately skilled professionals – translators with medical backgrounds handle lay texts differently from trained translators. The former may tend to produce less comprehensible and thus less lay-friendly texts as they use more terms of Latin and Greek origin and nominalizations – two features that detract from text readability [34]. Moreover, interpreters should not be asked to provide on-the-spot written translation, i.e., produce an instant written translation of a document they have just been presented (which should not be confused with sight translation when an interpreter reads a document and provides an oral account of its contents) [8].

Using images can help bridge communication gaps between patients and healthcare providers, and images can be helpful in translated texts. However, they need to be adequately selected in terms of focus on a given medical concept and sensitivity to cultural differences – various images, icons, or body language can be interpreted differently by different individuals and cultures [64]. Patients have been shown not to have confidence in healthcare materials if they do not reflect their identities [64].

Although the format in which original and translated health information is presented can also affect its accessibility, institutions often fail to ensure that patients receive their preferred format [65]. The majority of users prefer reading paper leaflets, but a considerable number of patients prefer them in large print, and some prefer a combination of large print and an audio recording, with groups of patients who would rather only use recordings [65]. That needs to be especially taken into consideration in the case of persons with visual impairment, speakers of languages that do not have written forms, or persons with low literacy. When such materials are prepared for blind patients, relevant audio description should be included, for example, to relate the shape of the medicine (e.g., an oval pill) or an image in the corresponding paper format for other patients. A significant amount of health information can be accessed online, which also opens access opportunities for persons with disabilities. Although patients seem to prefer, for instance, PILs in paper form, they are fairly positive toward reading them online [66].

In the absence of translated materials or translators who could prepare them, medical providers can and do seek other methods. There have been attempts to remove language barriers by using machine translation, and there is growing interest in machine translation of both speech to text and text to text. Most studies concern the English-Spanish language pair [67]. So far, the usability of machine translation for healthcare has proved problematic due to insufficient accuracy [68] and inconsistent results between languages, for example, producing better quality translation in the English-Spanish language pair than for the English-Armenian pair [69]. Consequently, at present, machine translation cannot be treated as an independent, fully reliable healthcare translation tool. Before it can be used in communication in multilingual healthcare settings, machine translation has to be improved in terms of accuracy and evaluation standards [67].

Recommendations for package information leaflets

The studies on leaflet usability show that patient comprehension of PILs is still a challenge [43]. On the one hand, the European Union regulations which define leaflet structure do not guarantee leaflet usability. On the other hand, leaflets can be improved by following Document Design principles within the existing regulatory framework [70]. The guidelines on PILs seem insufficiently detailed in terms of content and layout, and more attention could be paid to the translation of PILs and user testing in multiple languages [43]. The mandated structure should not only focus on understanding but also the ease of finding information [36].

The recommendations for improving PIL comprehensibility include reducing the visual length by means of reducing or deleting information that is not relevant to patients, such as information on all available pack sizes and doses, changing the design, and using landscape layout [43]. Other recommendations advise using booklet format and larger font [43]. The problems with length and font size are even more accentuated in the case of multilingual PILs used in countries with more than one official language – a separate leaflet is recommended for each language [43]. Including risk-benefit information is also listed as a vital issue in patients' decision-making process [43]. The language used to describe risks should be neutral and informative rather than activating or emotional [59].

The parties responsible for developing leaflets should design them based on valid data about the target readers' actual practical skills and the manner in which a leaflet is used, plan multiple versions to cater for the needs of patients that would find complex leaflets not usable, conduct consumer testing, introduce revisions to improve readability and usability [39]. Testing should also encompass evaluating the degree of anxiety provoked in patients when reading risk information as the negative emotional response may prevent patients from reading the leaflet carefully and retaining risk-benefit information [59].

Australian Consumer Medicine Information leaflets are also subject to evaluation and a fair amount of criticism – according to recommendations, changes should be made to the layout, style, and information design of the printed leaflet, lexicon and terminology should be updated and standardized, a template should be developed for over-the-counter medicines, and stakeholders should be more sensitive toward differences in health literacy across the patient spectrum [71].

Striving to improve the lay-friendliness, readability, and usability of translated texts for patients concerns other genres, too. In general, the expectation is that texts for patients, including websites and medicine labels, should be useful, desirable, findable, accessible, and credible [72]. That means that content should be original and fulfill a need, and websites must be easy to use and navigate and accessible to people with disabilities [72]. Regarding medicine labels, the content should be similar for drug products of the same class and should support safe and effective use of the product. Labels should be readable and understandable, with easy-to-find elements, and written in a manner that is suitable for patients with lower health literacy [72].

As demonstrated in studies, improving lay-friendliness of PILs and other materials for patients requires readability testing of templates and translated documents before they are used [73]. Readability can be checked in pilot studies with comprehension questions with participants representing diverse patients. Readability formulas are also used, for example, the Flesch-Kincaid formula or Simple Measure of Gobbledygook (SMOG), which are based on the length of words and sentences used in a particular text [24, 74]. Other metrics also include evaluating familiar versus unusual syllable types and stress patterns [75].

Intralingual translation

As already emphasized, complex medical texts are not lay-friendly, a problem that is aggravated by low literacy or low health literacy. That is why such texts should be and sometimes are adapted to the cognitive, communicative, and social needs of lay readers. This process can be referred to as intralingual translation [35, 76] or if the adaptation involves creating a different text type – intergeneric translation or genre shift [35, 37, 38]. One of the most prominent features of intralingual translation is determinologization [35], whereby a text is reformulated and recontextualized to make the concepts described in the text relevant and comprehensible to lay readers. Determinologization can be achieved through a range of strategies, including using synonyms (including more popular terms) or hyperonyms (words of a more general meaning), explanation, definition, exemplification, illustration, analogy, or comparison [35]. Intralingual translation also involves personalizing information through using personal pronouns and identifying the subject [35]. It is also connected with structural and syntactic simplification, using verbs instead of noun phrases, synthesizing information, or expanding relevant information for the target reader [35, 37, 38]. Health providers and medical translators also need to be sensitive to dialect variations and make sure that texts are adapted to fit specific geographical, social, and temporal contexts with which their recipients are familiar [64]. The strategies used in intralingual translation (within one language) can be applied in interlingual translation (between two languages) in producing lay-friendly target texts.

Conclusion

In the context of healthcare, translation bridges communication gaps between providers and linguistically diverse populations. That is why providers should be sensitive to potential problems in accessing healthcare experienced by patients with nondominant language preferences [77] and counteract them by employing adequate financing mechanisms to ensure language assistance from qualified medical translators [78]. In turn, the tasks of medical translators include adequately adapting text content, writing style, and format. What is also much needed is clear guidance and training for medical translators. Ensuring comprehensible and lay-friendly translation and formats usable by patients with nondominant language preference is a prerequisite to accessible healthcare. It also helps build patient-centered care where human dignity and rights are effectively respected.

Highlights

- Language discordance between patients and healthcare staff impedes access to healthcare services and affects clinical outcomes.
- Quality healthcare translation of written texts can help address the challenges arising from language discordance especially if it is complimented with interpreting or – whenever possible – language-concordant healthcare professionals for effective verbal communication.
- The challenges of healthcare translation include shifts in register (i.e., the use of less lay-friendly language), omissions of text which affect the comprehension of the text, and changes of meaning due to terminological errors.
- Healthcare translation training should cover genre-specific features of commonly encountered documents with emphasis on lay-friendliness of the translated texts.

REFERENCES

1. Al-Sharifi, F., Winther Frederiksen, H., Knold Rossau, H. et al. (2019). Access to cardiac rehabilitation and the role of language barriers in the provision of cardiac rehabilitation to migrants. *BMC Health Serv. Res.* 19 (1): 223.
2. Tip, L.K., Brown, R., Morrice, L. et al. (2019). Improving refugee well-being with better language skills and more intergroup contact. *Soc. Psychol. Personal. Sci.* 10 (2): 144–151.
3. Feinberg, I., O'Connor, M.H., Owen-Smith, A. et al. (2020). The relationship between

refugee health status and language, literacy, and time spent in the United States. *Health Lit. Res. Pract.* 4 (4): 230–237.
4. Shrestha-Ranjit, J., Payne, D., Koziol-McLain, J. et al. (2020). Availability, accessibility, acceptability, and quality of interpreting services to refugee women in New Zealand. *Qual. Health Res.* 30 (11): 1697–1709.
5. Saito, S., Harris, M.F., Long, K.M. et al. (2021). Response to language barriers with patients from refugee background in general practice in Australia: findings from the OPTIMISE study. *BMC Health Serv. Res.* 21 (1): 921.
6. Jaeger, F.N., Pellaud, N., Laville, B., and Klauser, P. (2019). The migration-related language barrier and professional interpreter use in primary health care in Switzerland. *BMC Health Serv. Res.* 19 (1): 429.
7. Bowen, S. (2001). *Language Barriers in Access to Health Care*. 120 p.
8. NCIHC (2009). *SIGHT TRANSLATION AND WRITTEN TRANSLATION Guidelines for Healthcare Interpreters [Internet]*. National Council on Interpreting in Health Care. https://www.ncihc.org/assets/documents/publications/Translation_Guidelines_for_Interpreters_FINAL042709.pdf.
9. Chesterman, A. (2016). *Memes of Translation*, 1–237.
10. Chesterman, A. (2017). The name and nature of translator studies. *HJLCB.* 42: 13–22.
11. Holmes, J. (1988). *The Name and Nature of Translation Studies*, Translated. Papers on literary translation and translation studies. 2, 67–80. Amsterdam and Atlanta: Rodopi.
12. Aixelá, J.F. (2010). Una revisión de la bibliografía sobre traducción e interpretación médica recogida en BITRA (Bibliografía de Interpretación y Traducción). *Panace.* 11 (32): 151–160.
13. Montalt, V., Zethsen, K.K., and Karwacka, W. (2018). Medical translation in the 21st century - challenges and trends. *MonTI.* (10): 27–42.
14. Fischbach, H. (ed.) (1998). *Translation and Medicine [Internet]*. Amsterdam: John Benjamins Publishing Company (American Translators Association Scholarly Monograph Series; vol. X). http://www.jbe-platform.com/content/books/9789027283269 (accessed 6 June 2022).
15. Sousa, V.D. and Rojjanasrirat, W. (2011). Translation, adaptation and validation of instruments or scales for use in cross-cultural health care research: a clear and user-friendly guideline: validation of instruments or scales. *J. Eval. Clin. Pract.* 17 (2): 268–274.
16. Karwacka, W. (2014). Quality assurance in medical translation. *J. Spec. Transl.* 21: 19–34.
17. Congost-Maestre, N. and Lor, M. (2020). Sociocultural issues in adapting Spanish health survey translation: The case of the Quality of Well-Being Scale (QWB-SA). In: *The Essential Role of Language in Survey Research*, 203.
18. Colina, S., Marrone, N., Ingram, M., and Sánchez, D. (2017). Translation quality assessment in Health Research: a functionalist alternative to back-translation. *Eval. Health Prof.* 40 (3): 267–293.
19. Han, C. (2020). Translation quality assessment: a critical methodological review. *Translator* 26 (3): 257–273.
20. Lauscher, S. (2000). Translation quality assessment: where can theory and practice meet? *Translator* 6 (2): 149–168.
21. Behr, D. (2017). Assessing the use of back translation: the shortcomings of back translation as a quality testing method. *Int. J. Soc. Res. Methodol.* 20 (6): 573–584.
22. Ozolins, U., Hale, S., Cheng, X. et al. (2020). Translation and back-translation methodology in health research – a critique. *Expert Rev. Pharmacoecon. Outcomes Res.* 20 (1): 69–77.
23. Colina, S. (2019). Quality, translation. In: *Routledge Encyclopedia of Translation Studies*, 458–463. Routledge.
24. Karwacka, W. (2021). Quality, accessibility and readability in medical translation. In: *The Routledge Handbook of Translation and Health*, 80–95. Routledge.
25. Honig, H.G. (1997). Positions, power and practice: functionalist approaches and translation quality assessment. *Curr. Issues Lang. Soc.* 4 (1): 6–34.

26. Chesterman, A. (1996). On Similarity. *Targets* 8 (1): 159–164.
27. Nida, E.A. (1964). *Toward a Science of Translation*. Brill Leiden.
28. Koller, W. (1995). The concept of equivalence and the object of translation studies. *Targets* 7 (2): 191–222.
29. Nord, C. (1991). Scopos, loyalty, and translational conventions. *Targets* 3 (1): 91–109.
30. House, J. (2014). Translation quality assessment: past and present. In: *Translation: A Multidisciplinary Approach*, 241–264. Springer.
31. Brelsford, K.M., Ruiz, E., and Beskow, L. (2018). Developing informed consent materials for non-English-speaking participants: an analysis of four professional firm translations from English to Spanish. *Clin. Trials* 15 (6): 557–566.
32. Zehnalová, J. (2013). Tradition and trends in translation quality assessment. In: *Tradition and Trends in Trans-Language Communication*, 41–58. Olomouc: Univerzita Palackého.
33. Nisbeth, B.M. (2017). When translation competence is not enough: a focus group study of medical translators. *Z. MetaIlkd.* 62 (2): 396–414.
34. Nisbeth Jensen, M. and Korning Zethsen, K. (2021). Translation of patient information leaflets: trained translators and pharmacists-cum-translators – a comparison. *LANS-TTS* 11: 31–49. https://lans-tts.uantwerpen.be/index.php/LANS-TTS/article/view/295.
35. Muñoz-Miquel, A., Ezpeleta-Piorno, P., and Saiz-Hontangas, P. (2018). Intralingual translation in healthcare settings: strategies and proposals for medical translator training. *MonTI.* (10): 177–204.
36. Pander Maat, H., Lentz, L., and Raynor, D.K. (2015). How to test mandatory text templates: the European patient information leaflet. Pappalardo F, ed. *PLoS One* 10 (10): e0139250.
37. Montalt, V. and González, D.M. (2007). *Medical Translation Step by Step: Learning by Drafting*, 297. Manchester: Saint Jerome Publishing (Translation practices explained).
38. Ezpeleta, P.P. (2021). An example of genre shift in the medicinal product information genre system. *LANS-TTS* 11: 167–187. https://lans-tts.uantwerpen.be/index.php/LANS-TTS/article/view/302.
39. Gal, I. and Prigat, A. (2005). Why organizations continue to create patient information leaflets with readability and usability problems: an exploratory study. *Health Educ. Res.* 20 (4): 485–493.
40. Askehave, I. and Zethsen, K.K. (2003). Communication barriers in public discourse: the patient package insert. *DD* 4 (1): 22–41.
41. Lambrechts, A. and Verplaetse, H. (2018). Science popularization in English and translated Dutch patient information leaflets: specialized versus lay terminology and explicitation. *Parallèles* 30 (2): 35–52. https://www.paralleles.unige.ch/en/tous-les-numeros/numero-30-2/lambrechts-verplaetse.
42. Product-information templates [Internet]. (n.d.). The European Medicines Agency's (EMA) Working Group on Quality Review of Documents (QRD). https://www.ema.europa.eu/en/human-regulatory/marketing-authorisation/product-information/product-information-templates-human.
43. van Dijk, L., Monteiro, S.P., Vervloet, M. et al. (2014). *Study on the Package Leaflets and the Summaries of Product Characteristics of Medicinal Products for Human Use*, 141. European Union.
44. Pym, A. (2011). Website localizations. In: *The Oxford Handbook of Translation Studies [Internet]*. Oxford University Press. http://oxfordhandbooks.com/view/10.1093/oxfordhb/9780199239306.001.0001/oxfordhb-9780199239306-e-028 (accessed 17 June 2022).
45. Piacentini, T., O'Donnell, C., Phipps, A. et al. (2019). Moving beyond the 'language problem': developing an understanding of the intersections of health, language and immigration status in interpreter-mediated health encounters. *Lang. Intercult. Commun.* 19 (3): 256–271.
46. Floyd, A. and Sakellariou, D. (2017). Healthcare access for refugee women with

limited literacy: layers of disadvantage. *Int. J. Equity Health* 16 (1): 195.
47. Ponce, N.A., Hays, R.D., and Cunningham, W.E. (2006). Linguistic disparities in health care access and health status among older adults. *J. Gen. Intern. Med.* 21 (7): 786–791.
48. de Moissac, D. and Bowen, S. (2019). Impact of language barriers on quality of care and patient safety for official language minority francophones in Canada. *J. Patient Exp.* 6 (1): 24–32.
49. Lam, Y., Broaddus, E.T., and Surkan, P.J. (2013). Literacy and healthcare-seeking among women with low educational attainment: analysis of cross-sectional data from the 2011 Nepal demographic and health survey. *Int. J. Equity Health* 12 (1): 95.
50. Stewart, M.J., Neufeld, A., Harrison, M.J. et al. (2006). Immigrant women family caregivers in Canada: implications for policies and programmes in health and social sectors. *Health Soc. Care Community* 14 (4): 329–340.
51. LeVine, R.A., LeVine, S.E., Rowe, M.L., and Schnell-Anzola, B. (2004). Maternal literacy and health behavior: a Nepalese case study. *Soc. Sci. Med.* 58 (4): 863–877.
52. Bischoff, A. (2020). The evolution of a healthcare interpreting service mapped against the bilingual health communication model: a historical qualitative case study. *Public Health Rev.* 41 (1): 19.
53. Berbel, E.C. (2020). Challenges and difficulties of translation and interpreting in the migration and refugee crisis in Germany. *Open Linguist.* 6 (1): 162–170.
54. Badziński, A. (2019). Problems in medical translation among professional and non-professional translators: collocations as a key issue. *Beyond Philol.* (16/4): 157–177.
55. Azari, R. and Halim, S.A. (2018). *Translating Vague Language in Patient Information Leaflets*. Second Swiss Conference on Barrier-free Communication. https://bfc.unige.ch/files/4915/5170/2356/Azari_Halimi_BFC2018.pdf.
56. Kotovicz, F., Getzin, A., and Vo, T. (2018). Challenges of refugee health care: perspectives of medical interpreters, case managers, and pharmacists. *J. Patient Cent. Res. Rev.* 5: 28–35.
57. Breiding, H.M. (2019). Sexual orientation and gender identity rights lost in translation? *lambda* 23 (3–4): 122–145.
58. Payne, S., Large, S., Jarrett, N., and Turner, P. (2000). Written information given to patients and families by palliative care units: a national survey. *Lancet* 355 (9217): 1792.
59. Herber, O.R., Gies, V., Schwappach, D. et al. (2014). Patient information leaflets: informing or frightening? A focus group study exploring patients' emotional reactions and subsequent behavior towards package leaflets of commonly prescribed medications in family practices. *BMC Fam. Pract.* 15 (1): 163.
60. Antal, H., Bunnell, H.T., McCahan, S.M. et al. (2017). A cognitive approach for design of a multimedia informed consent video and website in pediatric research. *J. Biomed. Inform.* 66: 248–258.
61. Quinn, S.C., Garza, M.A., Butler, J. et al. (2012). Improving informed consent with minority participants: results from researcher and community surveys. *J. Empir. Res. Hum. Res. Ethics* 7 (5): 44–55.
62. George, S., Duran, N., and Norris, K. (2014). A systematic review of barriers and facilitators to minority research participation among African Americans, Latinos, Asian Americans, and Pacific islanders. *Am. J. Public Health* 104 (2): e16–e31.
63. Guidance Memorandum (2000). *Title VI Prohibition against National Origin Discrimination – Persons with Limited English Proficiency*. Office for Civil Rights, Department of Health and Human Services.
64. Tercedor-Sánchez, M. and López-Rodríguez, C.I. (2021). Access to health in an intercultural setting: the role of corpora and images in grasping term variation. *LANS-TTS* 11: 247–268. https://lans-tts.uantwerpen.be/index.php/LANS-TTS/article/view/306.
65. Thurston, M., Thurston, A., and Henderson, C. (n.d.). *The Accessibility of Health Information for Blind and Partially Sighted People [Internet]*. Centre for Educational and Psychosocial Research for

RNIB Scotland. www.rnib.org.uk/sites/default/files/accessibility_healthcare_information.pdf.

66. Hammar, T., Nilsson, A.L., and Hovstadius, B. (2016). Patients' views on electronic patient information leaflets. *Pharm. Pract. (Granada).* 14 (2): 702–702.

67. Dew, K.N., Turner, A.M., Choi, Y.K. et al. (2018). Development of machine translation technology for assisting health communication: a systematic review. *J. iomed. Inform.* 1 (85): 56–67.

68. Patil, S. and Davies, P. (2014). Use of Google translate in medical communication: evaluation of accuracy. *BMJ* 15 (349): g7392.

69. Taira, B.R., Kreger, V., Orue, A., and Diamond, L.C. (2021). A pragmatic assessment of Google translate for emergency department instructions. *J. Gen. Intern. Med.* 36: 3361–3365. https://doi.org/10.1007/s11606-021-06666-z.

70. Pander Maat, H. and Lentz, L. (2010). Improving the usability of patient information leaflets. *Patient Educ. Couns.* 80 (1): 113–119.

71. ThinkPlace Australia, The University of Sydney (2019). *Usability Evaluation of Consumer Medicine Information (CMI) Documents. Insights and Recommendations Report [Internet].* Australian Government Department of Health The Therapeutic Goods Administration Report No.: 1.2. www.tga.gov.au/sites/default/files/improved-consumer-medicine-information-template-report.pdf.

72. Soller, R.W. (2015). Functionality of drug label warnings defined post-marketing by user experience. *SelfCare.* 6 (2): 5.

73. Wolf, A., Fuchs, J., and Schweim, H.G. (2014). Readability of the European QRD template the European QRD template version 8 in comparison to its predecessor and a shorter model template. *Pharm. Ind.* 76 (8): 1312–1322.

74. Wang, L.W., Miller, M.J., Schmitt, M.R., and Wen, F.K. (2013). Assessing readability formula differences with written health information materials: application, results, and recommendations. *Res. Soc. Adm. Pharm.* 9 (5): 503–516.

75. Pires, C., Cavaco, A., and Vigário, M. (2017). Towards the definition of linguistic metrics for evaluating text readability. *J. Quant. Linguist.* 24 (4): 319–349.

76. Zethsen, K.K. (2008). Beyond translation proper – extending the field of translation studies. *TTR.* 20 (1): 281–308.

77. Wolz, M.M. (2015). Language barriers: challenges to quality healthcare. *Int. J. Dermatol.* 54 (2): 248–250.

78. Chen, A.H., Youdelman, M.K., and Brooks, J. (2007). The legal framework for language access in healthcare settings: title VI and beyond. *J. Gen. Intern. Med.* 22 (S2): 362–367.

9 Health Literacy and Plain Language

SUAD GHADDAR

Introduction

The World Health Organization (WHO), along with many governmental health agencies around the world, recognizes limited health literacy as a serious public health issue with significant implications for the health of individuals, communities, and corresponding healthcare costs [1, 2]. One of the most widely used health literacy definitions is "the degree to which individuals have the capacity to obtain, process, and understand basic health information and services needed to make appropriate health decisions" [3]. It is generally classified into three types that reflect various levels of skills and abilities to participate effectively in the health system. These are: *basic/functional health literacy*, which refers to basic reading and writing skills necessary for functioning effectively in health situations; *communicative/interactive health literacy*, which refers to more advanced literacy and cognitive skills that, in combination with social skills, are used to actively participate in health situations; and *critical health literacy*, which refers to more advanced cognitive skills which, along with social skills, are needed to critically analyze health information and apply it to exert greater control over one's health [4].

More recently, the definition of health literacy was reevaluated to reflect the progress in health literacy research and practice and the growing recognition of health literacy as a byproduct of individual-level as well as system-level characteristics. The new definitions are [5]:

Personal health literacy is the degree to which individuals have the ability to find, understand, and use information and services to inform health-related decisions and actions for themselves and others.

Organizational health literacy is the degree to which organizations equitably enable individuals to find, understand, and use information and services to inform health-related decisions and actions for themselves and others.

The Handbook of Language in Public Health and Healthcare, First Edition.
Edited by Pilar Ortega, Glenn Martínez, Maichou Lor, and A. Susana Ramírez.
© 2024 John Wiley & Sons, Inc. Published 2024 by John Wiley & Sons, Inc.

Prevalence of limited health literacy

Limited health literacy is a worldwide public health issue. In the United States, the 2003 National Assessment of Adult Literacy [6] revealed that approximately 36% of American adults were estimated to have only basic or below basic health literacy skills. Health literacy levels were lower among adults who were older, had lower educational attainment, were living below the poverty level, were from racially/ethnically minoritized groups, and spoke languages other than English before starting school. In Europe, results from the 2011 European health literacy survey reveal that limited health literacy impacts close to half the population in eight countries, with substantial differences reported across countries (e.g., 29% in the Netherlands versus 62% in Bulgaria), and with a clear social gradient – low income, low social status, low education, and old age were strong predictors of limited health literacy [7]. A report from the Organization for Economic Co-operation and Development, which includes a wide range of European and non-European countries (e.g., Australia, Canada, Israel, Japan, and Turkey), paints a similar picture, with a third of the population in 18 countries and half in 12 countries being at risk of limited health literacy [8].

Health literacy and health outcomes

Research over the past three decades has established the association between limited health literacy and a myriad of poor health outcomes [9]. Individuals with limited health literacy report lower use of preventive health services [10–12], less knowledge about one's disease [13], worse disease management skills [14], lower medication adherence [15], higher utilization of unnecessary healthcare services [16], increased risk of hospitalization [17–19], higher medical costs [20], poorer health status [11, 16, 21], and higher all-cause mortality rates [22]. It is estimated that the poor health outcomes associated with limited health literacy translate into at least 3–5% of total healthcare costs per year in the United States [23]; this would amount to $123–205 billion based on the 2020 national health expenditure data [24].

The organization of this chapter reflects the evolving nature of health literacy given our growing understanding of its multidimensional nature (Historical Development and Theoretical Framework) and the rapidly changing contexts within which its impact can be felt (Critical Issues and Topics). The chapter concludes with a set of recommendations (Recommendations for Research, Education, and Practice). Integral to these recommendations is the recognition of the various stakeholders who can impact health literacy (individuals, health providers, health systems, and policymakers at local, state, national, and international health agencies). Throughout, the chapter highlights the role that plain language can play in addressing limited health literacy and the areas where the needs of culturally and linguistically diverse groups represent unique challenges and opportunities.

While health literacy is an international public health issue with no geographical boundaries, the information presented in this chapter focuses primarily on the United States context. This focus reflects the United States' leading role in producing the majority of health literacy research and in building collaborative international networks [25, 26]. This focus, however, should not take away from the large body of work and efforts taking place around the world [26]; Australia, Canada, and England are major contributors to health literacy research, [25] and their governments have led multiple national initiatives that recognize health literacy and its contribution to health outcomes.

Historical development and theoretical framework

The 1990s marked recognition of health literacy as an issue that warrants investigation and assessment, as evidence was mounting in support of its impact on a variety of health outcomes [18, 27–32]. The first decade of the new millennium built on that evidence as health literacy research expanded to further understand its multiple facets and to explore the causal pathways through which health literacy impacts health outcomes. In 2001, the WHO recognized health literacy as a key to increase one's control over their health and to improve disease management. The new millennium also marked various policy initiatives that moved health literacy to the mainstream of healthcare practice [33].

Health literacy initiatives

In the United States, one of the first major initiatives recognizing the importance of health literacy was Healthy People 2010 which identified health literacy as a pathway to improving health communication [34]. This triggered the first national assessment of health literacy which revealed that more than a third (36%) of adults had basic (22%) or below basic (14%) health literacy [6]. The publication of the Institute of Medicines' *Health Literacy: A Prescription to End Confusion* [1] marked a key national-level recognition of health literacy as a major public health issue. Healthy People 2020 further highlighted advancing health literacy skills as an objective that promises to exert "a positive impact on health, healthcare, and health equity" [35]. Healthy People 2030 more clearly articulated health literacy as a high-impact priority area and as an overarching goal to eliminate health disparities and achieve health equity [36].

Commitment to health literacy at the federal level was further supported by the release of the *National Action Plan to Improve Health Literacy* in 2010 [37]. The *Plan* recognized the need for a multisector/multistakeholder approach to address limited health literacy. Its goals reflected the need for (a) accurate, accessible, and actionable health information; (b) a transformed healthcare system environment that promotes access to health information and services; (c) accurate, standards-based, and developmentally appropriate health information and curricula in the education system; (d) partnerships and policy-level changes; and (e) research dissemination to support the use of evidence-based health literacy practices and interventions. The *Plan* further recognized that limited health literacy and limited English proficiency (LEP) often coexist and highlighted the need for culturally and linguistically appropriate interventions and health information services that focus on the intersection of health literacy *and* language [38].

The Patient Protection and Affordable Care Act (ACA) of 2010, which aims to increase access and affordability of healthcare coverage in the United States, acknowledged health literacy's role in accessing care and in ensuring the success of implementing healthcare reform [39]. This is reflected in multiple provisions with either direct or indirect reference to health literacy [40] and was supported by expert consensus and later evidence that highlighted the impact of limited health literacy on ACA awareness and on obtaining healthcare coverage [41–44]. In 2016, the ACA's final rule ensured enhanced protections for marginalized populations and clarified language access requirements for individuals with LEP, such as taking reasonable steps to provide professional language assistance services [45]. These protections, however, were later reduced under the Trump administration [46].

At the state and local levels, there has been a growing number of collaborations between different stakeholders in academia, state and local governments, and nonprofit organizations. A comprehensive list and corresponding links to health literacy activities by state are available on the website of the Centers for Disease Control and Prevention (CDC) [47].

Internationally, many countries have similar initiatives and policy statements. For example, in Australia, several initiatives explicitly include health literacy within their frameworks (e.g., Australia's Health 2020, National Safety and Quality Health Service Standards); in China, the government consistently targets the promotion of health literacy in its strategic plans (e.g., Healthy China Initiative [2019–2030]).

Plain language initiatives

Plain language is clear communication that one's audience can understand the *first time* they hear or read it [48]. Using plain language is recognized as a key strategy to address limited health literacy [49], especially as evidence is mounting on the effectiveness of this approach at improving medication comprehension and administration [50–52], enhancing understanding of informed consent materials in clinical trials [53], and at improving health professionals' communication skills [54–56], among others.

In the United States, the Plain Writing Act of 2010 [57] represents a major initiative to promote clear communication. The Act was further supported by the Federal Plain Language Guidelines designed to ensure that governmental agencies write clearly so that users can "find what they need, understand what they find, [and] use what they find to meet their needs" [58]. While the guidelines did not directly address the needs of culturally and linguistically diverse groups, the first guideline focused on identifying and writing for one's audience and on addressing separate audiences separately.

Several countries have supported plain language initiatives including England, Australia, Canada, Sweden, Finland, etc. Among the largest efforts is the European Commission's 2010 Clear Writing for Europe campaign [59] with a variety of resources to support shorter and simpler writing in multiple languages (e.g., the *How to write clearly* booklet [60]).

Health literacy conceptual frameworks

Several conceptual frameworks have been developed to describe the relationship between health literacy and health outcomes. The plurality of these frameworks reflects the multi-dimensional nature of health literacy, the variety of contexts within which it applies, as well as the growing body of evidence on the factors associated with health literacy skills and their effect on health outcomes. The following section presents only two frameworks that reflect two relatively distinct approaches to depicting this relationship. For a list of additional frameworks, see Sørensen et al. [61]; Squiers et al. [62], and Cudjoe et al. [63].

Paasche-Orlow and Wolf (Figure 9.1; [64]) present an evidence-based causal model that focuses on the pathways through which health literacy impacts health outcomes. The model identifies three pathways and the corresponding patient and system/provider/extrinsic factors for each. The three pathways are access and utilization of healthcare, provider-patient interaction, and self-care.

The Integrated Model of Health Literacy (Figure 9.2, [61]) incorporates prior health literacy research and evidence to arrive at a comprehensive framework. The model

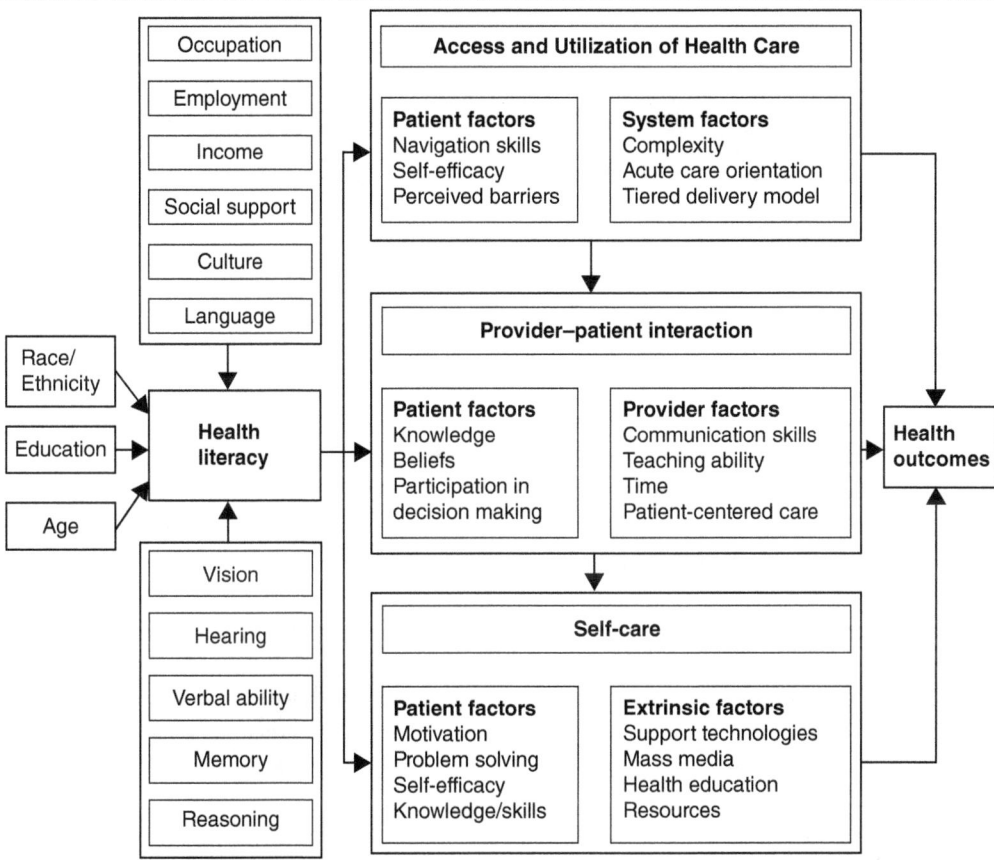

Figure 9.1 Health Literacy Framework as developed by Paasche-Orlow MK, Wolf MS. The causal pathways linking health literacy to health outcomes. *Source:* Paasche-Orlow and Wolf [61].

combines (a) the main dimensions of health literacy (the competencies of accessing, understanding, appraising, and applying health information); (b) distal (societal and environmental determinants) and proximal factors (personal and situational determinants) that impact health literacy; and (c) the pathways that link health literacy to health outcomes (health service use, health behavior, participation, and equity). These competencies are utilized in three domains in one's capacity as a patient in the healthcare setting, an at-risk person in the disease prevention system, and a citizen in relation to health promotion efforts in a variety of community, workplace, educational, and political settings. The model also takes into account that health literacy is a dynamic concept that evolves over the lifecourse as one's cognitive and psychosocial skills develop or deteriorate, as experiences with the healthcare setting expand, and as contextual demands change over time.

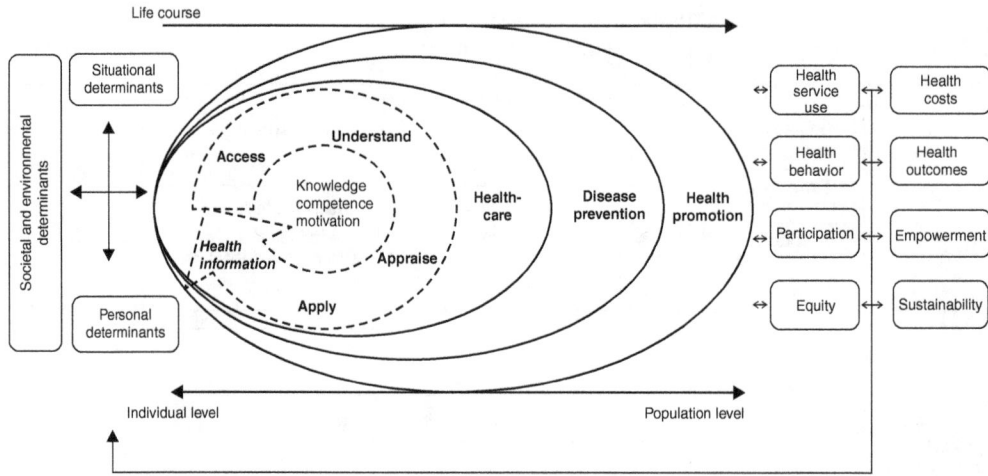

Figure 9.2 Integrated Model of Health Literacy. *Source:* Figure from Health literacy and public health: a systematic review and integration of definitions and models by Sørensen et al. [61], licensed under a Creative Commons Attribution License 2.0.

Critical issues and topics

While our knowledge of health literacy and its impact on health outcomes has considerably expanded over the past 30+ years, several critical issues remain. Some of these issues stem from the multitude of definitions and conceptual frameworks, each of which highlights different competencies, dimensions, and contexts. Others reflect the rapidly changing health environment which presents an ever-evolving set of demands on the healthcare consumer.

Health literacy measurement

Multiple measures exist to assess health literacy and its various dimensions [65–67]. Early tools focused on assessing reading abilities (e.g., Rapid Estimate of Adult Literacy in Medicine (REALM) [29]), numeracy skills (e.g., Newest Vital Sign [68]), and functional literacy in the healthcare setting (e.g., Test of Functional Health Literacy in Adults [69]). Later tools aimed to capture health literacy's various conceptual dimensions (e.g., Health Literacy Questionnaire [70]; Health Literacy Management Scale [71]) and/or the specific demands of a disease, sociodemographic group, or context (e.g., Health Literacy of Caregivers Scale – Cancer [72]). Over time, the most commonly used measurement tools were validated in different populations and across a wide spectrum of languages – alas with considerable variation and less-than-optimal quality evidence [73]. For a comprehensive list of health literacy measures, the Health Literacy Tool Shed provides an online database of over 100 measures, including each measure's description, source, and psychometric properties [74].

Among the main challenges for health literacy measurement is the tension between the need for a screening tool that is quick to administer in clinical settings yet comprehensive enough to capture the complex conceptual dimensions of health literacy. This has resulted in a wide spectrum of tools that range from a single question with less than a minute of administration time [75] to ones that are comprised of multiple questions/ activities requiring up to 60 min for administration. Other concerns relate to utilizing objective, performance-based measures (e.g., REALM) versus subjective, self-reported measures (e.g., Single Item Literacy Screener [75]). Reviews of health literacy measurement tools reveal: (a) variation in the underlying conceptual frameworks, if any; (b) poorly defined scoring categories; (c) variation in instrument association with existing measures; and (d) lack of reliability assessment for most instruments [65, 73, 76]. While newer tools have attempted to address some of these shortcomings, the continuing proliferation of tools makes it difficult to compare results across prevalence and intervention studies.

Most health literacy measurements, with a few exceptions, were developed in English. To meet the needs of linguistically diverse communities, tools have been translated from English into different languages, with Spanish as the most common non-English language in the United States. However, many of these translated tools fail to take into account that an individual's health literacy in their preferred language might be considerably different from their health literacy in English. For example, a commonly used screening question about a patient's confidence in filling out medical forms does not clarify the language of the forms; studies that clarified the languages of the forms have led to better identification of individuals with limited health literacy relative to studies that did not include the clarification [77].

To advance the science of health literacy measurement, recommendations include (a) developing a comprehensive unified health literacy conceptual framework; (b) aligning measures with health literacy definitions; (c) utilizing rigorous and robust research methods to empirically test frameworks and measures; (d) using a tiered approach to measuring health literacy; and (e) validating measures in linguistically and culturally diverse groups [78, 79].

Digital health

Recent years have witnessed rapid technological innovations that have allowed for the remote delivery of healthcare, use of web- and mobile-based applications for chronic disease self-management and monitoring, electronic communication with healthcare teams, electronic access to laboratory/test results, and among others. These innovations and corresponding system-level adoptions, however, have placed additional demands on both health consumers and health professionals and have assumed an engaged patient and caregiver with sufficient health literacy in the electronic health (eHealth) context.

To reflect the demands of these changes, the concept of eHealth literacy emerged to capture the skills needed to engage in the eHealth environment. It is commonly defined as "the ability to seek, find, understand and appraise health information from electronic sources and apply the knowledge gained to addressing or solving a health problem" [80]. Several frameworks capture the concept's additional dimensions. For example, the Lily model, in addition to traditional health literacy and numeracy skills, includes media, computer, science, and information literacies [80]; the Transactional Model of eHealth Literacy combines intrapersonal health literacy skills and eHealth task-oriented and user-oriented contextual factors [81].

Limited eHealth literacy and health literacy have been found to negatively impact the enrollment and use of eHealth services, including mobile technologies [82], patient portals [83–85], and online health information-seeking behavior [86]. For linguistically diverse populations, evidence reveals a digital language divide where LEP patients and their caregivers are less engaged in various eHealth service aspects; for example, they are less likely to utilize remote medication refill systems [87, 88], use mobile apps [89], electronically communicate with health professionals [90], have/use online patient portals [83, 91, 92]), and use video telemedicine visits [93].

Similar to health literacy measurement issues, eHealth literacy measurement tools capture a spectrum of skills, conceptual domains, and knowledge needed to engage in eHealth. Among the most widely used tools is the eHealth Literacy Scale (eHEALS), a self-administered eight-item scale where respondents rate their level of confidence in finding, evaluating, and using online health information [94]. The measure's psychometric properties have been extensively assessed in various languages, population groups, and contexts. However, since its publication in 2006, eHealth has considerably evolved to encompass more interactive dimensions that go beyond seeking health information online [95] and that require additional skills such as adding personal content, formulating and writing messages, assessing privacy implications, locating and interpreting health information in patient portals, etc. [96]. To capture these dimensions, new tools have been and continue to be developed (e.g., Transactional eHealth Literacy Instrument [97]) with different underlying conceptual frameworks, rendering comparability across studies problematic [67]. This is exacerbated by low-quality evidence supporting some of the instruments' validity and by inconsistencies in their factor structures [67].

Addressing the needs of limited eHealth/health literacy and linguistically diverse groups is essential to support an individual's ability to engage effectively with the eHealth environment. To our knowledge, there are currently no United States national policy initiatives that focus on the promotion of eHealth literacy. However, there are several opportunities that health organizations, health professionals, and communities can capitalize on to minimize the impact of limited eHealth literacy. For example, librarians are well positioned to provide eHealth literacy learning opportunities [98]; health professionals can capitalize on existing health literacy communication strategies and apply them within eHealth contexts; and health information website developers can apply plain language principles in designing website content, can engage target users during the development process, and can utilize visual aids and multimedia for a more engaging user experience [99]. Additionally, patient portals hold promise as a tool to promote health literacy through access to health information educational materials and facilitation of patient-provider communication [100, 101]. This, however, will require design features that support portal adoption and usability, especially by limited health literacy and LEP groups through user input, effective staff training, patient-centered and culturally tailored user training, multilingual portal platforms, compatibility of platforms for display on personal mobile devices, technological support, and discussion of privacy issues.

Public health emergency preparedness and response

Public health emergencies and their aftermath constantly highlight risk communication strategies as a key element that can mitigate or exacerbate the impact of such emergencies. Effective communication strategies and public health information campaigns require recognition of health literacy, language, and culture as integral components of emergency preparedness [102–104].

The disproportionate impact of natural disasters and public health emergencies on racially and ethnically minoritized populations, individuals with limited health literacy, and other marginalized groups highlights the inadequate preparedness in these communities and the failure of information dissemination strategies to consider culturally and linguistically appropriate communication tools. The aftermath of Hurricane Katrina led to the establishment of the National Consensus Panel on Emergency Preparedness and Cultural Diversity [105], which recognized factors related to culture, ethnicity, literacy, language, and trust as key to the effective implementation of public health preparedness programs [102]. The Panel published a diversity preparedness toolkit to provide guidance on integrating culturally and linguistically diverse communities into public health emergency preparedness [106].

The COVID-19 pandemic once again brought health literacy to the forefront as it underscored the importance of clear messaging, access to credible sources of health information, and the ability to critically appraise available information during public health crises. The large amount of misinformation propagated through social media and online platforms led the WHO to label the problem as an infodemic – overabundance of accurate and inaccurate information [107, 108]. The WHO's framework for managing infodemics during health emergencies advocated for programs and research agendas that boost critical thinking skills and promote health, eHealth, and media literacy across the population and throughout the life course [109–111]. An emerging body of research on COVID-19 supports health literacy as a cornerstone of pandemic preparedness, enabling people to critically assess the barrage of information during public health emergencies and facilitating the uptake of preventive actions [112–116].

Recommendations for research, education, and practice

Addressing limited health literacy requires a multipronged approach by multiple stakeholders. While earlier efforts have aimed to improve an individual's health literacy through health education interventions, more recent efforts have focused on ensuring a health-literate environment, systems, and workforce. These efforts recognize that health literacy is not only determined by individual competencies but that the healthcare environment's characteristics and demands determine to a great extent an individual's ability to navigate that environment, understand the information provided, and effectively interact with the healthcare system. Within such efforts, the special needs of linguistically diverse populations are frequently recognized and addressed.

At the individual level, research has established that well-designed single or multiple strategy interventions that are theoretically based and/or that emphasize skill building can be effective at improving the skills and knowledge to manage one's health and navigate the health environment and, in turn, can lead to changes in health behaviors [117, 118]. More recently, online health education interventions have also shown promise in improving health/eHealth literacy [119]. Most interventions, however, target functional health literacy and assess knowledge levels, with few assessing health outcomes [118, 120].

At the community level, several health literacy-based interventions have shown promise in improving the community's health knowledge. These interventions can be delivered in a variety of settings such as public libraries, adult education classes, schools, community centers, faith-based organizations, etc. [121]. However, the need remains for more systematically developed and experimentally designed interventions that are skills-based rather than task-based and that utilize valid and reliable health literacy tools suited for the community setting [122].

At the national level, policy initiatives constitute an important step in addressing limited health literacy. Primary among these in the United States are the Plain Writing Act of 2010 [57], the National Action Plan to Improve Health Literacy [37], and Healthy People 2030 [36]. In addition to the provisions related to linguistically diverse communities within these initiatives, the Department of Health and Human Services established in 2013 the Language Access Plan to ensure meaningful access by individuals with LEP to the Department's programs and activities [123]. The Plan outlines 10 essential elements related to oral language assistance services, written translations, policies and procedures, staff training, digital information, and among others.

At the hospital level, *The Health Literacy Environment of Hospitals and Health Centers* [124, 125] provides a comprehensive assessment tool to analyze and address health literacy-related structural barriers to healthcare access and navigation. The tool rates the hospital's organizational policies, practices, navigation, culture and language, and communication (print materials, forms, websites, and patient portals) through the lens of health literacy. The culture and language section focuses attention on the availability of prompt professional interpretation services and multilingual forms and webpages. It also highlights culturally competent communication and the rarely-addressed intersection of language and health literacy.

Other cultural and linguistic competence tools at the health system level include (a) the Cultural and Linguistic Competence Policy Assessment that aims to enhance service quality within culturally and linguistically diverse communities [126] and (b) the National Culturally and Linguistically Appropriate Services (CLAS) Standards that aim to provide a blueprint for implementing equitable, understandable, and respectful quality care and services that are responsive to the communication needs of culturally, linguistically, and health literacy-diverse communities [127].

At the practice level, the *Health Literacy Universal Precautions Toolkit* provides evidence-based guidance to primary care practices to ensure that systems are in place to promote understanding of health information by all patients [128]. The *Toolkit* includes 21 tools that aim to address and improve spoken communication, written communication, self-management and empowerment, and supportive systems. In terms of language-related health literacy issues, Tool 9 addresses language differences and provides several actions in this area (e.g., assessing language preferences and language assistance needs, using acceptable language assistance services, planning for interpreter services in advance, and providing written materials in patients' preferred languages).

Training the current and future health professions workforce in health-literate, culturally competent communication is key. Well-developed and well-delivered health literacy trainings have shown promise in improving health professional's verbal and written communication skills [54, 55, 129–131]. Rather than having standalone trainings, however, such trainings need to be integrated into health professions education and reinforced at multiple points in the curricula. Effective trainings are characterized by content that promotes clear communication strategies that use plain language and minimize medical jargon, fosters awareness of the needs of limited health literacy and linguistically and culturally diverse populations, promotes cultural competence skills, includes guidelines and strategies for communicating with persons with LEP, and employs interprofessional education activities that integrate communication professionals as team members. The *National Action Plan to Improve Health Literacy* [37] provides several strategies toward that end, highlighting the need for including coursework and training opportunities on health literacy as well as culturally and linguistically appropriate services in all health professions curricula. This needs to be supported by corresponding assessments and inclusion in licensure and continuing education requirements, respectively. In addition, diverse representation on the patient and provider ends is key to effective training along these dimensions. To support the existing health professions workforce, the CDC provides several online health literacy continuing education opportunities [132]. Similarly, there are a variety of continuing education opportunities through the Office of Minority Health in culturally and linguistically appropriate services [133].

Plain language tools

There are multiple plain language tools and guides to support people's understanding and to inform health literacy strategies in clinical and health settings. At the individual level, the Plain Language Medical Dictionary [134] provides plain language translations for high-level medical terms. At the practice and system levels, several tools (1) support the development of plain language materials (e.g., CDC's Simply Put [135], CDC Clear Communication Index [136], the Center for Medicare & Medicaid Services *Toolkit for Making Written Material Clear and Effective* [137]) and (2) allow organizations to quickly and objectively evaluate the audience suitability of their health information materials (e.g., Suitability Assessment of Materials [138], Patient Education Materials Assessment Tool [139], SMOG Readability Formula [140]). There are also various training opportunities such as those from the National Institutes of Health [141].

Conclusion

Health literacy is a complex multidimensional construct comprised of a set of functional, interactive, and critical thinking skills that enable an individual to find, understand, assess, and use information to support health-related decisions and actions and to navigate the health environment. Health literacy is not solely determined by individual abilities but by the demands of the healthcare environment as well.

Research has confirmed the high prevalence of limited health literacy and its association with a social gradient. Research has further established strong associations between limited health literacy and poor health outcomes highlighting the need for multisector interventions that simplify the demands of the healthcare environment as well as improve individual functional, interactive, and critical thinking skills.

While health literacy research has gained more prominence over the past three decades and has made important strides in advancing our knowledge, more nuanced work needs to (a) address the intersection of health literacy with language and culture; (b) implement theory-based, experimentally designed interventions that aim to improve health literacy and assess health outcomes; and (c) examine the cost-effectiveness of health literacy interventions.

The rapidly changing healthcare landscape and its corresponding demands require an engaged health consumer who can effectively navigate and interact with this environment and who can act as an informed participant in healthcare decisions. It also requires an environment that integrates health literacy, language, and culture in its delivery of quality health. Addressing these needs at the individual and system levels is key to reducing health disparities and achieving health equity and social justice for marginalized groups worldwide [142, 143].

Highlights

- Health literacy is an essential element to successfully navigate the healthcare environment, support sound health-related decisions, and ensure good health outcomes.
- National health literacy initiatives play an important role in championing health literacy and ensuring meaningful healthcare access for individuals with limited health literacy and those from linguistically and culturally diverse communities.
- Plain language tools in clinical practice and health system settings play an important role in addressing limited health literacy.
- Integrating health literacy training in health professions education ensures a healthcare workforce with health-literate, culturally competent communication skills that meet the needs of linguistically and culturally diverse groups.
- Health literacy research has to address the intersection of health literacy with language and culture and to support the identification of effective and cost-effective interventions through rigorous study design.

REFERENCES

1. Institute of Medicine Committee on Health L (2004). *Health Literacy: A Prescription to End Confusion* (ed. L. Nielsen-Bohlman, A.M. Panzer, and D.A. Kindig). Washington (DC): National Academies Press.
2. World Health Organization (2013). *Health Literacy the Solid Facts*. World Health Organization. https://apps.who.int/iris/bitstream/handle/10665/128703/e96854.pdf.
3. Ratzan, S., Parker, R., Selden, C., and Zorn, M. (2000). *National Library of Medicine Current Bibliographies in Medicine: Health Literacy*. Bethesda, MD: National Institutes of Health.
4. Nutbeam, D. (2000). Health literacy as a public health goal: a challenge for contemporary health education and communication strategies into the 21st century. *Health Promot. Int.* 15 (3): 259–267.
5. Office of Disease Prevention and Health Promotion (2022). *Health Literacy in Healthy People 2030 [Internet]*. U.S. Department of Health and Human Services. https://health.gov/our-work/national-health-initiatives/healthy-people/healthy-people-2030/health-literacy-healthy-people-2030.
6. Kutner, M.A. (2006). *The Health Literacy of America's Adults: Results from the 2003 National Assessment of Adult Literacy*. Washington, D.C: U.S. Dept. of Education, National Center for Education Statistics.
7. Sørensen, K., Pelikan, J.M., Röthlin, F. et al. (2015). Health literacy in Europe: comparative results of the European health literacy survey (HLS-EU). *Eur. J. Public Health* 25 (6): 1053–1058.
8. Moreira, L. (2018). *Health Literacy for People-Centred Care: Where Do OECD Countries Stand?* OECD Health Working Papers, No. 107. Paris: OECD Publishing. http://doi.org/10.1787/d8494d3a-en.
9. Dewalt, D.A., Berkman, N.D., Sheridan, S. et al. (2004). Literacy and health outcomes: a systematic review of the literature. *J. Gen. Intern. Med.* 19 (12): 1228–1239.
10. Scott, T.L., Gazmararian, J.A., Williams, M.V., and Baker, D.W. (2002). Health literacy and preventive health care use among Medicare enrollees in a managed care organization. *Med. Care* 40 (5): 395–404.
11. Bennett, I.M., Chen, J., Soroui, J.S., and White, S. (2009). The contribution of health literacy to disparities in self-rated health status and preventive health behaviors in older adults. *Ann. Fam. Med.* 7 (3): 204–211.
12. White, S., Chen, J., and Atchison, R. (2008). Relationship of preventive health practices and health literacy: a national study. *Am. J. Health Behav.* 32 (3): 227–242.

13. Gazmararian, J.A., Williams, M.V., Peel, J., and Baker, D.W. (2003). Health literacy and knowledge of chronic disease. *Patient Educ. Couns.* 51 (3): 267–275.
14. Mackey, L.M., Doody, C., Werner, E.L., and Fullen, B. (2016). Self-management skills in chronic disease management: what role does health literacy have? *Med. Decis. Making* 36 (6): 741–759.
15. Schönfeld, M.S., Pfisterer-Heise, S., and Bergelt, C. (2021). Self-reported health literacy and medication adherence in older adults: a systematic review. *BMJ Open* 11 (12): e056307.
16. Cho, Y.I., Lee, S.Y., Arozullah, A.M., and Crittenden, K.S. (2008). Effects of health literacy on health status and health service utilization amongst the elderly. *Soc. Sci. Med.* 66 (8): 1809–1816.
17. Baker, D.W., Gazmararian, J.A., Williams, M.V. et al. (2002). Functional health literacy and the risk of hospital admission among Medicare managed care enrollees. *Am. J. Public Health* 92 (8): 1278–1283.
18. Baker, D.W., Parker, R.M., Williams, M.V., and Clark, W.S. (1998). Health literacy and the risk of hospital admission. *J. Gen. Intern. Med.* 13 (12): 791–798.
19. Wu, J.R., Holmes, G.M., DeWalt, D.A. et al. (2013). Low literacy is associated with increased risk of hospitalization and death among individuals with heart failure. *J. Gen. Intern. Med.* 28 (9): 1174–1180.
20. Howard, D.H., Gazmararian, J., and Parker, R.M. (2005). The impact of low health literacy on the medical costs of Medicare managed care enrollees. *Am. J. Med.* 118 (4): 371–377.
21. Wolf, M.S., Gazmararian, J.A., and Baker, D.W. (2005). Health literacy and functional health status among older adults. *Arch. Intern. Med.* 165 (17): 1946–1952.
22. Baker, D.W., Wolf, M.S., Feinglass, J. et al. (2007). Health literacy and mortality among elderly persons. *Arch. Intern. Med.* 167 (14): 1503–1509.
23. Eichler, K., Wieser, S., and Brügger, U. (2009). The costs of limited health literacy: a systematic review. *Int. J. Public Health* 54 (5): 313–324.
24. CMS (2021). *National Health Expenditure Data 2020 [Internet]*. Centers for Medicare & Medicaid Services. https://www.cms.gov/Research-Statistics-Data-and-Systems/Statistics-Trends-and-Reports/NationalHealthExpendData.
25. Qi, S., Hua, F., Xu, S. et al. (2021). Trends of global health literacy research (1995-2020): analysis of mapping knowledge domains based on citation data mining. *PloS One* 16 (8): e0254988.
26. Roundtable on Health Literacy (2013). Board on population health and public health practice; Institute of Medicine. In: *Health Literacy: Improving Health, Health Systems, and Health Policy around the World: Workshop Summary*. Washington (DC): National Academies Press.
27. No authors listed (1999). Health literacy: report of the council on scientific affairs. Ad hoc committee on health literacy for the council on scientific affairs, American Medical Association. *JAMA* 281 (6): 552–557.
28. Davis, T.C., Michielutte, R., Askov, E.N. et al. (1998). Practical assessment of adult literacy in health care. *Health Educ. Behav.* 25 (5): 613–624.
29. Davis, T.C., Crouch, M.A., Long, S.W. et al. (1991). Rapid assessment of literacy levels of adult primary care patients. *Fam. Med.* 23 (6): 433–435.
30. Baker, D.W., Williams, M.V., Parker, R.M. et al. (1999). Development of a brief test to measure functional health literacy. *Patient Educ. Couns.* 38 (1): 33–42.
31. Gazmararian, J.A., Baker, D.W., Williams, M.V. et al. (1999). Health literacy among Medicare enrollees in a managed care organization. *JAMA* 281 (6): 545–551.
32. Williams, M.V., Parker, R.M., Baker, D.W. et al. (1995). Inadequate functional health literacy among patients at two public hospitals. *JAMA* 274 (21): 1677–1682.
33. Koh, H.K., Berwick, D.M., Clancy, C.M. et al. (2012). New federal policy initiatives to boost health literacy can help the nation move beyond the cycle of costly 'crisis care'. *Health Aff (Millwood)*. 31 (2): 434–443.
34. National Center for Health Statistics (2022). *Healthy People 2010*. Centers for Disease Control and Prevention. https://www.cdc.gov/nchs/healthy_people/hp2010.htm (accessed 1 January 2022).

35. National Center for Health Statistics (2022). *Healthy People 2020*. Centers for Disease Control and Prevention. https://www.cdc.gov/nchs/healthy_people/hp2020.htm (accessed 1 January 2022).
36. Office of Disease Prevention and Health Promotion (2022). *Healthy People 2030*. U.S. Department of Health and Human Services. https://health.gov/healthypeople (accessed 1 January 2022).
37. U.S. Department of Health and Human Services. (2010). *National Action Plan to Improve Health Literacy*. https://health.gov/sites/default/files/2019-09/Health_Literacy_Action_Plan.pdf (accessed 1 January 2022).
38. Sudore, R.L., Landefeld, C.S., Pérez-Stable, E.J. et al. (2009). Unraveling the relationship between literacy, language proficiency, and patient-physician communication. *Patient Educ. Couns.* 75 (3): 398–402.
39. Patient Protection and Affordable Care Act. 2010. Pub. L. No. 111–148. https://www.congress.gov/111/plaws/publ148/PLAW-111publ148.pdf (accessed 1 January 2022).
40. Somers, S.A. and Mahadevan, R. (2010). *Health Literacy Implications of the Affordable Care Act*. Center for Health Care Strategies, Inc.
41. Kostareva, U., Albright, C.L., Berens, E.M. et al. (2020). International perspective on health literacy and health equity: factors that influence the former Soviet Union immigrants. *Int. J. Environ. Res. Public Health* 17 (6): 1–20.
42. Ghaddar, S., Byun, J., and Krishnaswami, J. (2018). Health insurance literacy and awareness of the affordable care act in a vulnerable Hispanic population. *Patient Educ. Couns.* 101 (12): 2233–2240.
43. Braun, R.T., Barnes, A.J., Hanoch, Y., and Federman, A.D. (2018). Health literacy and plan choice: implications for Medicare managed care. *Health Lit Res Prac.* 2 (1): e40–e54.
44. National Academies of Sciences, Engineering, and Medicine (2017). *Health Insurance and Insights from Health Literacy: Helping Consumers Understand: Proceedings of a Workshop*. Washington, DC: National Academies Press https://doi.org/10.17226/24664.
45. Office of Civil Rights (2016). *Nondiscrimination in Health Programs and Activities [Internet]*. U.S. Department of Health and Human Services https://www.federalregister.gov/documents/2016/05/18/2016-11458/nondiscrimination-in-health-programs-and-activities (accessed 1 January 2022).
46. Musumeci, M., Kates, J., Dawson, L. et al. (2020). *The Trump Administration's Final Rule on Section 1557 Non-Discrimination Regulations under the ACA and Current Status 2020 [Internet]*. Kaiser Family Foundation. https://www.kff.org/racial-equity-and-health-policy/issue-brief/the-trump-administrations-final-rule-on-section-1557-non-discrimination-regulations-under-the-aca-and-current-status (accessed 1 January 2022).
47. Health Literacy (2021). *K-12 Literacy and Numeracy State Data [Internet]*. Centers for Disease Control and Prevention. https://www.cdc.gov/healthliteracy/statedata/index.html (accessed 1 January 2022).
48. plainlanguage.gov [Internet]. https://www.plainlanguage.gov/about/definitions (accessed 30 May 2022).
49. Stableford, S. and Mettger, W. (2007). Plain language: a strategic response to the health literacy challenge. *J. Public Health Policy* 28 (1): 71–93.
50. Smith, M.Y. and Wallace, L.S. (2013). Reducing drug self-injection errors: a randomized trial comparing a "standard" versus "plain language" version of patient instructions for use. *Res. Social Adm. Pharm.* 9 (5): 621–625.
51. Mohan, A., Riley, B., Schmotzer, B. et al. (2014). Improving medication understanding among Latinos through illustrated medication lists. *Am. J. Manag. Care* 20 (12): e547–e555.
52. Yin, H.S., Dreyer, B.P., van Schaick, L. et al. (2008). Randomized controlled trial of a pictogram-based intervention to reduce liquid medication dosing errors and improve adherence among caregivers of young children. *Arch. Pediatr. Adolesc. Med.* 162 (9): 814–822.
53. Kim, E.J. and Kim, S.H. (2015). Simplification improves understanding of informed consent information in clinical

trials regardless of health literacy level. *Clin. Trials* 12 (3): 232–236.
54. Sagi, D., Spitzer-Shohat, S., Schuster, M. et al. (2021). Teaching plain language to medical students: improving communication with disadvantaged patients. *BMC Med. Educ.* 21 (1): 407.
55. Bittner, A., Bittner, J., Jonietz, A. et al. (2016). Translating medical documents improves students' communication skills in simulated physician-patient encounters. *BMC Med. Educ.* 16: 72.
56. Goldsmith, J.V., Wittenberg, E., Terui, S. et al. (2019). Providing support for caregiver communication burden: assessing the plain language planner resource as a nursing intervention. *Semin. Oncol. Nurs.* 35 (4): 354–358.
57. Plain Writing Act of 2010. 2010. Pub. L. No. 111–274. https://www.govinfo.gov/app/details/PLAW-111publ274 (accessed 1 January 2022).
58. Plainlanguage.gov (2011). *Federal Plain Language Guidelines 2011 [Internet]*. Plainlanguage.gov https://www.plainlanguage.gov/media/FederalPLGuidelines.pdf (1 Janauary 2022).
59. European Commission (2021). *Clear Writing for Europe [Internet]*. European Commission https://ec.europa.eu/info/departments/translation/clear-writing-for-europe_en (accessed 30 May 2022).
60. Publications Office of the EU (2012). *How to Write Clearly [Internet]*. Luxembourg: Publications Office of the European Union https://op.europa.eu/en/publication-detail/-/publication/bb87884e-4cb6-4985-b796-70784ee181ce/language-en.
61. Sørensen, K., Van den Broucke, S., Fullam, J. et al. (2012). Health literacy and public health: a systematic review and integration of definitions and models. *BMC Public Health* 12: 80.
62. Squiers, L., Peinado, S., Berkman, N. et al. (2012). The health literacy skills framework. *J. Health Commun.* 17 (Suppl 3): 30–54.
63. Cudjoe, J., Delva, S., Cajita, M., and Han, H.R. (2020). Empirically tested health literacy frameworks. *Health Lit Res Prac.* 4 (1): e22–e44.
64. Paasche-Orlow, M.K. and Wolf, M.S. (2007). The causal pathways linking health literacy to health outcomes. *Am. J. Health Behav.* 31 (Suppl 1): S19–S26.
65. Haun, J.N., Valerio, M.A., McCormack, L.A. et al. (2014). Health literacy measurement: An inventory and descriptive summary of 51 instruments. *J. Health Commun.* 19 (Suppl 2): 302–333.
66. Okan, O., Lopes, E., Bollweg, T.M. et al. (2018). Generic health literacy measurement instruments for children and adolescents: a systematic review of the literature. *BMC Public Health* 18 (1): 166.
67. Lee, J., Lee, E.H., and Chae, D. (2021). eHealth literacy instruments: systematic review of measurement properties. *J. Med. Internet Res.* 23 (11): e30644.
68. Weiss, B.D., Mays, M.Z., Martz, W. et al. (2005). Quick assessment of literacy in primary care: the newest vital sign. *Ann. Fam. Med.* 3 (6): 514–522.
69. Parker, R.M., Baker, D.W., Williams, M.V., and Nurss, J.R. (1995). The test of functional health literacy in adults: a new instrument for measuring patients' literacy skills. *J. Gen. Intern. Med.* 10 (10): 537–541.
70. Osborne, R.H., Batterham, R.W., Elsworth, G.R. et al. (2013). The grounded psychometric development and initial validation of the health literacy questionnaire (HLQ). *BMC Public Health* 13: 658.
71. Jordan, J.E., Buchbinder, R., Briggs, A.M. et al. (2013). The Health Literacy Management Scale (HeLMS): a measure of an individual's capacity to seek, understand and use health information within the healthcare setting. *Patient Educ. Couns.* 91 (2): 228–235.
72. Yuen, E.Y., Knight, T., Dodson, S. et al. (2014). Development of the Health Literacy of Caregivers Scale - Cancer (HLCS-C): item generation and content validity testing. *BMC Fam. Pract.* 15: 202.
73. Jordan, J.E., Osborne, R.H., and Buchbinder, R. (2011). Critical appraisal of health literacy indices revealed variable underlying constructs, narrow content and psychometric weaknesses. *J. Clin. Epidemiol.* 64 (4): 366–379.
74. Boston University (2022). *Health Literacy Tool Shed [Internet]*. Boston University https://healthliteracy.bu.edu (accessed 1 January 2022).

75. Morris, N.S., MacLean, C.D., Chew, L.D., and Littenberg, B. (2006). The single item literacy screener: evaluation of a brief instrument to identify limited reading ability. *BMC Fam. Pract.* 7: 21.
76. Altin, S.V., Finke, I., Kautz-Freimuth, S., and Stock, S. (2014). The evolution of health literacy assessment tools: a systematic review. *BMC Public Health* 14: 1207.
77. Hadden, K.B., Prince, L.Y., Rojo, M.O. et al. (2019). Screening patients who speak Spanish for low health literacy. *Health Lit Res Pract.* 3 (2): e110–e116.
78. McCormack, L., Haun, J., Sørensen, K., and Valerio, M. (2013). Recommendations for advancing health literacy measurement. *J. Health Commun.* 18 (Suppl 1): 9–14.
79. Nguyen, T.H., Paasche-Orlow, M.K., and McCormack, L.A. (2017). The state of the science of health literacy measurement. *Stud. Health Technol. Inform.* 240: 17–33.
80. Norman, C.D. and Skinner, H.A. (2006). eHealth literacy: essential skills for consumer health in a networked world. *J. Med. Internet Res.* 8 (2): e9.
81. Paige, S.R., Stellefson, M., Krieger, J.L. et al. (2018). Proposing a transactional model of eHealth literacy: concept analysis. *J. Med. Internet Res.* 20 (10): e10175.
82. Bailey, S.C., O'Conor, R., Bojarski, E.A. et al. (2015). Literacy disparities in patient access and health-related use of internet and mobile technologies. *Health Expect.* 18 (6): 3079–3087.
83. Casillas, A., Cemballi, A.G., Abhat, A. et al. (2020). An untapped potential in primary care: semi-structured interviews with clinicians on how patient portals will work for caregivers in the safety net. *J. Med. Internet Res.* 22 (7): e18466.
84. Davis, S.E., Osborn, C.Y., Kripalani, S. et al. (2015). Health literacy, education levels, and patient portal usage during hospitalizations. *AMIA Annu. Symp. Proc.* 2015: 1871–1880.
85. Hemsley, B., Rollo, M., Georgiou, A. et al. (2018). The health literacy demands of electronic personal health records (e-PHRs): An integrative review to inform future inclusive research. *Patient Educ. Couns.* 101 (1): 2–15.
86. Lee, H.Y., Jin, S.W., Henning-Smith, C. et al. (2021). Role of health literacy in health-related information-seeking behavior online: cross-sectional study. *J. Med. Internet Res.* 23 (1): e14088.
87. Casillas, A., Moreno, G., Grotts, J. et al. (2018). A digital language divide? The relationship between internet medication refills and medication adherence among limited English proficient (LEP) patients. *J. Racial Ethn. Health Disparities* 5 (6): 1373–1380.
88. Moreno, G., Lin, E.H., Chang, E. et al. (2016). Disparities in the use of internet and telephone medication refills among linguistically diverse patients. *J. Gen. Intern. Med.* 31 (3): 282–288.
89. Hinami, K., Harris, B.A., Uriostegui, R. et al. (2017). Patient-level exclusions from mHealth in a safety-net health system. *J. Hosp. Med.* 12 (2): 90–93.
90. Khoong, E.C., Rivadeneira, N.A., Hiatt, R.A., and Sarkar, U. (2020). The use of technology for communicating with clinicians or seeking health information in a multilingual urban cohort: cross-sectional survey. *J. Med. Internet Res.* 22 (4): e16951.
91. Casillas, A., Abhat, A., Vassar, S.D. et al. (2021). Not speaking the same language- lower portal use for limited English proficient patients in the Los Angeles safety net. *J. Health Care Poor Underserved* 32 (4): 2055–2070.
92. Roy, M., Purington, N., Liu, M. et al. (2021). Limited English proficiency and disparities in health care engagement among patients with breast cancer. *JCO Oncol Pract.* 17 (12): e1837–e1845.
93. Hsueh, L., Huang, J., Millman, A.K. et al. (2021). Disparities in use of video telemedicine among patients with limited English proficiency during the COVID-19 pandemic. *JAMA Netw. Open* 4 (11): e2133129.
94. Norman, C.D. and Skinner, H.A. (2006). eHEALS: the eHealth literacy scale. *J. Med. Internet Res.* 8 (4): e27.
95. Norman, C. (2011). eHealth literacy 2.0: problems and opportunities with an evolving concept. *J. Med. Internet Res.* 13 (4): e125.

96. van der Vaart, R., Drossaert, C.H., de Heus, M. et al. (2013). Measuring actual eHealth literacy among patients with rheumatic diseases: a qualitative analysis of problems encountered using Health 1.0 and Health 2.0 applications. *J. Med. Internet Res.* 15 (2): e27.
97. Paige, S.R., Stellefson, M., Krieger, J.L. et al. (2019). Transactional eHealth literacy: developing and testing a multi-dimensional instrument. *J. Health Commun.* 24 (10): 737–748.
98. Chan, J. (2021). Exploring digital health care: eHealth, mHealth, and librarian opportunities. *J. Med. Libr. Assoc.* 109 (3): 376–381.
99. Kim, W., Kim, I., Baltimore, K. et al. (2020). Simple contents and good readability: improving health literacy for LEP populations. *Int. J. Med. Inform.* 141: 104230.
100. MacEwan, S.R., Gaughan, A., Hefner, J.L., and McAlearney, A.S. (2021). Identifying the role of inpatient portals to support health literacy: perspectives from patients and care team members. *Patient Educ. Couns.* 104 (4): 836–843.
101. Dendere, R., Slade, C., Burton-Jones, A. et al. (2019). Patient portals facilitating engagement with inpatient electronic medical records: a systematic review. *J. Med. Internet Res.* 21 (4): e12779.
102. Andrulis, D.P., Siddiqui, N.J., and Gantner, J.L. (2007). Preparing racially and ethnically diverse communities for public health emergencies. *Health Aff (Millwood).* 26 (5): 1269–1279.
103. Collins, T., Akselrod, S., Bloomfield, A. et al. (2020). Rethinking the COVID-19 pandemic: Back to public health. *Ann. Glob. Health* 86 (1): 133.
104. Vaughan, E. and Tinker, T. (2009). Effective health risk communication about pandemic influenza for vulnerable populations. *Am. J. Public Health* 99 (Suppl 2): S324–S332.
105. Andrulis, D.P. and Siddiqui, N.J. (2008). *National Consensus Panel on Emergency Preparedness for Racially and Ethnically Diverse Communities.* The Center for Health Equality, Drexel University School of Public Health. OMH.
106. Office of Minority Health (2011). *Guidance for Integrating Culturally Diverse Communities into Planning for and Responding to Emergencies: A Toolkit [Internet].* U.S. Department of Health and Human Services https://www.aha.org/system/files/content/11/OMHDiversityPreparednesToolkit.pdf (accessed 1 January 2022).
107. Zarocostas, J. (2020). How to fight an infodemic. *Lancet* 395 (10225): 676.
108. WHO (2020). *Munich Security Conference [Internet].* World Health Organization https://www.who.int/director-general/speeches/detail/munich-security-conference (accessed 1 January 2022).
109. Tangcharoensathien, V., Calleja, N., Nguyen, T. et al. (2020). Framework for managing the COVID-19 infodemic: methods and results of an online, crowdsourced WHO technical consultation. *J. Med. Internet Res.* 22 (6): e19659.
110. Calleja, N., AbdAllah, A., Abad, N. et al. (2021). A public health research agenda for managing infodemics: methods and results of the first WHO Infodemiology conference. *JMIR Infodemiology.* 1 (1): e30979.
111. Eysenbach, G. (2020). How to fight an infodemic: the four pillars of infodemic management. *J. Med. Internet Res.* 22 (6): e21820.
112. Li, S., Cui, G., Kaminga, A.C. et al. (2021). Associations between health literacy, eHealth literacy, and COVID-19-related health behaviors among Chinese college students: cross-sectional online study. *J. Med. Internet Res.* 23 (5): e25600.
113. An, L., Bacon, E., Hawley, S. et al. (2021). Relationship between coronavirus-related eHealth literacy and COVID-19 knowledge, attitudes, and practices among US adults: web-based survey study. *J. Med. Internet Res.* 23 (3): e25042.
114. Do, B.N., Tran, T.V., Phan, D.T. et al. (2020). Health literacy, eHealth literacy, adherence to infection prevention and control procedures, lifestyle changes, and suspected COVID-19 symptoms among health care workers during lockdown: online survey. *J. Med. Internet Res.* 22 (11): e22894.

115. Guo, Z., Zhao, S.Z., Guo, N. et al. (2021). Socioeconomic disparities in eHealth literacy and preventive behaviors during the COVID-19 pandemic in Hong Kong: cross-sectional study. *J. Med. Internet Res.* 23 (4): e24577.
116. Naveed, M.A. and Shaukat, R. (2021). Health literacy predicts Covid-19 awareness and protective behaviours of university students. *Health Info. Libr. J.* 39 (1): 46–58.
117. Berkman, N.D., Sheridan, S.L., Donahue, K.E. et al. (2011). Health literacy interventions and outcomes: an updated systematic review. *Evid. Rep. Technol. Assess. (Full Rep).* 199: 1–941.
118. Walters, R., Leslie, S.J., Polson, R. et al. (2020). Establishing the efficacy of interventions to improve health literacy and health behaviours: a systematic review. *BMC Public Health* 20 (1): 1040.
119. Claflin, S.B., Klekociuk, S., Fair, H. et al. (2022). Assessing the impact of online health education interventions from 2010-2020: a systematic review of the evidence. *Am. J. Health Promot.* 36 (1): 201–224.
120. Watkins, I. and Xie, B. (2014). eHealth literacy interventions for older adults: a systematic review of the literature. *J. Med. Internet Res.* 16 (11): e225.
121. National Academies of Sciences, Engineering, and Medicine (2018). *Community-Based Health Literacy Interventions: Proceedings of a Workshop.* Washington, DC: National Academies Press https://doi.org/10.17226/24917.
122. Nutbeam, D., McGill, B., and Premkumar, P. (2018). Improving health literacy in community populations: a review of progress. *Health Promot. Int.* 33 (5): 901–911.
123. Department of Health and Human Services. (2013). *Language Access Plan 2013* https://www.hhs.gov/sites/default/files/hhs-language-access-plan2013.pdf (accessed 1 Janaury 2022).
124. Rudd, R.E., Oelschlegel, S., Grabeel, K.L. et al. (2019). *HLE2: The Health Literacy Environment of Hospitals and Health Centers [Internet].* Boston: Harvard T. H. Chan School of Public Health https://cdn1.sph.harvard.edu/wp-content/uploads/sites/135/2019/05/april-30-FINAL_The-Health-Literacy-Environment2_Locked.pdf (accessed 1 Janaury 2022).
125. Rudd, R.E. and Anderson, J.E. (2006). *The Health Literacy Environment of Hospitals and Health Centers [Internet].* Boston: Harvard School of Public Health https://cdn1.sph.harvard.edu/wp-content/uploads/sites/135/2012/09/healthliteracyenvironment.pdf (accessed 1 January 2022).
126. National Center for Cultural Competence at Georgetown University. (2006). *Cultural and Linguistic Competence Policy Assessment [Internet].* https://nccc.georgetown.edu/assessments/clcpa.php (accessed 1 January 2022).
127. Office of Minority Health (2022). *National CLAS Standards [Internet].* U.S. Department of Health and Human Services https://thinkculturalhealth.hhs.gov/clas (accessed 1 January 2022).
128. Brega, A., Barnard, J., Mabachi, N. et al. (2015). *AHRQ Health Literacy Universal Precautions Toolkit*, Seconde. AHRQ Publication No. 15-0023-EF. Rockville, MD: Agency for Healthcare Research and Quality.
129. Mackert, M., Ball, J., and Lopez, N. (2011). Health literacy awareness training for healthcare workers: improving knowledge and intentions to use clear communication techniques. *Patient Educ. Couns.* 85 (3): e225–e228.
130. Green, J.A., Gonzaga, A.M., Cohen, E.D., and Spagnoletti, C.L. (2014). Addressing health literacy through clear health communication: a training program for internal medicine residents. *Patient Educ. Couns.* 95 (1): 76–82.
131. Hildenbrand, G.M., Perrault, E.K., and Keller, P.E. (2020). Evaluating a health literacy communication training for medical students: using plain language. *J. Health Commun.* 25 (8): 624–631.
132. Centers for Disease Control and Prevention *Health Literacy, Find Training [Internet].* Centers for Disease Control and Prevention https://www.cdc.gov/healthliteracy/gettraining.html (accessed 1 January 2022).

133. Office of Minority Health (2022). *Think Cultural Health, Education [Internet]*. U.S. Department of Health and Human Services https://thinkculturalhealth.hhs.gov/education (accessed 1 January 2022).
134. UMICH (2022). *Plain Language Medical Dictionary [Internet]*. University of Michigan Library https://apps.lib.umich.edu/medical-dictionary (accessed 30 May 2022).
135. Centers for Disease Control and Prevention (2009). *Simply Put; a Guide for Creating Easy-to-Understand Materials [Internet]*. Centers for Disease Control and Prevention https://stacks.cdc.gov/view/cdc/11938 (accessed 30 May 2022).
136. Centers for Disease Control and Prevention (2019). *The CDC Clear Communication Index [Internet]*. Centers for Disease Control and Prevention https://www.cdc.gov/ccindex/index.html (accessed 30 May 2022).
137. Centers for Medicare & Medicaid Services (2021). *Toolkit for Making Written Material Clear and Effective[Internet]*. Centers for Medicare & Medicaid Services https://www.cms.gov/Outreach-and-Education/Outreach/WrittenMaterialsToolkit (accessed 30 May 2022).
138. SAM (2008). *Suitability Assessment of Materials [Internet]*. Practice Development, Inc http://aspiruslibrary.org/literacy/SAM.pdf (accessed 30 May 2022).
139. AHRQ (2013). *The Patient Education Materials Assessment Tool (PEMAT) and User's Guide [Internet]*. Agency for Healthcare Research and Quality https://www.ahrq.gov/health-literacy/patient-education/pemat.html (accessed 30 May 2022).
140. THE SMOG Readability Formula. (2022). The *SMOG Readability Formula, a Simple Measure of Gobbledygook [Internet]*. Readability Formulas. https://www.readabilityformulas.com/smog-readability-formula.php.
141. National Institutes of Health (2016). *Plain Language: Getting Started or Brushing Up [Internet]*. National Institutes of Health https://www.nih.gov/institutes-nih/nih-office-director/office-communications-public-liaison/clear-communication/plain-language/plain-language-getting-started-or-brushing (accessed 30 May 2022).
142. Logan, R.A., Wong, W.F., Villaire, M. et al. (2015). *Health Literacy: A Necessary Element for Achieving Health Equity*. Washington, DC: National Academy of Medicine.
143. National Academies of Sciences, Engineering, and Medicine (2021). *Exploring the Role of Critical Health Literacy in Addressing the Social Determinants of Health: Proceedings of a Workshop*. Washington, DC: The National Academies Press.

Part III Language Concordance in Public Health and Healthcare

Introduction to Part III

Pilar Ortega and Glenn Martínez

Healthcare in multilingual settings occurs both through interpreter-mediated interactions, which were described in detail in the previous section, and through interactions that occur in the patient's preferred language when that language differs from the majority language. These direct interactions have been studied under the mantle of "language-concordant" care. Researchers have made great strides in determining the relative advantages and health-protective outcomes associated with language-concordant care when compared with language-discordant care. These studies reveal that language concordance is associated with both subjective and objective measures of improved performance including greater trust, less perceived discrimination, and improved measures of physical health.

Language concordance research is tied to other strands of health equity research including race/ethnicity concordance studies. Race/ethnicity concordance studies focus on clinical interactions where the clinician and patient share the same race/ethnicity. Race/ethnicity concordance has been shown to lead to improved communication between patients and their clinicians and a modest positive association with overall healthcare experience and patient satisfaction [1, 2]. Even so, in the United States, only 22% of Black patients have a race-concordant provider and only 29% of Hispanic/Latinx patients have an ethnically concordant provider [3]. This research has resulted in recommendations to widen the pathway for diverse racial and ethnic groups entering the health professions [4].

The Handbook of Language in Public Health and Healthcare, First Edition.
Edited by Pilar Ortega, Glenn Martínez, Maichou Lor, and A. Susana Ramírez.
© 2024 John Wiley & Sons, Inc. Published 2024 by John Wiley & Sons, Inc.

Language concordance may overlap with racial or ethnic concordance. In such cases, it may be difficult to disentangle the specific impact of race/ethnicity and language [5]. In cases where it does not overlap, many questions have arisen about the objectively measured language proficiency of the clinician. Does the clinician have sufficient command over the language or is the clinician merely "getting by"? [6] These questions have significant quality and safety implications. Aside from these concerns, there is currently no way to account for the number of fully proficient clinicians in a given language in the healthcare system making it difficult to assess the extent of inequities faced by patients with a non-English language preference.

The chapters in this section present a robust analysis of prior work on language concordance, outline critical issues, and propose strategies for advancing the field. Chapter 10 presents an overview of existing work regarding language concordance. After exploring the known effects of language concordance on health metrics including patient outcomes, patient satisfaction, healthcare costs and utilization, and clinician satisfaction, the authors provide recommendations for next steps needed in language concordance research.

Chapter 11 provides an in-depth analysis of what is meant by language concordance, including complex elements of pronunciation, pragmatics, and others to enrich current understanding of how language concordance in healthcare should be defined and evaluated. Importantly, this chapter presents an understanding of language concordance in healthcare as necessarily interactional, drawing from the varied linguistic and cultural practices of both interlocutors – patient and clinician.

Moving toward practical applications of language concordance in healthcare, Chapter 12 discusses language skills assessment as applied to clinicians' communication skills in a language different from their language of medical training. Moreover, the authors draw distinctions between language assessment for health professional purposes from general language proficiency assessment and discuss key considerations in health professional language test development, scoring, standard setting, and validity evaluation.

Chapter 13 contextualizes health professional language assessment within the health systems and explores the need for setting standards to confirm clinician language proficiency for safe patient care. The author also identifies challenges and opportunities for next steps in implementation and enforcement of language proficiency standards in healthcare.

Finally, in Chapter 14, the authors outline current gaps in language concordance research and policy, propose next steps to advance the field, and explore the public health and health policy impact of clinician language assessment.

REFERENCES

1. Shen, M.J., Peterson, E.B., Costas-Muñiz, R. et al. (2018). The effects of race and racial concordance on patient-physician communication: a systematic review of the literature. *J. Racial Ethnic Health Disparities* 5 (1): 117–140. https://doi.org/10.1007/s40615-017-0350-4.

2. Ku, L. and Vichare, A. (2023). The association of racial and ethnic concordance in primary care with patient satisfaction and experience of care. *J. Gen. Intern. Med.* 38: 727–732. https://doi.org/10.1007/s11606-022-07695-y.

3. Gonzalez, D., Kenney, G., McDaniel, M., and O'Brien, C. *Racial, Ethnic and Language Concordance Between Patients and Their Usual Health Care Providers*. Health Policy Center. Washington DC: Urban Institute. Retrieved May 25 2023 from: racial-ethnic-and-language-concordance-between-patients-and-providers.pdf (urban.org.
4. Institute of Medicine (2004). *Unequal Treatment: Confronting Racial and Ethnic disparities in healthcare*. Washington DC: National Academies Press.
5. Alegría, M., Roter, D.L., Valentine, A. et al. (2013). Patient–clinician ethnic concordance and communication in mental health intake visits. *Patient Educ. Counseling* 93 (2): 188–196. https://doi.org/10.1016/j.pec.2013.07.001.
6. Diamond, L.C. and Jacobs, E.A. (2010). Let's not contribute to disparities: the best methods for teaching clinicians how to overcome language barriers to health care. *J. Gen. Intern. Med.* 25 (Suppl 2): S189–S193. https://doi.org/10.1007/s11606-009-1201-8.

10 Language Concordance in Clinical Care

ALICIA FERNÁNDEZ AND FRANCINE RÍOS-FETCHKO

Evolution of the field of language-concordant healthcare

The growth in the number of patients with limited English proficiency (LEP) in the United States has been well documented. Since 2000, people with LEP have made up approximately 8% of the U.S. population, increasing in absolute numbers from 21.3 million in 2000 to 25.3 million in 2020 [1]. Less well recognized, however, is the change in linguistic diversity of the healthcare workforce, particularly the increase in physicians and nurses from immigrant backgrounds. Currently, about 28% of physicians and 15% of registered nurses are immigrants, up from 20% to 9% in 1990 [2]. Many of these healthcare professionals have skills in a language other than English [3]. Unfortunately, the growth in the United States population with non-English language preference far outstrips the supply of linguistically diverse clinicians and, as described below, there is a mismatch in the languages spoken by clinicians and those spoken by patients. There are currently no data tracking the number of patients receiving care in their preferred language.

National estimates of clinician language capabilities are sparse. One recent national study asked all certifying family physicians to self-report use of Spanish or another non-English language to communicate directly with their patients. About 22% of family physicians reported using Spanish, and about 15% reported at least occasional use of another non-English language [4]. The study did not ask the physicians how well they spoke the language, and it is quite likely that the range of proficiency varied substantially. Another study examined the language capabilities of physicians in California. California has many "well-represented languages," i.e., languages spoken by many physicians compared to the size of the population [5]. The most well-represented non-English language was Farsi, followed by Hindi, Korean, and "Chinese" (a category that contains many distinct languages). By contrast, Spanish, the most common non-English language in California, was the most underrepresented, with only 62 Spanish-speaking physicians/100,000 Spanish speakers compared to 344 English-speaking physicians/100,000 English speakers and 1627 Farsi-speaking physicians/100,000 Farsi speakers [5].

The Handbook of Language in Public Health and Healthcare, First Edition.
Edited by Pilar Ortega, Glenn Martínez, Maichou Lor, and A. Susana Ramírez.
© 2024 John Wiley & Sons, Inc. Published 2024 by John Wiley & Sons, Inc.

Despite the increase in linguistic and cultural diversity of the medical workforce, relatively few patients experience language-concordant care due to the mismatch between physician language capabilities and patient population needs.

What is language-concordant care?

Language concordance – when patients and clinicians communicate directly in the patients' preferred language – has no standard definition in clinical practice or research. It is important to note that encounters that are mediated through an interpreter are, by definition, not language-concordant and are not considered when discussing definitions of language concordance. In many states, physicians self-report to the state Medical Board what languages they speak [6]. However, language proficiency level (sometimes referred to as "fluency") is often not measured, nor are skills in reading, writing or using healthcare terminology, sometimes called medical language proficiency [7]. Lor and Martínez conducted a scoping review to understand how the term is being conceptualized in research and found that the majority of studies are using "speaks the same language" or "being fluent or proficient in the patient's language" as their measure of language concordance. These broad definitions make estimating the prevalence of language-concordant care difficult and, as stated above, do not capture the complexity of language skills in a healthcare setting. For example, someone who speaks fluent conversational Spanish, learned at home or in school, may not have the medical vocabulary required to say "your spleen is swollen," as they do not know the words for either spleen or swelling. Conversely, someone who knows the words for spleen or swelling because they learned a list of vocabulary may not necessarily have the Spanish language level to spontaneously produce an explanation about what the medical terms mean, why it is significant to the patient's health, and what the next steps in treatment are. In other words, a clinician or healthcare worker who reports speaking a non-English language may not have sufficient medical language proficiency to provide safe, effective, and medically accurate care for patients.

Asking physicians to rate their own language skills can have other pitfalls. The authors of this chapter conducted a study in which they asked physicians to rate their Spanish language skills on a 5-point Likert scale ranging from none to excellent [8]. Their patients were then asked, "does your doctor speak Spanish?" with either "yes" or "no" as possible answers. Patient and physician answers aligned well, with the exception of physicians who self-rated their Spanish as "fair," the middle and most common category. In that instance, only about half of the patients agreed that their physician did, in fact, speak Spanish [8]. Studies that compare physician self-rating of language level with other forms of assessment such as formal language tests or nuanced reports from patients also find that mid-level fluency is a broad range and is not consistently associated with passing a formal language test [7, 9]. In summary, self-report makes it easy to identify physicians who are highly proficient or those who do not speak the language. However, *self-report does not identify the capabilities of physicians with more intermediate levels of language proficiency.* This category is often enriched by physicians who learned Spanish in school, or by some heritage speakers (children of immigrants) who never studied the language formally or were never exposed to medical vocabulary.

Many health systems are now using formal language tests to establish healthcare language proficiency and certify clinicians and other health workers as not requiring interpreters. While much more expensive than self-report, and a possible unfair barrier for people with little experience with formal testing, language testing does assure certain levels of competency. For example, the widely available ALTA Language Services test certifies two levels – the lower level enables the certificate holder to provide services when knowledge of medical terminology is not required [10]. This can be particularly useful to certify bilingual healthcare workers who are sufficiently proficient to engage in relatively simple tasks (e.g., assisting with patient registration) yet lack the medical proficiency necessary to engage in the complexity of clinical care.

Language concordance and clinical care

Many studies have examined the impact of language concordance on clinical care; two recent systematic reviews are available with excellent syntheses of the literature [11, 12]. For this chapter, we will follow the conceptual framework used to guide assessment of the evidence in the Hsueh review (Figure 10.1) [12]. The authors grouped and evaluated studies examining patient behaviors (e.g., medication adherence and appointment care); interpersonal process of care (that we term patient experience of care); provider behavior (e.g., omitting counseling or important diagnostic questions); and clinical outcomes (e.g., glycemic or blood pressure control) [12]. The second recent systematic review focused on the associations of language concordance with quality of care, patient satisfaction, medical understanding, and mental health [11]. Below, we provide brief reviews of the evidence. Readers wishing more detail should consult the two systematic reviews and the original literature [11, 12].

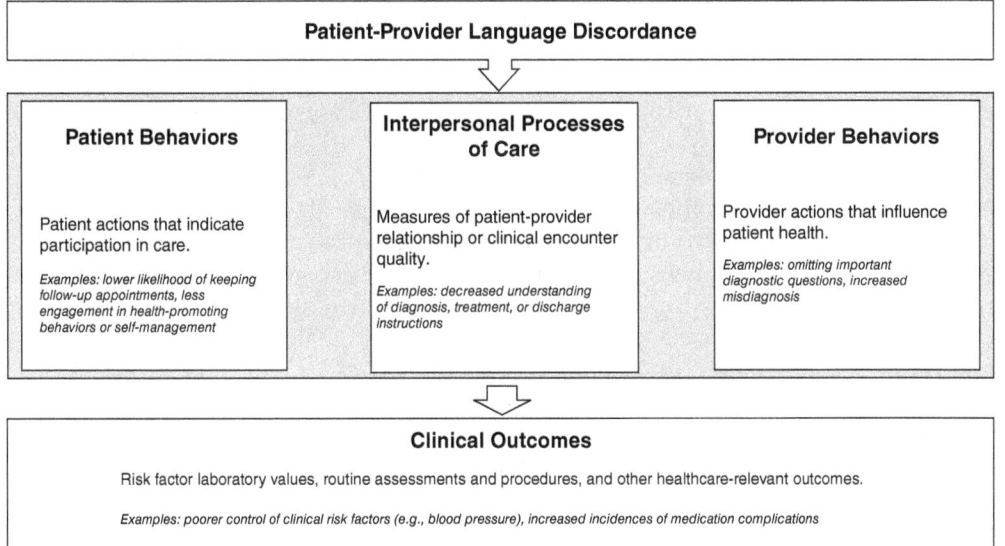

Figure 10.1 Conceptual Framework. Hsueh et al. [12]/With permission of Elsevier.

Language concordance and patient behaviors

The Hsueh review found nine studies that examined the association of language concordance and patient behaviors. Twenty-three unique patient behaviors were studied [12]. While some of the associations were positive, most were not. Medication adherence has been the most extensively studied. With the exception of one well conducted study from Kaiser Permanente in Northern California [13], most studies have not found an association between clinician-patient language concordance and medication adherence. Other studies that focused on specific aspects of patient adherence behavior found positive associations, such as one study that found an association between language-concordant care and decreased number of missed appointments [14]. At this point, more research is needed to understand the relationships between language concordance and specific patient behaviors, such as undergoing colonoscopy screening [15].

Language concordance and patient experience of care

Our understanding of the benefits of language concordance comes in part from studies that found difficulties with language discordant care. Patients consistently report difficulty with medical comprehension and less satisfaction with language discordant encounters, even when these encounters are mediated by a professional interpreter [16–22]. For example, patients who used interpreters were more likely than patients with a language-concordant clinician to report having unanswered questions about their care [23]. In a telling study conducted in the emergency department of Bellevue Hospital, the great public hospital of lower Manhattan, only 35–39% of patients who were randomized to one of two state-of-the-art professional interpreter systems reported that they understood the physician's care instructions as they left the ED. By contrast, 59% patients cared for by a language-concordant clinician reported understanding their ED follow-up instructions [24]. While this still leaves much room for improvement for both groups, this study and others like it confirm that patient understanding and satisfaction is better in language-concordant care. Unfortunately, *even high-quality medical interpretation does not provide patients as a group the same level of comprehension as language-concordant care does.*

Language concordance may help facilitate the types of clinical communication that enhance patient trust in their clinician. Certain clinician behaviors, such as making social comments at the start of the visit to put the patient at ease, eliciting the patient's point of view on a treatment or recommendation, or making an empathic comment when a patient reports a troubling symptom or life circumstance elicit trust in an encounter [25]. Busy physicians may not take the time to make social or empathic comments through the interpreter, leading to a more biomedical and ultimately less trust-eliciting visit. A study of Chinese and Spanish-speaking patients with diabetes found that patients with a language-concordant physician were less likely to report lack of confidence and trust in their physicians than patients whose encounter was mediated through interpreters (16% versus 35%, $p<0.0001$) [26]. Other studies have reported similar results [11]. Research studies on interpretation dynamics may offer a deeper understanding of this phenomenon. For example, a videorecording study of primary care encounters of Spanish and English-speaking patients compared the patient centeredness of the visits [27]. They found that in the interpreted visits, patients were less likely to offer up symptoms, thoughts, or feelings – and that physicians were more likely to ignore them when they did. The authors termed this a "double disadvantage" for Spanish-speaking patients [27]. A study of Spanish-speaking families in a pediatric surgery clinic also found that patients cared for by language-concordant providers asked more questions [21]. The ability to ask questions, receive sympathy, and express one's own point of view are critical to patient perceptions of the trustworthiness of their physicians; unfortunately, these opportunities appear more difficult to achieve in language-discordant care.

Language concordance and clinical outcomes

A 2019 review of the literature on language concordance and clinical outcomes found 33 studies that examined the relationship between language-concordant care and at least one clinical outcome [11]. Of those, 76% (25/33) found that at least one major outcome was better with language-concordant care. There are relatively few studies for any one disease, though several have examined glycemic, lipid and blood pressure control. A cross-sectional study by the authors of this chapter done with Kaiser Permanente patients in Northern California found that while both English and Spanish-speaking Latino patients were more likely to have poor glycemic control than their white counterparts, the glycemic control of Spanish speakers varied considerably depending on the Spanish skills of their primary care physician. Those with language-concordant physicians had rates of poor glycemic control similar to those of English-speaking Latinos, while those with language-discordant physicians were much more likely to have poor glycemic control (27.8% versus 16.1% p = 0.02) [26]. A follow-up study examined patient switches within the Kaiser Permanente system and compared outcomes of the patients with diabetes that switched from a language-discordant physician to a language-concordant physician while also examining all other switches, i.e., discordant to discordant, concordant to discordant, and concordant to concordant (Figure 10.2) [28]. At one-year, glycemic control was much improved among the group of patients that switched from a language-discordant doctor to one that spoke Spanish. After accounting for secular trends, the prevalence of glycemic control in this group increased by 10% (95% CI, 2–17%; p = 0.01), and poor glycemic control decreased by 4% (95% CI, −10–2%; p = 0.16) [28].

Implications for research

Two recent systematic reviews highlight the paucity of studies on language concordance [11, 12]. There are also methodological limitations worth noting. Most current studies are cross-sectional in nature and, like all cross-sectional studies, are subject to possible confounding. A few studies take advantage of natural experiments, such as switches from a language-concordant physicians to language-discordant physicians or vice versa. These quasi-experimental research designs are very valuable and more quasi experimental investigations of the impact of language barriers are needed. Even more valuable would be randomized clinical trials where patients with non-English language preference are assigned to bilingual or language-discordant clinicians. Recruitment for

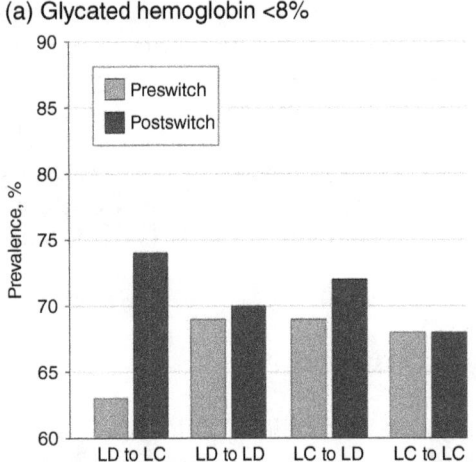 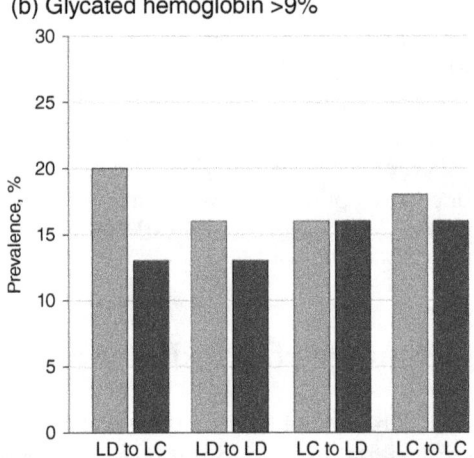

Figure 10.2 Glycated Hemoglobin Levels in Spanish-speaking Latino Patients With Diabetes Before and After Switching Primary Care Physicians. Switching PCPs is shown along the x-axis. For example, the LD to LC group consists of patients with a language-discordant PCP pre-switch and a language-concordant PCP post-switch. The prevalence (unadjusted) of glycated hemoglobin levels before and after switching PCPs is shown along the y-axis. Graph (a) displays the prevalence of glycated hemoglobin levels below 8%, and (b) displays the prevalence of glycated hemoglobin levels above 9%. Lower glycated hemoglobin levels indicate better glucose control. LC indicates language-concordant; LD, language-discordant; PCP, primary care physician. *Source:* Permission to publish granted from the American Medical Association [28].

these studies could be difficult, as many patients have a preference for language-concordant physicians when available. In addition, researchers may believe that the data on patient experience in language-concordant encounters are strong enough to rule out equipoise and find such a study unethical as well as impractical. Future studies should examine additional clinical outcomes using quasi-experimental designs and sophisticated statistical methods to account for as much confounding as possible. In addition, more research needs to be done in languages other than Spanish and with a diverse group of clinician specialties and clinical outcomes to more fully understand the role of language in clinical decision-making.

Finally, the definition of language concordance itself could benefit from additional research. What proficiency level is "enough" to foment trust, improve comprehension, and patient satisfaction? What level is enough to improve a clinical outcome such as glycemic control? These research questions have practical implications for both clinical care and workforce development.

Implications for education and training

Many medical schools offer some opportunities for students to learn medical Spanish. A 2015 study by Morales and colleagues found that 66% of medical schools reported offering a medical Spanish curriculum and that other medical schools were planning to do so in the near future [29]. A key question is about the implementation of these programs – who should they target and how should competency be assessed? One approach (advocated for by the authors of this chapter) is to provide "medical" language training for intermediate and advanced speakers of locally important languages (i.e., Medicaid threshold languages) [30, 31]. Trainees might be heritage speakers who learned the language informally from their immigrant parents and lack medical vocabulary, or second language speakers who studied the language in high school or college to intermediate or advanced level. Both groups of students would benefit from additional medical language training. Importantly, all students should be tested at the end of a course before being determined to be competent to deliver healthcare without an interpreter (see Section Implications for health systems and clinicians). While testing students and clinicians is increasingly common, the 2015 Morales study noted that not only was testing unusual but that many medical schools subsequently allowed students to function as interpreters without establishing their competence in Spanish or in interpretation – an entirely different skill set [29]. Additionally, medical students, like practicing physicians, tend to overestimate their language skills and underutilize professional interpreters [32, 33]. Establishing ethical norms around limitations of own language proficiency should be incorporated into the training of bilingual physicians. For example, a clinician who is qualified to deliver primary care in another language may still benefit from seeking out interpretation assistance for encounters that incorporate a distinct vocabulary, such as end-of-life discussions. Advocates for patients with non-English language preference are calling for increased access to courses in medical Spanish and other languages and highlight the importance of appropriately assessing medical students and physicians before allowing them to use their non-English language skills in clinical encounters [34]. Courses and continuing medical education opportunities are becoming increasingly common as practicing physicians recognize the need to maintain and improve their language skills.

Implications for health systems and clinicians

Millions of patients with non-English language preference struggle when navigating health systems and the complexities of clinical care. As both patient satisfaction and many clinical outcomes are better in language-concordant care, some health systems are doing more to recruit and retain bilingual physicians and healthcare workers. Some health systems have set up protocols to match patients with non-English language preference with clinicians who speak their preferred language at enrollment. In Southern California, for example, the Kaiser Permanente system will pay primary care clinicians and other health workers a bilingual salary differential [35] and use a formal assessment tool (Qualified Bilingual Staff Assessment) to determine the level of second language competence (basic or higher) and hence appropriate scope of practice for the bilingual staff member. This test is widely available, administered by telephone via prerecorded prompts, and scoring is quick. Testing is also useful in systems where the expected default is to use an interpreter if the clinician is not certified as sufficiently proficient in the patient's language. However, as of 2022, paying a bilingual differential or requiring all physicians to be tested before being allowed to opt out of interpreter use are still relatively uncommon health systems policies. Over time, these practices should increase as the number of non-English speaking patients grows, more become insured (e.g., via the Affordable Care Act) and more seek care outside of the safety net institutions that have long-standing experience in serving linguistically diverse populations. We also expect these health system changes to continue because of mounting evidence of the clinical importance of language-concordant care and because more payers are tying individual clinician and health system reimbursement to patient satisfaction ratings.

Clinicians with non-English language capabilities who care for a large number of patients who prefer non-English languages may suffer a form of minority tax if appropriate support is not in place. Relatively simple tasks such as explaining the way to the lab, ensuring after-visit summary communication, or setting up additional appointments may fall to the clinician with language capabilities if support staff are unable to do so readily. In addition, patients may resist referral to some specialties, particularly mental health or social work, if those clinicians do not speak the patient's preferred language, leaving the bilingual physician with more work and the patients at a disadvantage. Some systems have experimented with language pods or language days in order to fully staff a clinical service with bilingual healthcare workers. While successful for those systems, [36] the lack of widespread adoption may speak to the logistical burden involved in reorganizing services. Safety net clinics that care for a large number of patients with LEP but are unable to organize specific language days typically respond by hiring bilingual workers.

Conclusion

Communication is key to safe, effective, and high-quality patient care. Language-concordant care can improve patient experience and some clinical outcomes. While more research is needed to determine how and why language-concordant care improves outcomes, the evidence strongly suggests that increasing the number of multilingual clinicians would improve healthcare for patients from linguistically diverse and immigrant communities.

Highlights

- More research is needed to understand when and how language concordance benefits patient experience and care outcomes.
- Research examining the association between specific patient behavior and language concordance should be conducted in languages beyond Spanish.
- Medical Spanish and other courses should ensure testing of their graduates and caution graduates on the need for constant evaluation of skills.
- Health systems should institute formal language testing before students and clinicians waive use of interpreters.
- Language-concordant care is strongly associated with better patient experience of care, particularly higher patient comprehension and satisfaction, and greater trust in the treating physician; health systems should facilitate language-concordant care when possible.
- Health systems should continue to implement strategies to improve the satisfaction, safety, and clinical outcomes of patients with non-English language preferences by strengthening language access, including access to language-concordant clinicians and health professionals.

REFERENCES

1. United States Census Bureau (2000). *Ability to Speak English by Language Spoken at Home: 2000 [Internet]*. United States Census Bureau.
2. Bouvier, L.F. (1998). *A Demographic Profile of Doctors and Nurses*. https://cis.org/Report/Demographic-Profile-Doctors-and-Nurses#VII.
3. (ACS) MPIMtodftUSCBACS (2018). *Immigrant Health-Care Workers in the United States* http://migrationpolicy.org. Migration Policy Institute https://www.migrationpolicy.org/article/immigrant-health-care-workers-united-states-2018#:~:text=Immigrants%20are%20overrepresented%20among%20certain,percent%20of%20home%20health%20aides.
4. Eden, A.R., Bazemore, A., Morgan, Z.J., and Jabbarpour, Y. (2022). Family physicians increasingly deliver care in diverse languages. *J. Am. Board Fam. Med.* 35 (1): 5–6.
5. Paul Hsu, YB-MA., Anglin, L., and Hayes-Bautista, D.E. (2018). *California's Language Concordance Mismatch: Clear Evidence for Increasing Physician Diversity*. In: University of California SF, ed. http://latino.ucla.edu: UCLA Latino Policy and Politics Initiative.
6. Garcia, M.E., Bindman, A.B., and Coffman, J. (2019). Language-concordant primary care physicians for a diverse population: the view from California. *Health Equity* 3 (1): 343–349.
7. Chaufan, C., Karter, A.J., Moffet, H.H. et al. (2016). Identifying Spanish language competent physicians: the diabetes study of northern California (DISTANCE). *Ethn. Dis.* 26 (4): 537–544.
8. Rosenthal, A., Wang, F., Schillinger, D. et al. (2011). Accuracy of physician self-report of Spanish language proficiency. *J. Immigr. Minor. Health* 13 (2): 239–243.
9. Diamond, L., Chung, S., Ferguson, W. et al. (2014). Relationship between self-assessed and tested non-English-language proficiency among primary care providers. *Med. Care* 52 (5): 435–438.
10. Services AL. (2022) *Language Testing 2022*. https://www.altalang.com/language-testing.
11. Diamond, L., Izquierdo, K., Canfield, D. et al. (2019). A systematic review of the impact of patient-physician non-English language concordance on quality of care and outcomes. *J. Gen. Intern. Med.* 34 (8): 1591–1606.
12. Hsueh, L., Hirsh, A.T., Maupomé, G., and Stewart, J.C. (2019). Patient–provider language concordance and health outcomes: a systematic review, evidence map, and research agenda. *Med. Care Res. Rev.* 78 (1): 3–23.
13. Traylor, A.H., Schmittdiel, J.A., Uratsu, C.S. et al. (2010). Adherence to cardiovascular disease medications: does patient-provider race/ethnicity and language concordance matter? *J. Gen. Intern. Med.* 25 (11): 1172–1177.
14. Lor, M. and Martinez, G.A. (2020). Scoping review: definitions and outcomes of patient-provider language concordance in healthcare. *Patient Educ. Couns.* 103 (10): 1883–1901.
15. Chang, J., Fernandez, A., Thomas, J. et al. (2011). Adherence to colorectal cancer screening among culturally and linguistically diverse low-income patients—does patient-provider language concordance matter? *Gastroenterology* 140: S-21.
16. Wilson, E., Chen, A.H., Grumbach, K. et al. (2005). Effects of limited English proficiency and physician language on health care comprehension. *J. Gen. Intern. Med.* 20 (9): 800–806.
17. Baker, D.W., Hayes, R., and Fortier, J.P. (1998). Interpreter use and satisfaction with interpersonal aspects of care for Spanish-speaking patients. *Med. Care* 36 (10): 1461–1470.
18. Abdelrahim, H., Elnashar, M., Khidir, A. et al. (2017). Patient perspectives on language discordance during healthcare visits: findings from the extremely high-density multicultural State of Qatar. *J. Health Commun.* 22 (4): 355–363.

19. Cuevas, A.G., O'Brien, K., and Saha, S. (2017). What is the key to culturally competent care: reducing bias or cultural tailoring? *Psychol. Health* 32 (4): 493–507.
20. Zamudio, C.D., Sanchez, G., Altschuler, A., and Grant, R.W. (2017). Influence of language and culture in the primary care of Spanish-Speaking Latino adults with poorly controlled diabetes: a qualitative study. *Ethn. Dis.* 27 (4): 379–386.
21. Jaramillo, J., Snyder, E., Dunlap, J.L. et al. (2016). The hispanic clinic for pediatric surgery: a model to improve parent-provider communication for Hispanic pediatric surgery patients. *J. Pediatr. Surg.* 51 (4): 670–674.
22. Schenker, Y., Karter, A.J., Schillinger, D. et al. (2010). The impact of limited English proficiency and physician language concordance on reports of clinical interactions among patients with diabetes: the DISTANCE study. *Patient Educ. Couns.* 81 (2): 222–228.
23. Green, A.R., Ngo-Metzger, Q., Legedza, A.T. et al. (2005). Interpreter services, language concordance, and health care quality. Experiences of Asian Americans with limited English proficiency. *J. Gen. Intern. Med.* 20 (11): 1050–1056.
24. Gany, F., Leng, J., Shapiro, E. et al. (2007). Patient satisfaction with different interpreting methods: a randomized controlled trial. *J. Gen. Intern. Med.* 22 (Suppl 2): 312–318.
25. Frankel, R.M. and Stein, T. (2001). Getting the most out of the clinical encounter: the four habits model. *J. Med. Pract. Manage.* 16 (4): 184–191.
26. Fernandez, A., Schillinger, D., Warton, E.M. et al. (2011). Language barriers, physician-patient language concordance, and glycemic control among insured Latinos with diabetes: the Diabetes Study of Northern California (DISTANCE). *J. Gen. Intern. Med.* 26 (2): 170–176.
27. Rivadeneyra, R., Elderkin-Thompson, V., Silver, R.C., and Waitzkin, H. (2000). Patient centeredness in medical encounters requiring an interpreter. *Am. J. Med.* 108 (6): 470–474.
28. Parker, M.M., Fernández, A., Moffet, H.H. et al. (2017). Association of patient-physician language concordance and glycemic control for limited–English proficiency Latinos with type 2 diabetes. *JAMA Intern. Med.* 177 (3): 380–387.
29. Morales, R., Rodriguez, L., Singh, A. et al. (2015). National survey of medical Spanish curriculum in U.S. medical schools. *J. Gen. Intern. Med.* 30 (10): 1434–1439.
30. Fernández, A. and Pérez-Stable, E.J. (2015). Doctor, habla Español? Increasing the supply and quality of language-concordant physicians for Spanish-speaking patients. *J. Gen. Intern. Med.* 30 (10): 1394–1396.
31. Rittenhouse, D., Fernandez, A., Ament, A., Coffman, J. (2021). Health Professionals and Patients in California: Speaking the Same Language. http://healthforce.ucsf.edu/.
32. Diamond, L.C., Schenker, Y., Curry, L. et al. (2009). Getting by: underuse of interpreters by resident physicians. *J. Gen. Intern. Med.* 24 (2): 256–262.
33. Reuland, D.S., Frasier, P.Y., Olson, M.D. et al. (2009). Accuracy of self-assessed Spanish fluency in medical students. *Teach. Learn. Med.* 21 (4): 305–309.
34. Molina, R.L. and Kasper, J. (2019). The power of language-concordant care: a call to action for medical schools. *BMC Med. Educ.* 19 (1): 378.
35. SEIU (2016). *United Health Care Workers West Collective Bargaining Agreement*. Kaiser Permanente Northern and Southern California. https://www.seiu-uhw.org/wp-content/uploads/2019/09/UHW-Kaiser-Local-Agreement-2012-2016-04152013_with-cover.pdf.
36. Meyers, K., Tang, G., and Fernandez, A. (2009). Responding to the language challenge: Kaiser Permanente's approach. *Perm. J.* 13 (3): 77–83.

11 Language Concordance as Interactional Concordance in Multilingual Clinical Consultations

CAROLINE H. VICKERS
AND RYAN A. GOBLE

Introduction

Language-concordant (LC) healthcare has been defined as a clinical interaction in which the healthcare professional is proficient in the language the patient prefers to use [1]. Lor and Martínez problematize such definitions, stating, "typically defined as the provision of healthcare in a shared non-dominant, minority language. In this way, LC care is embedded in the larger social linguistic order that normalizes or domesticates one or more languages while labeling other languages as abnormal or foreign" (p. 1884). In most cases, LC healthcare for patients who prefer to use a minoritized language has been shown to lead to positive health outcomes and experiences [1, 2]. Diamond et al. [1] completed a comprehensive review of 33 studies of language concordance in healthcare that looked at primary care, diabetes care, pain management, cancer care, hospital care, mental healthcare, as well as studies that examined satisfaction with care and medical understanding. Overall, their review found that 75% of the studies indicated that language concordance most often led to better health outcomes. Fifteen percent of the studies showed that language concordance led to no difference in outcomes, and 9% of studies found that language concordance led to worse health outcomes. Interestingly, all of the studies they reviewed indicated that LC care led to higher levels of patient satisfaction and higher levels of medical understanding.

In another comprehensive review of 50 studies, Lor and Martínez [2] found six emergent themes concerning the effects of LC healthcare. As the authors stated, "These outcomes included (1) interpersonal relationships, (2) access to health information, (3) access to care, (4) healthcare decision-making, (5) satisfaction and healthcare

The Handbook of Language in Public Health and Healthcare, First Edition.
Edited by Pilar Ortega, Glenn Martínez, Maichou Lor, and A. Susana Ramírez.
© 2024 John Wiley & Sons, Inc. Published 2024 by John Wiley & Sons, Inc.

experience, and (6) patient-related health outcomes" (p. 1885). LC care was overwhelmingly associated with positive effects in all six areas with very few exceptions.

One recommendation that Lor and Martínez [2] made was to ensure that studies of language concordance more consistently define the language proficiency of healthcare professionals so that study findings can be generalized. They asked two important questions that future research on LC care must address: "What criteria determines if a healthcare provider is LC [in a given patient care situation]? What type of assessments are needed to consider healthcare providers LC?" (p. 1899).

As Lor and Martínez [2] noted, language concordance is not a well-defined construct in terms of the linguistic features that lead to or detract from concordance. Given the lack of a clear definition of concordance, it is difficult to assess concordance in patient and healthcare professional interactions [3]. However, language concordance does not only involve the level of language proficiency of the healthcare professional. Language proficiency is, of course, crucial as a shared code to achieve mutual understanding, but as we will demonstrate in this chapter, healthcare interactions are LC when the clinician *and* the patient interactionally align in the meaning-making process. Through the analysis of data from multilingual healthcare consultations, the purpose of this chapter is to examine interactional processes involved in multilingual clinical consultations to enrich current understandings of how language concordance in healthcare should be defined and evaluated and to offer implications for healthcare professional training. As we will show, language concordance is at its basis interactionally achieved.

Deconstructing language proficiency

In the United States, a pervasive English-only monolingual ideology becomes a lens through which people understand possibilities in education, public services, and healthcare. The metric becomes how much like the gold standard of "native" you seem, and if you are deemed to be less than this gold standard, you are considered to be limited. The label of limited appears quite vividly in the term *limited English proficient* (LEP), and the ideology can affect people's interactions in institutional contexts in subtle and not-so-subtle ways. In the United States, these effects include limited healthcare access leading to health disparities for LEP people [4].

Problematizing limited proficiency

But what happens if we deconstruct this monolingual ideology? What happens if we reimagine institutional spaces as multilingual? The term LEP was first used in the 1974 court case, *Lau v. Nichols* [5], which ruled that school districts that receive federal funding must "rectify the language deficiency" of students who use English as a second language. As this phrasing makes clear, the term LEP was tied to notions of second English language users as deficient because it was rooted in an ideologically monolingual conception of the United States. There was no acknowledgment that the 2800 students of Chinese ancestry whose families brought the case *did* use Chinese – only that they did *not* use English – which the court ruled put them at a disadvantage compared to the "English-speaking majority."

In 1999, linguist Cook [6] argued that second language (L2) users are not failed native speakers; rather, L2 users are multicompetent language users. As Cook stated, "L2 users should be treated as people in their own right, not as deficient native speakers" (p. 195). Cook's concept of multicompetence focuses on the fact that if someone has an L2, then by definition, they also have a first language (L1). Therefore, the addition of an L2 must be considered a gain. It is only through the lens of normative monolingualism that an *additional* language could be considered a deficit. By contrast, in contexts of productive multilingualism, like most of the world, being monolingual is the deficit [7].

If we reimagine the monolingual orientation toward language in the healthcare setting through a lens of normative multilingualism, the issue is that monolingual professionals who serve a multilingual clientele have a linguistic deficit (i.e., they are not multilingual). If we reimagine many healthcare settings as productive multilingual sites, it becomes clear that using only one language is the source of the limitation. Ortega et al. [8] recognized that it is the ideologically monolingual healthcare setting serving multilingual patients that has the language deficit rather than the patient. They took issue with labels often provided for the multilingual patient experience in the healthcare setting, including "primary language," "limited ability," and "language assistance," as these labels focus on patient deficiencies instead of the professional deficiencies in healthcare organizations.

Ortega and colleagues suggested an alternative label for multilingual patients, *non-English language preference* (NELP), and recommended assessments of healthcare professionals' non-English skills and training on when to ask for interpreters. According to Ortega et al. and Showstack [9], healthcare professionals, not patients, have deficits when operating in multilingual contexts. Such a shift in orientation[1] – from patient deficits toward the responsibility of healthcare professionals to linguistically accommodate their patients – is an essential step toward more equitable and higher quality healthcare for multilingual people. As Ortega et al. argued, it focuses the narrative on patients' strengths rather than their marginalization. Of course, overcoming deficits in the provision of language-appropriate care means developing multilingual clinicians.

Multilingualism and translanguaging in professional practice

Second language acquisition (SLA) and bilingualism research have questioned the general preparedness and capacity of US collegiate language learners to use a non-English language in professional settings beyond formal, instructed SLA. Magnan [10], for example, argued that ever-influential American Council on the Teaching of Foreign Languages (ACTFL) World-Readiness Standards for Language Learning perpetuates an ideology that languages are *first* learned *and then* applied. She asserted that this ideology is problematic because it constructs participation in multilingual communities of practice as a byproduct of language study rather than the *sine qua non* for multilingual development as informed by sociocultural theories of learning. In ethnographic work on the intersection between multilingual and professional development, Goble [11] demonstrated how the learn-then-apply ideology circulates multilingual students' career advising appointments and complicates their expectations, linguistic insecurity, and self-confidence, and identity work in exploring and cultivating bi/multilingual-professional trajectories.

Furthermore, Pomerantz [12] observed the dismay among collegiate L2 Spanish students who realized that language proficiency – defined as passing scores on standardized proficiency and grammar/vocabulary examinations by the department – had not prepared them to participate in Spanish-language interactions. Nevertheless, Pomerantz examined how such passing scores institutionally positioned these L2 students as legitimate and competent Spanish users who could commodify the target language, despite limited linguistic expertise and participation in Spanish-speaking communities. As Pomerantz pointed out, such favorable institutional positioning when it comes to evaluating language proficiency contrasts considerably with the experiences of U.S. Latinos and Spanish heritage speakers, whose bilingualism is societally viewed from a deficit perspective. In this respect, serious concerns have been raised about *whose* multilingual development is nurtured, celebrated, and valued in academic and professional environments [13–15]. Therefore, it is important to deconstruct what effective multilingualism and language use look like in localized, professional practice.

While it is crucial to conceptualize healthcare settings as multilingual spaces, it is equally necessary to deconstruct what it means to be multilingual and the consequences for meaning-making. Early work on the use of multiple languages among multilinguals came from the assumption that multilingual people were competent users of multiple codes and that alternation between codes occurred in a rule-governed way. As Gumperz [16] asserted, previous sociolinguistic work on codeswitching "does not attempt to account for the listener's ability to assign speakers to social categories, to place them within the spectrum of known social categories, and to assess shared social background" (p. 9). Gumperz argued that such social work was an essential part of language use. Gumperz asserted that when people switch codes, they create contextualization cues, which allow people to make inferences about social categories. Such work planted the seed for understandings of linguistic form as an index of social category.

One significant development in understandings of multilingualism as a social process has been the complication of the notions of essentialized language codes and essentialized social categories. Work on translanguaging [17] has contributed strong arguments that the complexity of language choices can index infinite possibilities for social categories. Several scholars have reconceptualized notions of code-switching in ways that focus on a single linguistic repertoire rather than knowledge of multiple discrete whole language systems [18–21]. In work on translanguaging, the question is whether multilingual people interacting in localized multilingual contexts adhere to essentialized notions of discrete languages at all, and empirical data seems to indicate that in some contexts of use, they do not.

Importantly, translanguaging emphasizes individual performance. Otheguy et al. [22] argued that *named languages* such as English, Japanese, and German are social constructions. They asserted that language use is comprised of individuals enacting idiolects to employ their linguistic repertoires and make meaning in the world. Named languages, they maintained, have social meaning and value as social realities that carry ideological weight. Similarly, the work of Otsuji and Pennycook demonstrates how people in superdiverse contexts use linguistic resources to accomplish social needs. It seems that in any multilingual context, including new media [23, 24], multinational workplaces [25, 26], multilingual education [17, 27, 28], and healthcare [29], people make use of linguistic resources to define, create, and co-construct social spaces and identities.

Ortega and Prada [29] advocated for the importance of incorporating emergent, community-based linguistic practices into medical language education. In addition, we would assert the importance of understanding how translanguaging functions as an emergent interactional phenomenon that creates language concordance on the ground in the process of face-to-face interaction between the clinician and the patient.

Conversely, it is also essential to attend to the discordance when clinicians and patients miss the mark on making emergent meaning within the medical consultation. In the section that follows, we draw on interactional data in the healthcare setting to demonstrate language concordance in clinical interactions.

Data

The data we analyze here was collected in a small community clinic located in a low-income urban neighborhood in California where many Spanish-speaking people live. The clinic is intentionally a Spanish-English bilingual context with clinic materials available in the two languages and clinic staff who use both Spanish and English. The data comes from a corpus of 50 medical consultations in which the patients mostly preferred Spanish but would occasionally use English or translanguage. The five excerpts that we analyze below contain consultations with three healthcare professionals and their patients. Dr. Thomas[2] is an L1 English user and L2 Spanish user. Her patient, Arturo, is a monolingual Spanish user. Laura, a nurse practitioner, is an L1 Spanish user and L2 English user, and she interacts with Bea, an L1 Spanish user and L2 English user. Carrie, a nurse practitioner, is an L1 English user and L2 Spanish user, and she interacts with Ana, an L1 Spanish and L2 English user, and Roberto, an L1 Spanish and L2 English user.

The clinic was part of a vibrant religious community, which ran sewing classes, English language classes, after-school tutoring, and Spanish-language religious services. The community also served free daily lunches and housed a homeless shelter and food bank. In addition, community members collaborated to maintain a community garden, organize a weekly thrift store, and play volleyball matches.

Data analysis: Occasioned membership categories

Ultimately, data from this clinical context indicates that language concordance in multilingual interaction must be understood as emergent. As people engage in interaction, their ways of making meaning are fluid, developing in the process of interaction. Vickers [30] developed the concept of occasioned membership categories to examine how identities emerge through sequential interaction. The concept of occasioned membership category is derived from Sacks' [31] membership categories, which he defines are societal roles, such as mother, doctor, or teacher, that people assume in interaction. Occasioned membership category complicates this static notion of membership category to allow for the analysis of interactionally achieved membership categories. At its core, the medical consultation is a category-bound activity [31] involving interaction between a clinician and a patient. However, as Vickers [30] demonstrated, this core relationship becomes complicated through the process of face-to-face interaction as the clinician and patient identities become refined, and occasioned membership categories emerge. As we will demonstrate in our findings, such occasioned membership categories become the basis for meaning-making as language becomes refined to communicate with the particular *type* of healthcare professional and patient that emerges interactionally.

In the analysis of data samples in this chapter, we demonstrate that language concordance is at its basis a process of designing language to meet the occasioned membership categories that emerge in interaction. Through sequential analysis, we examine how the clinician and the patient align and the associated linguistic features that make meaning in the context of the occasioned membership categories that emerge. As we will show, clinician orientations toward patient membership categories create discordance at times, while the consultations do meet the mark as LC at other times.

Findings

Below, we present a series of data excerpts with the language used, Spanish (left column) and English translations (right column). These excerpts demonstrate particular orientations that healthcare professionals and patients take toward each other as interlocutors. We will look at the interactional moves that position the interactants in particular ways and consider how these moves affect language concordance. We will also attend to the patient's and clinician's alignment toward each other's contributions to identify instances of the kind of flexibility with language that contributes to concordance as well as instances when concordance is not linguistically achieved.

Alignment

Arturo was a relatively new patient to the clinic, having just one previous consultation with Dr. Thomas prior to the one analyzed below in Table 11.1. Arturo had come to the clinic with uncontrolled diabetes, as well as high triglycerides, high cholesterol, and high blood pressure. Dr. Thomas had begun treating these conditions in the previous consultation, but it was unclear which medications Arturo was taking when Dr. Thomas met with him before. Sorting out his medications was one purpose of the excerpted dialog in Table 11.1.

As Dr. Thomas elicits Arturo's health history, occasioned membership categories become co-constructed, whereby Arturo is a very ill patient who has lost control over his health because of not following a prescribed treatment regimen, and Dr. Thomas is a very concerned clinicians.

In line 2, Arturo expresses concern about his health, showing the doctor a physical symptom, a sore on his swollen foot. Dr. Thomas indicates distress, uttering with a breathy, sigh "ah:: oh geez," demonstrating an emotional, concerned reaction to the state of his foot. In lines 4–8, Arturo expresses fear and further describes the worrying symptoms related to the foot. Dr. Thomas nails it down as a problem in line 9, asking Arturo why he had said that he did not have any of those symptoms the week before when she had consulted with him. In line 10, Arturo gives an emphatic, lengthened "no::," perhaps indicating that the foot was not symptomatic then but is now. In line 11, Dr. Thomas indicates that the foot is warm, a little red, and somewhat swollen before asking Arturo how long he had been living with diabetes, and in line 12, Arturo indicates 13 years.

In lines 14 and 15, Arturo indicates that he needs refills of his prescriptions, but he does not know the dosage. After Arturo asks "¿por qué tanto?" in line 18, Dr. Thomas states in line 19 that she does not know how to buy all of the medicine that Arturo needs, followed by a distressed "oh geez." In lines 32 through 40, Arturo shows Dr. Thomas records of his blood sugar measurements, explaining that his blood sugar came under control when he was taking insulin. In line 41, Dr. Thomas asks about now. Arturo

Table 11.1   Arturo.[a,b]

Excerpt 1.
<T = 1:09:57>

1.	DT:	¿cómo se siente?	how do you feel?
2.	A:	ahora ando preocupado porque me salió una herida ((xxx)) con el zapato y se me pone bien hinchado el pie ((sounds of furniture moving))	now I'm worried because I have a wound ((xxx)) with the shoe and my foot's become quite swollen ((sounds of furniture moving))
3.	DT:	(4.0) (Hx) ah:: oh geez (Hx) ((sounds distressed))	(4.0) (Hx) ah:: oh geez (Hx) ((sounds distressed))
4.	A:	(3.0) y tengo miedo que	(3.0) and I'm afraid that
5.	DT:	(1.6) y tiene razón. ¿cuando empezó?	(1.6) and you're right. when did it start?
6.	A:	me la descubrí el sábado	I discovered it on Saturday
7.	DT:	(1.0) le duele cuando toca?	(1.0) does it hurt when you touch it?
8.	A:	no: no tengo sensibilidad en el pie [no tengo mucha pena	no: it's not sensitive [I don't have a lot of pain
9.	DT:	[yeah:: y esta es la problema (3.4) porque me dijo la semana pasada que: (2.2) no ha tenido nada de heridas? [no	[yeah:: and this is the problem (3.4) because you told me last week tha:t (2.2) you haven't had any wounds [no
10.	A:	[no:: pero esta pena	[no:: but this pain
11.	DT:	yeah:..no es caliente es un poquito rojo un poquito hinchada. . .no mucho. . .(Hx)(1.5) dígame otra vez ¿cuántos años de diabetes tiene?	yeah:..it's not hot it's a little red a little swollen..not much (Hx) (1.5) tell me again how many years of diabetes do you have?
12.	A:	aproximadamente. . .noventa y siete tres..¿trece años?	approximately..ninety-seven three..thirteen years?
13.	DT:	Yeah	Yeah
14.	A:	(3.5) qué cree que le pedí la prescription..¿la receta se llama?	(3.5) what do you think that I asked you for the prescription ..the prescription..what's it called?
15.	DT:	(TSK)	(TSK)
16.	A:	de la medicina que me dieron ((xxx)) cuánto cree que me cobro ((xxx)) de ese me daban	of the medicine that you gave me ((xxx)) how much do you think it'll cost me ((xxx)) of the one you gave me
17.	DT:	(2.5) oh geez	(2.5) oh geez
18.	A:	y ¿ese mil ah? ¿por qué tanto?	and that of a thousand? why so much?

(Continued)

Table 11.1 (Continued)

Excerpt 1.
<T = 1:09:57>

19.	DT:	(8.0) yo no sé como compra todas sus medicinas...oh geez (Hx) (5.0) (Hx)	(8.0) I don't know how you buy all your medicines...oh geez (Hx) (5.0) (Hx)
20.	A:	y le traje la muestra de la insulina	and I brought you the sample of insulin
21.	DT:	(2.0) bueno excelente	(2.0) good excellent
22.	A:	y también le traje pero estos estudios yo me los hacia antes..el ((xxx xxx)) corriente	and I also brought but these studies you did before the ((xxx xxx)) the current
23.	DT:	(Hx) okay	(Hx) okay
24.	A:	(11.5) mire..aquí empecé yo..empecé la insulina [mil	(11.5) look..here I started.. I started insulin [thousand
25.	DT:	[okay.. [mhm	[okay..mhm
26.	A:	[mil 19 de marzo del 2009 y esto eran los estudios que yo tenia el azúcar así mire...a las 8 de la mañana en ayunas..257..después de almorzar 268..203 y 241 y mire como cuando empecé pero..ya desde hace un año.. con la insulina empecé el 19 y aquí esta empecé el 19 el 20 empecé a checarlo..168 130	[a thousand march 19 2009 and this those were the studies that I had the sugar so look...at 8 in the morning fasting..257..after lunch 268..203 and 241 and look how when I started but..a year ago..with the insulin I started the 19 and here this I started the 19 the 20 I started to check it..168 130
27.	DT:	okay ese es más aceptable..esta no tanto..pero ahora solo me uh me ayuda para entender..uh <u>ese</u> es de esta año..¿sí?	okay this is more acceptable .. this isn't so high..but now just uh help me me to understand.. uh <u>that</u> is from this year..yeah?
28.	A:	sí=	yes=
29.	DT:	=de hace poco..y estuvo poniendo la:=	=recently..and you were putting the:=
30.	A:	=no: esto es de hace poco (2.0) es de 2009	=no: this is recent (2.0) it's from 2009
31.	DT:	eso es 2009 <u>esta</u> es 2009	that es 2009 <u>this</u> is 2009
32.	A:	sí pero esto es antes de insulina	yes but this is before insulin
33.	DT:	<u>ah</u>:: okay okay	<u>ah</u>:: okay okay
34.	A:	aquí aquí es	here here is
35.	DT:	do—[cuando empezó	wh—[when did you start?
36.	A:	[18 y 19	[18 and 19
37.	DT:	oh [okay	oh [okay
38.	A:	[yo empecé aquí [19	[I started here [19
39.	DT:	[okay	[okay
40.	A:	pero ya tenía un año entonces [us—	but I already had one year [us—

Table 11.1 (Continued)

Excerpt 1.
<T = 1:09:57>

41.	DT:	[¿y ahora?	[and now?
42.	A:	no ahorita no tengo control no tengo aparato ya..y este: pero la medicina no me la dieron aquí ustedes	no now I don't have control I don't have a device anymore:... and thi:s but the medicine you didn't give it to me here

<T = 1:13:27>
Excerpt 2.
<T = 1:23:51>

43.	A:	pero aquí yo lo estoy surtiendo en Costco ((DT typing)) y me cuesta 23	but here I was getting it at Costco ((DT typing)) and it costs me 23
44.	DT:	(1.0) y:: u:m. . .¿lo cortizó e:n Walmart?	(1.0) a::nd u:m. . .did you get a quote at Walmart?
45.	A:	esa insulina no. . .porque no tenía prescription. . .y en Costco me la dieron sin presc—sin receta	that insulin no. . .because I didn't have a prescription. . .and at Costco they gave it to me without a pre—prescription
46.	DT:	sí pero yo le he dado receta:	yeah but I gave you a prescriptio:n
47.	A:	pero de esa no	but not that one
48.	DT:	¿ellos no lo tienen?	they didn't have it?
49.	A:	no [lo—	no [it—
50.	DT:	[en Walmart?	[in Walmart?
51.	A:	no lo he buscado..no he llevado receta	I haven't looked for it..I haven't taken the prescription
52.	DT:	Kay	Kay
53.	A:	(2.3) pero aquí tengo:. . .mire. . .por ejemplo (10.0) ((papers shuffling))	(2.3) but here I ha:ve..look..for example (10.0) ((papers shuffling))
54.	DT:	okay (2.8) no tenemos sus resultados de su colesterol entonces no podemos hablar bien de esto. . .u::m su presión esta bien controlado con esto	okay (2.8) we don't have your cholesterol results so we can't talk very well about this. . .u::m your blood pressure is well controlled with this
55.	A:	(1.0) sí	(1.0) yes
56.	DT:	(1.8) pero sabe uh:: e:stoy (10.0) ((papers shuffling and mouse clicking audible)) okay=	(1.8) but you know uh:: I:'m (10.0) ((papers shuffling and mouse clicking audible)) okay=
57.	A:	=mire..por ejemplo..¿cuántas?. . . surtié yo..pero no sé las cantidades.. aquí me costó ese ((xxx)) es este..y me costó 9	=look..for example..how many?. . .I got..but I don't know the quantity..here it cost me that ((xxx)) it's this..and it cost me 9

(*Continued*)

Table 11.1   (Continued)

<T = 1:13:27>
Excerpt 2.
<T = 1:23:51>

58.	DT:	Mhm	Mhm
59.	A:	y ¿pero cuantas son? aquí no dice [¿cuántas pastillas?	and but how many are there? here it doesn't say [how many pills?
60.	DT:	[oh uh ahí dice dice 30?	[oh uh there it says it says 30?
61.	A:	30 pastillas?	30 pills?
62.	DT:	30 cues—uh cuesta 9	30 cos—uh costs 9
63.	A:	9..y ¿acá me costó? ¿veinticuatro son?	9..and here it cost me? 24 is it?
64.	DT:	eh: 120	eh: 120
65.	A:	ciento [¿veinte?..((xxx))	one hundred [twenty?..((xxx))
66.	DT:	[entonces 4 veces <u>más</u> por menos cuenta	[so 4 times <u>more</u> for less cost
67.	A:	pero aquí son..180 y me cuesta..85 dólares	but here are..180 and it costs me..85 dollars
68.	DT:	(4.0) pero esta es porque era en Stater Brothers	(4.0) but this is because it was in Stater Brothers
69.	A:	¿es mas caro?	is it more expensive?
70.	DT:	@@ oh..yeah (1.0) ((pills in bottle shaking)) eh probamente en la primera cosa es sinceramente prob'mente siempre seria bueno cotizarlo en Wal[mart	@@ oh..yeah (1.0) ((pills in bottle shaking)) eh probably in the first thing is sincerely probably it always would be good to get a quote at Wal[mart
71.	A:	[Walmart	[Walmart
72.	DT:	(H) eh: y si no:..eh allá..Walmart Target tiene más o menos lo mismo precios pero:..eh:. . .K-Mart..ta—tambien más o menos..esos tres. . .uh Walgreens CVS. . .ellos tienen una programa..pero tiene que pagar..y uh: se me olvido cual es cual..um yo creo que uh Walgreens..paga:: ..10 dólares uh: al año. . .con esto se puede lograr por doce dólares . . .u::m..uh sus recetas	(H) eh: and yes no:...eh there.. Walmart Target has more or less the same prices bu:t..eh: K-mart..t—too more or less.. those three. . .uh Walgreens CVS. . .they have a program..but you have to pay..and uh: I forgot which is which..um I think that Walgreens..you pay::...10 dollars uh: a year. . .with this you can get for 12 dollars. . . u::m..uh your prescriptions
73.	A:	oh=	oh=
74.	DT:	=¿okay?..pero tiene que pagar algo anual..¿CVS?..yo entiendo es como 25 dolares por..persona o 35 por familia.. para entrar igual y para tener um	=okay?..but you have to pay something annually..CVS?..I understand it's like 25 dollars per..person or 35 per family..to enter and have um

Table 11.1 (Continued)

<T = 1:13:27>
Excerpt 2.
<T = 1:23:51>

75.	A:	descuentos=	discounts=
76.	DT:	=descuentos..(H) seria bueno eh:: tal vez voy a hacer receta de todo..y hacer dos copias que puede guardar un copia..para cotizar en diferente lugares (H) pero es cierto esta Walmart y supues—yo sé que era en otra ciudad pero supuestamente Walmart es Walmart (H) eh tal vez subio un poquito solo porque es un año después pero en todos modos (H) u:m...uh..esta parece mucho más:...económico ¿no? es tres veces menos	=discounts..(H) it would be good eh:: maybe I'm going to make the prescription for everything.. and make two copies..to get a quote a different places (H) but it's true that Walmart and supos—I know that you were in another city but supposedly Walmart is Walmart (H) and possibly it increases a little only because it's one year later but anyway (H) u:m...uh...this seems much more:...economic right? it's three times less
77.	A:	mucho menos	much less

[a] Occasional deviations from standard orthography in the Spanish transcript are intentional to reflect the way the interlocutor spoke.
[b] Transcription Conventions. Adapted from Du Bois (2005).

1. Turn Sequence   Left to right and top to bottom order
2. Overlap   [ ]
3. Hold (short closure/pause) ..
4. Pause, untimed   ...
5. Timed Pause   (1.0)
6. Truncated word   wor-
7. Laugh   @
8. Laugh voice   @word
9. Inhale   (H)
10. Exhaled release   (Hx)
11. Utterance final question ?
12. Emphatic   word
13. Unintelligible string   ((xxx))
14. Uncertain word   #word
15. Linked utterances   ==

responds in line 42 that he currently has no control over his diabetes. He neither has the machine to measure his blood sugar nor the means to buy the medicine he needs.

Thus far, Dr. Thomas is able to elicit from Arturo a situation in which he had had control over his health when he had access to healthcare. And though it is not clear how he stopped receiving health treatment, it appears that his ability to afford the treatment was a factor. In line 18, Arturo asks why the cost of his prescription was so high, to which Dr. Thomas responds in line 19 that she does not know how he goes about purchasing his medicines. It becomes evident that cost is a barrier to Arturo's health, which becomes even clearer in Excerpt 2. But it is noteworthy in Excerpt 1 that Dr. Thomas has managed to cede the floor to Arturo, which allowed Arturo to lead the conversation and Dr. Thomas to determine the cause of Arturo's failure to follow the prescribed treatment regimen from another clinic – that is, cost.

Approximately 10 minutes later into the consultation, Dr. Thomas moves on to prescribing treatment. In doing so, she aligns with cost as the barrier to Arturo taking care of his health.

In lines 43–53, Arturo orients toward the cost of the insulin, mentioning the cost at Costco, while Dr. Thomas recommends going to Walmart to get a quote for the cost of the medicine. Then in line 54, Dr. Thomas changes the topic to discuss the fact that Arturo's cholesterol results are not available yet and that his blood pressure is under control. In line 56, Dr. Thomas begins an utterance followed by a 10 seconds pause, typically, in the context of our data, indicative of attention to information on the computer screen [32].

However, in line 57, Arturo retopicalizes the cost of the medications. In lines 58–66, Dr. Thomas clarifies the quantity of pills available as well as the cost for each quantity, advising that Costco is the most expensive option to buy insulin, charging $120 for 24 units rather than $9 for 30 units, presumably at Walmart. In lines 67–68, Arturo indicates that he paid $85 for 30 units, and Dr. Thomas states that he paid $85 because he filled the prescription at Stater Brothers, which the interactants establish as one of the more expensive options in turns 69–70.

From turns 70 through 76, Dr. Thomas clearly aligns with Arturo's concern with the cost of the medications and demonstrates her own stock of knowledge for navigating affordable medicine (for the uninsured). And we see Arturo register understanding of this vital information in turn 77, saying that the alternative means of filling his prescription that Dr. Thomas laid out would be more affordable. Furthermore, when Arturo returned to the clinic for a follow-up consultation three weeks later, we observed that his health had improved dramatically after this consultation with Dr. Thomas because, as he reported, the affordable path to obtaining his prescriptions allowed him to comply with the treatment regimen.

What Dr. Thomas did in Excerpt 2, in response to prompting from Arturo, was to realign her role as a doctor, and in tune with Arturo, occasioned membership categories were co-constructed in which she became a consumer resource for an uninsured patient. This ability to realign her role in response to an obvious barrier to a good health outcome for Arturo is an example of an essential move that made this consultation LC. Dr. Thomas aligned with the patient and re-constructed her role in the interaction to meet the patient's particular needs. It was not necessarily language at the levels of morpho-syntax and phonology that created the concordance. Rather, it was Dr. Thomas's ability to align with the social circumstances of consultation that afforded concordance. Dr. Thomas' Spanish phonology was not ideologically standard, but she was adept as interactionally aligning with the linguistic and social needs of the patients.

In fact, if we were to evaluate Dr. Thomas' Spanish use prescriptively, one might say that her Spanish pronunciation was heavily Anglicized; for instance, she repeatedly would replace Spanish-language vowels with the English-language schwa. In addition, instances of her anomalous Spanish morpho-syntax were evident through the transcript (e.g., incorrect article-noun agreement in terms of gender: "la problema" (the problem) in line 11; incorrect use of *ser* instead of *estar* (to be): "es un poquito rojo" (it's a little red).

Regardless, her ability to align with the social circumstances of the patient and to reimagine her role as a healthcare professional were the key elements of concordance. And though Dr. Thomas could improve her Spanish-language pronunciation and grammatical accuracy, the fact that she could use Spanish was critical. That is, the quality of her language use in terms of concordance with the patient rested in her ability to align with the patient rather than in the morpho-syntactic and phonological quality.

Nonalignment

Conversely, in Table 11.2, Laura does not seem to have the same ability to align with her patient, Bea, a patient with diabetes who came in to review the results of her blood work. Though Bea had seen Laura before, her health was not improving, and as we will demonstrate, the lack of improvement can be tied to language discordance.

In lines 1 and 3, Laura explains that Bea's triglycerides and bad cholesterol are too high, prompting Bea to ask Laura what the solution is in turn 4. Laura's immediate response in turn 5 is to exercise daily. Bea indicates that daily exercise is difficult for her in turn 6; however, Laura does not align with Bea's concern. Instead, in line 7, Laura proceeds to list several food items that Bea must not eat. Laura's delivery style is quite authoritarian here in terms of how she structures the utterance grammatically and emphatically with "nada de. . ." (no...). The authoritarian style is also constructed prosodically with falling intonation and a slight pause after each food item. Most importantly, Laura never uptakes Bea's contribution that she would find daily exercise challenging, as was a clear move of resistance on Bea's part, which Laura never addresses throughout the consultation.

In turn 8, Bea overlaps with Laura to elicit confirmation that it is indeed "nada" (nothing) that she must not eat from this list of food items, a list that Laura expands upon in turn 9. In turn 10, Bea uptakes Laura's suggestion that she entirely avoid certain foods by repeating some of the dairy options before asking if she should avoid milk as well. In turn 11, Laura explains that she can have nonfat milk, which Bea seems to understand in turn 12 before clarifying food items that she should avoid in turn 14, followed by Laura's confirmation and authoritative repetition that Bea should avoid fried food in turns 13 and 15. After a 1-s pause, Bea says very quietly in line 23, "okay..'sta bien," indicating that she understands Laura's directive, but the whispered tone of the utterance indicates some resistance, which Laura does not acknowledge or uptake.

Although Laura authoritatively communicates several food items that Bea needs to avoid, there is no indication of what Bea *can* eat. This discursive move, or lack thereof, follows Bea's contribution in turn 5 that daily exercise would be difficult for her, which Laura ignored. In other words, Laura does not seem concerned with Bea's input on these dietary restrictions given her life circumstances. Laura does not ask what Bea *does* eat or about her access to food. Perhaps Bea cannot comply with Laura's dietary regimen because she does not actually cook for herself, or perhaps she eats leftovers from meals she prepares for others, or perhaps she lives in a food desert where fresh produce is not readily available. Regardless, suppose Bea's diet and cooking skills currently consist of only the foods that Laura listed as forbidden. In that case, any other food may seem unimaginable, and here and throughout the consultation, Bea does not receive the information and resources needed to comply with regimen.

Laura changes the topic in turn 19 to Bea's blood sugar, which Bea expresses that she is ready to discuss in turn 20. In turns 21 through 25, Laura explains why Bea's blood

202 Language Concordance in Public Health and Healthcare

Table 11.2 Bea.[a]

Excerpt 3.
<T = 0:37:28>

1.	L:	se nota que necesitas:..bajar solamente los triglycerides..lo necesitas <u>má:ximo</u> 150..tú estás 167..el colesterol ma:lo [má:ximo	it's noted that you nee:d..to lower the triglycerides..you need it at <u>maximum</u> 150..you're 167.. bad cholesterol [maximum
2.	B:	[uhuh	[uhuh
3.	L:	130..estás 164..entonces esos están causando que colesterol <u>total</u>..te suba a 248=	130..you're 164..so those are causing your <u>total</u> cholesterol ..to increase to 248=
4.	B:	=eh ¿<u>cómo lo soluciono</u>?	=eh <u>what's the solution</u>?
5.	L:	ejercicio diario	daily exercise
6.	B:	aye doctora [me lo pone difícil	aye doctor [that's difficult
7.	L:	[nada— (Hx) @. . .<u>nada</u> de frituras..<u>queso</u>.. mayonesa.. mantequilla.. [carne de res	[nothing— (Hx) @. . .<u>no</u> fried foods..cheese ..mayonnaise..butter [beef
8.	B:	[¿nada de eso?	[nothing of that?
9.	L:	y de puerco..esos son los que son más altos	and pork..those are what are highest
10.	B:	ok..no mantequilla queso..n::o ¿leche tampoco?	ok..no butter cheese..n:o milk either?
11.	L:	que sí de leche puedes tomar ah yo prefería que tomes la de non-fat [es—no tiene <u>nada</u> de grasa=	yes you can drink milk ah I'd prefer that you drink non-fat [it's—it does<u>n't</u> have fat=
12.	B:	[oh okay =uhuh..y carne de::	[oh okay =uhuh ..and mea::t
13.	L:	de puerco [ni de res	pork [or beef
14.	B:	[ni de res..uhuh okay=	[or beef..uhuh okay=
15.	L:	=¿okay?..nada de fri<u>turas</u>	=okay?..no <u>fried</u> foods
16.	B:	(1 .0) °okay..'sta bien°	(1.0) °okay..that's fine°
17.	L:	okay..esos son los que te van a ayudar para el colesterol..<u>ah:</u>ora=	okay..those are what's going to help your cholesterol..<u>no:w</u>=
18.	B:	=mhm=	=mhm=
19.	L:	=vamos a ir a la <u>azúcar</u>	=let's go to the sugar
20.	B:	ándale..¿hay una cosa adelante?=	go on..there's another thing?=
21.	L:	=la azúcar..135 por ese día..pero si nos fijamos la azúcar por los últimos tre:s meses eh que es esto aquí hemoglobin A1C=	=the sugar..135 for that day..but if we adjust for the last 3 months eh that is this here hemoglobin <u>A1C</u>=

Table 11.2 (Continued)

Excerpt 3.
<T = 0:37:28>

22.	B:	=ah::=	=ah::=
23.	L:	=estamos 9.3..eso me enseña que está completamente..<u>no</u> tenemos control de la azúcar..no es que no tenemos control esa sem<u>a</u>na: o: o ese día que te sacaron la sangre..pero los últimos tres [meses la azúcar	=we're 9.3..this shows me that it's completely..we <u>don't</u> have control of the sugar..it's not we don't have control that <u>wee:k</u> o:r or that day we took blood..but the last three [months the sugar
24.	B:	[oh	[oh
25.	L:	está descontrolada...[¿okay?	it's not controlled...[okay?
26.	B:	[porque no estaba tomando medicamento	[because I wasn't taking medicine
27.	L:	okay ¿cuánto tiempo estuviste sin la medicina?=	okay how much time were you without medication?=
28.	B:	=oh:: estuve como como: uno:::s ocho meses	=oh:: I was like li:ke so::me eight months
29.	L:	okay..entonces eso puede haber sido la razón déjame fijarme mis notas de la última vez..entonces lo que hicimos es te pusimos en el metformin	okay..so that may have been the reason..let me fix my notes from the last time..so what we did is we put you on metformin
30.	B:	Mhm	Mhm
31.	L:	no: (1.5) aquí me dijiste tú que estabas tomando metfo:rmin=	no: (1.5) here you told me that you were taking metfo:rmin=
32.	B:	=uhuh	=uhuh
33.	L:	<u>por</u>:que: aquí en mis notas yo estoy poniendo que continúes con el metformin..pero si no lo estuviste tomando por 8 meses [entonces	<u>be</u>:cause: here in my notes I was putting you continue with metformin..but if you weren't taking it for 8 months [then
34.	B:	[mhm	[mhm
35.	L:	nunca va a mejorar eso	it's not going improve that
36.	B:	oh:: y como	oh:: and like
37.	L:	porque las únicas prescripciones que te di fue ibuprofen y la moxifloxacina..(H) [pero en mis notas aquí dicen	because the only prescriptions that I gave you was ibuprofen and moxifloxacin..(H) [but in my notes here the say
38.	B:	[uhuh	[uhuh
39.	L:	(1.0) que hay que continuar con el metformin..porque aquí dicen que estás tomando el metformin..entonces neces[itamos	(1.0) it's necessary to continue with metformin.. because here it says you're taking metformin..so [we need

(*Continued*)

Table 11.2 (Continued)

Excerpt 3.
<T = 0:37:28>

40.	B:	[ah::	[ah::
41.	L:	ese metformin lo e<u>stás</u> tomando? o no lo [estás tomando?	that metformin <u>you're</u> taking it? or you're not [taking it?
42.	B:	[sí sí no..lo empecé a tomar..[como 3 mes—3 semana'	[yes no ..I started to take it.. [like 3 mon—3 weeks
43.	L:	[right	[right
44.	B:	4 semana' como lo e'taba tomando por allí cuando vine a verle=	4 weeks like I was taking it around then when I came to see you=
45.	L:	=mhm (1.5) entonces <u>sí</u> lo estabas tomando cuando viniste a vernos=	=mhm (1.5) so <u>yes</u> you were taking it when you came to see us=
46.	B:	=sí [estaba tomando	=yes [I was taking
47.	L:	[metformin ¿<u>dónde</u> lo empezaste a tomar?	[metformin <u>where</u> did you start to take it?
48.	B:	¿dónde?=	where?=
49.	L:	=ah=	=ah=
50.	B:	=o cuán[—	=or whe[—
51.	L:	[quién te lo—¿quién te lo dio?=	[who—who gave it to you?=
52.	B:	=eh: hicieron una feria de salud=	=eh: they did a health fair=
53.	L:	=de salud y hay feria	=and there was a health fair
54.	B:	y el [doctor..me la dio	and [the doctor..gave me it
55.	L:	[okay	[okay
56.	B:	y me recomendaron que viniera aquí [((xxx))	and they recommended to come here [((xxx))
57.	L:	[excelente..entonces ¿cuánto tiempo estuviste a tomando la—el metformin? <u>antes</u> de [venir a vernos	[excellent..so how much time were you taking metformin <u>before</u> [coming to see us
58.	B:	[antes oh: yo llevaba como unos:: 6 años. . .y cuando perdí mi seguranza	[before oh: I was taking it like so::me 6 years. . .and when I lost my insurance
59.	L:	Uhuh	Uhuh
60.	B:	hoy no:: no tuve: más metformin	today no:: I didn't ha:ve more metformin
61.	L:	Okay	Okay
62.	B:	(.5) y tomaba..medicina natural	(.5) and I was taking..natural medicine

[a] Occasional deviations from standard orthography in the Spanish transcript are intentional to reflect the way the interlocutor spoke.

sugar is not under control, which prompts Bea to state turn 26 that she was not taking her medicine. In lines 27 and 28, the interactants establish that Bea had taken medicine for eight months. In turn 29, Laura indicates that Bea's not taking medicine could be the reason and that she needs to adjust her notes, but Laura indicates that metformin, a common medication to treat type 2 diabetes, was in her notes. In turn 31, Laura says, "aquí me dijiste tú que estabas tomando metfo:rmin" (here you told me that you were taking metformin), a statement with which Bea seems to agree in turn 32.

Laura continues in turn 33 to reiterate that her notes indicate that Bea was taking metformin when Laura last consulted with her, and in turn 35, Laura states that Bea's health is not going to improve this way. Bea wonders about the reason in turn 36, and Laura reads what she had prescribed when they last met in 37. After a back-channel cue from Bea in turn 38, Laura repeats in turn 39 that her notes reveal that Bea was taking metformin at the time and that she should have continued to do so. Then, in turn 40, overlapping with Laura, Bea says, "aw::" in a tone as though she is being scolded. Laura then asks in turn 41 whether or not Bea is taking the metformin. Bea clarifies in turn 42 that she did not start taking metformin after their last consultation and in turn 44 that she had been taking it for a few weeks when she consulted with Laura the last time. In turns 46 through 51, after two clarification requests from Bea in turns 48 and 50, Laura asks Bea who gave her the metformin. Bea explains in turns 52 through 56 that she obtained the metformin at a health fair, which is also where she was recommended to visit the clinic – information that Laura then evaluates positively.

In turn 57, Laura asks how long Bea had been taking the metformin before coming to that clinic, to which Bea responds in turn 58 around 6 years. However, in turns 58 and 60, she informs Laura that she had lost her insurance then and that today she does not take the metformin anymore. While we do not have access to the consultation in which Laura missed Bea's health history concerning metformin, it seems that the health history style that we see in Table 11.2 would be conducive to such missed information. As evidenced by Laura's delivery of the dietary regimen, she leaves no room for the patient to narrate her actual experience or life circumstances. This lack of patient input into the conversation creates discordance as the clinician misses the patient's health narrative, which some indicate constitutes 60–80% of the diagnosis [33].

It is noteworthy that Laura is a native Spanish speaker from Peru, and though her variety of Spanish is different from Bea's Puerto Rican variety, the quality of the morphosyntax or phonology is not at issue in this consultation. Rather, the issue is that Laura does not leave room discursively to understand Bea's health history. Laura never leaves room for the creation of nuanced roles in this clinician-patient interaction. Bea is a patient like any other, and Laura is the authoritative clinician throughout. This lack of more nuanced alignments with the patient as a unique actor is the basis of the discordance that we see in Excerpt 3.

Another interesting feature of Laura's consultation is that she primarily uses the informal tú form with patients. She was the only clinician in the clinic to use the tú form so consistently. Although it does not contribute to or detract from concordance in terms of meaning-making, it does contribute to her authoritative style along with other linguistic features such as the unhedged directives with falling intonation on each food item Bea should avoid, as discussed above. This authoritative style generally discourages patient agency as Laura relies on test results to diagnose, as opposed to patient narratives, and then to direct the patient to follow a regimen.

Alignment, translanguaging helping to establish the alignment

In Table 11.3 below, Carrie interacts with Ana and Roberto, a couple of Carrie's regular patients. In the extracted dialog, we see Carrie not only align with the patients' social circumstances but also with their language preferences through translanguaging, as both Ana and Roberto are multilingual users of Spanish and English. The interaction below begins with Carrie treating Ana for an earache.

In turns 1 through 10, Carrie asks Ana a series of health history questions in Spanish. In line 11, Carrie switches to English to say, "let's take a look," switching back to Spanish to joke whether Ana has a cockroach in the ear – a joke that Ana finds funny through laughter, as evidence in turn 12. In Carrie's consultations, it is not uncommon for her to switch to English when she talks through a procedure out loud, and in Vickers et al. [34], we extensively discussed discourse moves that instigate such switches to English from Spanish. We see Carrie switch again to Spanish in turn 16 to ask if she is scratching the ear. It could be that Carrie's use of English in previous turns motivated Ana to use English in her response in turn 18, but Ana was responding directly to a question that Carrie posed in Spanish.

The conversation returns to Spanish in turn 19 when Ana describes her symptoms. Carrie expresses surprise in turn 20, which prompts joint laughter from Ana and Roberto in turn 21, followed by Carrie's playful, empathetic reaction in turn 22 and more laughter from the patients in turns 23 and 24. In turn 25, Carrie continues to elicit health history information in Spanish, to which Ana responds in turn 26 in Spanish. In turn 27, Carrie starts to diagnose Ana's ear ailment in Spanish and then in English in the same utterance. Carrie continues to use English in turn 29 before switching to Spanish to ask for additional health history information in turn 31 and then back to English in turn 33 to confirm where Ana is experiencing the pain.

Maintaining orientation to English, Carrie topicalizes Ana's and Roberto's puppy in turn 35, and the sidebar chat remains in English with the exception of Roberto's "como eh eh" in turn 39, which is followed by his own switch to English, and then his contribution of "chiquito" in turn 49. In this conversation, all participants are users of Spanish and English, and Carrie and Ana align with each other as bilingual, maintaining the use of English through turn 52 during the talk of the dog. The three interactants draw on the entirety of their respective linguistic repertoires to construct meaning and to align with each other by way of translanguaging.

In the first part of Table 11.3, the participants select words and phrases from their repertoire to co-construct Ana's ailment. It is notable that Carrie aligns with Ana not just as a patient but as a person with a life outside of the clinic when she asks about her puppy (in English). It is hard to say what motivates Carrie's use of English at this point. Perhaps given that all interactants were multilingual, Carrie is more comfortable using English for everyday conversation, but interestingly, Carrie's switches to English are often followed by Ana also switching to English.

Several minutes later in the same consultation, Carrie tends to Roberto's health issues, which include high blood pressure, diabetes, loss of appetite, and weight loss. After co-constructing his health history with him earlier, Carrie explains Roberto's treatment regimen, which is included in Table 11.3. Although this second excerpt is from the same consultation, Carrie mainly uses Spanish with Roberto, with the exceptions of "what else?" in turn 56, "right_right_right" in 62, and "that's alright" in 75. That is, Carrie's use of language is considerably different than when her attention

Table 11.3 Ana and Roberto.[a]

Excerpt 4.
<T = 0:18:20>

1.	C:	no..no estaba [enferma	no..you weren't [sick
2.	A:	[no:: [no:	[no:: [no:
3.	C:	[no le duele la garganta	[your throat doesn't hurt?
4.	A:	no:	no:
5.	C:	¿ni corre la nariz?	and your nose isn't runny?
6.	A:	no:	no:
7.	C:	¿nada de eso?	nothing of that?
8.	A:	No	no
9.	C:	(TSK) okey doke (H) ¿no hacía vómitos?	(TSK) okey doke (H) you haven't been vomiting?
10.	A:	n:oo no	n:oo no
11.	C:	okey doke..let's take a look (1.0) a ver..si tiene cucaracha=	okey doke..let's take a look (1.0) let's see..if you have a cockroach=
12.	A:	=@@@@@	=@@@@@
13.	R:	((xxx)) [((xxx))	((xxx)) [((xxx))
14.	A:	[ouch	[ouch
15.	R:	[eh eh	[eh eh
16.	C:	[oh ¿le duele huh? (1.0) ok I'll be more gentle (2.0) hm:: (1.0) ¿está rascando?	[oh it hurts huh? (1.0) ok I'll be more gentle (2.0) hm:: (1.0) are you scratching?
17.	A:	(.5) uh maybe yeah	(.5) uh maybe yeah
18.	C:	hm: yeah (TSK) (H) okay=	hm: yeah (TSK) (H) okay=
19.	A:	=eh eh..a a veces que me..me ((xxx xxx)) se duele ((xxx xxx xxx)) el oído	=eh eh..a sometimes that ((xxx xxx)) me..me it hurts ((xxx xxx xxx)) my ear
20.	C:	((surprised)) hmm:↑	((surprised)) hmm:↑
21.		((Ana and Roberto laughing))	((Ana and Roberto laughing))
22.	C:	qué malo	how bad
23.	A:	@@[@@	@@[@@
24.	R:	[@@@	[@@@
25.	C:	(1.3) y esta le duele también o solamente [la—	(1.3) and does this hurt too or only [the—
26.	A:	[no no más de esa	[no no more than that
27.	C:	okay..okay (9.0) (TSK) (Hx) no hay mucho cerumen you don't have a bunch of..ear [wax	okay..okay (9.0) (TSK) (Hx) there isn't much ear wax you don't have a bunch of..ear [wax
28.	A:	[¿no?=	[no?=
29.	C:	=no:..let's see but there's a little bit (1.0) say ah	=no:..let's see but there's a little bit (1.0) say ah
30.	A:	=ah:=	=ah:=
31.	C:	=mkay (TSK) (4.8) y ¿le duele aquí?	=mkay (TSK) (4.8) and does it hurt you here?

(Continued)

Table 11.3 (Continued)

Excerpt 4.
<T = 0:18:20>

32.	A:	No	No
33.	C:	nothin' huh? just this ear	nothin' huh? just this year
34.	A:	Yeah	Eah
35.	C:	okay:: (2.7) so your puppy's big now?=	okay:: (2.7) so your puppy's big now?=
36.	A:	=oh yeah	=oh yeah
37.	C:	Uhuh	Uhuh
38.	A:	[((xxx))	[((xxx))
39.	R:	[como como nine nine [months	[like like nine nine [months
40.	A:	[uhuh=	[uhuh=
41.	C:	=<u>yeah</u>?=	=<u>yeah</u>?=
42.	R:	=yeah=	=yeah=
43.	C:	-and what kind dog is it? do you know?	-and what kind dog is it? do you know?
44.	R:	it's—	it's—
45.	A:	it's a ch_ch eh ha_half terrier uh wu with a ha_half weenie	it's a ch_ch eh ha_half terrier uh wu with a ha_half weenie
46.	C:	(TSK) so how big? not too big=	(TSK) so how big? not too big=
47.	A:	<u>no</u>::	<u>no</u>::
48.	C:	[mhm	[mhm
49.	R:	[chiquito	[small
50.	A:	(.5) weenie [@@@	(.5) weenie [@@@
51.	C:	[@@weenie dog..mhm=	[@@weenie dog..mhm=
52.	A:	=mhm	=mhm

Excerpt 5.
<T = 0:41:20>

56.	C:	what else? vamos a sacar poco sangre hoy [(TSK)	what else? we're going to draw a little blood today [TSK
57.	R:	[ah	[ah
58.	C:	y voy a darle un u:::n orden por rayo equis del pecho..but..no necesita cita para hacer una rayo equis	and I'm going to give you an order for a chest x-ray..but..you don't need an appointment for the x-ray
59.	R:	ah [okay	ah [okay
60.	C:	[solamente cuando..puede llegar a:: ((location name))	[only when..you're able to go to:: ((location name))
61.	R:	entonces en [((city name))	so in [((city name))
62.	C:	[right_right_right	[right_right_right
63.	R:	Okay	Okay
64.	C:	uhuh..entonces solamente va	uhuh..so just go
65.	R:	ah ok[ay	ah ok[ay
66.	C:	[porque no necesita cita por el rayo [equis	[because you don't need an appointment for the x-[ray

Table 11.3 (Continued)

Excerpt 5.
<T = 0:41:20>

67.	A:	[oh	[oh
68.	R:	oh [okay	oh [okay
69.	C:	[y entonces..quiero verle otra vez en::..(TSK) (.5) una semana [((xxx)) okay?	[so then..I want to see you again in:: (TSK) (.5) a week [((xxx)) okay?
70.	R:	[ah: bien	[ah: okay
71.	C:	Okay	Okay
72.	R:	porque..por—porque esta semana que viene=	because..be—because this next week=
73.	C:	=yeah	=yeah
74.	R:	yo estoy un poquito ocupado=	I'm a little busy=
75.	C:	that's alright	that's alright
76.	R:	Ah	Ah
77.	C:	va la otra	you come the other week
78.	R:	ah okay	ah okay
79.	C:	okay? cundo puede=	okay? when you can=
80.	R:	=ah okay	=ah okay

[a] Occasional deviations from Spanish orthography in the Spanish transcript are intentional to reflect the way the interlocutor spoke.

was focused on Ana's diagnosis. As we have discussed previously in detail [34], Carrie often switched to English with monolingual patients when thinking aloud and evaluating patient contributions and actions, which is what we see here in her interaction with Roberto. However, Carrie's uses of English were *not* accompanied by Roberto's uses of English, as was the case with Ana. And Carrie's few turns in which she used English were surrounded by Spanish contributions that served to align with Roberto as a Spanish user. In Vickers et al. [35], we demonstrated what happens when Carrie uses English with a bilingual third party leaving the monolingual Spanish-speaking patient as a nonparticipant in her own consultation. However, in this consultation, Carrie is aligned with Roberto as a person who prefers to use Spanish. Carrie's uses of English index her status as a dominant English speaker, but there is no multilingual alignment with Roberto because they are not creating meaning together in English.

Table 11.3 demonstrates that translanguaging can be a means of achieving concordance when both the clinician and the patient are comfortable with translanguaging, as in the case of Ana. It is notable that Carrie does not attempt to translanguage with Roberto and that Roberto does not attempt to translanguage with Carrie, and that somehow Carrie knows not to with Roberto. Concordance is interactionally achieved using aspects of the linguistic repertoire that best align with the needs of the patient. Monolingual language use is not the only means of concordance. Rather, concordance can be achieved through using all aspects of the multilingual repertoire.

Discussion

The excerpts analyzed in this chapter demonstrate that alignment between the patient and the clinician is at the heart of language concordance as they co-construct occasioned membership categories. In terms of proficiency, Dr. Thomas would undoubtedly test lower than Laura in an ACTFL Oral Proficiency Interview that rates speaking proficiency on a scale of (sub-)levels from Novice to Intermediate, Advanced, Superior, and Distinguished. However, Dr. Thomas's consultation with Arturo was more interactionally concordant than Laura's consultation with Bea because of the specific linguistic choices that each clinician made that either contributed to or detracted from interactional concordance.

Meanwhile, Carrie and Ana were aligned through their interactional choices and willingness to draw upon their full linguistic repertoires, orienting to each other bilingually as people who can use both English and Spanish codes. In line with productive multilingual practice, Carrie and Ana were translanguaging [17]. Carrie's astute ability to translanguage was further evident in her alignment with Roberto as a Spanish user, demonstrating the flexibility that multilingual people have to align with their interactants' language preferences. It is not as though Carrie had to ask about language preference. Instead, language preference emerged interactionally. Similarly, Dr. Thomas and Arturo "let it pass" [36] in a way that is very natural for multilingual people. Arturo was in tune with Dr. Thomas linguistically even though her Spanish phonology was heavily Anglicized and morpho-syntax was somewhat anomalous, and they were in tune with each other interactionally. As Ortega and Prada [29, p. 254] state:

> Medical translanguaging reminds us to adjust our words and communication styles to respectfully acknowledge individual patients' histories and the dynamic natures of language and medicine, and in so doing, encourages us to contribute to a push for the inclusion and recognition of subjects whose discursive practices have been historically left out of professional spaces . . .

However, language concordance is not simply a matter of understanding the individual words; rather, it is an interactional achievement. Language concordance with a patient who prefers to use a minoritized language in the context of any particular healthcare setting necessitates the clinician's and patient's abilities to understand the sentence-level language, of course. However, our data caution against noninteractional evaluation of clinician language through language proficiency tests, such as monologic oral proficiency tests and written proficiency examinations. See Knoch and Fan (this volume) for an extensive discussion of assessment of clinical language skills. Any assessment of language concordance must occur by examining the interaction between the healthcare professional and the patient to assess how concordance (or discordance) emerges in interactional processes lest we risk institutionally positioning someone as capable of concordance on a false basis, as discussed by Pomerantz [12].

Implications for training

Ultimately, language learning and multilingual development alongside university students' non-linguistic specializations, responsibilities, and aspirations can coincide or compete with language development, as observed by Goble [11]. In particular, Goble documented a pattern whereby study abroad was perceived as the peak of target language development, which impedes prolonged multilingual development beyond higher education and into graduate school, law school, or medical school, for instance.

However, one focal participant in Goble's study, Javed, narrated having developed his target language, Japanese, through a biomedical engineering summer internship in Japan ahead of his plan to apply to medical school [11]. In his career advising appointment and post-advising interview, Javed described the particulars of the work he performed *through* Japanese and how he negotiated meaning with Japanese-monolingual lab mates and the bilingual Principal Investigator. According to Goble's narrative analysis, Javed's story was not one of merely *applying* acquired language; it was one of situated language socialization where Javed drew upon and expanded his linguistic repertoire to align himself with the social environment.

Javed's internship was notable because he was both a language learner and a STEM student. Language learners tend to study rather than intern abroad, and STEM students tend to carry unit-heavy course loads and work hours, as Javed reported in Goble [11]. Goble argued that experiences such as Javed's, in addition to service-learning and volunteer opportunities, are crucial for prolonged bilingual development because they afford localized opportunities to negotiate meaning, develop linguistic self-confidence, and perform aspects of identity beyond that of "language learner." Javed's experience brings to mind the importance of developments, such as bilingual tracks for both medical and nursing students. The University of California, Irvine Medical School's PRIME-LC program is a good example of a productive bilingual track to develop multilingual physicians. This program provides a medical school curriculum designed to develop Spanish speaking people into Spanish-speaking doctors to serve underserved Latino communities.

On that note, healthcare professionals need to understand multilingual interaction and interactional alignment more generally to develop the capacity to effectively achieve language concordance with their patients. To achieve this ability, clinicians need sustained opportunities to practice and obtain feedback in actual multilingual clinical practice. Future research should address effective means of training multilingual clinicians to be interactionally concordant with their patients. It is also important to note that LC care is contextual, so such training needs to be designed and implemented with particular contextual needs in mind. It is not only the ability to use a particular language proficiently that contributes to LC care but the ability to micro-interactionally align with the patient interpersonally, socially, and linguistically that becomes the basis for LC care.

Conclusion

Language concordance is not easily measurable in terms of monologic linguistic knowledge of morpho-syntax and phonology. Indeed, there are plenty of language proficiency exams that allow for the assessment of one's L2 linguistic knowledge (e.g., ACTFL Oral Proficiency Interview, Computerized Oral Proficiency Instrument, and Simulated Oral Proficiency Interview). However, such test-based evaluations should be accompanied by evaluations of the clinician's ability to achieve interactional concordance through alignment and situated joint meaning-making with the patient. In other words, we should not assess potential language concordance by measuring someone's proficiency level alone through an inorganic, decontextualized language examination. The proficiency level measured through language testing represents a potential rather than actual interactional performance during a clinical consultation. Actual language concordance is observable through careful analysis of clinician-patient interaction as it emerges on the ground in practice with the actual patients that healthcare professionals serve.

Highlights

- Actual language concordance is observable through careful analysis of clinician-patient interaction as it emerges on the ground in practice with the actual patients that healthcare professionals serve.
- Future research should address effective means of training multilingual clinicians to be interactionally concordant with their patients.
- Healthcare professionals need to understand multilingual interaction and interactional alignment more generally to develop the capacity to effectively achieve language concordance with their patients.
- LC care is contextual, so such training needs to be designed and implemented with particular contextual needs in mind.
- Clinicians need sustained opportunities to practice and obtain feedback in actual multilingual clinical practice.

NOTES

1 This flipped orientation began in education with George I. Sanchez who opposed his mentor's use of the term "language handicap" and offered instead the term "dual language handicap" to reflect the deficits of the school system. See Martinez and Train (2020) pp 71–73.
2 All names used are pseudonyms.

REFERENCES

1. Diamond, L., Izquierdo, K., Canfield, D. et al. (2019). A systematic review of the impact of patient–physician non-English language concordance on quality of care and outcomes. *J. Gen. Intern. Med.* 34: 1591–1606.
2. Lor, M. and Martinez, G. (2020). Scoping review: definitions and outcomes of patient-provider language concordance in healthcare. *Patient Educ. Couns.* 103: 1883–1901.
3. Ortega, P. (2018). Spanish language concordance in U.S. medical care: a multifaceted challenge and call to action. *Acad. Med.* 93: 1276–1280.
4. Foiles Sifuentes, A., Robledo Cornejo, R., Chen Li, N. et al. (2020). The role of limited English proficiency and access to health insurance and health care in the affordable care act era. *Health Equity* 4: 509–517.
5. Lau V. Nichols. Lau V. Nichols. 414 U.S. 563, 1974.
6. Cook, V. (1999). Going beyond the native speaker in language teaching. *TESOL Quart.* 33: 185–209.

7. Canagarajah, S. (2007). Lingua Franca English, multilingual communities, and language acquisition. *Mod. Lang. J.* 91: 923–939.
8. Ortega, P., Shin, T., and Martinez, G. (2021). Rethinking the term "Limited English Proficiency" to improve language-appropriate healthcare for all. *J. Immigr. Minor. Health* 5: 1–7.
9. Showstack, R. (2019). Patients don't have language barriers; the healthcare system does. *Emerg. Med. J.* 0: 1–2.
10. Magnan, S. (2008). Reexamining the priorities of the national standards for foreign language education. *Lang. Teach.* 41 (3): 349–366.
11. Goble, R. (2022). *The Construction of Language Learners' Multilingual-Professional Identities and Trajectories in Career Advising Appointments: A Figured Worlds Perspective [Dissertation]*. Madison, WI: The University of Wisconsin-Madison.
12. Pomerantz, A. (2002). Language ideologies and the production of identities: Spanish as a resource for participation in a multilingual marketplace. *Multilingua* 21: 275–302.
13. Da Silva, E. (2007). Humor (re)positioning ethnolinguistic ideologies: "You tink is funny?". *Lang. Soc.* 44: 187–212.
14. Heller, M. (2003). Globalization, the new economy, and the commodification of language and identity. *J. Socioling.* 7 (4): 473–492.
15. Block, D. (2018). What on earth is 'language commodification'? In: *Sloganization in Language Education Discourse: Conceptual Thinking in the Age of Academic Marketization* (ed. B. Schmenk, S. Breidbach, and L. Küster), 121–141. Bristol: Multilingual Matters.
16. Gumperz, J. (1977). The sociolinguistic significance of conversational code-switching. *RELC J.* 8: 1–20.
17. Otheguy, R., García, O., and Reid, W. (2018). A translanguaging view of the linguistic system of bilinguals. *Appl. Linguistics Rev.* 10: 1–27.
18. Blommaert, J. (2010). *The Sociolinguistics of Globalization*. Cambridge: Cambridge University Press.
19. Jorgensen, J. (2008). Polylingual languaging around and among children and adolescents. *Int. J. Multiling.* 5: 161–176.
20. García, O. and Wei, L. (2014). *Translanguaging: Language, Bilingualism and Education*. London: Palgrave Macmillan Pivot.
21. Pennycook, A. and Otsuji, E. (2015). *Metrolingualism: Language in the City*. New York: Routledge.
22. Otheguy, R., García, O., and Reid, W. (2015). Clarifying translanguaging and deconstructing named languages: a perspective from linguistics. *Appl. Linguistics Rev.* 2015 (6): 281–307.
23. Lo, A. and Park, J. (2017). Metapragmatics of mobility. *Lang. Soc.* 46: 1–4.
24. Reyes, R. (2014). Translanguaging in multilingual third grade ESL classrooms in Mindanao, Philippines. *Int. J. Multiling.* 16: 1–15.
25. Gunnarsson, B. (2013). Multilingualism in the workplace. *Annu. Rev. Appl. Linguist.* 33: 162–189.
26. Otsuji, E. and Pennycook, A. (2010). Metrolingualism: fixity, fluidity, and language in flux. *Int. J. Multiling.* 7: 240–254.
27. Canagarajah, S. (2011). Translanguaging in the classroom: emerging issues for research and pedagogy. *Appl. Linguistics Rev.* 2: 1–28.
28. Creese, A. and Blackledge, A. (2015). Translanguaging and identity in educational settings. *Annu. Rev. Appl. Linguist.* 35: 20–35.
29. Ortega, P. and Prada, J. (2020). Words matter: translanguaging in medical communication skills training. *Perspect. Med. Educ.* 9: 251–255.
30. Vickers, C. (2020). Occasioned membership categorization in a transnational medical consultation: interaction, marginalization, and health disparities. *J. Socioling.* 24: 1–19.
31. Sacks, H. (1992). *Lectures on Conversation*. New York: Wiley Blackwell.
32. Goble, R. and Vickers, C. (2015). 'Shift' 'n 'control': the computer as a third interactant in Spanish-language medical consultations. *Commun. Med.* 12: 171–185.
33. Peterson, M., Holbrook, J., Von Hales, D. et al. (1992). Contributions of the history,

physical examination, and laboratory investigation in making medical diagnoses. *Western J. Med.* 156: 163–165.
34. Vickers, C., Deckert, S., and Goble, R. (2014). Constructing language normativity through the animation of Stance in Spanish-language medical consultations. *Health Commun.* 29: 1–10.
35. Vickers, C., Goble, R., and Deckert, S. (2015). Third party interaction in the medical context: code-switching and control. *J. Pragmat.* 84: 154–171.
36. Firth, A. (1996). The discursive accomplishment of normality. On "lingua franca" English and conversation analysis. *J. Pragmat.* 26: 237–259.

12 Assessing Clinician Language Skills

UTE KNOCH AND JASON FAN

Introduction

Assessing clinician language skills, as part of language assessment for professional purposes [1], has been gaining significant attention due to the pivotal role that language ability plays in successful healthcare communication, which is in turn intrinsic to high-quality healthcare [2]. Questionable language ability or workplace communication skills have been argued to be the cause of unsatisfactory healthcare outcomes, healthcare safety concerns, and even incidents [3], which have attracted media attention and policy debates. The importance of assessing clinician language skills is significantly amplified by the massive and accelerating global movement of overseas-trained clinicians in recent decades, most of whom emigrated from contexts where English is not the principal language and where the cultural norms and styles of communication and models of patient care are not aligned with the local context. Such movement of professional personnel is vital to countries such as Australia, New Zealand, the United States, and United Kingdom whose shortfalls in the healthcare workforce need to be filled [4].

The purpose of language assessment for professional purposes is to make inferences about a test taker's ability to communicate effectively in professional contexts, termed as target language use domain in language assessment [5]. Depending on the context, the target language may refer to the dominant language in a particular country or region, or the patient's preferred language, or both. In this chapter, we examine several key issues surrounding the assessment of clinician language skills. We use "clinician" here to broadly encompass a wide range of medical and health professionals who practice in different clinical specializations in a jurisdiction, including, for example, doctors, nurses, and pharmacists. We will first discuss the distinct features of language assessment for professional purposes which distinguish it from assessment of general language abilities, with an emphasis on assessing clinician language skills. Next, we focus on a few fundamental considerations in developing and using a test to measure clinician language skills. Finally, we introduce the argument-based validation approach to interrogate the validity of such a test.

The Handbook of Language in Public Health and Healthcare, First Edition.
Edited by Pilar Ortega, Glenn Martínez, Maichou Lor, and A. Susana Ramírez.
© 2024 John Wiley & Sons, Inc. Published 2024 by John Wiley & Sons, Inc.

Approaches to the assessment of clinician language skills: Distinguishing language assessments for professional purposes from general language proficiency tests

There are various approaches to assessing the linguistic readiness of clinicians seeking professional registration/licensing in English-speaking countries [6]. Two key distinctions need to be considered: (1) whether a separate language assessment is used in combination with an assessment of professional skills; and (2) whether the language assessment is of general nature or specifically designed to assess language skills of clinicians.

The licensing model to practice as a physician in the United States includes several steps – language proficiency is not separately assessed in the United States Medical Licensing Examination (USMLE) but integrated into one of the steps, the medical school's competency exams (which simulate through standardized patients). This is similar to the recently discontinued Clinical Skills examination. It, therefore, comprises one aspect that is scored by simulated patients, who are laypeople and not trained as physicians. Integrating the assessment of language proficiency into an assessment of clinical knowledge is not without its difficulties. Assessment designers as well as policymakers need to consider whether various components of language proficiency are sufficiently captured in such an assessment, who makes the judgment of language proficiency, and what criteria they draw on when doing this. Whether different medical schools actually include a focus on language proficiency is less clear, since the Clinical Skills examination was discontinued. In other jurisdictions, for example, in the United Kingdom, Australia, and New Zealand, language proficiency is assessed separately from clinical competence. Professional registration (licensing) authorities (which cover a range of 13 healthcare professions, including physicians, nurses, physical therapists, optometrists, dentists, etc.) accept proof of English language competency from a variety of different assessments, which can be broadly classified as either general English assessments or language assessments for professional purposes, each of which we describe in more detail now.

The development of a language test starts with a sound understanding of the language ability to be assessed, known in the language testing literature as "test construct" [5]. The test construct that a language assessment for professional purposes assesses is the language ability and/or communication skills deemed essential to a professional context or the target language use domain (e.g., doctor–patient consultation in the case of assessing physician language skills). The construct for a general language proficiency test, on the other hand, is language ability in less specialized and more general contexts (e.g., listening to a news report). In other words, compared with a general language test, the language samples that a language assessment for professional purposes is designed to elicit from test takers are more relevant and contextualized, thus making it possible to draw more accurate inferences about a test taker's linguistic readiness for workplace communication [7, 8]. We discuss both test types here because both of them are often accepted for professional registration/licensing of clinicians who have trained overseas and are seeking professional registration/licensing in an English-speaking country.

We can use two examples of language tests, that is, the International English Language Testing System (IELTS) and the Occupational English Test (OET) to illustrate the distinctive features of language assessment for professional purposes. Both tests are accepted for professional registration/licensing of clinicians in Australia, New Zealand, and the United Kingdom. Designed to assess a test taker's readiness to study in an English-medium tertiary program, the IELTS is a test of general academic English proficiency, comprising four components of listening, reading, writing, and speaking. In the listening and reading modules of the IELTS, task formats such as multiple-choice questions, matching, and short-answer questions are used to assess a test taker's listening and reading comprehension ability in the context of academic study. In the writing module, test takers are required to complete two writing tasks that they are likely to encounter in academic settings, including describing visual information (e.g., graph, table, and diagram) and writing on a topic in a rhetorically discursive style. The speaking module is a face-to-face oral proficiency interview between a test taker and an IELTS examiner, focusing on very generic, preselected topics (e.g., a performance that the test taker enjoyed watching, a time when someone apologized to the test taker, or a person who taught the test taker).

The OET, by contrast, is a language assessment for professional purposes designed to evaluate the English ability of overseas trained or certified clinicians who plan to study or practice in certain English-speaking countries [9]. The OET covers 12 health professions, including medicine, nursing, dentistry, physiotherapy, veterinary science, pharmacy, occupational therapy, dietetics, radiography, speech pathology, podiatry, and optometry. Like the IELTS, it is a four-skill test. Different from the IELTS, however, all test takers complete the same components for receptive skills, that is, listening and reading, whereas the writing and speaking skills are tailored to the specific requirements of each health profession. The writing tasks for doctors, for example, are different from those for pharmacists. As a performance test, the OET tasks and content are designed to simulate workplace communication for healthcare professionals. For example, in the speaking subtest of the OET, test takers are required to perform in a healthcare roleplay scenario where they play clinical roles such as a doctor or nurse and interact with an interlocutor who takes the role of a patient. Though the listening and reading modules are the same for all test takers, the topics of the texts used in these modules are health-related and selected in light of their relevance across different clinical specializations [8].

Though designed as a general academic English proficiency test, the IELTS has been commonly used by regulatory bodies in countries such as the United Kingdom, Australia, and New Zealand to assess clinicians' English language proficiency. For example, the General Medical Council (GMC), a regulatory body responsible for registering doctors to practice medicine in the United Kingdom, uses the IELTS to assess applicants' English proficiency, though it should be noted that they are also required to pass a follow-up test of professional competence to fulfill the registration/licensing requirements [3, 6]. The value of using a general proficiency test like the IELTS to assess clinicians' language skills has been criticized as dubious and inadequate primarily due to the ostensible lack of alignment between its test construct and associated target language use domain (i.e., academic domain) and medical communication [4, 10]. The OET, however, was developed through a careful needs analysis characterized by collaboration between language specialists and domain experts to ensure that the test tasks and content adequately reflect communication demands in the healthcare profession. By drawing on insights from both language experts and healthcare professionals, subsequent research has further refined the rating criteria used to evaluate test takers' performance on the OETe [11], an aspect which is considered vital to the authenticity of a language assessment for professional purposes [12]. Despite the efforts to simulate medical communication in terms of both test design and rating criteria, it is worth noting that the OET is essentially a language test, as opposed to a test of professional competence. Indeed, as indicated by McNamara [9], it is legal requirement in Australia that the OET should not assess a test taker's professional competence. This claim about the OET relates to the challenge of *inseparability* in language assessment for professional purposes, that is, whether language knowledge and specific-background knowledge (e.g., medical knowledge) are "inextricably entwined" [7].

Assessing clinician language skills: Key considerations

In this section, we focus on several key considerations in the design and use of a language assessment for professional purposes, namely test development, scoring test takers' performances, setting appropriate passing standards, and establishing its validity.

Test development

Language assessments for professional purposes are designed to collect evidence about test takers' ability to cope with the linguistic demands of a certain domain, in this case, the ability to function linguistically in a healthcare workplace. As developers of language tests are usually not insiders to the language domain of clinicians, test design usually starts with a careful needs analysis designed to provide test developers with information about, among others, the language tasks common to the domain, the language that is used to accomplish these tasks, the aspects of language that are valued in the domain (target language use domain criteria) and the specific needs and challenges of typical test taker populations required to take the assessment. Knoch and Macqueen [1] also add other components to a needs analysis for a language assessment for professional purposes, including undertaking a policy analysis (to gain an understanding of the policy environment in which the testing requirements will be embedded), a means analysis (to understand the resources available to deliver an assessment) and a test requirement analysis (any specific requirements of what a language test needs to look like and what resources are available for its development and administration). The most crucial component is the analysis of domain tasks and the language required to successfully complete these tasks. Such an analysis can provide information about the tasks and subtasks that are used by a specific community of users, task frequency, the steps that are typical of a standard performance of these tasks, assessability (i.e., whether the language in the tasks is assessable or worth assessing), the language used to accomplish the tasks, those that are involved in accomplishing such tasks in the domain (e.g., doctors, patients, families, and other clinicians), the importance of tasks to minimizing risks in the domain, the criteria for assessing acceptable completion of the tasks and the standards used to assess such accomplishment [1, 13].

A needs analysis carried out in a healthcare domain is likely to show a list of tasks that can be further categorized according to different layers in terms of their "saturation of specialist content" [1], where intra-professional communication (e.g., at a nursing handover) may include more specialist content than inter-professional communication (e.g., medical professional communicating with a physiotherapist), and those that involve communication within the wider workplace community (e.g., doctor–patient consultation or doctor–family member discussion). Sampling tasks from across this spectrum of workplace tasks is likely to result in a language assessment for professional purposes that is more authentic, and therefore likely to result in more accurate predictions about how test takers may be able to cope with the language demands of the domain.

A key decision for test developers is the specificity of the content to be included in a language assessment for professional purposes. Should an assessment be generalist in content, so it applies to all health professionals, or should the content be focused on specific professions, such as doctors, or specializations, such as neurologists? These are key decisions that need to be made at the outset.

Authenticity in language assessments for professional purposes is more than a simulation of language tasks to make test takers feel comfortable. When test tasks and the preparation materials and courses for a test reflect real-world tasks test takers are likely to encounter in the workplace in the future, this is likely to result in a positive flow-on effect (also known as positive washback [14]) in that the test helps workforce entrants to set appropriate expectations about their future roles. Test preparation will then likely engage the relevant abilities by test takers and will likely result in benefits to them, and the receiving workplace. Authenticity includes the situational authenticity of test tasks that test takers encounter, the authenticity of their interaction with the test tasks, as well as authenticity in scoring [12, 15] (see the section on scoring performances below).

Authenticity is not an all-or-nothing property of tasks in language assessments but rather a question of degree. All language assessments are somewhat inauthentic purely because tasks are in an assessment context [16]. Certain speaking tasks also involve interlocutors/examiners, which creates situations and is likely to change how test takers interact with tasks. A carefully designed needs analysis with input of healthcare professionals is likely to increase task authenticity. Employing interlocutors with suitable backgrounds or ensuring adequate training of interlocutors in speaking assessments can also add to authenticity. In the next section, we examine how authenticity in scoring criteria can be created.

Scoring performance

Authentic language assessments typically include tasks in which test takers need to produce language. For example, for a language assessment for professional purposes in the context of healthcare, test takers might be required to write a letter of referral or they might be asked to perform a role play with a simulated colleague or patient. The scoring of such performances is more complicated than the scoring of more restricted language tasks which may draw on multiple-choice item types. Historically, the scoring criteria used to judge such performances were generally linguistic in nature. They represented what language test developers and/or applied linguists thought mattered in spoken or written performances. This has been challenged recently by a number of studies that set out to establish the criteria that mattered to those working in healthcare contexts and termed the resultant criteria, the "indigenous" criteria to the domain. The first group of studies [17–19] focused on the writing subtest of the OET in which test takers are asked to write a letter of referral or discharge based on a set of simulated patient notes they are given. Elder and McNamara [17] set out to establish the indigenous criteria of physiotherapy educators reviewing video recordings of students interacting with simulated patients to inform the criteria used for the OET speaking subtest. The physiotherapists commented on the strengths and weaknesses in these interactions (e.g., on the student's awareness of/sensitivity to a patient's ideas and concerns, the student's interactional resources, such as sign-posting in interaction, or their nonverbal communication skills). In the second phase, the study examined the routinely occurring feedback provided by clinical educators during students' clinical placement (which focused on very similar strengths and weaknesses in communication). A parallel study undertaken by Pill [11], the author focused on the indigenous criteria of doctors and nurses when reviewing student doctors' and nurses' interactions with patients or simulated patients. Based on the findings of these studies, Pill proposed two new criteria for the spoken subtest of the OET: "clinician engagement" and "management of interaction" and created a list of checklist indicators that can be used to train raters/markers, who generally do not have a background in healthcare, in applying these new criteria [11].

A more recent study by Knoch et al. [20] aimed to create indigenous criteria for the writing subtest of the OET. The authors recruited three groups of informants for the study, all selected because they regularly interact with written patient records: doctors, nurses, and health information managers. The authors showed the informants' referral letters and discharge summaries extracted from real patient records from two large Australian hospitals. The informants commented on the strengths and weaknesses of these documents in small focus groups. All comments that related directly to the texts were coded and grouped, and based on these groupings, a new set of indigenous criteria were created. Knoch et al. [21] showed in a detailed paper the challenges of applying these indigenous criteria to a language testing context, including what aspects valued by the three groups of informants could not be included in the criteria used for the language test. This included items such as whether the writing was considered suitable for multiple audiences or future uses (as this is not in line with the design of the OET writing task), or whether the document was written in a way that showed the clinical ability of the writer (not part of the OET's brief). A follow-up study conducted by Knoch et al. [22] explored the challenges of training OET raters, who are not from healthcare backgrounds but usually have a background in language teaching (or similar) and are used to applying linguistic criteria to use the new indigenous criteria. The study showed some of the challenges language assessment providers may encounter when intending to use indigenous criteria, which add authenticity to the assessment [12].

Methodologically, eliciting indigenous criteria from domain experts in health is not without its challenges. Studies eliciting indigenous criteria in various professional domains have drawn on different methodological choices. Knoch and Macqueen [1] review these choices and present these options visually in a series of discs, which can be turned to create various combinations of methodological considerations, which are described in Table 12.1.

Knoch and Macqueen describe each of these in more detail and consider the likely outcome on the indigenous criteria resulting from the data. The authors argue that more research is needed to understand the effect of particular combinations of methodological choices.

Standard setting

Language assessments generally produce a score or a score band based on test takers' responses. However, in many contexts, particular pass-fail distinctions need to be made, or different score meaning is attributed to different score levels. Therefore, how the

Table 12.1 Methodological considerations when eliciting indigenous criteria.

Methodological consideration	Description
Purpose of verbalization	This considers whether the criteria were verbalized in a naturally occurring setting or whether this was for research or test development purposes.
Timing of verbalization	This considers whether the criteria were verbalized at the same time the performance occurred or later on when, for example, reviewing a video or audio recording of the performance.
Audience of verbalization	This considers who the criteria were verbalized to – for example, whether the audience were colleagues, students, or domain laypeople.
Type of stimulus materials	Stimulus material may be drawn from the domain (real patient-clinician interaction), from the training domain (e.g., interaction of student with simulated patient), from a language test domain, or criteria may be elicited without using stimulus material.
Producers of stimulus material	This criterium considers who the speakers or writers of the performance are that is used for stimulus material. For example, is the performance produced by a senior physician or a student?
Background of stimulus material selector	It is also important to consider who selects the stimulus material and whether this person's background (for example domain layperson or domain expert) may focus on particular features in the performances selected.
Feature selection	Particular features in the performances selected as the stimulus material may influence the criteria that are subsequently verbalized. For this reason, it is important to include a spread of particular performance features and discuss the justifications for their inclusion. For example, specific features in written handover letters could include whether the writer followed an expected letter structure, used paragraphs, provided sufficient background information about the patient, etc.

score of a language assessment for professional purposes is interpreted is specific to a particular policy context. Score meaning is ideally established through a process of standard-setting "by which qualified panelists, following carefully developed and documented procedures that mitigate against arbitrariness, assign interpretative meaning to performances on tests" [23]. In the context of language assessments for healthcare contexts, panelists may be asked to decide at which language proficiency threshold test takers may be ready to cope with the language demands of their chosen profession. This results in a cut score on the range of possible test scores that is used to establish if a test taker's score is sufficient or not for a certain purpose (e.g., professional registration/licensing in a new country).

Knoch and Macqueen [1] argue that in the case of language assessments for professional purposes, which are often used as high-stakes gatekeepers for internationally-trained clinicians, a lot can depend on the defensibility of this standard.

Setting cut scores too high or too low can have significant consequences, as Pill and McNamara [19] argue. If cut scores are set too high, and therefore bar many competent health professionals from registration/gaining licensing, the health system may be disadvantaged. On the other hand, if the cut score is set too low, and overseas-trained clinicians are able to register and practice who are not yet linguistically ready, this might pose a risk to patient safety. The standards set on language assessments therefore need to balance the needs of the public, test takers, and health workforce policymakers.

Defensible passing standards are clearly important; however, what constitutes an acceptable standard is a values judgment that "reflects the values of the professionals who take part in its definition and adoption, and different professionals may hold different values" [24]. To ensure the defensibility of standards adopted in high-stakes contexts (such as the registration/licensing standards for overseas clinicians), standard-setting workshops must follow clearly defined, principled procedures. Procedural rigor is one aspect of the validation of such standard-setting exercises [23]. Another key aspect for the setting of standards on language assessment for professional purposes is the involvement of domain experts as participants in the standard-setting activities [25, 26].

In the context of setting standards on language assessments used in the registration/licensing of overseas-trained clinicians, Knoch and Macqueen [1] divide existing standard-setting studies of language assessments for clinicians into three groups:

- Studies that set standards on general or academic language assessments for a specific workplace purpose
- Studies in which a cut score was set on a language assessment designed for workplace purposes
- Studies that set out to pinpoint a standard on a language framework (such as the Common European Framework of Reference, or CEFR) for specific workplace purposes.

A number of studies set out to set principled, empirically-based standards on general academic language assessments, including the International English Language System (IELTS), Test of English as a Foreign Language (TOEFL), and the Pearson Test of English (PTE). The studies varied in the particular professions they focused on and the standard-setting methodologies they drew on. For example, O'Neill [24] and O'Neill et al. [27] recommended passing standards for nurses in the United States for the TOEFL paper-based test. Also in the context of the United States, O'Neill et al. [28] set standards for nurses on the IELTS test. Drawing on the performance profile method, Qian et al. [29] set standards for nurses on the Michigan English Language Assessment Battery (MELAB). What all these studies have in common is that they involved nurses as informants in the workshops that were conducted to set the passing standards. Focusing on international medical graduates (i.e., physicians) in the United Kingdom, Berry et al. [3] conducted a study to set passing standards on the IELTS for physicians migrating to the United Kingdom. Unlike previous studies, the authors not only involved physicians in their panels (i.e., domain experts from the same profession), but also nurses, allied healthcare professionals and patients (i.e., groups commonly interacting with physicians).

Studies setting standards on a language test for healthcare professionals are less common in comparison. The only studies we are aware of focused on setting standards on the OET. One group of studies focused on the speaking subtest [18, 19, 26] and explored both quantitative and qualitative aspects of the judgments made by healthcare professionals on the panels. More recently, Knoch et al. [20] and Davidson [25] conducted research setting cut-offs for doctors and nurses on the OET writing subtest. These studies show what aspects of the performances were seen as key in deciding on minimum standards by the panelists. These aspects included, among others, the participants' consideration of overall task fulfillment, the appropriateness of the language used, the comprehension of the stimulus material, control of linguistic features, and how well the writer recognized the intended audience.

Research is clearly still needed to get a better understanding of the most suitable standard-setting methodologies for professional contexts, how to best sample a representative panel of health professionals, and how to ensure procedural validity. Validity of passing standards is, however, just one aspect of validation that language assessment specialists are concerned with in the case of language assessment for professional purposes used in healthcare contexts. In the following section, we outline broader considerations for establishing the validity of language assessments for professional purposes.

Establishing the validity of language assessments for professional purposes

Validity is the primary consideration for any assessment. It concerns the meaningfulness and fairness of test score interpretation and use in relation to the target language use domain. The process of establishing the validity for a test is known as validation. In test validation, both evidence and theory can be drawn on to support test score interpretation and use [30]. While aware that there are different approaches to test validation [31], we introduce the argument-based approach to test validation in this chapter to establish the validity of language skills for clinicians. This validation framework represents a more recent development of validation theory in language testing and educational measurement more broadly [32, 33], and has been widely applied to language test validation research [34, 35]. By adopting this validation framework, test developers and researchers need to build a validity argument for a language test through specifying a series of inferences, together with their associated warrants and assumptions, to interrogate test score interpretation and use. To examine the plausibility of each inference, its underlying warrants and assumptions need to be formulated. Evidence needs to be collected, and relevant theories, if necessary, need to be consulted to examine these warrants and assumptions. The plausibility of an inference depends on the support from both evidence and theoretical rationales. In the context of assessing clinician language skills, we refer to Knoch and Macqueen [1] by specifying seven inferences for establishing the validity for a test: domain description, evaluation, generalization, explanation, extrapolation, decision, and consequence. A generic structure of this validation framework is presented in Figure 12.1.

We briefly explain each inference as it relates to the assessment of clinician language skills. The first inference, domain description, concerns whether the design and delivery of the test tasks mirror language use in the context of healthcare communication. Next, the evaluation inference examines whether the elicited language samples from prospective clinicians are properly evaluated to yield their observed scores on the test of clinician language skills. The third inference, generalization, considers whether test takers' observed scores represent their expected scores across parallel test tasks, raters, and test

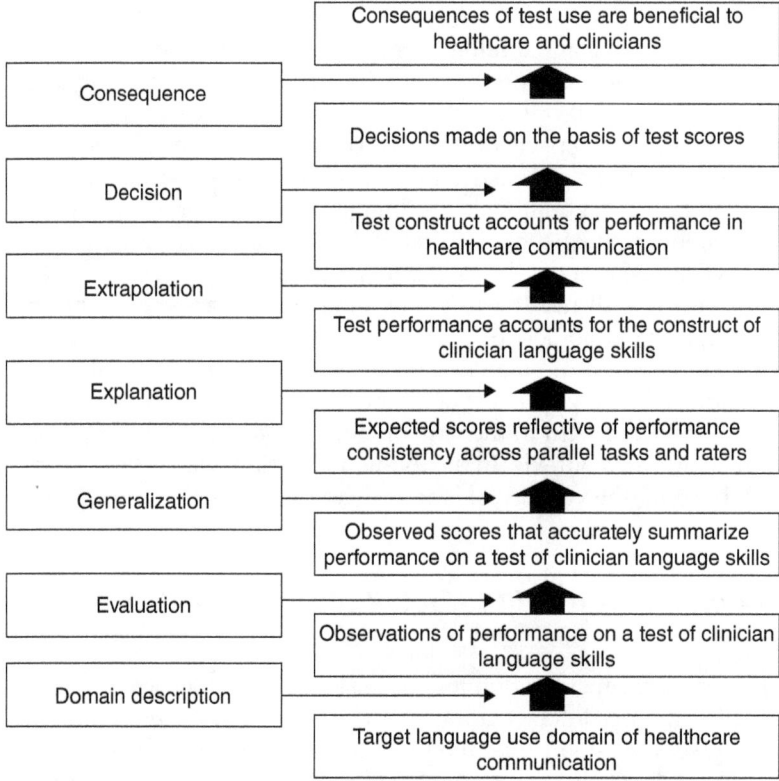

Figure 12.1 Inferences in a validity argument.

administrations. For example, if a test taker (i.e., a prospective clinician) takes a test of clinician language skills, will they get the same score if they take a parallel form of the test, or if the test is administered at a different time or location? The next inference, that is, explanation, interrogates whether test takers' expected scores are attributed to the construct of clinician language skills or healthcare communication that the test claims to measure. In other words, does a test taker get a higher score on the test because they have a higher level of proficiency in clinician language skills? The focus of the next inference, extrapolation, is that the language abilities assessed in the test accounts for the quality of linguistic performance in healthcare settings. We would expect a test taker with a higher score on a test of clinician language skills to demonstrate higher quality of linguistic performance in their clinical practices. The decision inference concerns whether the decisions made by test takers based on their test results are appropriate. That is, if a test taker passes the test, can they function adequately in healthcare communication? The last inference is a consequence which examines whether the consequences of developing and using a test are beneficial to healthcare workplace and clinicians. Interested readers can refer to Kane [33] for a detailed account of this validation framework, Knoch and Macqueen [1] for an elaboration of applying this framework to conducting validation activities in the context of language assessment for professional purposes. In this chapter, we use the first inference in this validation framework, that is, domain description, as an example to illustrate how this inference could be justified in the context of assessing clinician language skills, and to demonstrate how test developers and researchers could use this framework to plan and conduct validation activities for a test of clinician language skills.

The domain description inference can be justified by examining the correspondence between the design and delivery of test tasks and the communication demands in the target language use domain of healthcare communication. As noted previously, an important feature of a language assessment for professional purposes lies in that the language samples that it elicits from test takers are more relevant and contextualized so that an accurate inference could be drawn about their linguistic readiness for workplace communication. As such, the domain description inference is particularly pertinent to establishing the validity of a language assessment for professional purposes. This inference is typically justified by careful needs analysis, aiming to gain a sound understanding of the communication demands at the healthcare workplace. As demonstrated in the previous section, needs analysis, typically involving both language specialists and domain experts, plays a significant role in the development and subsequent revisions or refinement of a language assessment for professional purposes. Table 12.2

Table 12.2 Domain description inference: claim, warrant, assumptions, and backing.

Claim: Selection, design, and delivery of the test tasks take healthcare communication into consideration.

Warrant	Assumptions	Possible sources of backing
Test tasks and their administration conditions reflect language use and communication at healthcare workplace.	• Test tasks mirror what clinicians do in healthcare communication.	Analysis of clinicians' communication at workplace; interviews, focus groups, and/or surveys with healthcare experts and test takers
	• Test tasks elicit and are sufficiently representative of language skills, knowledge, and processes that clinicians need for healthcare communication.	Analysis of clinicians' communication at workplace; interviews, focus groups, and/or surveys with healthcare experts and test takers
	• Task administration conditions mirror how language is used in healthcare communication.	Analysis of clinicians' communication at workplace; observations of the test in use; interviews, focus groups, and/or surveys with healthcare experts and test takers

below summarizes the claim, warrant, assumptions, and possible sources of backing or evidence that we have identified to support the domain description inference for a test of clinician language skills.

The warrant underlying this inference states that test tasks and their administration conditions reflect language use and communication at healthcare workplace. Three assumptions can be identified that underpin this warrant. The first assumption states that test tasks mirror what clinicians do in healthcare communication. To support this assumption, evidence can be collected through a careful analysis of clinicians' communication at workplace; it can also be collected through interviews, focus groups, or surveys with healthcare experts and test takers. Take reading demands at healthcare workplaces. If evidence emerges that clinicians often need to find specific information through skimming and scanning techniques across several texts [6], tasks that tap into these reading techniques need to be included. Conversely, a lack of such tasks would weaken the plausibility of the domain description inference.

Different from the first assumption which focuses on the correspondence between test tasks and healthcare communication, the second assumption evaluates the representativeness of the elicited language samples of the domain of healthcare communication. Evidence in support of this assumption can be collected through a detailed analysis of language use in healthcare communication as well as interviews, focus groups, or surveys with healthcare experts and test takers. Pill, in a study that we cited previously, demonstrates how this assumption is addressed [11]. It aimed to investigate whether the rating criteria for the OET speaking subtest were adequately representative of those at the healthcare workplace. Five aspects of performance were included in the OET rating criteria, including overall communicative effectiveness, fluency, intelligibility, appropriateness of language, and resources of grammar and expression, representing a generalized view of language. Data were collected through workshops with both educators who provided training to clinicians and clinician supervisors. During the workshops, the researcher interacted with these two groups of stakeholders and solicited their comments on the criteria of evaluating spoken communication at workplace. The findings provided empirical basis for adding two professionally relevant criteria (i.e., clinical engagement and management of interaction) to the rating criteria for the OET speaking subtest.

The third assumption states that task administration conditions mirror how language is used in healthcare communication. This can be similarly investigated through a detailed analysis of the domain in focus, in this case, healthcare communication. Feedback collected through interviews, focus groups, or surveys with healthcare experts and test takers can also shed light on this assumption. The findings can then be put vis-à-vis observations of how the test is administered to test takers. For instance, if research uncovers very few instances of clinicians writing referral letters by hand and reveals that the majority of them produce those on the computer [36], this should be reflected in the administration conditions of the writing tasks in the test.

Here we use the domain description inference as an example to illustrate how the argument-based validation framework could be utilized to establish the validity of a test of clinician language skills. Other inferences in the framework can be justified in a similar fashion by specifying the associated warrants and assumptions and identifying the potential sources of backing. It should be noted that the warrants and assumptions that we have listed in relation to the domain description inference in Table 12.2 are not applicable to all assessment contexts. We recommend that test developers and researchers use them as a point of reference and specify warrants and assumptions that are more pertinent to the purpose and context of their tests. We also suggest that when planning validation agendas and activities, test developers, and researchers should carefully examine the warrants and assumptions underlying each inference in the argument-based validation framework, assess which ones might be most questionable in light of their testing context, and prioritize those accordingly as they might be the weakest links in the validity argument [33]. For example, if a test developer feels uncertain about whether the test tasks are sufficiently representative of the language skills, knowledge, and processes in the target language use domain, priority should be given to collecting the backings to interrogate the plausibility of this assumption.

Conclusion

In this chapter, we examine several key considerations in designing and developing language assessments for professional purposes, with an emphasis on assessing clinician English language skills, including test development, scoring test takers' performance, standard setting, and test validation. While we have mainly focused on assessing English language skills in this chapter, the fundamental considerations in developing, using, and validating a test of clinician language skills outlined in this chapter are also applicable to the contexts where languages other than English are used for healthcare communication. For example, in the United States, there is a need to assess clinicians' language skills in using languages such as Spanish, Polish, Vietnamese, Korean, and Chinese with patients who have limited proficiency in English. Test developers in these contexts can follow the concepts and methods delineated here for test development and validation. There is, however, a further consideration in such contexts. Often designing a standardized language test is not necessarily practical, in particular in the case of lesser-used languages. Physicians or clinicians speaking languages other than those of the dominant culture should, however, be trained in awareness of when it is not appropriate to discuss health issues with a patient in another language, but rather to call in an interpreter.

Language assessment for professional purposes differs from general language proficiency assessment in terms of its purpose, test construct, and the target language use domain. A test of clinician language skills is designed with the express purpose to draw accurate inferences about a test taker's linguistic readiness for healthcare workplace communication, based on the elicited language samples. It is therefore essential for test developers to clearly delineate the language abilities, skills, and processes which are valued in successful healthcare communication. A careful needs analysis, involving both language specialists and clinicians, has proven an effective procedure to gain a comprehensive and nuanced understanding of the domain of healthcare communication. Scoring spoken and written performances is another important consideration for a language assessment for professional purposes. In the case of assessing clinician language skills, the involvement of clinicians in establishing the indigenous criteria has been recognized as a viable means to maintain test authenticity. Given that many language assessments for professional purposes are used as a mechanism to regulate professional registration/licensing and international mobility, the importance of standard setting is worth highlighting, as the cut scores have clear implications for the validity and fairness of these assessments. As we have argued in this chapter, this exercise must follow rigorous and well-defined procedures to establish its procedural validity. Finally, we also demonstrate how to interrogate the validity of a language assessment for professional purposes by applying the argument-based approach to test validation. Test developers and researchers can effectively utilize this framework to guide test development, map out test validation agendas and activities, and set priorities in their validation endeavors. Due to the significance of this topic, we expect to see more research in the future aiming at addressing key issues in assessing clinician language skills.

Highlights

- Language assessment for professional purposes differs in significant ways from assessment of general language abilities.
- Various approaches have been adopted to assessing the linguistic readiness of clinicians seeking professional registration/licensing in English-speaking countries.
- Some fundamental considerations in developing a test of clinician language skills include a careful needs analysis, the establishment of scoring criteria, and rigorous standard-setting procedures.
- The argument-based validation approach provides an effective approach to interrogating the validity of a test of clinician language skills.

REFERENCES

1. Knoch, U. and Macqueen, S. (2020). *Assessing English for Professional Purposes*. Routledge.
2. Elder, C., Pill, J., Woodward-Kron, R. et al. (2012). Health professionals' views of communication: implications for assessing performance on a health-specific English language test. *TESOL Q.* 46 (2): 409–419.
3. Berry, V., O'Sullivan, B., and Rugea, S. (2013). *Identifying the Appropriate IELTS Score Levels for IMG Applicants to the GMC Register. Report Submitted to the General Medical Council*. (150 pp). UK: Centre for Language Assessment Research (CLARe), University of Roehampton.
4. Wette, R. (2011). English proficiency tests and communication skills training for overseas-qualified health professionals in Australia and New Zealand. *Lang. Assess. Q.* 8 (2): 200–210.
5. Bachman, L.F. and Palmer, A.S. (1996). *Language Assessment in Practice: Designing and Developing Useful Language Tests*. Oxford: Oxford University Press.
6. Taylor, L. (2014). General language proficiency (GLP): reflections on the "Issues Revisited" from the perspective of a UK examination board. *Lang. Assess. Q.* 11 (2): 136–151.
7. Douglas, D. (2000). *Assessing Languages for Specific Purposes*. Cambridge University Press.
8. Pill, J. and Woodward-Kron, R. (2012). How professionally relevant can language tests be?: a response to Wette (2011). *Lang. Assess. Q.* 9 (1): 105–108.
9. McNamara, T. (1996). *Measuring Second Language Proficiency*. Longman.
10. Whelan, G.P., McKinley, D.W., Boulet, J.R. et al. (2001). Validation of the doctor–patient communication component of the educational Commission for Foreign Medical Graduates Clinical Skills Assessment. *Med. Educ.* 35 (8): 757–761.
11. Pill, J. (2016). Drawing on indigenous criteria for more authentic assessment in a specific-purpose language test: health professionals interacting with patients. *Lang. Test.* 33 (2): 175–193.
12. Elder, C. (2016). Exploring the limits of authenticity in LSP testing: the case of a specific-purpose language test for health professionals. *Lang. Test.* 33 (2): 147–152.
13. Malicka, A., Gilabert Guerrero, R., and Norris, J.M. (2019). From needs analysis to task design: insights from an English for specific purposes context. *Lang. Teach. Res.* 23 (1): 78–106.

14. Basturkmen, H. and Elder, C. (2004). The practice of LSP. In: *The Handbook of Applied Linguistics* (ed. A. Davies and C. Elder), 672–694. Blackwell.
15. Lewkowicz, J.A. (2000). Authenticity in language testing: some outstanding questions. *Lang. Test.* 17 (1): 43–64.
16. Spolsky, B. (1985). The limits of authenticity in language testing. *Lang. Test.* 2 (1): 31–40.
17. Elder, C. and McNamara, T. (2016). The hunt for "indigenous criteria" in assessing communication in the physiotherapy workplace. *Lang. Test.* 33 (2): 153–174.
18. Elder, C., McNamara, T., Woodward-Kron, R. et al. (2013). *Towards Improved Healthcare Communication: Development and Validation of Language Proficiency Standards for Non-native English Speaking Health Professionals*. University of Melbourne.
19. Pill, J. and McNamara, T. (2016). How much is enough? Involving occupational experts in setting standards on a specific-purpose language test for health professionals. *Lang. Test.* 33 (2): 217–234.
20. Knoch, U., Elder, C., Woodward-Kron, R. et al. (2017). *Towards Improved Quality of Written Patient Records*. University of Melbourne.
21. Knoch, U., Zhang, B.Y., Elder, C. et al. (2020). "I will go to my grave fighting for grammar": exploring the ability of language-trained raters to implement a professionally-relevant rating scale for writing. *Assess. Writ.* 46: 100488.
22. Knoch, U., Elder, C., Woodward-Kron, R. et al. (2020). Capturing domain expert perspectives in devising a rating scale for a health specific writing test: how close can we get? *Assess. Writ.* 46: 100489.
23. Kenyon, D. and Romhild, A. (2014). Standard setting in language testing. In: *The Companion to Language Assessment* (ed. A.J. Kunnan), 1–14. John Wiley & Sons.
24. O'Neill T. The Minimum Proficiency in English for Entry-Level Nurses. Retrieved September. 2004;30:2009.
25. Davidson, S. (2018). *How Valid Are Domain experts' Judgements of Workplace Communication? Implications for Setting Standards on the Occupational English Test (OET) Writing Sub-Test*. University of Melbourne.
26. Manias, E. and McNamara, T. (2016). Standard setting in specific-purpose language testing: what can a qualitative study add? *Lang. Test.* 33 (2): 235–249.
27. O'Neill, T.R., Tannenbaum, R.J., and Tiffen, J. (2005). Recommending a minimum English proficiency standard for entry-level nursing. *J. Nurs. Meas.* 13 (2): 129–146.
28. O'Neill, T.R., Buckendahl, C.W., Plake, B.S. et al. (2007). Recommending a nursing-specific passing standard for the IELTS examination. *Lang. Assess. Q.* 4 (4): 295–317.
29. Qian, H., Woo, A., and Banerjee, J. (2014). *Setting an English Language Proficiency Passing Standard for Entry-Level Nursing Practice Using the Michigan English Language Assessment Battery*. National Counsel of State Boards of Nursing–NCLEX Technical Brief.
30. AERA, APA, and NCME (2014). *Standards for Educational and Psychological Testing*. AERA.
31. Chalhoub-Deville, M. and O'Sullivan, B. (2020). *Validity: Theoretical Development and Integrated Arguments*. Equinox Publishing Limited.
32. Chapelle, C.A., Enright, M.K., and Jamieson, J. (2010). Does an argument-based approach to validity make a difference? *Educ. Meas. Issues Pract.* 29 (1): 3–13.
33. Kane, M.T. (2013). Validating the interpretations and uses of test scores. *J. Educ. Meas.* 50 (1): 1–73.
34. Chapelle, C.A., Enright, M.K., and Jamieson, J.M. (2008). *Building a Validity Argument for the Test of English as a Foreign Language*. NY and London: Routledge, Taylor & Francis Group.
35. Knoch, U. and Chapelle, C.A. (2018). Validation of rating processes within an argument-based framework. *Lang. Test.* 35 (4): 477–499.
36. Macqueen, S., Yahalom, S., Kim, H. et al. (2012). *Exploring Writing Demands in Healthcare Settings*. University of Melbourne.

13 Setting Standards for Clinician Language Use in Patient Care

JOHN D. COWDEN

Introduction

For healthcare professionals, serving patients with diverse language needs is a fact of life worldwide, where more than 7000 languages are spoken in just under 200 countries [1, 2]. Because communication lies at the heart of competent clinical practice, standards for providing safe, effective care should be expected for clinicians using multiple languages in practice. Yet, multilingual communication traditionally has been given less attention than other clinical skills by the healthcare professions (e.g., medicine, nursing, psychology, and pharmacy) and by healthcare policymakers and regulators. In addition, support for clinicians in developing, measuring, and maintaining language skills at the level required by ethical and professional expectations should be fundamental to training and practice but instead is uncommon. Without standards and support for such clinicians, healthcare systems provide an uncertain quality of care to culturally and linguistically diverse populations.

In many countries, healthcare regulatory bodies such as professional boards have long required clinicians trained outside the country to prove their proficiency in the dominant language(s) of the nation's healthcare training and delivery systems. These standards require clinician language testing and set a minimum level of proficiency to be allowed to train or practice as a healthcare professional. Such dominant language standards will not be the focus of this chapter. Instead, the standardization and regulation of *nondominant* language skills – those used to communicate directly with patients who speak a language other than the dominant language(s) in a healthcare system – will be outlined, including the justification and practical guidance for setting such standards and creating the systems needed to support them.

This chapter begins with a description of theoretical frameworks and historical efforts related to the ongoing movement for "professionalization" of nondominant language proficiency in healthcare (particularly in the United States), followed by a discussion of topics critical to advancement in this area, including how to build a professional approach to bilingualism, elements of qualification systems, and roles for bilingual clinicians. The chapter ends by offering recommendations for policy and practice to readers in a position to influence progress in these areas. While the chapter is written from a United States perspective, international examples and lessons are given where available.

Theoretical frameworks

Concepts from diverse theoretical frameworks apply to clinicians' use of multiple languages to communicate with patients. These concepts provide a rationale to guide and support policymakers, healthcare leaders, and individual clinicians working to promote access to equitable, high-quality care for culturally and linguistically diverse communities.

Professionalism

The healthcare professions are characterized by commitments and responsibilities that set them apart from other occupations. For example, the preamble of "Physician Charter on Professionalism" [3] states:

> Professionalism is the basis of medicine's contract with society. It demands placing the interests of patients above those of the physician, setting and maintaining standards for competence and integrity, and providing expert advice to society on matters of health.

In addition to these demands, healthcare professionals must complete specialized education and training culminating in certification of their abilities and adhere to strict ethical obligations to those they serve, to their peers, and to the profession. How do the demands of professionalism relate to clinicians' use of nondominant languages to give care?

In healthcare communication, a hallmark of prioritizing patient interests is determining a patient's preferred language and providing language-appropriate services that support full expression and comprehension for everyone involved in an interaction. Clinicians who develop job-specific language proficiency in multiple languages address this demand, assuming they do so at the level of communicative competence determined by the profession at large. Clinicians with substandard language proficiency cannot adequately provide the expert advice expected by society and may cause harm because of miscommunication. To be treated as a professional competency, job-specific proficiency in a nondominant language must be taught as a specialized skill and measured as part of professional certification. Where healthcare professions have failed to provide specialized training or set a measurable standard for nondominant language use, clinicians are left unsure of whether they are abiding by their ethical duties to do no harm, to practice only in areas of proven competence, and to protect patients' interests.

The Charter for Professionalism for Healthcare Organizations [4] proposes that in addition to the individual actors in a healthcare system, hospitals, clinics, and other organizations also bear responsibility for upholding professional standards. Commitments in four domains are described: patient partnerships, organizational culture, community partnerships, and operations and business practices. Setting organizational standards for clinicians' use of nondominant languages supports commitments in all four domains and reflects an organizational dedication to safe, effective care based on clear communication.

Health equity

In 2017, a Robert Wood Johnson Foundation report defined "health equity" as follows [5]:

> Health equity means that everyone has a fair and just opportunity to be as healthy as possible. This requires removing obstacles to health such as poverty, discrimination, and their consequences, including powerlessness and lack of access to good jobs with fair pay, quality education and housing, safe environments, and health care.

A common obstacle to health in the clinical setting is the lack of meaningful access for patients who speak a nondominant language. Within a health equity framework, the removal of language-related obstacles is a question of fairness and justice, making it not only a technical challenge but also a struggle against structural discrimination that traditionally centers on the dominant language and culture. The goal of such pursuits could be termed "language equity" in healthcare, meaning that everyone has a fair and just opportunity to communicate as fully as possible with healthcare team members using the language they prefer.

Providing quality care in the context of linguistically diverse populations raises the question: How do the demands of health and language equity relate to clinicians' use of nondominant languages to give care? Fair and just access to language-appropriate care for patients speaking nondominant languages cannot be achieved if clinicians use substandard language skills in the clinical setting, as the patient is denied the opportunity to fully understand and be fully understood. Applying regulatory and professional standards only to dominant language proficiency among healthcare professionals creates a two-tiered system, where some patients (i.e., dominant language speakers) are treated to a different level of communication competence than others (i.e., speakers of nondominant languages). Patients unable to communicate in the system's dominant language can become powerless, marginalized, and unable to advocate for their needs. The result puts patients at risk of poorer health outcomes related to differential, unfair treatment.

Historical development

The history of standard-setting for language proficiency in clinical practice can be divided into (1) long-standing national efforts to assure international graduates in healthcare professions speak and read the dominant language of a healthcare system well enough to be licensed and (2) more recent efforts to assure bilingual clinicians already licensed in a healthcare system are able to communicate safely and effectively with patients who speak nondominant languages. Although their proximate purposes differ, the ultimate goal is the same – clear, safe communication between clinicians and patients. Examples of national licensing efforts related to dominant language use, where decades of experience have accumulated across numerous jurisdictions, cultures, and languages, can provide lessons for the standardization of nondominant language use, a field still poorly defined at the professional and systemic scale.

Dominant language proficiency policy

Regulatory bodies around the world have created language proficiency requirements for internationally trained healthcare professionals seeking licensure. In some countries, language standards are set at the national level for all healthcare professions (e.g., Australia, France, Japan, Spain, and United Kingdom), while others use a combination of national and regional standards, depending on the profession (e.g., Canada and United States). Required assessments vary along a spectrum of language specificity from general language proficiency to broad healthcare proficiency to narrow, profession-specific proficiency. Examples of healthcare-specific assessments include the Occupational English Test (OET), developed and continually adapted in Australia since the 1980s and now used for up to 12 healthcare professions in multiple English-speaking countries [6], the Canadian English Language Benchmark Assessment for Nurses (CELBAN) [7], and the telc Deutsch exams for physicians and nurses in Germany [8]. In the United States, requirements vary by profession – physicians must pass the OET as part of certification through the Educational Council for Foreign Medical Graduates (ECFMG), while nurses and pharmacists typically can use a general language exam, such as the Test of English as a Foreign Language (TOEFL) or the International English Language Test System (IELTS). In some states, nurses can select from multiple general or specific assessments.

The rationale for such standards rests on the need to ensure that professionals trained outside of the country's educational and healthcare systems meet the expected level of competency to practice safely and effectively, including the ability to speak the dominant language of the healthcare system. The primary concern is that patients who speak the system's dominant language are at risk of receiving inadequate care from a professional who cannot communicate well with them.

Nondominant language proficiency policy

The rationale for regulating nondominant language use is the same as for dominant language use, but the concern is that patients who do *not* speak the system's dominant language are at risk of receiving inadequate care from a professional who cannot communicate well due to use of inadequate nondominant language skills. In the last 20 years, two developments in guidance from the federal government have set the stage for improved standard-setting in the United States related to nondominant language by healthcare professionals: the National Standards for Culturally and Linguistically Appropriate Services and Section 1557 of the Patient Protection and Affordable Care Act.

Culturally and linguistically appropriate services

In 2001, the Office of Minority Health, part of the United States Department of Health and Human Services, published the first edition of the National Standards for Culturally and Linguistically Appropriate Services (National CLAS Standards), including guidance specific to bilingual healthcare professionals. In this original version, CLAS Standard 6 stated that "health care organizations must assure the competence of language assistance provided to limited English proficient patients/consumers by interpreters and bilingual staff" [9]. Explanatory text included the following:

> Bilingual clinicians and other staff who communicate directly with patients/consumers in their preferred language must demonstrate a command of both English and the target

language that includes knowledge and facility with the terms and concepts relevant to the type of encounter. Ideally, this should be verified by formal testing. Research has shown that individuals with exposure to a second language, even those raised in bilingual homes, frequently overestimate their ability to communicate in that language, and make errors that could affect complete and accurate communication and comprehension [9].

In 2013, an updated edition called the enhanced National CLAS Standards was published [10], with detailed treatment of bilingual staff largely removed. Enhanced CLAS Standard 7 stated that organizations should "ensure the competence of individuals providing language assistance, recognizing that the use of untrained individuals and/or minors as interpreters should be avoided." In an accompanying document called "A Blueprint for Advancing and Sustaining CLAS Policy and Practice," a note on assessment was given:

> Before one can be considered qualified to interpret, translate, or provide other communication assistance, he/she must be assessed to determine his/her competence. Language ability alone does not qualify an individual to provide language assistance [11].

Neither "language assistance" nor "communication assistance" were defined in the enhanced Standards or the Blueprint, resulting in guidance that was more ambiguous than in the original CLAS Standards. In the enhanced CLAS Standards, bilingual staff were specifically mentioned only in the context of who should be allowed to interpret between healthcare providers and patients.

Four of the original 14 CLAS Standards (including Standard 6) were considered mandates for all federally-funded organizations. When the enhanced CLAS Standards were announced in 2013, the United States government specified that they were "not statutory or regulatory requirements" but could help organizations avoid violating the nondiscrimination requirements of Title VI of the Civil Rights Act of 1964 [12].

Affordable care act, Section 1557

In 2016, ideas expressed as guidance in the National CLAS Standards took the force of law when they were included in the final rule implementing Section 1557 ("Nondiscrimination") of the United States federal Patient Protection and Affordable Care Act (ACA) [13]. As in the original National CLAS Standards, the responsibility of healthcare organizations to qualify bilingual healthcare professionals was addressed specifically. A new final rule in 2020 maintained wording from the 2016 rule under "Meaningful access for individuals with limited English proficiency," stating that required language services may include "the use of qualified bilingual or multilingual staff to communicate directly with individuals with limited English proficiency." In addition, organizations "shall not rely on staff other than qualified bilingual/multilingual staff to communicate directly with individuals with limited English proficiency" [14]. Removed from the 2020 rule was a definition of qualified bilingual/multilingual staff from 2016:

> Qualified bilingual/multilingual staff means a member of a covered entity's workforce who is designated by the covered entity to provide oral language assistance as part of the individual's current, assigned job responsibilities and who has demonstrated to the covered entity that he or she: (1) Is proficient in speaking and understanding both spoken English and at least one other spoken language, including any necessary specialized vocabulary, terminology and phraseology, and (2) is able to effectively, accurately, and impartially communicate directly with individuals with limited English proficiency in their primary languages [13].

Because each presidential administration has the authority to modify regulations under the ACA, further changes could restore the definition above or otherwise change the current final rule for Section 1557 (from 2020). Enforcement of Section 1557 is the responsibility of the Office for Civil Rights in the Department of Health and Human Services, which acts primarily in response to complaints of possible civil rights violations.

State policies

In the United States, authority to regulate many aspects of the healthcare system lies with individual states. While all states must follow the federal policies outlined above, they may create additional healthcare standards beyond federal requirements. As of 2019, all 50 states and the District of Columbia had passed laws related to language access in healthcare (ranging from 3 to 257 provisions, depending on the state) [15]. While "qualified interpreters" are mentioned extensively throughout state provisions (including specific definitions of "qualified"), only four states had a provision mentioning "qualified" or "authorized" bilingual staff, and none included definitions or standards for qualified competency. These provisions relate to specific health-related programs rather than a broad standard for bilingual clinicians.

Nongovernmental standard-setting

Language access has long been promoted by advocates for health equity, first through the professionalization of healthcare interpreters starting in the 1990s [16, 17], and more recently through the professionalization of language use by bilingual healthcare professionals. Leaders and advocates from healthcare systems, accrediting bodies, and other organizations in the United States have promoted and created an evolving set of language equity standards that have informed and responded to governmental guidance. The interaction between policymakers and nongovernmental organizations has advanced the field significantly since the appearance of the original National CLAS Standards in 2001.

Healthcare systems

Early efforts to set standards for bilingual clinicians in healthcare organizations relied on rudimentary methods to determine who should use nondominant language skills to give care, such as "self-qualification" (each clinician deciding on their own), informal or structured interviews of clinicians by staff interpreters, or the use of general proficiency or interpreter tests (despite the clinician only intending to give direct services in the target language). Not until the last 10–15 years have organizations been able to incorporate non-English language assessments specific to clinical healthcare roles.

In 2003, Kaiser Permanente, a large healthcare provider and nonprofit health plan, launched the Qualified Bilingual Staff (QBS) Program to take advantage of the language skills of their clinicians and staff [18, 19]. Program development included the creation and validation of two tests, the QBS Assessment and the Clinician Cultural and Linguistic Assessment (CCLA). The QBS Assessment was designed as a broad test of language for specific purposes (LSP), measuring the ability of diverse types of healthcare workers to communicate directly with patients in the healthcare setting about a range of topics. Possible passing results included level 1 (non-clinical proficiency) and level 2 (clinical proficiency). The CCLA was designed as a narrow LSP test specific to a clinician's ability to interact with patients in a primary care setting, with a single cutoff score of 80%. In addition to being used in the Kaiser Permanente system, the tests were made commercially available in 2008 through a partnership with ALTA Languages, Inc. (http://altalang.com), currently offering each test in 30 languages.

For several years after the program launch, Kaiser Permanente held training workshops in QBS program development for healthcare organizations throughout the United States, and the model has continued to spread throughout the country. Other assessments have appeared in recent years, including the Bilingual Fluency Assessment from LanguageLine [20] and the Canopy Credential from Canopy Innovations [21], offering healthcare organizations new options for both broad and narrow healthcare-specific language proficiency assessments. As compliance with federal regulations related to language access has become a growing priority, new assessment options and qualification models have set the stage for organizational qualification systems to become more robust and gain stronger support from organizational leaders.

Accrediting bodies

Accrediting bodies play a central role in putting federal standards, such as those related to language access, into action at the organizational and individual levels. Two such bodies are the Joint Commission and the National Committee for Quality Assurance (NCQA), both with standards related to bilingual clinicians. The Joint Commission began to place special emphasis on language access challenges after its 2007 report, "Hospitals, Language, and Culture: A Snapshot of the Nation," outlined the gap between policy expectations and the reality in healthcare organizations around the country [22]. Over time, visits by surveyors have increasingly focused on how hospitals assure the competence of interpreters and bilingual staff. In 2023, the Joint Commission began offering organizations a voluntary Healthcare Equity certification including a requirement that the organization have a process to assess the language proficiency of bilingual staff [23]. The NCQA has recently transitioned its former Distinction in Multicultural Healthcare to the new Health Equity Accreditation opportunity, which specifies that the organization uses competent bilingual staff whose language capabilities are assessed [24]. The pressure on organizations to become and remain accredited has allowed accrediting bodies to effectively communicate and enforce language access regulations while providing support through detailed training and education on meeting their standards of care.

Organizations related to accreditation in healthcare education are optimally positioned to create and implement standards for students and trainees related to nondominant language use. Such bodies in the fields of medicine (Liaison Committee on Medical Education [LCME], American Association of Medical Colleges [AAMC], Accreditation Council for Graduate Medical Education [ACGME]), nursing (Accreditation Commission for Education in Nursing [ACEN]), and pharmacy (Accreditation Council for Pharmacy Education [ACPE]) have yet to offer standards related to clinician multilingualism or guidance for programs on the incorporation of professional training in nondominant language use.

Other organizations

National coalitions including major health professional groups have advocated for language access standards through statements of principles, policy and issue briefs, and resource guides. Key publications included the 2006 "Language Access in Health Care Statement of Principles: Explanatory Guide" (31 organizations), which stated that "mechanisms should be developed to establish the competency of those providing language services, including interpreters, translators and bilingual staff/clinicians," [25] and the Commission to End Health Disparities (75 organizations) report, "Promoting Appropriate Use of Physicians' Non-English Language Skills in Clinical Care: Recommendations for Policymakers, Organizations and Clinicians" [26]. This document provides a rare example of a detailed discussion specifically related to clinicians' use of nondominant language to give care. Historically, language access advocacy has been dominated by questions of interpretation and translation, with occasional mention of bilingual staff, but often only in the context of whether they should play the role of interpreter. This trend is mirrored in the way the professionalization of bilingualism has lagged well behind that of healthcare interpretation and translation, both of which have well-established specialized training opportunities, pathways to national certification, and professional codes of ethics.

Critical issues and topics

Building a professional approach to multilingualism

Despite the theoretical rationale and historical developments described above, clinician multilingualism has yet to be consistently treated as a professional competency at the individual, organizational, and systemic levels. Opportunities exist at all levels to advance the movement toward professionalization.

Individual level

Responsibility begins with individual clinicians, who have a duty to use only those skills for which they have been specially trained and proven competent. This longstanding professional standard provides the foundation for ethical clinical practice throughout healthcare. So why do some clinicians use inadequate bilingual skills to provide care? They may overestimate their abilities [27–30], unaware that they put patients at risk through potentially ineffective communication. Or they may be motivated by expediency, feeling the pressure of limited time or lack of interpreter access [31, 32], assuming that some language skill is better than nothing. Perceived need for interpreter support may differ by job role [33, 34] or complexity of the communication task [30, 32, 35]. All these situations reflect a potential disconnect between a clinician's professional responsibility and communication choices.

Awareness of the professional nature of language use can be taught from the outset of a clinician's professional schooling, where classes on patient-clinician communication, health equity, and professionalism are natural settings for this topic. In addition, the flourishing of medical Spanish courses in medical schools [36, 37] offers the opportunity to address professional standards for multilingualism, including the incorporation of standardized proficiency assessment early in a clinician's career. Such training can continue throughout the clinical phase of training (e.g., residency and fellowship for physicians) and be reinforced through organizational expectations and standards upon starting professional practice. For individual clinicians to avoid the disconnects described above, the structures they move through must consistently communicate the message that multilingualism is a professional matter and that language access for patients is a civil right.

Actions by individual clinicians reflect the standards they set for themselves as professionals, which can either reinforce or undermine language access standards set at a higher level. Because clinician decisions impact patient well-being most directly, the cultivation of personal standards merits inclusion in efforts to regulate and support bi/multilingual clinicians.

Organizational level

Organizations providing healthcare, such as health systems, hospitals, and clinics, are in an ideal position to advance the professionalization of clinician language skills because of their responsibility for clinician oversight, commitment to quality and safety, and need to comply with accreditation and regulatory requirements. Following the lead of Kaiser Permanente's QBS model [18, 19], healthcare organizations have begun to develop more sophisticated programs for the qualification and support of bilingual staff. Where such staff was once evaluated through a brief conversation with a staff interpreter or through self-report, they are increasingly assessed through formal language proficiency testing under policies that clearly define who is allowed to use language skills in their clinical role.

In addition to setting standards and assessing language competency, organizations can also advance professionalized bilingualism through developmental support for bilingual clinicians, such as education on language access, proficiency test preparation, 1:1 culture and language coaching [38], formation of QBS peer groups, and connection to outside language development resources. Creation of a maintenance of qualification expectation, including continuing education (discussed below), would further solidify the professional culture related to nondominant language use.

While many organizations are moving forward, progress is patchy. Without consistent, formal reporting of QBS policies through professional or accrediting organizations, it is difficult to know where the larger healthcare system stands. National language access surveys published in 2006 and 2008 showed that 87% of 861 United States hospitals and 59% of 650 community health centers used bilingual clinical staff to provide care to patients with limited English proficiency [39, 40]. Fifty-seven percent of the community health centers assessed bilingual staff skills, but only 16% required formal competency testing or outside accreditation; most relied on their own evaluation. Much has changed since then – the creation of Section 1557 regulations, increased attention from accrediting bodies, and the spread of ideas among peer organizations have increased the momentum among healthcare organizations. There is a need for reliable data on how healthcare organizations comply with federal QBS regulations, including QBS policies, approach to assessment, and proportion of staff who are qualified bilingual. Sharing these data makes an organization's professional treatment of multilingualism visible, normalizing it within and beyond the organization.

Systemic level

As individual clinicians and organizations on the front lines work through challenges to making multilingualism a professional responsibility, groups that oversee major components of the larger health system have the opportunity to make a clear commitment to standards for nondominant language use. Professional and trade groups have formed coalitions to address health disparities and language access in general, but not the need to fully professionalize bilingualism. The relationship between accrediting bodies and policymakers at the national and state levels presents an opportunity to create a national body dedicated to the qualification of bilingual healthcare professionals, similar to the ECFMG. Such a body could consolidate assessment efforts and set standards for various healthcare professions, using either a broad LSP approach (e.g., the Occupational English Test) or a set of narrow assessments. This would provide a reliable source of assessment support for the states, where licensing authority rests, and individual healthcare organizations, who currently shoulder the responsibility of selecting assessment approaches (an expertise that is lacking in almost all organizations).

Elements of a qualified bilingual staff program

Creating a QBS program at the organizational level involves consideration of policy, assessment, post-qualification expectations, incentives and compensation, and marketing and promotion.

Organizational policy

The foundation of a bilingual qualification system lies in organizational policy, where rules about nondominant language use by clinical and non-clinical staff may appear in at least two areas: (1) language services, including language access planning, and (2) credentialing and privileging processes used for licensed independent practitioners (i.e., physicians, nurse practitioners, and physician assistants).

The inclusion of bilingual clinicians in language services policy allows a healthcare organization to define how bilingual competency is determined and compensated, how qualified bilingual skills may be used, and the consequences for staff members who violate policy. In addition, policy can establish authority and responsibility for qualification program updates and explicitly demonstrate how the organization meets regulatory requirements by referring to applicable national and state standards (e.g., Section 1557 of the ACA, the National CLAS Standards). Because bilingual clinician qualification is a young, dynamic field where research and programming are expanding rapidly, organizational policy should be written with flexibility in mind, balancing general principles (e.g., that bilingual staff must be qualified) with specific details that might change more frequently (e.g., what language proficiency assessments are accepted as proof of competency). In organizations where policy review and approval occur on a timescale of multiple years, this balance may be achieved by creating a broad, general policy document accompanied by separate, modifiable protocols that outline assessment, compensation, and maintenance of qualification processes.

For licensed independent practitioners (i.e., physicians, nurse practitioners, and physician assistants), the ability to provide care using a nondominant language might ideally be included in credentialing and privileging, well-established processes used by medical staff or other administrators to verify appropriate professional preparation and grant specific clinical practice privileges. While proof of bilingual preparation and ability could be similar to that required in an organization's QBS policy, inclusion in the privileging process would send a clear signal to clinicians that using inadequate or unproven nondominant language skills is a question of professional ethics and responsibility, as described above in Theoretical Frameworks. It also would make bilingual competency subject to the professional oversight given to all other independent practitioner skills. Policies should also be clear with regard to how qualified bilingual skills may be used (and, conversely, how they must not be used).

Assessment

Theoretically, assessment of clinician language proficiency is a straightforward question – can a given healthcare professional speak a language well enough to carry out their job duties effectively and safely? In practice, answering this question confidently is perhaps the most significant challenge facing the movement to professionalize bilingualism in healthcare. As described above, assessments of English for specific purposes (ESP) have been developed for various areas of healthcare, but validated LSP tests for non-English languages in healthcare are scarce and young. Designers of bilingual qualification systems have addressed the challenge of assessment in diverse ways, relying on one or more of the following: self-report, internal assessment, tests of language for general purposes, broad and/or narrow tests of healthcare-specific language proficiency, tests of interpretation skills, internal language assessment by staff interpreters, and exemption for certain clinicians (e.g., those whose professional training occurred in the target language). As the professionalization of bilingualism has progressed, the question of an assessment's validity has become more prominent, with decreasing tolerance for approaches that rely on informal evaluation by untrained assessors, on self-report alone, or on mismatched testing (for example, using an interpreter test for bilingual clinicians giving direct care). Table 13.1 lists pros and cons of various approaches, including examples from the field. As we wait for research-informed development of a broader range of valid assessment tools, compromises will be unavoidable and should be acknowledged transparently by the organization.

To date, bilingual assessment has focused primarily on oral language skills (expression and comprehension) rather than written language skills (writing and reading). The QBS and CCLA exams, used widely in the United States for qualifying bilingual clinicians, do not assess writing or reading ability (except for a sight translation exercise at the end of the QBS) [41, 42]. The CanopyCredential [21], a newer LSP test of medical Spanish and medical English, includes reading exercises but does not assess a physician's ability to perform job-specific written tasks, such as writing patient instructions or communicating electronically (e.g., emails and patient portal messages). Those designing a qualification process should consider the need to assess written skills for each clinical role (e.g., physician versus nurse versus pharmacist) and the available means for assessment. For job-specific written tasks, an evaluation created by the organization may be necessary.

Prior to completing an assessment, a candidate should be oriented to the QBS role. In some organizations, qualified bilingual staff are considered dual-role interpreters, while in others, interpreting is forbidden unless they have separately completed the process for healthcare interpreter certification. If a candidate were uncomfortable with a dual-role expectation, the ability to opt out of the interpreter role (if applicable) should be discussed. Candidate preparation for the assessment also may include access to a detailed description of how the assessment will occur and the opportunity to practice with a coach or through mock testing.

Table 13.1 Approaches to Bilingual Clinician Language Proficiency Assessment in Standard-Setting.

Approach	Opportunities and Examples	Pros, Cons, and Suitability for Standard-Setting
Self-assessment	Clinicians at the extremes of the language proficiency spectrum (very low and very high proficiency) have been shown to accurately assess their own abilities using a standard scale [50, 51], leading to the use of self-assessment as part of a qualification system in some organizations, either to screen for testing or to become qualified directly. **Standardized scales that have been used for self-assessment** Employee Languages Self-Assessment Tool [52] Adapted Interagency Language Roundtable (ILR) Scale [27, 50, 51] ALTA Performance Levels Description (combination of ILR and ACTFL)	**Pros** Low cost, applicable to multiple healthcare professions **Cons** Uncertain validity and reliability, especially at middle levels, open to intentional misreporting (especially if financial incentive involved) **Suitability** Proceed with caution – may be suitable if evidence-based and combined with testing for clinicians in the middle self-rated categories
General language proficiency test	As with dominant language assessments required for international graduate licensing in many healthcare professions, general language assessments have been used to determine a clinician's general proficiency. Such use might be combined with further assessment of language skills in a specific clinical setting. **Examples of tests in non-English languages:** Arabic – Arabic Language Proficiency Test (ALPT) Mandarin – Hanyu Shuiping Kaoshi (HSK) Spanish – Diploma de Español como Lengua Extranjera (DELE) *Diploma of Spanish as a Foreign Language – general* Spanish – Servicio Internacional de Evaluación de la Lengua Española (SIELE) *International Evaluation Service of the Spanish Language – academic and professional*	**Pros** Assessments widely available, often validated, many have a long track record, many include assessment of reading and writing **Cons** Do not include vocabulary and tasks specific to healthcare interactions, may give a false sense of ability **Suitability** Proceed with caution – may be suitable if combined with further assessment (e.g., by observation of communication skills in clinical setting)

Broad healthcare-specific language proficiency test	The long-established Occupational English Test (OET), used for clinicians in 12 healthcare professions, has been adopted in multiple English-speaking countries for licensing. Nothing with the same research track-record exists for non-English languages, but there are emerging options for QBS program administrators to consider. **Examples of broad healthcare-specific tests in non-English languages:** Qualified Bilingual Staff (QBS) Assessment (30 languages) Bilingual Fluency Assessment (BFA) Medical Spanish Certification for Healthcare (in development)	**Pros** Can be used for all or most types of clinicians in an organization, specific to healthcare content and tasks **Cons** Current tests do not assess writing and reading, may be tempting to use for clinicians outside of test's ideal scope (e.g., QBS for psychologists, clinical social workers, and dentists) **Suitability** Best used for healthcare professionals not assessable using a narrow healthcare-specific test; check validation process and content match with candidate job roles
Narrow healthcare-specific language proficiency test	The specificity of a test is relative – a test for physicians in general practice is narrower than one for clinicians in general, but it may not feel specific enough for subspecialty contexts. The impracticality of creating validated assessments for every clinical role in healthcare means that narrower tests may cover several clinician types. QBS program administrators can consider whether one or more narrow tests will provide the right balance between specificity and feasibility. **Examples of narrow healthcare-specific tests in non-English languages:** Clinician Cultural and Linguistic Assessment (CCLA) (30 languages) *Physicians, nurse practitioners, physician assistants in primary care* Bilingual Fluency Assessment for Clinicians (BFAC) (26 languages) *Available in nine specialty versions, e.g., "Pediatrics," "Mental Health," "Pharmacy"* CanopyCredential (Spanish) *Physicians, nurse practitioners, physician assistants*	**Pros** Specific to job role **Cons** Current tests do not assess writing and reading, not available for most clinician types, tend to be newer tests with a shorter track-record than general language assessments **Suitability** Best option for clinicians included in test's target scope; check validation process and content match with candidate job roles

(Continued)

Table 13.1 (Continued)

Approach	Opportunities and Examples	Pros, Cons, and Suitability for Standard-Setting
Combined approach	In practice, a combination of two or more of the above approaches has proved popular for QBS programs. A common combination has been the CCLA for physicians, nurse practitioners, and physician assistants and the QBS Assessment for other clinicians, such as registered nurses, technicians, pharmacists, etc. At least one program certifies clinicians with the highest self-rating without testing (after signing an attestation) and uses the CCLA to test those in lower self-rated categories. As further healthcare-specific assessments are created and validated, QBS programs will be able to minimize mismatches between test content and clinician roles, closing gaps in assessment coverage.	**Pros** Flexible, covers a wider range of clinician types, less risk of mismatch between assessment and clinician role **Cons** More complicated to administer **Suitability** Currently most suitable option in many healthcare contexts, check for gaps in test coverage where any of the included assessment methods does not adequately cover a clinical role

Post-qualification expectations

Once qualified, bilingual clinicians should be trained in detail on the scope of their role, including expectations and responsibilities. Requirements for maintenance of qualification (e.g., continuing education or periodic re-testing, if required) should be presented, and compensation explained. Common challenges can also be explored and guidance given on how to navigate them.

Continuing education (CE) is a hallmark of professional healthcare licensing (including for healthcare interpreters), raising the question: As a professional competency, should bilingualism be subject to CE requirements? The answer may differ based on how a clinician gained their bilingual skills. For example, a bilingual qualification system might require a second language or heritage speaker to show ongoing maintenance of skills in a nondominant language (e.g., Spanish) through CE (and perhaps periodic re-testing), while a clinician who completed professional training in the nondominant language (e.g., graduated from a Spanish-language medical or nursing school) might be exempt. After all, native English speakers who completed training in English in the United States are not required to prove maintenance of English proficiency over time. Alternatively, a system could treat all bilingual clinicians equally, recognizing that even native speakers can improve their communication abilities through CE, particularly considering the cultural and linguistic diversity presented by patients who speak many varieties of the same nondominant language (e.g., Spanish from all over Latin America in the United States).

The primary challenges for including CE requirements in an organization's bilingual qualification system are practical. What would the costs be, in staff and clinician time, to administer a CE credit system? How would activities be approved and verified, particularly for multiple qualified languages (see the elaborate, resource-intensive systems in place for CE in medicine, nursing, and other professions)? And what would the unintended consequences be? Would requirements discourage participation in the qualification system? How much would it contribute to CE fatigue? Realistically, a robust CE system for bilingual clinicians will need to be developed at a level above the individual organization, likely under the current CE authority of each healthcare profession. In the meantime, organizations can consider alternatives, such as an annual universal CE module completed by all QBS as a requirement to be paid their differential compensation, periodic observation of bilingual clinicians by trained observers (e.g., senior interpreters) in their regular work or in a simulation environment, provision of voluntary educational opportunities, formal culture and language coaching [38], and creation of a QBS peer support network. Although periodic re-testing may be considered, its usefulness would depend on the development of validated assessments designed for repeated use with the same individual over time.

Incentives and compensation for qualification

Compensating qualified bilingual clinicians in the form of an hourly rate differential or a one-time or periodic bonus reflects the value an organization places on multilingual skills and promotes a sense of professional pride in having such skills recognized. It also rewards the clinician for organizational savings in interpreter costs and expected improvements in quality, safety, and patient satisfaction with care, all of which are positively associated with language concordance [43–45]. From a practical standpoint, compensation also incentivizes engagement with the qualification system, a challenge system administrators should anticipate. Clinician motives for avoiding a qualification system can vary – native speakers may feel insulted, second language and heritage speakers may feel intimidated, and everyone is likely to feel inconvenienced. Being paid to engage can lighten the burden of participation and encourage satisfaction and pride in taking part in an important organizational pursuit. Finally, a compensated, QBS program can help recruit multilingual candidates to the organization.

Other incentives, such as test preparation support and culture and language coaching, can be used to identify and encourage bilingual staff who may be uncertain if they can pass the qualification assessment. For those who come close, but do not pass, ongoing support of language development from the organization may allow them to pass on a subsequent attempt, further increasing the capacity to provide language-concordant care.

Marketing and promotion of a QBS program

Marketing and promotion of a QBS program can advance diverse organizational goals related to language access, among them: (1) increased awareness among bilingual and non-bilingual staff of the QBS program, leading to increased participation, (2) patient and family identification of clinicians who speak their language, resulting in language-concordant care (3) demonstration of the organization's commitment to language equity and quality and safety of care for all patients, (4) attraction of bilingual job candidates, and (5) organizational culture change through normalizing multilingualism as a professional competency.

Qualified bilingual clinicians may be identified by wearing badges or pins that state the language(s) they speak (displayed in both English and the non-English language) and including their qualified languages on the organizational website. The QBS program can share reports internally and externally about the outcomes of qualification efforts (e.g., number and types of qualified staff by language and department), as well as stories about individual qualified bilingual clinicians and the patients they serve. Presentations throughout the organization can spread awareness to all staff, who can then become empowered to advocate for language-appropriate care. Finally, the organization can share with the community that language access is essential to delivering high-quality care. An appeal for partnership can lead to members of communities who speak languages other than English giving input on the QBS program and its impact on their access to care.

Recommendations for policy and practice

Policy recommendations

The current federal requirement that bilingual clinicians be qualified to give care in a nondominant language provides a solid foundation for the development of a more robust and consistent set of professional practices related to multilingualism. Because federal and state guidance often changes along with administrations and legislatures, there is a continuous need for attentive advocacy at all levels where standards for healthcare professionals are defined. The following recommendations address areas of opportunity for strengthening regulations and professional standards on multilingualism:

Federal and state government

- **Use specific, detailed descriptions of qualified bilingual staff giving direct care to patients in a language other than English (including a definition of "qualified bilingual staff") when creating federal or state guidance on culturally and linguistically appropriate care**

  The loss of specific guidance on QBS between the original and the enhanced National CLAS Standards shows how such guidance can complement (in the original) or be overshadowed by (in the enhanced) discussion of interpreter qualification when language access guidelines are created. For regulations to be followed consistently, users must understand what key terms mean operationally. The current final rule on Section 1557 of the ACA [14] and some state provisions addressing qualification of language service providers (including bilingual clinicians) [15] do not define "qualified," leaving those responsible for complying with the regulations uncertain about how to do so.

- **Create state-level policies tied to professional licensing that require bilingual clinicians to be formally assessed before being allowed to practice in a non-English language**

  The model for dominant language proficiency assessment (e.g., English in the United States) could be used, with the creation of a national body similar to the ECFMG to provide the credentialing needed to ensure appropriate language assessment. The main difference would be the need for assessment in multiple languages. There would be an opportunity through this national body to create an assessment similar to the Occupational English Test (a broad healthcare-specific assessment) [6], starting with Spanish, the most common non-English language in the United States, then expanding to other languages.

- **Consider qualified bilingual staff in reimbursement models for language services**

  Federal and state regulations on language access can be tied to reimbursement opportunities, especially for the costs of interpretation [46, 47]. Including QBS in reimbursement models from state or private insurers could offset the organizational costs of creating and administering a QBS program. The rationale for such payments would be based on increased quality, safety, and efficiency of language-concordant care, in addition to relieving the burden of what is currently an unfunded mandate to qualify bilingual staff.

Accrediting bodies

- **Include qualification of bilingual staff in language access standards from healthcare accrediting bodies**

  As a requirement for all healthcare organizations receiving federal funding (which includes most healthcare organizations in the United States), language access is commonly included in standards published by accreditation bodies – especially those given deeming authority by the Centers for Medicare and Medicaid Services (e.g., the Joint Commission) [48]. Including specific standards related to QBS in the accreditation process heightens awareness and compliance and allows healthcare organizations to explore approaches to compliance with the support of an accreditation team.

Advocacy groups

- **Include qualification of bilingual staff in statements from coalitions promoting language access and health equity**
  Language access coalitions have formed at the national and state levels to promote language equity, especially related to adequate interpretation and translation [49]. Their educational and policy advocacy materials rarely address the role of QBS, focusing instead on the qualification of interpreters and translators. Incorporating the qualification of bilingual staff in the provision of healthcare and other services in such advocacy would help complete the language access picture for state and federal policymakers. Policy advocacy related to language equity also should include representation from the communities speaking languages other than English.

Practice recommendations

The actions of clinicians and the organizations where they work determine whether the use of nondominant language skills conforms to professional and regulatory expectations. Where it does not, the following recommendations can help establish a consistent approach to achieving effective language-concordant care:

Individual clinician

- **Ensure that language skills are adequate and safe for patient interaction through formal assessment and principled communication choices**
  In addition to seeking assessment through validated measures (see Table 13.1 for examples), clinicians should determine in what clinical situations they are or are not comfortable using their language skills and should prepare for each encounter, considering possible challenges related to their language abilities. Best practices include routine use of plain language and checking for patient understanding in every encounter using teach-back [53] and related health literacy techniques to achieve effective communication.
- **Continually maintain and improve language skills**
  Clinicians should consider whether their language use is frequent enough to maintain an adequate proficiency level for clinical situations commonly encountered in their practices. They also can identify and pursue CE opportunities for cultural and linguistic improvement, for example, through online curricula, immersion experiences, or individualized coaching.
- **Advocate for treatment of bilingualism as a professional competency**
  When they notice a colleague or other staff member using unqualified language skills to provide clinical care, clinicians should address the issue with the individual (e.g., asking if they are aware of the organization's QBS process) or with appropriate leaders. They also can discuss their experiences as a bilingual clinician, including facilitators and barriers to treating bilingualism as a professional skill, with leaders in the organization and with other bilingual clinicians to build momentum toward creation or improvement of organizational standards and support systems.
- **Teach trainees that multilingualism is a professional skill subject to the same ethical responsibilities as other clinical competencies**
  Clinicians who supervise trainees should provide guidance on bilingual qualifications to students and trainees who work in clinical settings as part of their

education. If no qualification system exists for those settings, advocate for a policy (and qualification system, if possible) that clearly describes which students and trainees are allowed to use bilingual skills in their clinical roles.

Organization

- **Create an organizational qualification system for bilingual staff founded in organizational policy and based on available models and assessments**
  Built-in flexibility will allow organizations to accommodate innovations in this rapidly evolving area of professional practice. One such innovation could be the incorporation of bilingualism into the credentialing and privileging process for independent licensed practitioners (i.e., physicians, nurse practitioners, and physician assistants).
- **Support bilingual staff and trainees aspiring to become qualified with educational and training opportunities**
  Starting with orientation, organizations should outline professional responsibilities, including ethical and regulatory obligations, related to clinician bilingualism. They should also include training related to communication, health equity, language access, and patient rights, and provide opportunities for assessment [54].

System

- **Create a system-wide certification system for bilingual clinicians and other healthcare staff**
  Although professionalization could continue to be pursued in a piecemeal manner within individual organizations (and states) by choosing from competing assessment products, ideally the healthcare professions would be able to access a valid, reliable source of assessment for multiple clinician roles. The OET, created in Australia for use with multiple healthcare professions [6], could serve as a model for the development of a system-wide approach to assessment. In the United States, the National Association of Medical Spanish is a non-profit professional organization with the goal of standardizing education and assessment of language proficiency for clinicians who wish to provide direct medical care for Spanish-speaking patients.

Next steps

Increased attention to language access in healthcare has led to growing research efforts in clinician second language learning and proficiency assessment (see Chapter 12 and Part IV in this volume). Studies of standard-setting and policy impact are rare, though, given that governmental policies regulating the qualification of bilingual staff have been in effect for less than a decade, and early implementation models (e.g., the QBS model at Kaiser Permanente) have been created and disseminated only recently. Formal evaluation in the following areas would benefit the move to professionalize multilingualism in healthcare through standard-setting:

- **Healthcare professionals' attitudes toward treating nondominant language skills as a professional competency subject to specialized training and formal assessment**

Of particular benefit would be studies of facilitators and barriers to clinician engagement in bilingual qualification across the spectrum of bilingualism and by different types of speakers (e.g., native, heritage, and second language speakers). Comparative studies of attitudes in various healthcare professions (e.g., medicine, nursing, pharmacy, psychology, social work, interpretation, and translation) could highlight opportunities for customizing training and engagement strategies to specific disciplines.

- **QBS program evaluation, including case study descriptions, cost–benefit analyses, and reports of process and outcome metrics**
  Language access planners in all healthcare organizations need examples of effective QBS program design and implementation, ideally based on evidence from formal studies. Such studies should consider effects on clinicians and the organization, as well as patients and their communities.
- **Uptake of policy provisions, with a focus on education of healthcare leaders and clinicians, empowerment of affected communities, and reporting by organizations**
  Compliance with regulations depends on leaders and clinicians being aware of requirements. How effective are current approaches to education? How can advocates for affected communities best advise organizations and hold them accountable to language access requirements? How can policymakers take advantage of existing data collection systems to measure uptake of policy provisions on qualification of bilingual staff (e.g., national or state hospital association surveys of member hospitals, de-identified data from accrediting bodies, commercial "best hospital" surveys including diversity, equity, and inclusion measures)?

Conclusion

Setting standards for bilingualism in clinical practice, grounded in theories of professionalism and health equity, is essential to achieving effective language access in healthcare. Despite some advances in elements of standard-setting in the last 20 years, clinicians' use of nondominant languages to directly care for patients remains poorly regulated at the level of the individual practitioner, the healthcare organization, and the healthcare professions. In addition to more consistent policy and programming in the clinical setting, a coordinated movement of leaders in the healthcare professions would provide an opportunity to set broad standards for the use of nondominant languages and outline system-wide strategies to advance policy, practice, education, and research. In the meantime, there are concrete steps that clinicians and organizations can take to assure that nondominant language use is safe and effective, providing culturally and linguistically diverse populations with care based in language equity.

Highlights

- The imperative to professionalize nondominant language use by healthcare clinicians arises from ethical obligations related to patient-centered care and health equity.
- Although early examples of the standard setting and specialized training required for professionalization have appeared, policymakers, organizational leaders, and individual clinicians must act to create healthcare-wide improvement.

- Policymakers should incorporate nondominant language use by clinicians in the growing movement to encode health equity into regulatory and accreditation expectations.
- Healthcare organizations should use emerging best practices to build formal qualification systems for their bilingual clinicians.
- Individual clinicians should treat their use of a nondominant language as they treat all other professional skills, seeking specialized training and formal assessment of their competency.

REFERENCES

1. Eberhard, D.M., Simons Gary, F., and Fennig, C.D. (2021). *Ethnologue: Languages of the World*. Twenty-fourth edition. [Internet]. SIL International. www.ethnologue.com (accessed 13 January 2022).
2. SIL International. Languages of the World [Internet]. https://www.sil.org/worldwide (accessed 13 January 2022).
3. Blank, L. (2002). Medical professionalism in the new millennium: a physician charter. *Ann. Intern. Med.* 136 (3): 243–246.
4. Egener, B.E., Mason, D.J., McDonald, W.J. et al. (2017). The charter on professionalism for health care organizations. *Acad. Med.* 92 (8): 1091–1099.
5. Braveman, P., Arkin, E., Orleans, T. et al. (2017). *What Is Health Equity? and What Difference Does a Definition Make?* Princeton (NJ): Robert Wood Johnson Foundation.
6. Elder, C., Mcnamara, T., Woodward-Kron, R. et al. (2013). *Towards Improved Healthcare Communication: Development and Validation of Language Proficiency Standards for Non-native English Speaking Health Professionals*. Melbourne (AU): Occupational English Test Centre.
7. Lewis, C. and Kingdom, B. (2016). CELBAN™: a 10-year retrospective. *TESL Canada J.* 33 (2): 69–82. http://dx.doi.org/1018806/tesl.v33i2.1236 (accessed 12 February 2022).
8. telc – Language examinations [Internet]. https://www.telc.net/en/candidates/language-examinations (accessed 12 February 2022).
9. US Department of Health and Human Services and Office of Minority Health (2001). *National Standards for Culturally and Linguistically Appropriate Services in Health Care*. Washington (DC): US Department of Health and Human Services.
10. US Department of Health and Human Services and Office of Minority Health (2013). *National Standards for Culturally and Linguistically Appropriate Services (CLAS) in Health and Health Care Engagement, Continuous Improvement, and Accountability* [Internet]. Washington (DC): US Department of Health and Human Services. http://www.ahrq.gov/downloads/pub/evidence/pdf/minqual/minqual.pdf.
11. US Department of Health and Human Services and Office of Minority Health (2013). *National Standards for CLAS in Health and Health Care: A Blueprint for Advancing and Sustaining CLAS Policy and Practice*. Washington (DC): US Department of Health and Human Services.
12. US Federal Register Vol 78 No 185. (2013). National Standards for Culturally and Linguistically Appropriate Services (CLAS) in Health and Health Care.
13. US Federal Register Vol. 81 No. 96. (2016) Nondiscrimination in Health Programs and Activities; Final Rule.
14. US Federal Register Vol. 85 No. 119. (2020) Nondiscrimination in Health and Health Education Programs or Activities, Delegation of Authority.
15. Youdelman, M. (2019). *Summary of State Law Requirements Addressing Language Needs in Health Care*. Washington (DC): National Health Law Program.
16. The National Board of Certification for Medical Interpreters. History.

https://www.certifiedmedicalinterpreters.org/history (accessed 12 February 2022).
17. Certification Commission for Healthcare Interpreters. CCHI timeline – CCHI [Internet]. https://cchicertification.org/about-us/cchi-timeline (accessed 12 February 2022).
18. Tang, G., Lanza, O., Marinely Rodriguez, F., and Chang, A. (2011). The Kaiser Permanente clinician cultural and linguistic assessment initiative: research and development in patient-provider language concordance. *Am. J. Public Health* 101 (2): 205–208.
19. Kaiser Permanente Institute for Health Policy (2014). *Kaiser Permanente's Qualified Bilingual Staff Model*. Aurora (CO): Kaiser Permanente Institute for Health Policy.
20. LanguageLine Solutions. Language Proficiency Test [Internet]. https://www.languageline.com/s/LanguageProficiency (accessed 2 March 2022).
21. Canopy Innovations. Canopy Credential, Canopy Innovations [Internet]. https://www.withcanopy.com/canopy-credential (accessed 13 February 2022).
22. Wilson-Stronks, A. and Galvez, E. (2007). *Hospitals, Language, and Culture: A Snapshot of the Nation Exploring Cultural and Linguistic Services in the nation's Hospitals*. Washington (DC): The Joint Commission.
23. The Joint Commission. New Health Care Equity Certification Program [Internet]. https://www.jointcommission.org/standards prepublication-standards/new-health-care-equity-certification-program/ (accessed 16 January 2022).
24. National Committee for Quality Assurance. Health equity accreditation – NCQA [Internet]. https://www.ncqa.org/programs/health-equity-accreditation (accessed 14 February 2022).
25. Martinez, E.L., Hitov, S., and Youdelman, M. (2006). *Language Access in Health Care Statement of Principles: Explanatory Guide*. Washington (DC): National Health Law Program.
26. Regenstein, M., Andres, E., Wynia, M., and for the Commission to End Health Care Disparities (2013). *Promoting Appropriate Use of physicians' Non-English Language Skills in Clinical Care: A White Paper of the Commission to End Health Care Disparities with Recommendations for Policymakers, Organizations and Clinicians*. Chicago (IL): American Medical Association.
27. Diamond, L., Toro Bejarano, M., Chung, S. et al. (2019). Factors associated with accuracy of self-assessment compared with tested non-English language proficiency among primary care providers. *Med. Care* 57 (5): 385–390.
28. Reuland, D.S., Frasier, P.Y., Olson, M.D. et al. (2009). Accuracy of self-assessed Spanish fluency in medical students. *Teach. Learn. Med.* 21 (4): 305–309.
29. Rosenthal, A., Wang, F., Schillinger, D. et al. (2011). Accuracy of physician self-report of Spanish language proficiency. *J. Immigr. Minor. Health* 13 (2): 239–243.
30. Lion, K.C., Thompson, D.A., Cowden, J.D. et al. (2013). Clinical Spanish use and language proficiency testing among pediatric residents. *Acad. Med.* 88 (10): 1478–1484.
31. Diamond, L.C. and Reuland, D.S. (2009). Describing physician language fluency: deconstructing medical Spanish. *JAMA* 301 (4): 426–428.
32. Hsieh, E. (2015). Not just "getting by": factors influencing providers' choice of interpreters. *J. Gen. Intern. Med.* 30 (1): 75–82.
33. Schenker, Y., Pérez-Stable, E.J., Nickleach, D., and Karliner, L.S. (2011). Patterns of interpreter use for hospitalized patients with limited English proficiency. *J. Gen. Intern. Med.* 26 (7): 712–717.
34. Diamond, L.C., Tuot, D.S., and Karliner, L.S. (2012). The use of Spanish language skills by physicians and nurses: policy implications for teaching and testing. *J. Gen. Intern. Med.* 27 (1): 117–123.
35. Würth, K.M., Reiter-Theil, S., Langewitz, W., and Schuster, S. (2018). "Getting by" in a Swiss tertiary hospital: the inconspicuous complexity of decision-making around patients' limited language proficiency. *J. Gen. Intern. Med.* 33 (11): 1885–1891.
36. Morales, R., Rodriguez, L., Singh, A. et al. (2015). National survey of medical Spanish curriculum in US medical schools. *J. Gen. Intern. Med.* 30 (10): 1434–1439.

37. Ortega, P., Francone, N.O., Santos, M.P. et al. (2021). Medical Spanish in US medical schools: a national survey to examine existing programs. *J. Gen. Intern. Med.* 36 (9): 2724–2730.
38. Cowden, J.D., Martinez, F.J., Dickmeyer, J.J., and Bratcher, D. (2022). Culture and language coaching for bilingual residents: the first 10 years of the CHiCoS model. *Teach. Learn. Med.* 1–12. https://doi.org/10.1080/10401334.2022.2092113.
39. Hasnain-Wynia, R., Yonek, J., Pierce, D. et al. (2006). *Hospital Language Services for Patients with Limited English Proficiency: Results from a National Survey*. Chicago (IL): Health Research and Educational Trust.
40. National Association of Community Health Centers (2008). *Serving Patients with Limited English Proficiency: Results of a Community Health Center Survey*. Bethesda (MD): National Association of Community Health Centers.
41. ALTA Language Services (2022). Qualified Bilingual Staff assessment [Internet]. https://www.altalang.com/language-testing/qbs.
42. ALTA Language Services (2022). Clinician Cultural and Linguistic Assessment [Internet]. https://www.altalang.com/language-testing/ccla.
43. Diamond, L., Izquierdo, K., Canfield, D. et al. (2019). A systematic review of the impact of patient-physician non-English language concordance on quality of care and outcomes. *J. Gen. Intern. Med.* 34 (8): 1591–1606.
44. Cano-Ibáñez, N., Zolfaghari, Y., Amezcua-Prieto, C., and Khan, K.S. (2021). Physician–patient language discordance and poor health outcomes: a systematic scoping review. *Front. Public Health* 9: 158.
45. Reaume, M., Batista, R., Talarico, R. et al. (2022). In-hospital patient harm across linguistic groups: a retrospective cohort study of home care recipients. *J Pat Safety.* 18 (1): E196–E204.
46. Ku, L. (2006). *Paying for Language Services in Medicare: Preliminary Options and Recommendations*. Washington (DC): Center on Budget and Policy Priorities.
47. Youdelman, M. (2017). *Medicaid and CHIP Reimbursement Models for Language Services*. Washington (DC): National Health Law Program.
48. Centers for Medicare and Medicaid Services. (2021). *Accreditation of Medicare certified providers & suppliers [Internet]*. https://www.cms.gov/Medicare/Provider-Enrollment-and-Certification/SurveyCertificationGenInfo/Accreditation-of-Medicare-Certified-Providers-and-Suppliers.
49. http://LEP.gov. Community organizations [Internet]. https://www.lep.gov/community-organizations.
50. Diamond, L.C., Luft, H.S., Chung, S., and Jacobs, E.A. (2012). "Does this doctor speak my language?" improving the characterization of physician non-English language skills. *Health Serv. Res.* 47 (1 Pt 2): 556–569.
51. Diamond, L., Chung, S., Ferguson, W. et al. (2014). Relationship between self-assessed and tested non-English-language proficiency among primary care providers. *Med. Care* 52 (5): 435–438.
52. Health Industry Collaboration Effort C and LW (2010). Introduction for Healthcare Professionals [Internet]. http://www.iceforhealth.org/library/documents/ICE_C&L_Provider_Toolkit_7.10.pdf (accessed 14 February 2022).
53. Talevski, J., Wong Shee, A., Rasmussen, B. et al. (2020). Teach-back: a systematic review of implementation and impacts. *PLoS One* 15 (4): e0231350.
54. Ortega, P. and Shin, T.M. (2021). *Language is not a barrier – it is an opportunity to improve health equity through education*. Health Affairs Blog https://www.healthaffairs.org/content/forefront/language-not-barrier-opportunity-improve-health-equity-through-education.

14 Current Gaps and Future Directions in Language Concordance Research and Policy

GEORGE S. CORPUZ, DAVID A. CHIRIKIAN, AND LISA C. DIAMOND

Introduction on language concordance in healthcare

Language-appropriate healthcare occurs when clinicians are either proficient in a patient's preferred language or use trained interpreters [1]. Good communication between patients and their clinicians is an integral part of patients' experiences. This important aspect of care is hindered for patients with limited English proficiency (LEP) when they are unable to receive language-concordant care. When unable to speak in their patients' primary languages themselves, clinicians often turn to interpreter-mediated care via the assistance of professional interpreters or ad hoc interpreters (e.g., other patients, family members [often including minors], friends, uncertified interpreters, or bilingual employees) [2]. Recently, as immigration trends become more complex, linguistic diversity has become increasingly common, particularly in English-speaking countries [3, 4]. In 2000, the United States recorded more than 46 million people whose preferred language was not English, 21 million of whom reported speaking English less than "very well," connoting LEP [2]. By 2018, this number rose to 58 million, 25 million of whom reported having LEP [4–6]. The fact that an estimated one in five people in the United States speaks a non-English language at home has inevitably led to a large number of crosslinguistic encounters in the healthcare setting. This, combined with the structural barriers in health systems when clinicians try to use professional interpreters, can lead clinicians to use their own, non-proficient language skills or untrained interpreters, resulting in health disparities [5]. An important distinction is that some clinicians choose to forgo interpreter-mediated care in favor of direct communication in the patient's preferred language [2]. Language concordance, for the

---

The Handbook of Language in Public Health and Healthcare, First Edition.
Edited by Pilar Ortega, Glenn Martínez, Maichou Lor, and A. Susana Ramírez.
© 2024 John Wiley & Sons, Inc. Published 2024 by John Wiley & Sons, Inc.

purposes of this chapter, refers to when clinicians are proficient in their patient's preferred language [5]. However, the term "language concordance" has not been clearly defined [7, 8]. In fact, this lack of specificity demonstrates that language concordance might even exist on a continuum of language-appropriate care, which encompasses fully interpreter-mediated care, partial interpreter assistance, and fully clinician-executed language-concordant care. In this chapter, we will survey the existing research on language concordance to understand opportunities and highlight future directions of the field and their implications for health policy.

Several studies have demonstrated that patients who prefer to communicate in non-dominant languages in the healthcare setting are more likely to experience health disparities [9]. The use of the term LEP is common in the United States and some other English-language dominant countries to describe patients who have difficulties with "speaking, reading, writing, [and/or] understanding" the English language [1, 5]. Research has extensively demonstrated decreased access to preventive and screening measures and poorer quality of care and outcomes for patients with LEP [1, 5]. Additionally, LEP is associated with less access to medical treatments, lower treatment adherence, and longer lengths of hospital stays and higher readmission rates for some conditions, poorer quality of chronic care, more medical complications, and compromised informed consent procedures [4, 6, 9]. When a patient and clinician do not share a common language, the care may be compromised, leading to potential misunderstandings, unforeseen errors, and poorer outcomes [1, 5]. Patients with LEP who have neither a language-concordant clinician nor a professional interpreter are often less satisfied with their care [2].

While good quality communication is an essential aspect of the patient–clinician relationship, patients with LEP often lack this key element. Effective patient–clinician communication is defined as "creating a good interpersonal relationship, facilitating exchange of information, and including patients in [shared] decision making" [10]. Effective communication has been positively correlated with "increased medical literacy, and improved recognition of a patient's needs, opinions, and expectations with respect to healthcare" [10]. Immigrant patients are better cared for when language-concordant care is made available [10]. Language concordance is associated with better quality of care for LEP patients in the preventive, diabetes, pain management, cancer, mental health, and inpatient settings [5]. Unfortunately for many patients with non-English language preference, there are fewer clinicians with multilingual skills suitable for medical practice, and many institutions have inadequate language assistance services [5].

Research has shown that structural barriers to linguistically appropriate care serve as direct and indirect pathways to health disparities across different modalities as depicted by Terui in Figure 14.1 [9]. One direct mechanism is that LEP restricts a patient's network, which may lead to a perpetuation of culturally ingrained, unhealthy behaviors (such as lack of physical activity or consuming high amounts of nonnutritious foods) [9]. Additionally, these communication barriers can lead to a lack of knowledge about when to seek medical attention for concerning symptoms [9]. Stigma and discrimination can also be a direct source of stress for patients with non-dominant language preference thus causing adverse health outcomes [9]. Indirect mechanisms encompass ways in which language discordance decreases healthcare access either via lack of available resources or by their association with limited health literacy [9]. Furthermore, indirect mechanisms can also manifest when communication-related impediments occur either due to language discordance or third-party interpretive errors [9].

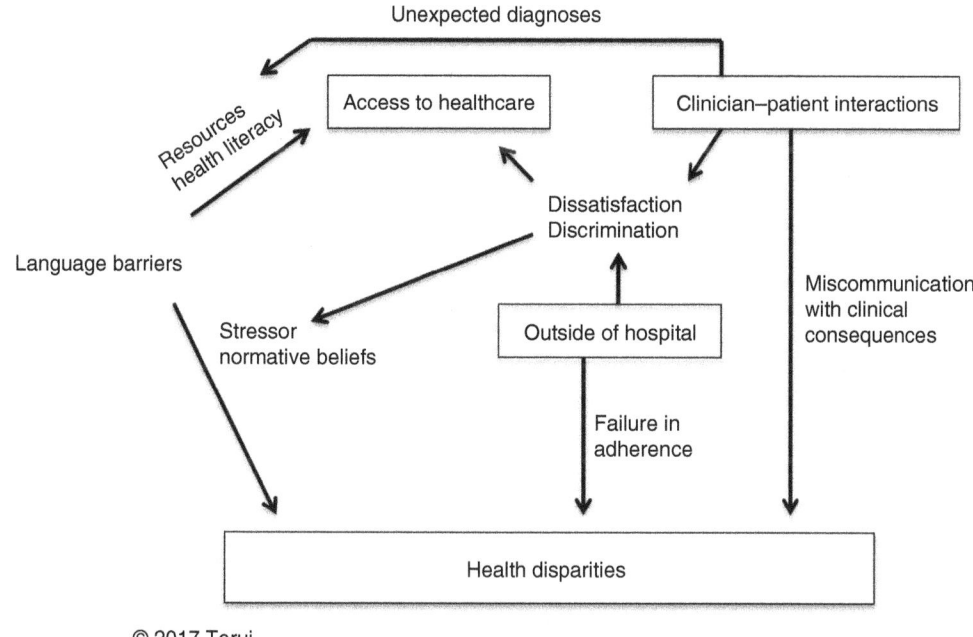

Figure 14.1 Pathways and Processes Between Structural Barriers to Language-Appropriate Care and Health Disparities. *Source:* Sachiko Terui [9]/ Springer Nature.

In the United States, there are relevant policies and regulations that dictate how healthcare organizations approach the issue of language concordance. Federal regulations, including Title VI of the Civil Rights Act of 1964 and Section 1557 of the Affordable Care Act, require healthcare organizations to provide language access services, including qualified interpreters, to patients with LEP. Title VI of the Civil Rights Act requires that institutions with any funding from federal sources provide "meaningful linguistic access" [2, 11–13]. Section 1557 of the Affordable Care Act stipulates that qualified plans "incentivize providers for implementation of activities to reduce health and healthcare disparities, including the use of language services" in an effort to make preferred-language care more accessible [14]. It further defines "qualified interpreter" and specifies that simply being bilingual does not qualify a person as an interpreter. State and local policies, along with regulatory agencies, also have some role in enforcing the provision of linguistically appropriate resources in healthcare settings [2, 5, 15]. Similarly, various guidelines including the Culturally and Linguistically Appropriate Services (CLAS) Standards guide healthcare organizations to assure the competence of anyone providing language access, which include bilingual clinicians (CLAS). Despite federal policies and regulatory agency requirements, there is poor compliance among healthcare organizations, further exacerbating disparities in care for patients with non-English language preference [2, 5, 15]. Simultaneously, these policies and guidelines vaguely center around the access of language resources rather than multilingual providers who could facilitate language-concordant care themselves. Language-concordant care provides an important point of discussion for healthcare policy in directing when and how multilingual clinicians can optimally improve communication for patients from linguistically diverse communities.

In this chapter, we will address several important aspects of language concordance research beyond what systematic reviews have demonstrated [5]. These pertain to which healthcare worker is providing language-concordant care, geographic areas where language concordance is more relevant (and needed), how language barriers have been (and need to be) studied, and future directions of language concordance as a field. First, we will discuss research related to language concordance conducted in clinician populations that are less commonly studied (e.g., nurses and other care team members) given that the majority of language concordance research has studied physicians' interactions with patients. Second, we will address language concordance research outside of the United States and other more commonly studied areas. Third, we will address language concordance research in surgical fields. Fourth, we introduce the notion of measuring clinician proficiency and its implication for language instruction for the health professions. Finally, we discuss elements that are missing from language concordance research, such as ways in which language concordance can be better measured.

Language concordance in the context of the interdisciplinary healthcare team

It is important to discuss the language-related research that is conducted in relatively understudied groups of clinicians. The entire interdisciplinary team involved in the care of a patient with LEP, including nurses, social workers, speech therapists, dieticians, occupational therapists, physical therapists, pharmacists, and interpreters, contribute to the patient's experience. As such, research must expand upon the definition of clinicians beyond physicians to other members of the interdisciplinary care team.

While healthcare language research has gradually increased within the last two decades, this surge in the United States context tends to focus on physicians, with a lack of attention to other types of clinicians, such as nurses [3, 6]. Such work is particularly important, as nurses are often the first member of the care team to come into contact with patients and can improve patient outcomes, safety, and satisfaction as they also work alongside physicians to address patients' communication needs [3]. Gerchow et al. conducted a scoping review of the literature on the impact of language on the patient–nurse relationship [3]. Especially for nurses, language, and culture are directly connected to the role they play in the setting of patient care as they are commonly the first team member to initiate clinical interaction and ultimately spend larger amounts of time with patients [3]. Research has found that nurses in various countries face language-related challenges in discordant clinical encounters across settings, languages, and regions [3]. For example, nurses have observed that patients who prefer non-English languages do not fully comprehend the importance of their bedside call light in the inpatient setting and, thus, use it less frequently [3]. In addition, existing studies demonstrate that nurses spend less time with patients with LEP [3]. In fact, like research on patient-physician relationships, nursing research has shown that communication is an important aspect of a nurse's care delivery regardless of their clinical specialty and setting. Several qualitative studies highlight language as a challenge for nurses providing care to patients with non-English language preference [3]. Furthermore, language discordance has been shown to negatively impact the nurse–patient relationship, more so in certain clinical environments including psychiatry units, intensive care units, prehospital settings, ambulances, prisons, and "maternal child community health centers" [3].

As is the case with nurses, relatively few studies have been conducted on the impact of language in occupational therapy. Occupational therapy-related research has dealt with themes related to "the professions' [evidence-based] clinical practice and the development of cultural sensitivity and attitudes from occupational therapy students" [16]. A scoping review of the literature on conducting occupational therapy research in ethnically minoritized groups noted challenges that included a lack of validated, translated tools and data collection that used interpreters to help in analyzing data [16]. "Culturally relevant occupational therapy" has been a growing theme in this sector of research as worldwide migration has created a demand for scholarship and delivery of occupational therapy in crosslinguistic and cross-cultural encounters [16]. It would be reasonable that – given the need for appropriate crosslinguistic occupational therapy care – that more research within occupational therapy settings begin to turn their attention to language concordance between occupational therapists and their patients.

Research on language concordance among clinicians who are not physicians is limited [3]. In a study conducted by Diamond et al., nurses were shown to use interpreters to a varying degree, largely dependent on their Spanish language proficiency [17]. Specifically, nurses with low language proficiency used professional interpreters and ad hoc interpreters at a higher rate than nurses with medium or high language proficiency [17]. This was consistent among all information presentation types including discharge instructions, explaining the plan of care, symptom management, and patient education [17]. Medium proficiency nurses showed more variability, when compared to the low and high proficiency groups, in selecting a professional interpreter, selecting an ad hoc interpreter, or using their own Spanish skills [17]. Another study by Squires and colleagues explored language concordance among home health nurses and other home healthcare team members in a population of 18,132 LEP patients [18]. The authors determined that only 20.2% of nurse and physical therapist visits were language-concordant [18]. This further illustrates the need to expand the number of language-concordant clinicians in the healthcare system. Researchers should shift their focus on what clinicians at all levels can do to provide care in their patients' preferred languages. Kaiser Permanente is an example of one healthcare organization that has implemented strategies to improve language concordance within their own system [19]. Specifically, their strategies include (1) appointment matching by language, (2) hiring strategies for bilingual staff and clinicians, (3) incentive programs for staff with bilingual skills, (4) monitoring and evaluation of language-concordant services, (5) training and educational development for clinicians, and (6) upstream approaches to inform pipelines for bilingual clinicians in medical education [19]. Although these measures have not been widely implemented and represent the efforts of a single healthcare system, similar efforts should be the focus of the future directions of language-concordant care and intervention studies.

Equally important to understanding the role of language concordance in patient care is comprehending how to navigate situations in which the provision of language-concordant care is not possible. Clinicians (including physicians) at all levels of care who are not proficient in the preferred languages of their patients must know their limitations and use professional interpreters to facilitate communication. Because interpreters provide language-appropriate care when the clinician is not proficient in the patient's preferred language, interpreters should be considered members of the interdisciplinary healthcare team and thus, included in the context of nonphysician clinicians. Despite the many advances in modern medicine and technology, interpretation carried out by third-party professionals is far from perfect, and literature provides a conflicting picture on its role in fostering trust. On one hand, the presence of professional interpreters in clinical encounters is associated with increased physician visits and use of preventative care, among several other benefits [3, 20]. Yet, sociolinguistic discourse studies that examine transcripts of medical encounters have shown that interpreters show bias in their role by "selectively [translating] in non-random" ways to prioritize the provider's busy schedule; in this manner, interpreters censor and guide parts of their interactions with patients while often mistranslating or indirectly editorializing patient's dialogue through adding their own comments [3, 21–23]. Additionally, interpreters have been shown to deliver fewer statements than directly dictated by patients and clinicians during first oncology visits [24]. Furthermore, clinical studies have shown that drawbacks to using interpreters include longer interaction times, cost to healthcare organizations, disruption in the flow of discussion between patients and clinicians, lost information, issues with patient confidentiality, and disruption in patient–clinician rapport building [3, 20]. Ultimately, these barriers to interpreter use lead to underuse of interpreters by clinicians [3, 25]. Despite studies showing that clinicians do not adequately use interpreter services, these obstacles can be overcome to cultivate collaborative working arrangements with interpreters and improve patient–clinician relationships when consistency of interpreter personnel is prioritized [3, 26]. Encouraging consistent interpreter use would also decrease the burden on multilingual staff who are often called on to serve as ad hoc interpreters at a moment's notice. To address clinician complaints that interpreters are either not readily available or difficult to incorporate into patient communication without detracting from building rapport, research in language concordance must address these concerns while balancing quality of care and patient safety [27].

In addition, research should focus on characterizing which clinical circumstances actually need an interpreter [3]. For example, it would be unrealistic to expect a nurse to use a professional interpreter for every clinical interaction in the inpatient setting. Not all interactions with patients carry the same communicative weight and, in fact, Squires goes so far to report in a review that crucial instances in which nurses should be prioritizing the use of an interpreter include admission, patient teaching sessions, and discharge in order to prevent medical errors and future rehospitalization [18]. If these circumstances were defined, (e.g., which kinds of interactions might be adequately served by "basic communication" without an interpreter), research could be conducted to determine whether the patient experience, quality of care, and outcomes were affected [3]. Surprisingly, preliminary research on this topic from the patient's perspective has revealed that factors they consider warrant the use of an interpreter include (1) their self-reported proficiency in English and (2) the estimated complexity of information to be conveyed in their encounters [6]. Additional research could focus on incorporating interpreters into the care team, designing training for clinicians on recognizing their own limitations in non-English language proficiency, and fostering seamless care with interpreters [3, 22, 27]. Delineating where exactly an interpreter best fits in, during which specific circumstances they are needed, and what they add to or detract from clinical communication will provide important insight on currently nonexistent guidelines on what clinicians must consider when trying to decide if and how to provide language concordance amidst a

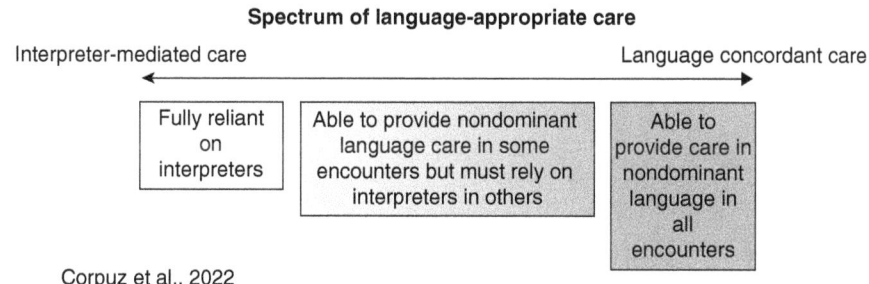

Figure 14.2 Spectrum of Language-Appropriate Care Depicting Language Concordance as a Continuum Instead of as a Discrete Notion. More research is required to elucidate mechanisms of language concordance at all levels of this spectrum.

continuum of language proficiency levels. Future directions in research and policy on language in medicine should focus on the complementary nature of language assistance, which can range from fully language-concordant clinicians to partially language-concordant clinicians using professional interpreters to supplement the discussion and confirm accuracy of clinician statements, to monolingual English speakers relying solely on professional interpreters for communication (Figure 14.2) [21]. Future directions, strategies to address shortcomings, and policy implications are outlined in Table 14.1 at the end of the chapter.

Although less research exists on language concordance between nonphysician clinicians and their patients, the unique relationships developed between these clinicians and their patients are equally important to study [6]. Priorities for future research include interventions to increase cultural humility and communication competence in nurses, physical and occupational therapists, advanced practice providers, and other clinicians (Table 14.1). This literature gap stems from a failure of organizations to recognize how clinicians are affected by cultural and linguistic differences with their patients [6, 28, 29]. This research could result in a program to train clinicians to become champions in the realm of cultural and linguistic competence and train colleagues accordingly [28]. In addition, there is a need for cultural and linguistic competence training for clinical trainees (e.g., nursing students, physical and occupational therapy students) to establish this awareness and knowledge before they transition to fully-independent clinicians [30]. The differences in clinical responsibilities among care team members call for individualized streams of research specific to each profession that are related to language concordance. This research would serve to improve communication between LEP patients and clinicians at all levels of care while guiding larger-scale policy discussions to address language disparities [3]. Theoretical questions that remain unaddressed among bilingual clinicians include whether research can identify which member(s) of the care team are able to communicate in a language-concordant manner, and which clinicians in a care team can serve as a communicative liaison for LEP patients. As such, the commonalities that these future priorities share are that they envision – more than simply measure the effects of language discordance – the optimal interventions for each specific member of the healthcare team to create a cohesive approach to promoting language concordance [3].

Table 14.1 Missing Elements in Language Concordance and their Respective Strategies and Policy Implications.

Missing Element in Language Concordance	Strategies to Address Shortcoming	Implications for Health Policy
Language concordance research among nonphysician members of the care team	Increasing research and intervention studies among nurses, physical and occupational therapists, and other clinicians (i.e., pharmacists and social workers)	Further insight will lead to improved guidance on how to craft language concordance policies for nonphysician clinicians
Recommendations regarding which levels of proficiency and specific scenarios that necessitate the use of professional interpreters (i.e., knowing when to rely on one's bilingual skills and when to use an interpreter)	Investigating which circumstances can adequately be served by "basic communication" (without an interpreter) and how they related to patient experience, quality of care, and outcomes	We will have evidence to develop guidelines delineating where interpreters best fit into the clinical care team to foster (and not detract from) communication with culturally and linguistically diverse (CALD) patients
Research within rural, indigenous, and remote settings as well as within CALD populations	Prioritizing research within less commonly studied settings and populations of CALD patients	Focused research on CALD populations will help develop interventions and best practices when providing care to CALD patients within contexts that are difficult to generalize from research in more commonly studied counterparts
Research on language concordance within surgical fields	Designing studies and interventions to improve communication with CALD patients and their families within surgical, procedural, and intensive care settings. Utilizing property of patient reported outcome measures (PROMs) to evaluate language-related surgical disparities	Improved understanding at the intersection of language and surgery will provide insight into implementing frameworks and practices to optimize communication and limit language-based errors within surgical settings

Table 14.1 (Continued)

Missing Element in Language Concordance	Strategies to Address Shortcoming	Implications for Health Policy
Prioritization by training programs to foster formalized language instruction programs to teach future language-concordant clinicians	Advocating and lobbying for training programs to implement formalized and credit-bearing language training programs that adhere to the basic standards at minimum	Prioritizing proper training for future language-concordant clinicians will address the communicative gap in caring for CALD communities and their cumulative health inequalities
Validated tools in nondominant languages as well as non-English language teaching materials	Performing assessments to validate any nondominant language tool or teaching material for patients and trainees	Validation of the tools used to study language concordance will assure quality in medical language instruction to those in CALD communities
Standardized definitions of terms such as language concordance, variable relating to the language concordance studies, and strategies to measure clinician proficiency	Investigating which parameters are most appropriate and validated to serve as standardized "gold standards" for language concordance studies	Standardizing the terminology used within language concordance research will allow researchers to compare different studies to develop more cohesive policies to improve CALD communication

Language concordance research outside of the United States and in less commonly studied settings

While the United States has released most of the current research on language barriers and language concordance, most studies outside of the United States have been conducted in Australia, Canada, and the United Kingdom [6]. Inside the United States, the majority of research has taken place in the West and Northeast regions, although there has been an increase in the Midwest and South [6]. It seems that increasing publication of healthcare language research follows immigration patterns and occurs in areas that have the largest LEP populations [6]. Most of the research carried out in the United States has been descriptive in design and has examined the impact of language in healthcare for Spanish speakers, who comprise the majority of the United States population with non-English language preference. Relatedly, the distribution of languages studied in this type of research domestically has paralleled the number of speakers belonging to each respective nondominant language [6]. Outside of the United States, the broad scope of research on social and medical science research has been noted to take place in western, industrialized societies [16].

The majority of these studies are conducted in academic and/or urban medical centers [5]. Consequently, there is a lack of research on language concordance in rural, indigenous, and remote settings. One such example is the rural Latino population in the American agricultural industry, which may have different healthcare needs compared to an urban population [31–33]. An additional underexplored healthcare setting includes nonacademic healthcare systems [1]. As research and policy advance to introduce new measures to providing language-concordant care, specific considerations and more attention must be paid to include these less commonly studied settings, particularly from a wider array of geographic regions, that have historically been overlooked and less studied [3]. Clinicians who practice in environments outside of the conventional settings of language concordance research should be aware of the generalizability limitations of the current work, until more research relevant to the cultural and linguistic enclaves of their communities is thoroughly available or lead the campaign to conduct this research themselves [34].

As noted, much of the research on language in healthcare, let alone language concordance, has taken place in settings largely confined to urban or academic environments. These studies typically exclude patients outside of these traditionally defined settings. Australian researchers have introduced the term Culturally and Linguistically Diverse (CALD) to describe those "who were born overseas, speak languages other than the official national languages and/or have lower proficiency of native or national languages, and or who have parents who were born overseas" [35]. In the context of language concordance, the term CALD can include refugees and other transnational settings as well as nonurban and nonacademic foci of healthcare [35]. In fact, the field of language research in healthcare has already begun to adopt the term CALD to define understudied populations of interest examples including an Australian study that examined "cultural and linguistic diversity" and its effects in the experiences of "CALD women" demonstrating LEP within the prison population [36]. A Swiss research group looked at language concordance in healthcare interactions with a diverse asylum-seeking population [37]. This was the first effort to assess the quality of language-concordant care in this setting based on clinician proficiency and adjunctive interpreter use. The researchers reported that language concordance was directly correlated with better-quality encounters [37]. Additionally, it was found that inadequate language concordance, which was defined as an encounter with a non-proficient provider or no interpreter, was associated with "the underreporting of important symptoms and a risk indicator for under-referral to psychological and medical care" [37]. Conversely, adequate language concordance, which was defined as an encounter with a proficient clinician or trained interpreter, improved appropriate referrals to facilitate care [37]. Within the United States, limited work has shown that language concordance within a rural Hispanic/Latinx population in Northern California was correlated with better diabetes control [31]. These examples highlight the need for further work on language concordance to explore the unmet needs of linguistically diverse populations in these less commonly studied settings [31].

Language concordance extending beyond primary care into surgical fields

As language concordance refers to communication between clinicians and patients, most language concordance research takes place in medical specialties with greater time spent in communication between patients and clinicians. As a result, much of what has been reviewed on this topic takes place in primary care, hospital medicine, cancer care, pain management, and psychiatry settings [3, 5, 29]. Disparities in care for patients with non-English language preference are well studied and acknowledged within primary care [38]. This falsely imparts the notion that language differences only affect the care of linguistically diverse populations in chronic care settings and/or in settings that involve longitudinal relationships with patients. However, there is an emerging body of literature regarding language-appropriate care in surgical and procedural settings. The surgical studies that have been done have demonstrated that agnostic of language, general communication errors within surgical teams were the most common cause of adverse events and accounted for double the number of deaths as inadequate clinical management [39]. Consequently, effective communication is likely to play a principal role in patient safety errors in surgery, anesthesiology, and intensive care settings [39].

Surgical specialties lag behind other medical disciplines in evaluating the impact of language concordance on patient care, satisfaction, and outcomes [38]. Given that communication is a central tenet to providing adequate care, developing exemplary trust with patients and their families positively increases compliance and understanding of medical illnesses and treatments [38]. In a surgical context, dissimilarities in language, ethnicity, and culture all can contribute to a patient's decision to not proceed with a surgery, as they result in not fully understanding their clinician [40]. Furthermore, surgical patients have been shown to prefer when clinicians are culturally competent, which ultimately yields higher patient satisfaction levels [40]. It is clear that, despite the relative lack of research on language concordance in surgical settings, there exists a relevant obligation to examine how language concordance affects each step of surgical care.

Before any medical or surgical procedure takes place, obtaining informed consent from the patient is a requirement at all healthcare organizations within the United States as both an ethical and legal requirement [41]. Despite this requirement, few studies have assessed understanding of informed consent by patients with non-English language preference and physician behavior around this important interaction. A study conducted by Patel et al. evaluated the preoperative informed consent process for patients with LEP [15]. Surgeons were asked to complete a 32-item survey covering topics including demographics, level of medical training, non-English language skills and their clinical use, language learning experiences, and hypothetical scenarios with LEP patients undergoing informed consent. The authors set out to determine surgeons' preoperative consenting processes with LEP patients, describe surgeons' self-assessed non-English language proficiency levels, and understand the relationship between surgeons' self-assessed non-English language proficiency levels and their use of interpreters during preoperative informed consent. The study found that: (1) surgeons often deferred to perceived patient or family preferences to forgo interpreters and (2) surgeons had their own thresholds for inquiring about a professional interpreter rather than following a standard protocol. Additionally, the authors summarized that surgeons reported using bilingual hospital staff members, family members, and even children as ad hoc interpreters when obtaining preoperative informed consent, contrary to their hospital's written policy. Among surveyed surgeons, 32% reported using their own language skills to obtain surgical consent. Surgeons reported using their own limited language abilities or engaging ad hoc untrained interpreters when professional services were not promptly available. In hypothetical scenarios, surgeons weighed the clinical urgency and the speed at which a professional interpreter could arrive to determine whether they used their non-proficient language skills or a professional interpreter to obtain informed consent. These findings have significant implications for surgical care as clinicians are tasked with the duty of making sure that their patients understand the purposes, risks, benefits, and alternatives to proposed procedures [15].

Like research findings in other medical specialties, studies in surgical settings have found that ethnically and racially marginalized patients prefer to receive their care from racially and ethnically concordant clinicians [38, 42]. Few studies exist to evaluate the impact of language-concordant surgical care on understanding and satisfaction of care for LEP patients and their families [38]. A study by Dunlap et al. explored the impact of language-concordant care on Hispanic patients' satisfaction and understanding [38]. Participants in the study were placed into one of three groups: (1) an English-speaking group, agnostic to race/ethnicity, (2) a Spanish-speaking group that used interpreters with an English-speaking clinical team, and (3) a Spanish-concordant clinician team called the Hispanic Center for Pediatric Surgery (HCPS) [38]. The authors reported that participants in the HCPS group had higher levels of satisfaction with care compared to the English-speaking group or Spanish-speaking interpreter group [38]. Additionally, participants in the HCPS group showed better understanding of the information presented during a patient visit compared to the English-speaking group or Spanish-speaking interpreter group [38]. In a related study, Jaramillo and colleagues further studied the HCPS clinic and found that participants in the HCPS clinic rated communication quality higher than those who did not have access to language-concordant care. Similarly, patients with LEP who did not have language-concordant care appeared to be less engaged with their providers, as they asked fewer questions and reported that they felt the desire to ask more questions but were limited by language [43]. Importantly, the study found that participants in both the Spanish-concordant and Spanish-discordant groups preferred language-concordant care [43]. Jaramillo et al. suggest that disparities in access to health information may arise from language discordance between patients and physicians [43]. The collective work of Dunlap and Jaramillo demonstrates that the HCPS model of care is a feasible way to provide language-concordant care from language-concordant front desk staff, medical assistants, nurses, advanced practice providers, physicians, and other members of the care team. The HCPS was associated with higher satisfaction levels for patients with LEP because they were able to actively engage in their care [38].

Dunlap and Jaramillo's findings demonstrate that further studies are needed to address ways to standardize non-English language concordance among surgeons. In one such study, Solomon et al. studied language proficiency among surgical residents [44]. The authors reported that non-English language certification increased from 1.5% to 15.4% among surgical residents when they were tested using the Clinician Cultural and Linguistic Assessment (CCLA), a commonly used oral examination [19]. It is critical to test the proficiency levels of surgeons or other clinicians who report non-English language skills and the CCLA is one such tool to accomplish this. However, as associated editorial by Diamond cautions that further research is needed to ensure language concordance among surgeons and other clinicians. The CCLA is designed for primary care interactions and has not been validated by surgeons [45]. Further research on making language-concordant care more accessible must include valid measures of clinician language proficiency.

Studies of surgical outcomes have focused less on patient satisfaction and quality of care, although patient-reported outcomes measures (PROMs) are an emerging trend in surgery research and may provide a mechanism to evaluate language-related surgical disparities. PROMs take into account factors including a patient's health status, experience, and quality of life [38, 46]. PROMs have become particularly resonant in plastic surgery, which previously employed qualitative measures in research, and can provide an opportunity to study language concordance in the surgical setting. While PROMs have offered fields like plastic surgery tools to examine outcomes from the patient perspective, applying these to linguistically diverse populations poses unique challenges. PROMs are calibrated for "cross-cultural validity," in which the semantic phrasing of questions is maintained across different languages and cultures [46, 47]. Nonetheless, what surgery patients and families with non-English language preference desire in their surgical experiences has been an elusive topic [38]. Surgical research on language concordance, particularly focusing on the patient experience, has yet to uncover the extent to which patients value language concordance in a surgical setting and what benefits to the surgical experience language and cultural competence might offer, particularly in offering patients more of a participatory role in their surgical care [38]. Increasingly, PROMs are being collected electronically and both availability and use of translated PROMs and/or translation of electronic data collection platforms for PROMs vary widely [48, 49]. This leads to the possibility that family members will complete the PROM instead of patients, potentially altering the outcomes observed for surgical patients with LEP due to over or underestimation of symptoms by family members/caregivers. Incorporating these considerations into surgical research on PROMs could result in important ways to reduce language-related disparities in surgical outcomes.

Future studies in the surgical setting must identify how language concordance facilitates good quality communication between clinicians, patients, and their caregivers. It is also important to understand how language concordance impacts access to care, quality of care, trust, and surgical outcomes [38]. Due to the needs of surgical patients, which may be complex, language concordance in surgery may be ever more important in helping patients with LEP navigate through the entire surgical process [38].

Measuring language concordance

There is no current consensus about how language proficiency among healthcare professionals should be measured, which is a critical component to enforcing concordance in healthcare settings. Historically, the field of language concordance has utilized three approaches to assess provider proficiency in nondominant languages, which include (1) patients' assessments of their clinicians, (2) formalized language competency testing (i.e., oral proficiency interviews), and (3) clinicians' self-assessment of their own language capabilities [50]. Each strategy has its own advantages and drawbacks. Patient assessment of their clinicians and formalized language competency testing are more costly and time-consuming [50]. Furthermore, while patient assessment strategy allows the patient's voice to play a role in assessment, gathering these measures from patients has proven cumbersome [50]. As such, self-assessment measures are advantageous in terms of efficiency and cost-effectiveness, but these measures are less accurate than formal testing.

Prior studies have compared measures of language proficiency. One study compared self-reported measures of Spanish proficiency by physicians to Hispanic/Latinx patient assessments of those physicians' language proficiency levels [51]. Physicians' self-assessment of their Spanish proficiency was well-correlated with their patients' assessments except for when physicians reported their abilities as "fair," in which case the patient would report a lower assessment than the physician's own [51]. Another study compared physician self-assessment of language proficiency (the Interagency

Language Roundtable [ILR] scale modified for healthcare) to an oral proficiency examination (the CCLA) [52]. This study concluded that the self-assessment by physicians correlated to the CCLA at the low and high ends of the ILR healthcare scale and that the middle categories of ILR healthcare scale scores demonstrated a wider variability in CCLA scores [52]. Despite these collective findings, most studies investigating this topic, however, focus on clinicians who report advanced self-assessment in language proficiency. More research is needed to inform policy implications on how clinicians should be measured for language concordance, particularly in the middle of the proficiency spectrum [52].

How we measure clinician language proficiency carries tremendous weight in the policy discourse of language concordance. The absence of consistency in how clinician language proficiency is reported hinders progress in addressing healthcare disparities [53]. Some scholars have proposed that healthcare organizations need to implement a standard, such as the ILR healthcare scale, that is already widely used [53]. Introducing a more consistently applied measure for clinician language proficiency would then guide policy in healthcare organizations to identify which clinicians can and cannot provide language-concordant care and which clinicians should use an interpreter [53]. Clinicians demonstrating lower-levels of proficiency could be required to document their use of professional interpreters, particularly during important interactions with language-discordant patients [53]. Policies should not be overly explicit in dictating when language-concordant care can and cannot be administered (other than for clinicians at either end of the proficiency spectrum), as more research is needed to understand the differential levels of language proficiency needed to provide adequate care across various clinical situations [53]. As language concordance research better characterizes these scenarios, more granular policies can be introduced to guide decision-making about participating in language-concordant communication [53].

One important goal of identifying the best ways to measure nondominant language proficiency is in the training of future language-concordant clinicians in medical and other clinical training programs. This is important because prior work has found that United States residency applicants, while demonstrating diverse linguistic backgrounds, have proficiency in languages that do not match the languages spoken by patient populations. Future directions of language concordance research and policy need to examine whether expanding the number of multilingual residents and implementing medical nondominant language instruction programs to supplement interpreter use would improve care for linguistically diverse communities [54]. While many United States medical schools offer some type of medical Spanish instruction, more training programs should offer such opportunities. In a survey completed by 125 medical schools, several barriers to instituting formalized language instruction programs included limited course length, lack of student body diversity, and a lack of faculty support [55]. While basic standards of a medical Spanish curriculum include having (1) a formal curriculum, (2) a faculty advocate and instructor, (3) post-course assessments, and (4) credit-bearing status, the same survey concluded that only 21% of United States medical schools with medical Spanish offerings met all four basic standards [55]. Promoting the adoption of these basic standards is an important way to foster bilingual education in medical schools. Medical Spanish courses with a formalized curriculum that grants students credit more often contain a student language-skills assessment [55]. Training programs must go beyond language education in the form of student clubs and clinical exposure and supplement these modalities with faculty-supervised formal education to ensure various competencies can be attained [55]. Additional future directions to enhance language instruction in medical schools should include interdisciplinary perspectives that combine medical and linguistic expertise. Themes that language professionals might emphasize include teaching contextual grammar and technical vocabulary that is suited for clinical practice to address practical applications and clinical context [56]. As efforts turn toward making language concordance medical education more relevant to patients, it would be important to include the perspective of patients to guide how such efforts might alleviate healthcare inequities stemming from language discordance [56].

Promoting language concordance within healthcare interactions involves characterizing proficiency at the policy level which, in turn, will influence how language skills should be taught to future language-concordant clinicians while empowering medical training programs at the grassroots level.

Future directions for the field of language concordance

Although research on language concordance has employed a variety of study designs and approaches, there are some key factors that could improve the quality of language concordance studies. First, studies must provide a clear definition for how they define the language proficiency levels of clinicians being included. Second, controlling for confounders that could be associated with language discordance must be addressed. Third, we must disentangle the role that culture plays in language concordance research as it may confound findings and misattribute them solely to language. Fourth, we must standardize definitions being used in language concordance research. Finally, validation of tools in nondominant languages must be addressed.

A common shortcoming of language concordance research is that many studies do not use a standardized measure of the language proficiency levels of the clinicians included. This makes the findings of these studies difficult to compare and interpret, particularly those that demonstrate marked trends in positive or negative directions. The lack of a standard measure of clinician language proficiency leads to concerns that clinicians classified as language-concordant in research studies are not actually proficient in their patient's preferred language, which, in its simplest form, would be a standardized proficiency assessment that can be utilized universally across different healthcare organizations [5]. Having a unified measurement of language proficiency is especially crucial to understanding whether communication quality in non-English language-concordant encounters is on par with that of English-language concordant patient–clinician pairs [5]. Complicating this is the fact that there are no standards for measuring clinician language proficiency [2, 57, 58]. As a result, studies have often used non-validated, self-reported measures by clinicians [57]. This raises both reliability and validity issues. Research has shown that clinicians may over- or underestimate their self-reported non-English language skill levels [58]. Developing a standardized assessment for clinician non-English language proficiency would also have clinical implications, as patients prefer language-concordant clinicians, and a standardized assessment would help healthcare organizations match patients with clinicians proficient in their preferred languages [2, 51].

Although several studies have documented the impact of language concordance on quality of care and outcomes, it is important to control for possible confounding variables [2]. These include a patient's age, insurance, comorbidities, acuity of illness, acculturation level, and literacy [2]. Other factors that could be more extensively studied are country of origin, occupation, years of education, years lived in the country to which the patient immigrated, religion, and degree to which the patient speaks the dominant language [16]. Adopting an intersectional approach to identify factors associated with poor outcomes for patients with non-English language preference will help us gauge which subsets of the linguistically diverse population are more vulnerable to language-related disparities and which groups would benefit the most from language-concordant interactions with clinicians.

In addition to controlling for confounding factors in language concordance research, studies need to attempt to disentangle culture-specific beliefs and behaviors from misunderstandings due to language differences [59]. While culture likely contributes to disparities in care, it may not necessarily be related to language discordance [59]. The apparent lack of clarity on what defines and discerns language preference from race, ethnicity, and culture is a prominent source of confusion in language concordance research [16]. Culture is well defined in anthropological spheres (largely associated with qualitative research) to encompass "the shared set of (implicit and explicit) values, ideas, concepts, and rules of behavior that allow a social group to function and perpetuate itself" [60]. The concept of culture is complicated to measure, at least within clinical research [16]. Even when well defined in qualitative fields, it is not easily measured, especially in quantitative settings. Furthermore, a lack of clear measures can cause difficulties in comparing work across different regions and challenges in defining what constitutes a "minority" or "minoritized group" – as it relates to ethnicity, culture, language and other social markers of interest [16]. Finding a way to quantitatively measure culture can also reveal moments in clinical care in which cultural discordance may be contributing to language discordance. Because language is an integral part of culture, cultural discordance could contribute to health disparities that are related to, although distinct from, those observed in patient-clinician pairs who are language-discordant. It would be important to measure the differences in benefit between a patient with a clinician who is language-concordant but not culturally concordant (e.g., a United States-born Asian-American physician who is fully proficient in Spanish) compared to a clinician who is both language- and culturally concordant (e.g., a Hispanic/Latinx physician proficient in Spanish). Even more granularly, examining the differences between a Dominican patient interacting with a Chilean physician compared to a Mexican patient with a Mexican physician would be crucial to understanding the role of culture within language. As language concordance research advances, we must continue to prioritize featuring a diverse range of experiences for racial and ethnic groups with large populations with non-English language preference. It is particularly important to understand the attitudes and opinions of patients from linguistically diverse communities who have been historically disadvantaged and excluded from research [4]. We must realize that a particular challenge remaining in this field is separating preferred language from cultural identity, while simultaneously understanding their interaction [59].

Another important missing factor in language concordance research is the lack of definitions for important variables. These include measures of how often interpreters are used, how to identify language-concordant patient–clinician pairs in data sets, and which clinician in a care team should be designated as the language-concordant clinician in a data set. One ambiguity is that research that compares language-concordant clinicians to professional interpreters does not take into account the interpreter quality (e.g., professional versus ad hoc, nationally certified versus not certified). Often, the type of interpreter is not mentioned in the study or professional and ad hoc interpreters are combined into one category as a comparison group, making results difficult to compare [2]. Another issue is that studies often do not explicitly define the linguistic population being studied and may conflate patient self-reported preferred language (the gold standard), clinician perception of patients' language needs, and/or interpreter use [2, 9]. The fundamental notion of language concordance has been defined differently across studies to either refer to providers speaking their patients' preferred nondominant language, demonstrating proficiency in the nondominant language of their patients, possessing the capability to carry out a conversation, or identifying themselves from the same ethnic enclave as their patients [8]. It is imperative that future directions within language concordance research and policy explicitly define what constitutes a concordant provider, how language concordance and a clinician's role relate to one other, and what can be deemed as a sufficient level of concordance for linguistically displaced patients [8]. The lack of definitions for these important variables impairs the ability to compare studies and, thus, design effective interventions to reduce disparities.

Finally, language concordance studies must use validated tools as much as possible and, in the absence of such measures, use appropriate translation methods to assure face validity at a minimum [3, 9]. Despite employing the traditional translation and back-translation technique for surveys and questionnaires, study tools are often translated literally and thus do not convey the intended themes of the tool, thus making it difficult to draw comparisons between groups and collect the desired data [16]. These methodological discrepancies again speak to the need to address a general lack of standards [61]. One commonly used method that has been successfully employed is transcreation, a process that changes a survey tool into the target language while maintaining the intended message [62]. One research and clinical area where transcreation has been employed is within health information technology. One study described the transcreation of nondominant language tools to develop a linguistically and culturally appropriate mobile health application intervention. The purpose of the intervention was to better prepare Hispanic patients with Spanish-language preference before seeing their primary care providers [63]. As we scrutinize elements of language concordance research in the hopes of generating randomized controlled trials for interventions to improve care, these identified elements will lead to higher-quality studies.

Conclusion

There are millions of patients whose preferred languages do not match the dominant languages of the healthcare systems in which they receive care. The growing numbers of language-concordant, interdisciplinary clinicians present an opportunity to enhance healthcare access and quality for linguistically diverse populations. Research in language concordance draws from clinical science, applied social science, linguistics, and the humanities. By exposing the gaps remaining in this field of research, we proposed future directions to advance the field (Table 14.1). Eliminating structural barriers to language-appropriate healthcare involves the entire care team, across a multitude of settings, and in all disciplines of medicine. The study of language concordance begins with research that first documents the presence of language-related disparities in a specific context and they affect quality of care and outcomes. Then, research should focus on interventions that involve language-concordant clinicians in a variety of settings, disease states, healthcare professionals, and associated outcomes, before ultimately guiding policies directed at increasing access to language-concordant clinicians for patients who need them. Promoting scholarship and policy change at every stage of this continuum represents the future directions of language concordance research.

Highlights

- Language concordance improves healthcare access and quality for linguistically diverse populations.
- Eliminating structural barriers to language-concordant care involves the entire care team, across a multitude of settings, and in all disciplines of medicine.
- Language instruction in the medical field should include interdisciplinary perspectives, particularly that of patients, to guide efforts to alleviate healthcare inequities stemming from language discordance.
- Promoting language concordance within healthcare interactions involves characterizing proficiency at the policy level which, in turn, will influence how language skills should be taught to future language-concordant clinicians while empowering medical training programs at the grassroots level.
- Research in language concordance is a continuum that first documents language-related disparities, then assesses various interventions to promote concordance, and finally guides policy discussions toward increasing language-concordant healthcare access.
- Research in language concordance must coalesce around a common definition and measure for language proficiency so that findings from studies across various fields can be compared.

Acknowledgements

This work was supported by the National Institute of Minority Health and Health Disparities of the National Institutes of Health (NIH) under Award Number T37MD014220. The content is solely the responsibility of the authors and does not necessarily represent the official views of the National Institutes of Health.

REFERENCES

1. Al Shamsi, H., Almutairi, A.G., Al Mashrafi, S., and Al Kalbani, T. (2020). Implications of language barriers for healthcare: a systematic review. *Oman Med. J.* 35 (2): e122.
2. Jacobs, E., Chen, A.H.M., Karliner, L.S. et al. (2006). The need for more research on language barriers in health care: a proposed research agenda. *Milbank Q.* 84: 111–133. https://doi.org/10.1111/j.1468-0009.2006.00440.x.
3. Gerchow, L., Burka, L.R., Miner, S., and Squires, A. (2021). Language barriers between nurses and patients: a scoping review. *Patient Educ. Couns.* 104 (3): 534–553.
4. Yeheskel, A. and Rawal, S. (2019). Exploring the "patient experience" of individuals with limited English proficiency: a scoping review. *J. Immigr. Minor. Health* 21 (4): 853–878.
5. Diamond, L., Izquierdo, K., Canfield, D. et al. (2019). A systematic review of the impact of patient-physician non-English language concordance on quality of care and outcomes. *J. Gen. Intern. Med.* 34 (8): 1591–1606.
6. Schwei, R.J., Del Pozo, S., Agger-Gupta, N. et al. (2016). Changes in research on language barriers in health care since 2003: a cross-sectional review study. *Int. J. Nurs. Stud.* 54: 36–44.

7. Molina, R.L. and Kasper, J. (2019). The power of language-concordant care: a call to action for medical schools. *BMC Med. Educ.* 19 (1): 378.
8. Lor, M. and Martinez, G.A. (2020). Scoping review: definitions and outcomes of patient-provider language concordance in healthcare. *Patient Educ. Couns.* 103 (10): 1883–1901.
9. Terui, S. (2017). Conceptualizing the pathways and processes between language barriers and health disparities: review, synthesis, and extension. *J. Immigr. Minor. Health* 19 (1): 215–224.
10. Ha, J.F. and Longnecker, N. (2010). Doctor-patient communication: a review. *Ochsner J.* 10 (1): 38–43.
11. Culturally and Linguistically Appropriate Services [Internet]. http://hhs.gov. https://thinkculturalhealth.hhs.gov/clas/standards (accessed 10 February 2022).
12. Civil Rights Requirements- A. Title VI of the Civil Rights Act of 1964, 42 U.S.C. 2000d et seq. ("Title VI") [Internet]. http://hhs.gov. https://www.hhs.gov/civil-rights/for-individuals/special-topics/needy-families/civil-rights-requirements/index.html#:~:text=Title%20VI%20of%20the%20Civil%20Rights%20Act%20of%201964%2C%2042,or%20other%20Federal%20financial%20assistance (accessed 10 February 2022).
13. Section 1557 of the Patient Protection and Affordable Care Act [Internet]. http://hhs.gov. https://www.hhs.gov/civil-rights/for-individuals/section-1557/index.html#:~:text=The%20Office%20for%20Civil%20Rights,in%20covered%20health%20programs%20or (accessed 10 February 2022).
14. Kornack, J., Cernius, A., and Persicke, A. (2019). The diversity is in the details: unintentional language discrimination in the practice of applied behavior analysis. *Behav. Anal. Pract.* 12 (4): 879–886.
15. Patel, D.N., Wakeam, E., Genoff, M. et al. (2016). Preoperative consent for patients with limited English proficiency. *J. Surg. Res.* 200 (2): 514–522.
16. Morville, A.L. and Erlandsson, L.K. (2016). Methodological challenges when doing research that includes ethnic minorities: a scoping review. *Scand. J. Occup. Ther.* 23 (6): 405–415.
17. Diamond, L.C., Tuot, D.S., and Karliner, L.S. (2012). The use of Spanish language skills by physicians and nurses: policy implications for teaching and testing. *J. Gen. Intern. Med.* 27 (1): 117–123.
18. Squires, A., Peng, T.R., Barrón-Vaya, Y., and Feldman, P. (2017). An exploratory analysis of patient-provider language-concordant home health care visit patterns. *Home Health Care Manag. Pract.* 29 (3): 161–167.
19. Tang, G., Lanza, O., Rodriguez, F.M., and Chang, A. (2011). The Kaiser Permanente clinician cultural and linguistic assessment initiative: research and development in patient-provider language concordance. *Am. J. Public Health* 101 (2): 205–208.
20. Ali, P.A. and Watson, R. (2018). Language barriers and their impact on provision of care to patients with limited English proficiency: nurses' perspectives. *J. Clin. Nurs.* 27 (5–6): e1152–e1160.
21. Davidson, B. (2000). The interpreter as institutional gatekeeper: the social-linguistic role of interpreters in Spanish-English medical discourse. *J. Sociolog.* 4: 379–405. https://doi.org/10.1111/1467-9481.00121.
22. Seale, C., Rivas, C., and Kelly, M. (2013). The challenge of communication in interpreted consultations in diabetes care: a mixed methods study. *Br. J. Gen. Pract.* 63 (607): e125–e133.
23. Seale, C., Rivas, C., Al-Sarraj, H. et al. (2013). Moral mediation in interpreted health care consultations. *Soc. Sci. Med.* 98: 141–148.
24. Roter, D.L., Gregorich, S.E., Diamond, L. et al. (2020). Loss of patient centeredness in interpreter-mediated primary care visits. *Patient Educ. Couns.* 103 (11): 2244–2251.
25. Barnes, J., Ball, M., and Niven, L. (2011). Providing the family-nurse partnership programme through interpreters in England. *Health Soc. Care Community* 19 (4): 382–391.
26. Suurmond, J., Lieveld, A., van de Wetering, M., and Schouten-van Meeteren, A.Y.N. (2017). Towards culturally competent

paediatric oncology care. A qualitative study from the perspective of care providers. *Eur. J. Cancer Care* 26 (6): e12680. https://doi.org/10.1111/ecc.12680.

27. Diamond, L.C., Schenker, Y., Curry, L. et al. (2009). Getting by: underuse of interpreters by resident physicians. *J. Gen. Intern. Med.* 24 (2): 256–262.

28. Chae, D. and Park, Y. (2019). Organisational cultural competence needed to care for foreign patients: a focus on nursing management. *J. Nurs. Manag.* 27 (1): 197–206.

29. Li, S., Pearson, D., and Escott, S. (2010). Language barriers within primary care consultations: an increasing challenge needing new solutions. *Educ. Prim. Care* 21 (6): 385–391.

30. Savio, N. and George, A. (2013). The perceived communication barriers and attitude on communication among staff nurses in caring for patients from culturally and linguistically diverse background. *Int. J. Nurs. Educ.* 5: 141. https://doi.org/10.5958/j.0974-9357.5.1.036.

31. Detz, A., Mangione, C.M., Nunez de Jaimes, F. et al. (2014). Language concordance, interpersonal care, and diabetes self-care in rural Latino patients. *J. Gen. Intern. Med.* 29 (12): 1650–1656.

32. Ross, L., Harding, C., Seal, A., and Duncan, G. (2016). Improving the management and care of refugees in Australian hospitals: a descriptive study. *Aust. Health Rev.* 40 (6): 679–685.

33. Meuter, R.F.I., Gallois, C., Segalowitz, N.S. et al. (2015). Overcoming language barriers in healthcare: a protocol for investigating safe and effective communication when patients or clinicians use a second language. *BMC Health Serv. Res.* 15: 371. https://doi.org/10.1186/s12913-015-1024-8.

34. Davies, S.E., Dodd, K.J., and Hill, K.D. (2017). Does cultural and linguistic diversity affect health-related outcomes for people with stroke at discharge from hospital? *Disabil. Rehabil.* 39 (8): 736–745.

35. Harrison, R., Walton, M., Chitkara, U. et al. (2020). Beyond translation: engaging with culturally and linguistically diverse consumers. *Health Expect.* 23 (1): 159–168.

36. Watt, K., Hu, W., Magin, P., and Abbott, P. (2018). "Imagine if I'm not here, what they're going to do?"—Health-care access and culturally and linguistically diverse women in prison. *Health Expectations* 21 (6): 1159–1170.

37. Bischoff, A., Bovier, P.A., Rrustemi, I. et al. (2003). Language barriers between nurses and asylum seekers: their impact on symptom reporting and referral. *Soc. Sci. Med.* 57 (3): 503–512.

38. Dunlap, J.L., Jaramillo, J.D., Koppolu, R. et al. (2015). The effects of language concordant care on patient satisfaction and clinical understanding for Hispanic pediatric surgery patients. *J. Pediatr. Surg.* 50 (9): 1586–1589.

39. Nagpal, K., Vats, A., Lamb, B. et al. (2010). Information transfer and communication in surgery. *Ann. Surg.* 252: 225–239. https://doi.org/10.1097/sla.0b013e3181e495c2.

40. Iuzzolino, E. and Kim, Y. (2020). Barriers impacting an individuals decision to undergo bariatric surgery: a systematic review. *Obes. Res. Clin. Pract.* 14 (4): 310–320.

41. Clark, S., Mangram, A., Ernest, D. et al. (2011). The informed consent: a study of the efficacy of informed consents and the associated role of language barriers. *J. Surg. Educ.* 68 (2): 143–147.

42. Zhao, C., Dowzicky, P., Colbert, L. et al. (2019). Race, gender, and language concordance in the care of surgical patients: a systematic review. *Surgery* 166 (5): 785–792.

43. Jaramillo, J., Snyder, E., Dunlap, J.L. et al. (2016). The Hispanic Clinic for Pediatric Surgery: a model to improve parent-provider communication for Hispanic pediatric surgery patients. *J. Pediatr. Surg.* 51 (4): 670–674.

44. Solomon, A., Calotta, N., Kolarich, A. et al. (2020). Surgical residents as certified bilingual speakers: a quality improvement initiative. *Jt. Comm. J. Qual. Patient Saf.* 46 (6): 359–364.

45. Diamond, L.C. (2020). Testing bilingual clinicians: an important part of providing comprehensive language Services for Patients with limited English proficiency. *Jt. Comm. J. Qual. Patient Saf.* 46 (6): 311–313.

46. Wormald, J.C.R. and Rodrigues, J.N. Outcome measurement in plastic surgery. *J. Plast. Reconstr. Aesthet. Surg.* 71: 283–289. https://doi.org/10.1016/j.bjps.2017.11.015.
47. Sharma, K., Steele, K., Birks, M. et al. (2019). Patient-reported outcome measures in plastic surgery: an introduction and review of clinical applications. *Ann. Plast. Surg.* 83 (3): 247–252.
48. Yu, J.Y., Goldberg, T., Lao, N. et al. (2021). Electronic forms for patient reported outcome measures (PROMs) are an effective, time-efficient, and cost-minimizing alternative to paper forms. *Pediatr. Rheumatol. Online J.* 19 (1): 67.
49. Slade, A.L., Retzer, A., Ahmed, K. et al. (2021). Systematic review of the use of translated patient-reported outcome measures in cancer trials. *Trials* 22 (1): 306.
50. Chaufan, C., Karter, A.J., Moffet, H.H. et al. (2016). Identifying Spanish language competent physicians: the diabetes study of Northern California (DISTANCE). *Ethn. Dis.* 26 (4): 537–544.
51. Rosenthal, A., Wang, F., Schillinger, D. et al. (2011). Accuracy of physician self-report of Spanish language proficiency. *J. Immigr. Minor. Health* 13 (2): 239–243.
52. Diamond, L., Chung, S., Ferguson, W. et al. (2014). Relationship between self-assessed and tested non-English-language proficiency among primary care providers. *Med. Care* 52 (5): 435–438.
53. Diamond, L.C. and Reuland, D.S. (2009). Describing physician language fluency: deconstructing medical Spanish. *JAMA* 301 (4): 426–428.
54. Diamond, L., Grbic, D., Genoff, M. et al. (2014). Non-English-language proficiency of applicants to US residency programs. *JAMA* 312 (22): 2405–2407.
55. Ortega, P., Francone, N.O., Santos, M.P. et al. (2021). Medical Spanish in US medical schools: a national survey to examine existing programs. *J. Gen. Intern. Med.* 36 (9): 2724–2730.
56. Ortega, P., Avila, S., and Park, Y.S. (2022). Patient-reported quality of communication skills in the clinical workplace for clinicians learning medical Spanish. *Cureus* 14 (2): e22222.
57. Lion, K.C., Thompson, D.A., Cowden, J.D. et al. (2012). Impact of language proficiency testing on provider use of Spanish for clinical care. *Pediatrics* 130 (1): e80–e87.
58. Diamond, L., Toro Bejarano, M., Chung, S. et al. (2019). Factors associated with accuracy of self-assessment compared with tested non-English language proficiency among primary care providers. *Med. Care* 57 (5): 385–390.
59. Yeo, S. (2004). Language barriers and access to care. *Annu. Rev. Nurs. Res.* 22: 59–73.
60. Hudelson, P.M. (2004). Culture and quality: an anthropological perspective. *Int. J. Qual. Health Care* 16 (5): 345–346.
61. Squires, A. (2009). Methodological challenges in cross-language qualitative research: a research review. *Int. J. Nurs. Stud.* 46: 277–287. https://doi.org/10.1016/j.ijnurstu.2008.08.006.
62. Díaz-Millón, M. and Olvera-Lobo, M.D. (2023). Towards a definition of transcreation: a systematic literature review. *Perspectives* 31: 347–364. https://doi.org/10.1080/0907676x.2021.2004177.
63. Ruvalcaba, D., Nagao Peck, H., Lyles, C. et al. (2019). Translating/creating a culturally responsive spanish-language mobile app for visit preparation: case study of "trans-creation". *JMIR Mhealth Uhealth* 7 (4): e12457.

Part IV   Pedagogy of Medical Language Education

Introduction to Part IV

Pilar Ortega

Language is the principal tool that health professionals use for patient care. For instance, health professionals interview patients to gather information about the presenting problem and to understand their medical history. They explain next steps needed to evaluate the patient's symptoms. They counsel patients and families about healthy lifestyle choices. They comfort patients in times of stress or grief. Medical history-taking alone has been found to yield the correct diagnosis 75% of the time [1], without need for blood tests or imaging studies. For this reason, communication skills with patients are a core learning objective for health professions education throughout the globe. Research regarding communication skills training in healthcare education is extensive across multiple health professions and countries and ranges in scope from broad to highly specialized clinical topics. Some recent examples include a Swiss study regarding longitudinal communication skills training in medical school [2], a United States study to improve resident physicians' discharge communication [3], a dental school survey involving German-speaking countries in Europe regarding communication skills curricula [4], an Australian study of nursing communication skills [5], a South African study of community health worker communication training [6], and a study of oncologists in Mexico and their skills for delivering serious news [7].

Despite the worldwide recognition of the importance of communication skills in health professional education, these skills are typically taught exclusively in the dominant language of instruction. As a result, when individuals who prefer non-dominant languages need healthcare services, they may not benefit from the diagnostic or therapeutic power of language. Patients who experience language discordance with their clinician experience worse health outcomes and less satisfaction of care [8]. Thus, medical language educational initiatives – programs that teach clinicians or clinicians-in-training to effectively communicate with patients in a non-dominant language – present an opportunity to improve health equity for linguistically diverse populations.

The Handbook of Language in Public Health and Healthcare, First Edition.
Edited by Pilar Ortega, Glenn Martínez, Maichou Lor, and A. Susana Ramírez.
© 2024 John Wiley & Sons, Inc. Published 2024 by John Wiley & Sons, Inc.

Historically, efforts to improve healthcare communication for marginalized linguistic groups have most commonly been student-led, extracurricular, and unsupervised. In the recent years, there is a growth in research and publications related to health professional communication skills training in non-dominant languages. For example, in the United States, where the most common non-English language spoken is Spanish, an interprofessional group of experts established a consensus document in 2020 establishing guidelines and core competencies for medical Spanish educational programs in medical schools [9]. A growing number of United States-based medical education curricular publications address pedagogical issues in training clinicians on language-appropriate healthcare. Medical Spanish education has seen the most significant growth [10–13], but educators have similarly applied language-appropriate communication training for specific cultural groups in which language identity plays a key role, such as Arab and Muslim patients [14] and Puerto Rican patients [15] as well as teaching clinicians to work with medical interpreters [16, 17]. In the field of nursing, several European countries have evaluated the role of multilingual education to prepare nurses-in-training for linguistically diverse populations [18, 19]. Significant gaps remain in medical language education. Recent research shows that despite the increasing prevalence of medical Spanish programs in the United States, a majority of programs do not meet basic quality standards [20].

The chapters in this section present a robust historical and theoretical framework, outline critical issues, and propose actionable recommendations related to pedagogy of medical languages. A considerable amount of the published literature on medical language pedagogy has focused on physicians and physicians-in-training, which is reflected in the content of this section. Authors have taken care to incorporate available data regarding medical language education published in other health professions, consider educational implications that may apply across multiple health fields, and propose steps needed for broad advancement of clinician training in language-appropriate healthcare communication. To begin the section, Chapter 15 presents a linguistic perspective on pedagogy for second language acquisition for healthcare purposes and addresses issues in distinguishing learner proficiency levels in healthcare language courses. The author also identifies gaps and proposes strategies to raise quality expectations for medical language education.

Chapter 16 explains that communities who speak non-dominant languages are often multilingual and, as a result, individuals from these communities spontaneously incorporate the mixed use of more than one language into their day-to-day linguistic practices, a concept known as translanguaging. The authors discuss multilingualism around the world, present evidence incorporating translanguaging in medical language pedagogy, and explore the unique characteristics of heritage speakers can bring to the medical language classroom.

Next, Chapter 17 focuses on medical Spanish education and explores similarities and differences between educational initiatives that target specific competencies in medical Spanish compared to those that target more generalizable crosslinguistic communication skills. In this context, crosslinguistic skills refer to the skillset needed by a clinician to effectively communicate with patients who have any non-dominant language preference. These include skills to self-assess their non-dominant language skills as well as their ability to work with a medical interpreter.

Chapter 18 discusses the unique aspects, benefits, and challenges of medical language education in languages besides Spanish, the ad hoc development of medical language courses, the supervision of students seeking to gain or enhance communication skills in specific languages, assessing proficiency in language acquisition, and the cultural nuances that may play an important role in medical language training for specific communities. The authors present several examples of medical language educational interventions in a United States medical school, including courses that teach medical Mandarin and medical Portuguese, and their potential application to other languages, health professions, and countries.

Chapter 19 presents strategies for teaching clinical communication skills in minoritized languages including: service-learning, clinical skills, interpersonal communication training and assessment, simulation training, and local versus study abroad programs. The authors present practical recommendations for sustainable medical language programs across the continuum of medical education.

Finally, Chapter 20 addresses faculty development and institutional leadership for developing and teaching medical language courses. The lack of faculty available, trained, and institutionally supported to teach medical language courses remains an unresolved challenge for sustainable programs. The authors present strategies for improving medical language faculty development and support. Each chapter ends with actionable recommendations for research and advancements needed in medical language education.

REFERENCES

1. Lown, B. (1999). *The Lost Art of Healing: Practicing Compassion in Medicine*. New York: Ballantine Books.
2. Junod Perron, N., Klöckner Cronauer, C., Hautz, S.C. et al. (2018). How do Swiss medical schools prepare their students to become good communicators in their future professional careers: a questionnaire and interview study involving medical graduates, teachers and curriculum coordinators. *BMC Med. Educ.* 18 (1): 285. https://doi.org/10.1186/s12909-018-1376-y.
3. Trivedi, S.P., Kopp, Z., Tang, A.J. et al. (2021). Discharge communication: a multi-institutional survey of internal medicine residents' education and practices. *Acad. Med.* 96 (7): 1043–1049. https://doi.org/10.1097/ACM.0000000000003896.
4. Rüttermann, S., Sobotta, A., Hahn, P. et al. (2017). Teaching and assessment of communication skills in undergraduate dental education - a survey in German-speaking countries. *Eur. J. Dent. Educ.* 21 (3): 151–158. https://doi.org/10.1111/eje.12194.
5. Kerr, D., Ostaszkiewicz, J., Dunning, T., and Martin, P. (2020). The effectiveness of training interventions on nurses' communication skills: a systematic review. *Nurse Educ. Today* 89: 104405. https://doi.org/10.1016/j.nedt.2020.104405.
6. Laurenzi, C.A., Gordon, S., Skeen, S. et al. (2020). The home visit communication skills inventory: piloting a tool to measure community health worker fidelity to training in rural South Africa. *Res. Nurs. Health* 43 (1): 122–133. https://doi.org/10.1002/nur.22000.
7. Platas, A., Cruz-Ramos, M., Mesa-Chavez, F. et al. (2021). Communication challenges among oncologists in Mexico. *J. Cancer Educ.* 36 (5): 1098–1104. https://doi.org/10.1007/s13187-020-01703-7.
8. Diamond, L., Izquierdo, K., Canfield, D. et al. (2019). A systematic review of the impact of patient-physician non-English language concordance on quality of care and outcomes. *J. Gen. Intern. Med.* 34 (8): 1591–1606. https://doi.org/10.1007/s11606-019-04847-5.

9. Ortega, P., Diamond, L., Alemán, M.A. et al. (2020). Medical Spanish standardization in U.S. medical schools: consensus statement from a multidisciplinary expert panel. *Acad. Med.* 95 (1): 22–31. https://doi.org/10.1097/ACM.0000000000002917.
10. Ortega, P., López-Hinojosa, I., Park, Y.S., and Girotti, J.A. (2021). Medical Spanish musculoskeletal and dermatologic educational module. *MedEdPORTAL* 17: 11071. https://doi.org/10.15766/mep_2374-8265.11071.
11. Almanzar, A., Martinez, D., Vega, E. et al. (2022). COVID-19 education for health professionals caring for Spanish-speaking patients. *MedEdPORTAL* 18: 11240. https://doi.org/10.15766/mep_2374-8265.11240.
12. Alzate-Duque, L., Sánchez, J.P., Marti, S.R.M. et al. (2021). HIV pre-exposure prophylaxis education for clinicians caring for Spanish-speaking men who have sex with men (MSM). *MedEdPORTAL* 17: 11110. https://doi.org/10.15766/mep_2374-8265.11110.
13. Ortega, P., González, C., López-Hinojosa, I. et al. (2022). Medical Spanish endocrinology educational module. *MedEdPORTAL* 18: 11226. https://doi.org/10.15766/mep_2374-8265.11226.
14. Sarsour, N.Y. and Hammoud, M.M. (2021). Integration of Arab and Muslim health education into a medical school curriculum. *MedEdPORTAL* 17: 11188. https://doi.org/10.15766/mep_2374-8265.11188.
15. Díaz, D.H.S., Garcia, G., Clare, C. et al. (2020). Taking care of the Puerto Rican patient: historical perspectives, health status, and health care access. *MedEdPORTAL* 16: 10984. https://doi.org/10.15766/mep_2374-8265.10984.
16. Zdradzinski, M.J., Backster, A., Heron, S. et al. (2019). A novel simulation to assess residents' utilization of a medical interpreter. *MedEdPORTAL* 15: 10853. https://doi.org/10.15766/mep_2374-8265.10853.
17. Pinto Taylor, E., Mulenos, A., Chatterjee, A., and Talwalkar, J.S. (2019). Partnering with interpreter services: standardized patient cases to improve communication with limited English proficiency patients. *MedEdPORTAL* 15: 10826. https://doi.org/10.15766/mep_2374-8265.10826.
18. Garone, A. and Van de Craen, P. (2017). The role of language skills and internationalization in nursing degree programmes: a literature review. *Nurse Educ. Today* 49: 140–144. https://doi.org/10.1016/j.nedt.2016.11.012.
19. Garone, A., Van de Craen, P., and Struyven, K. (2020). Multilingual nursing education: nursing students' and teachers' interests, perceptions and expectations. *Nurse Educ. Today* 86: 104311. https://doi.org/10.1016/j.nedt.2019.104311.
20. Ortega, P., Francone, N.O., Santos, M.P. et al. (2021). Medical Spanish in US medical schools: a national survey to examine existing programs. *J. Gen. Intern. Med.* 36 (9): 2724–2730. https://doi.org/10.1007/s11606-021-06735-3.

15 Second Language Acquisition for Healthcare Purposes

KAROL J. HARDIN

Introduction

Language is a social determinant of health [1]. Studies consistently demonstrate that when clinicians use professional interpreters or communicate proficiently in a patient's preferred language, they reduce disparities in treatment and health outcomes [2, 3]. In contrast, brief, intensive language training of clinicians results in underuse of interpreters and an increase in significant errors [4, 5]. Hence, the way healthcare professionals acquire and are taught language may directly impact patients' quality of care and their experience.

This chapter presents an applied linguistics perspective on teaching methods in second language acquisition for healthcare purposes, specifically focusing on second language learners and issues when distinguishing proficiency levels for healthcare language courses. Strikingly, when it comes to medical practitioners speaking another language, there is a general belief that "something is better than nothing" and that "getting by" is good enough [6], yet we would never say this about the standards and rigor needed for medical education. We need to aim higher.

Applied linguistics and key terms

Why is an applied linguistics perspective important for healthcare communication? Applied linguistics has two common definitions: (1) the study of learning and teaching another language and (2) the application of language and linguistics to practical problems [7]. Both definitions can apply to language for healthcare. The applied linguist relates research on how we learn other languages to ways language should be taught and also connects language analysis to solving real-life problems, such as improving communication during healthcare encounters. Although many applied linguists are also language teachers, the reverse is not necessarily true. Language instructors often have literary, cultural, translation, or interpreter training without a background in second language acquisition or linguistics. Additionally, educators who teach LHP are often bilingual healthcare professionals with no language-teaching experience at all [8]. Consequently, language experts and others who teach Language for Health Purposes (LHP) can also benefit from the insights applied linguistics offers.

To effectively teach another LHPs, we need to know how a language is learned, who the learners are, and what teaching methods are appropriate. Situated within applied linguistics, second language acquisition (SLA) encompasses a broad area of study, focusing on how another language (L2) is acquired in the classroom, as well as in non-instructed, naturalistic contexts [9]. Although there is considerable individuality and variability, particularly for adults, SLA addresses the aspects of language learning that are relatively stable and can be generalized to many learners [9]. (Chapter 16 focuses on heritage language learning, as distinct from L2.)

This chapter addresses four foundational concepts in SLA for healthcare purposes:

1. *language proficiency* – a basis for understanding learners, designing curricula, and teaching courses
2. *language acquisition theories* – major approaches to language learning
3. *pedagogy* – teaching methods and activities
4. *pedagogy for healthcare purposes* – language teaching for healthcare contexts and recommended approaches

Historical development and theoretical framework

Language proficiency

Who is acquiring another language? Although language instructors often have classes with mixed groups of learners (both L2 and heritage learners [10] or mixed levels of proficiency), learners can also be grouped by proficiency level to target learner needs [11]. In SLA parlance, language proficiency is viewed as fundamental to understanding the language learner [12]. The term is a complex construct, referring to what an individual "can do" with language [13]. While the terms "fluency" and "proficiency" are often used interchangeably in healthcare literature, language specialists differentiate between "proficiency" to designate different levels of language performance, versus "fluency" to describe how easily or fluidly one uses language. That is, an individual can speak fluidly without having advanced proficiency. Both national and international standards can be used to determine proficiency.

The American Council on the Teaching of Foreign Languages (ACTFL) presents guidelines describing language levels for "speaking, writing, listening, and reading in real-world situations in a spontaneous and non-rehearsed context" [14]. In their terms, proficiency is determined through an interactive oral proficiency interview (OPI) by a certified examiner, and interviewees are graded based on function (e.g., ability to narrate or persuade), accuracy and comprehensibility, contextual appropriateness, and text type (elaboration and organization) [15]. The OPI has some limitations regarding range of tasks, validity for certain types of language speakers, and underemphasis on conversation and interactional strategies [16, 17]. The ACTFL OPI also does not address language for health professional settings.

ACTFL's scale provides benchmarks, or "can-do" statements, describing speakers' consistent performance in three different language modes: interpretive, interpersonal, and presentational [13]. For example, at the novice level in the interpersonal mode (two-way communication), a speaker can "communicate in spontaneous spoken, written, or signed conversations on both very familiar and everyday topics, using a variety of practiced or memorized words, phrases, simple sentences, and questions" [13]. At the intermediate level, speakers are able to create a series of sentences on familiar topics. Advanced speakers are able to communicate using more complex topics and structures and across major time frames. Superior speakers can fully participate in a broad range of topics, including abstraction. The distinguished level is equivalent to that of highly educated native speakers. Untrained instructors in language for healthcare may find it helpful to access The Center for Open Educational Resources and Language Learning website [18] to practice ascertaining learners' proficiency levels using the ACTFL scale. The modules are available for English and Spanish and offer video examples explaining identifiers at each skill level.

The ACTFL guidelines also purportedly correspond to skill level descriptions in the United States government's Interagency Language Roundtable (ILR) [19] and the Common European Framework of Reference for Languages (CEFR) [20]. Perhaps because it is user-friendly, less detailed than the other frameworks, offers self-assessment checklists, and has been modified for healthcare contexts, the ILR healthcare scale has been used to self-assess proficiency in medical schools and residencies [3]. As an example, the American Medical College Application Service (AMCAS) for entry into medical schools [21] and the Electronic Residency Application Service (ERAS), for entry into residency, identify five language levels, "Basic, Fair, Good, Advanced, or Native/Functionally Native" [22], which correspond to the five-point ILR healthcare scale [3]. The ILR also provides level descriptions for competence in intercultural communication [19].

The European framework (CEFR) provides a holistic reference table with three general proficiency levels: A (basic user), B (independent user), and C (proficient user). CEFR offers extensive detail with scales for listening, reading, speaking, oral interaction, and writing activities. It also offers self-assessment descriptors in many languages and qualitative descriptors (range, accuracy, fluency, interaction, and coherence) for spoken-language use [20].

Since there is no definitive equivalence between the validated ACTFL, ILR, and CEFR frameworks, Table 15.1 presents only a tentative estimated mapping of overall productive language proficiency levels for speaking (or writing) [19, 23, 24] along with AMCAS and ERAS designations [19, 21, 22, 25]. Shading represents estimated similarity to language levels between the three major language frameworks. The correspondence between frameworks would differ, however, when specifically examining receptive skills (reading/listening comprehension) versus productive skills (speaking/writing) since they involve different types of proficiencies.

Even though the proficiency frameworks provide extensive guidance for overall (global) language skills, they do not adequately address languages for specific purposes, such as business or healthcare. This is a crucial issue in languages for healthcare purposes since program designers need to assess *both* global and specific healthcare proficiency in order to appropriately design curricula.

In response to the need for bilingual healthcare personnel and the lack of domain-specific proficiency assessments, ALTA Language Services, working with Kaiser Permanente, created language-specific standardized LHP exams, the Clinician and

Table 15.1 Estimated mapping of language proficiency frameworks for overall proficiency.

ACTFL	CEFR	ILR	ILR for healthcare	AMCAS/ERAS
Distinguished	Proficient user C2+ (mastery)	Functionally native fluency 5	Excellent 5	Native/ functionally native
Superior	Proficient user C2 (mastery)	Advanced professional proficiency 4/4+		
Advanced-high	Proficient user C1 (advanced)	General professional proficiency 3/3+	Very good 4	Advanced
Advanced-mid	Independent user B2 (vantage)	2+	Good 3	Good
Advanced-low	Independent user B1+ (threshold)	Limited working proficiency 2		
Intermediate-high	Independent user B1 (threshold)	1+		
Intermediate-mid	Basic user A2+ (waystage)	1	Fair 2	Fair
Intermediate-low	Basic user A2 (waystage)	Elementary proficiency 1		
Novice-high	Basic user A1 (breakthrough)	Memorized proficiency 0+	Poor 1	Basic
Novice-mid	Pre-A1	No proficiency 0		
Novice-low	Pre-A1	0		

Note: ACTFL, American Council on the Teaching of Foreign Languages [14]; CEFR, Common European Framework of Reference for Languages [20]; ILR, Interagency Language Roundtable [19]; AMCAS, American Medical College Application Service [21]; ERAS, Electronic Residency Application Service [22].

Cultural Linguistic Assessment (CCLA) for bilingual clinicians and the Qualified Bilingual Staff Assessment (QBS) for other healthcare employees [26]. Priced at $110, the CCLA is a language-specific, 40-minute phone exam requiring responses to medical situations. The QBS telephone exam includes customer service, diagnosis and instructions, medical terminology, and sight translation. A QBS passing score at Level 1 allows employees to interpret general information, and Level 2 corresponds to the ability to interpret during a medical provider-patient encounter. On the CCLA, 80% corresponds to a passing score, qualifying a clinician to communicate directly with patients without an interpreter, yet it is unclear how scores correspond to the major proficiency frameworks above. The CCLA is the only validated OPI that specifically evaluates clinicians' abilities for language-concordant care [3]. Nevertheless, researchers and practitioners suggest issues with the exam regarding unintended consequences (such as a bias against heritage speakers), validity in predicting success in actual healthcare communication with patients, systematic biases against certain dialects or bilingual speakers, consistency in grading, a lack of transparency about validity, and changes in the test format over time that make it difficult to compare test results and success rates for the test longitudinally [16, 27, 28].

Studies on proficiency levels in healthcare indicate the importance of advanced proficiency in healthcare workplace settings [29] and consistently illustrate benefits of starting specialized healthcare language instruction at the intermediate level or higher [2, 30, 31]. Self-assessment of proficiency by healthcare personnel continues to be problematic, especially for heritage speakers and individuals at the intermediate level [31, 32].

Language acquisition theories

Before discussing teaching, it is important to understand how a second language is actually acquired. What follows is a simplified, yet broad panorama of five major theoretical approaches to language teaching and principles that evolved from them. Examples are offered to illustrate how these principles might look in LHP settings.

The first theoretical approach arose from the belief that learners should move from their first language (L1) to a second language (L2), or vice versa, in the traditional Grammar-Translation Method [33]. The approach imitated the way classical languages were taught but failed to take into account that modern languages extend far beyond words and sentences in a written text. This prescriptive method also emphasized standard language varieties, grammar rules, and written precision, rather than what real speakers actually say. The method might be utilized for certain aspects of healthcare translation courses but has generally fallen out of use in language teaching.

A second theory with roots in structuralism and behaviorism maintained that learners should directly learn the L2, without reference to the L1. This approach, known as the Direct Method, can be seen in language courses that used the then popular "Berlitz Method" to emphasize and memorize vocabulary [34]. The approach led to another common method in the 1950s and 1960s, the Audiolingual Method, widely used in the United States Army and at universities [33]. Learners listened to a model sentence and orally repeated increasingly complex drills in order to purportedly internalize grammatical structures and create language habits. The method focused on pronunciation and speaking in sentences, rather than extended discourse, and it did not overtly teach grammar. Current online resources in languages for health professions sometimes employ similar methods in drill and repeat sequences; however, this method fails to take into account the interactional and relational nature of communication and is not well-supported in SLA research.

A third method, popular in the 1960s, is also related to structuralism and behaviorism. Contrastive Analysis was used to highlight comparisons and contrasts between the L1 and L2. This error-analysis classified similarities (positive transfer) and dissimilarities (negative transfer) from the L1 [9], assuming that mistakes were evidence of interference in the language-learning process. The method has been criticized for focusing on learners' deficiencies rather than what they are able to do with language. This approach is sometimes used very briefly in explicit grammar instruction, for example, to illustrate similarities and differences between English and Spanish past tenses or to contrast pronunciation but is seldom used in current SLA instruction [9].

A fourth approach stemming from sociocultural theory in the 1980s views language as collaborative social achievement. The Zone of Proximal Development (ZPD) describes what learners can do without help as compared to their potential with help. Applying this idea of collaboration between novices and experts, the teacher uses scaffolding activities to build onto successively more complex tasks, and the process allows the learner to be more successful [33, 35]. The ZPD has been criticized for being difficult to apply in classroom teaching and for reducing the learner's role to passive reliance on an instructor [36].

Finally, a fifth major approach, based on cognitive theory, is the Communicative Competence Model. Indirectly extending Chomsky's "innatist" argument that competence (cognitive capacity) precedes performance (actual production) [37], Krashen's Natural Approach distinguishes between the more desirable *acquisition* (acquiring language unconsciously, similarly to L1) and *learning* (knowledge gained from explicit instruction) [38]. Learners purportedly acquire language in a natural order, with the teacher as a facilitator in the process. The teacher should provide language input just one level above the learner's comprehension level, or "input+1," so that learners can gradually increase in proficiency. Krashen also stressed that learners actively monitor their speech and that they have an "affective filter," the idea that the environment should be positive to lower the filter and allow comprehensible input. In this view, individuals should not be forced to use language until they are ready. Critics argue that the communicative competence model is too implicit and fails to show students the patterns and systems within a language. Others maintain that it is not supported by empirical research [39].

Communicative language teaching

Various learner tendencies have been identified in language research. Interlanguage – the language spoken by L2 learners – is an important SLA concept that has evolved over the years [40]. Researchers noted patterns in interlanguage development such as fossilization, simplification, overgeneralization, transfer, the one-to-one principle, and U-shaped learning [39]. Fossilization refers to the ongoing use of non-L2 constructions in learners' interlanguage [40], whereas simplification and overgeneralization refer to tendencies to either oversimplify or overuse a particular form. For example, language learners might simplify by omitting "the" before a noun even when required. Similarly, after learning that there are two verbs meaning "to be" (*ser* and *estar*) in Spanish, an individual might overgeneralize *estar* in contexts where *ser* would be appropriate. The one-to-one principle describes how learners tend to map just one form to a single meaning, assuming that there is only one possible vocabulary item [41]. U-shaped learning describes how learners may grasp a memorized concept early on and then proceed to overgeneralize and overproduce as they begin to analyze the concept (as in the case of *estar*), before returning to a high level of accuracy again [39]. Initially, interlanguage was viewed from a deficit perspective, comparing learners to native speakers, but eventually, it came to be viewed as part of normal language development. Language researchers also began to study individual differences in the way learners acquired language. For example, learners' age, context (e.g., classroom or natural immersion), ability, and motivation appeared to influence proficiency outcomes [9]. This variationist approach is evident, for example, in some study abroad research emphasizing different contexts and their impact on acquisition [42].

As an example of interlanguage, ACTFL's Can-Do statements describe what learners are able to do with language. Created by a consortium of language-related organizations, they describe three modes of communication: interpersonal, interpretive, and presentational [13]. The statements identify proficiency benchmarks along a continuum, provide performance indicators, and offer examples at each level. They are not intended as a checklist for a course or a comprehensive description of what learners do, but they can guide goal-setting and performance rubrics [13].

Although not strictly adhering to Krashen's naturalist approach, Communicative Language Teaching (based on the notion of communicative competence) is the leading language-teaching approach today. The approach follows many of Krashen's principles, especially the communicative function of language [43]. In this view, language instruction should be almost exclusively in the target language, using gestures, drawings, rephrasing, or other context clues to clarify, rather than defaulting to the learner's L1. A widely accepted extension of the theory emphasizes face-to-face interaction as the best way to promote language proficiency, for example, through a two-way information gap [44] and negotiation of meaning [45]. Such principles are evident in LHP teaching, for example, in conversational pair work, role-play activities, Objective Structured Clinical Examinations (OSCE), or standardized patient interviews. A two-way information gap might be used when learners work together to solve a problem where one lacks information that another learner has. Negotiation of meaning takes place when individuals work together to co-construct an interaction. In a medical school language course, it might include a role-play conversational medical interview where the medical student and "patient" dialogue in a natural way, both participating and adding to the informational exchange.

Another key concept in communicative language instruction is the "noticing hypothesis," the idea that learners must first notice a form before they can acquire it [46]. This concept is especially true for acquiring pragmatics – the use of language in context – where students receive explicit instruction about linguistic devices speakers use to convey implicit information. For instance, the question *Do not you have any batteries for your insulin pump?* might sound like a reproach in English due to the negation, but the equivalent form in Spanish, *¿No tienes pilitas para la bomba de insulina?* could be a conventionally implied suggestion without any sense of reproach, despite the negation [47].

Many L2 researchers emphasize that language input should focus on meaning before focusing on specific forms or details [48]. Others argue that learners should receive structured language input so that they can both focus on meaning and also understand patterns of use [9]. Output is also important, especially in LHP contexts where providers and personnel must talk to each other. "Pushed output" is a way for learners to increase their oral proficiency, emphasizing that instructors should compel students to produce language by speaking or writing [49].

Another useful concept is the importance of feedback [9], and the various ways that feedback is conveyed to learners. For instance, a language teacher may rephrase or repeat in order to reinforce natural language without overtly correcting a learner. Summative feedback is sometimes practiced separately from teaching itself but should be integrated in pedagogy. It may include written tests, performance evaluation, or oral coaching (e.g., after an oral interview). Student-centered assessments via portfolios, class discussions, or written reflections comprise other forms of feedback where learners explain and evaluate their own learning [50].

In summary, SLA research is rooted in cognitive, functional, and sociocultural theories that account for language acquisition. Collaborative communication is a primary objective in language learning, focusing on language use, rather than only grammar or individual language components.

Critical issues and topics

Pedagogy

To achieve the goal of communicative competence, we now turn to teaching methods. What are some organizational design principles for language curricula especially for healthcare purposes? ACTFL's *World Readiness Standards*, the standards most commonly used by language teachers in the United States, include five language-learning goals [51]:

- Communication (in more than one language)
- Cultures (cultural competence and understanding)
- Connections (with other disciplines)
- Comparisons (between L1 and L2)
- Communities (interaction in L2 beyond the classroom)

These standards advocate learning a language beyond the confines of the classroom and continuing lifelong learning.

Curricula and teaching methods

One of the most influential curricular design models is backward design, where educators identify desired outcomes, design performance-based tasks to measure proficiency, and create activities to develop language skills [52]. Unlike traditional set programmatic goals that focus on structured vocabulary and grammar, backward design begins with the learner's goals, context, and proficiency level. It also requires taking into account the acquisition context, whether via self-study, classroom learning, online coursework (asynchronous, synchronous, or hybrid formats), immersive settings, study abroad (and its differing contexts), on-the-job mentoring and coaching, or some other format. Curricula and lessons are then tailored to learners' needs. This type of student-centered content planning and pedagogy is practical in LHP contexts where a needs analysis should be performed before designing course goals and activities [53].

Activities

What are some examples of teaching activities to achieve communicative competency? Total Physical Response (TPR) has existed since the 1970s as part of the previously mentioned Direct Method of language acquisition [33]. It is still used today to help students recognize vocabulary [54]. The activity involves listening and responding with gestures or physical actions, and the process is intended to mimic the way learners acquire their first language. For example, in an LHP classroom, the instructor might give commands during a simulated medical exam that students perform to show comprehension, or students might draw vocabulary they hear or act it out as charades [55]. A related method,

TPR Storytelling allows students to learn vocabulary and then practice in the context of a spoken story [56, 57]. Learners help expand the story by adding details, retelling, or reading aloud. This storytelling method might be modified in an LHP classroom, for example, by having learners retell a patient history or anecdote in the target language or by using a digital storytelling mode.

Situated within communicative pedagogy, other activities include task-based learning, role-play, simulation, and spontaneous conversation. Task-based learning defines a "task" as daily behavior using L2 [58]. Instead of focusing on discrete structures like grammar or vocabulary, a syllabus would evolve from a needs analysis of the sorts of tasks the learner needs to perform. In LHP, it might consist of incrementally scaffolded modules focusing on specific tasks, such as inquiring about a patient's chief complaint or obtaining informed consent [58].

Authentic materials are encouraged within a communicative pedagogy. Applied to LHP, examples might include real-life videos of language-concordant patient-physician conversations, instructional leaflets for patients with diabetes, or consent forms for medical procedures. More recently the move toward online and computer-assisted learning has spawned a number of pedagogical resources and methods including gamification – such as use of Escape Rooms – to solve a problem [59], virtual reality to simulate interactive experiences, TalkAbroad for Healthcare to provide interaction with native speakers who are medical professionals in other countries [60], and supplementary online platforms. Unfortunately, the proliferation of resources does not always ensure quality standards or actual gains in proficiency, so materials should be critically reviewed prior to course implementation [61]. The Center for Open Resources in Language Learning provides a useful module on teaching methods for new language educators [18].

In summary, communicative pedagogy suggests that instructed SLA requires "doing" rather than "talking about" language and that the goal of language is two-way communication. Many L2 instructors utilize an eclectic methodology within a communicative teaching framework with a variety of methods, activities, and materials to accomplish the goal of interaction.

Pedagogy for healthcare purposes

Language for Healthcare Purposes (LHP) is a relatively new field of research and teaching within the broader discipline of Language for Specific Purposes (LSP), which began in the 1960s in the United Kingdom [62]. It initially focused on English but has continued to grow in a variety of courses in different languages. In such courses, SLA research is applied to meet learners' needs for their specific professional areas. Course design begins with a needs analysis focusing on the context, student proficiency levels, and desired outcomes [53]. LSP courses in university and career settings fall into two different categories: (1) those with broad emphases, such as Language for the Professions, where students are presented with language samples from a variety of career contexts, and (2) Language for Specific Contexts, where the focus is on a particular context, such as social work, healthcare, or law [16]. LSP assessment of domain-specific proficiency presents challenges since language used in a specific domain (profession) also interacts with the general domain of language use (global language use), which cannot be rigidly defined [63].

This chapter is oriented toward L2 adult learners. Historically, LHP courses encompassed a wide variety of goals, curricular design, methods, tasks, and resources [30].

Rather than applying SLA communicative pedagogy, early courses emphasized vocabulary and grammar or independent research projects on health-related topics. Course design historically tended toward instructor goals and preference, rather than student needs, which are fundamental to LSP [53]. However, even when tailored to students, learners do not necessarily know what it is they need to learn for healthcare careers, and instructors do not necessarily have the training or experience to teach the healthcare content. The following section discusses resources, instructor training, and curricular design as it relates to LHP pedagogy.

Didactic LHP resources

Research on textbooks and online courses suggests a misalignment between instructional needs and offerings. In particular, current textbooks and online resources often lack content to teach the healthcare competencies and also lack appropriate language content [64]. For example, an interdisciplinary study of online resources suggested that medical and language specialists need to collaborate in creation and periodic evaluation of LHP materials [61]. Online resources did not adequately present core competencies in medicine, targeted mostly beginning proficiency, emphasized noncommunicative activities, and inadequately addressed culture.

The following comprises recommendations for textbook content when teaching healthcare language [65]:

- target intermediate proficiency level or higher
- organize vocabulary in context around medical themes relevant to learners and incorporate dialectal variation
- target oral/aural communication and nonstandard varieties used by patients
- apply grammar to communicative activities for healthcare interaction
- include significant cultural and sociolinguistic information
- include pragmatic information, such as politeness, levels of formality, areas of miscommunication, and how to effectively work with interpreters
- utilize authentic materials and situations for role-play and interaction.

Grammar and vocabulary should be presented in the context of discourse beyond the sentence level (e.g., dialogues and video conversations) and organized around themes central to learners' tasks (e.g., discussing organ systems, taking a social history). Certain grammatical structures tend to align well with certain tasks (e.g., questions, past, and perfect tenses for taking a history; command forms when performing a physical exam; subjunctive mood for giving recommendations). Stories, dialogues, social-dimension exercises, and cultural vignettes can be effective for cultural content and application. Ultimately, the efficacy of textbooks and resources depends on their actual use and appropriate adaptation to learners.

LHP instructor training

The extant literature on LHP demonstrates a need for an interprofessional approach; both language and healthcare professionals need each other's expertise to teach effectively. Few instructors receive training in SLA and LSP [63] or LHP and healthcare, which presents a key challenge, leading to variable and possibly ineffective pedagogy.

Being a native speaker does not guarantee an ability to teach a language. That is, without training, many native speakers have difficulty explaining or knowing how to effectively teach their own language. Similarly, bilingualism does not necessarily endow a person with skills to teach either language. Training as a language instructor may not confer skills to specifically teach medical language; in fact, it is quite unlikely without considerable exposure or education in healthcare contexts. Even then, an instructor might not have an applied linguistics background to know how to design curricula and implement pedagogy based on SLA principles. Without adequate contextual experience using language in healthcare settings, even training as an applied linguist does not suggest the ability to teach healthcare language.

Conversely, physician education does not include skills to teach a language, much like a language specialist could not teach biology or chemistry (without training). Experience as an educator does not automatically confer the ability to teach language, a domain with specific set of methods and outcomes. While a medical interpreter or translator understands healthcare language, and in some ways, can cross the divide between language and healthcare disciplines, even interpreters and translators do not necessarily have training or skills to teach LHP, since language teaching is very different from language use. Finally, being a student – even a medical student or resident physician – does not imply teaching competency in medicine or language. Students do not necessarily understand what they need to know since they have yet to complete training themselves and are likely to lack competency in teaching a language.

At this point, it should be clear that effective language pedagogy and adequate content instruction require interdisciplinary collaboration. LHP instructor training would benefit from apprenticeships similar to language-teacher training and other methods involving a stepwise approach [66]: (1) studying SLA, (2) observing language classes to see applied methods, (3) assisting language instructors, and (4) teaching with supervision and constructive feedback.

LHP curricular design

LHP has yet to develop evidence-based curricula. Despite the proliferation of healthcare Spanish courses in the United States, programs are variable [67]. In the United States, students must first attend a four-year university and complete pre-medical/pre-health course requirements for entry into medical schools or other doctoral-level health professions programs. At the pre-medical/pre-health level, courses tend to target beginning or intermediate proficiency levels; however, calls have been made for curricular design based on specific contexts and needs analysis, an intermediate level or higher, collaboration with other disciplines, replicability, and longitudinal emphasis [30]. Objectives need to extend to sociolinguistic and pragmatic competencies required for adequate conversation with patients in the healthcare setting [68].

Course content, design, and teaching should be situated within SLA research, focusing on communicative goals and principles, proficiency levels, and development. Additionally, LSP design principles and transferrable skills, such as critical thinking, adaptability, intercultural competence, and collaboration, should be applied to LHP [69]. By identifying target-language goals for the specific purpose within healthcare and understanding learner proficiency levels at onset of instruction, instructors can match methods to goals and tasks to methods via backward design. As an example, if the learners' goal was oral interaction with Chinese-speaking patients, a library assignment on lupus would not match the stated goal, although it might increase passive vocabulary and an understanding of the disease. Similarly, vocabulary memorization could expand passive (or even productive) knowledge but would not relate to the goal of patient interaction unless vocabulary was implemented in contextual, oral, task-based conversation such as role-play or simulation. A reimagined assignment on lupus to match the stated goal of communication and oral/aural proficiency could instead include watching a video about lupus to become familiar with key terms, then viewing a simulated conversation about lupus modeled by the instructor and a Chinese-speaking patient, later practicing the interaction through role-play with another learner or a simulated patient, and finally reflecting on observations about culture and discourse.

Recently, there has been a movement to standardize the way that LHP is taught, particularly at the medical school level [70]. While individuals should be encouraged to acquire language, regardless of their proficiency levels, an intermediate proficiency level or higher is the suggested minimal starting level for coursework involving patient-provider communication [2, 31, 65]. Also, language classes are most effective when they are small, grouped by proficiency level, and meet frequently [30].

Medical and health professional schools, such as physician assistant [71], physical therapy [72], pharmacy [73], and nursing schools [74], have had mixed outcomes since methodology differs, the amount of contact time in the target language varies considerably, and evaluation has been difficult to compare or replicate, especially since few programs report longitudinal data [2, 30, 75]. Curricular content also fails to emphasize crucial sociolinguistic and pragmatic competencies beyond the scope of medical-language content itself, such as regional dialects, euphemisms, language register, and politeness norms [68].

To improve LHP, the National Association of Medical Spanish is making efforts to study existing curricula. A recent consensus statement [70] emphasized five core competencies for medical school language courses:

1. knowledge regarding organ systems and medical interviewing
2. knowledge regarding common disease entities
3. patient-centered explanation of medical diagnoses/assessment
4. patient-centered explanation of treatment/evaluation plan
5. determination of self-assessed confidence and limitations

Skill assessment via standardized patient encounters and standardized program evaluation were also recommended.

A handful of medical residency programs have offered bilingual language programs, but most were brief, focused on a particular goal (number of words, number of errors, and mini-immersion), and did not target long-term proficiency goals [67]. In contrast, very few medical residencies and continuing medical education programs have attempted longitudinal bilingual physician education [75]. At the residency and post-residency levels, curricular recommendations include on-the-job training and standardized language credentialing [6].

In summary, there is a growing LHP emphasis on standardized proficiency-based assessment, communicative pedagogy consistent with educational-level content and contexts, longitudinal program evaluation, interdisciplinary collaboration, and continued research on best practices.

Recommendations for research and practice

Proficiency levels

What are recommended methods from model LHP programs? Scant research has been devoted to evidence-based research on pedagogy in LHP settings [58]; however, one common consensus is emphasis on oral/aural interaction with patients [76] and cross-cultural communication [16]. Additionally, valid and reliable standardized proficiency assessments are recommended to appropriately place learners in courses and teach more effectively [67]. Unfortunately, LHP-specific language proficiency is different from global proficiency, and valid LHP proficiency-rating tools are scarce. Standardized evaluation is especially important at the medical/professional level where instructors (e.g., physicians) are less likely to have experience and training in assessing language levels or applying proficiency-level information. Reliance on self-assessment – a common tool in medical school and graduate levels – has mixed results in determining proficiency levels, especially for bilinguals and learners at the intermediate level [77, 78]. Language learners demonstrate moderate success self-evaluating their proficiency over time; however, novice and advanced learners tend to be more accurate than intermediate learners, who tend to over-evaluate their abilities [31]. Self-assessment is best reserved for low-stakes situations [79].

The following section outlines proficiency-specific content using ACTFL's major divisions of novice, intermediate, and advanced levels [14]. At the novice proficiency level, individuals should acquire the basics of communication, rather than focusing on specialized healthcare terminology. For this reason, Dejbord Sawan (2019), drawing from experience teaching communicative language pedagogy in a hospital setting, advocates an emphasis on rapport-building and cultural humility [80].

Intermediate level is the lowest appropriate starting point for more specialized vocabulary, but an emphasis on vocabulary at the expense of two-way communication is counterproductive to increasing proficiency [81]. Practice with interactive strategies such as circumlocution, rephrasing, and paraphrasing is important at this level [82], since learners have limited vocabulary but can learn strategies to "get by." The intermediate level is challenging because it occurs over an extended period of time. At this level, students should learn how to appropriately work with interpreters, rather than relying exclusively on their own language abilities [4]. Additionally, exposure to naturally occurring LHP interactions can model pragmatic concepts, miscommunication, and culturally implied information, for example, through video and actual LHP encounters [83–85].

Advanced proficiency level classes are appropriate for more complex interactions: clinical observations [6], service-learning interactions with patients [86], standardized clinical assessments [87], and healthcare immersions abroad [88]. At the advanced level, learners should be exposed to imperfect, naturally occurring discourse, demonstrating professional and informal registers, co-constructed dialogue, negotiated meaning, back-channeling, use of plain language, teachback, and other communication strategies. This level is also appropriate for demonstrating ways that politeness and rapport can be missed through interpretation [84].

Finally, sociolinguistic and cultural discussions are essential at all proficiency levels. Complex authentic interactions provide excellent models to improve communication with patients and therefore trust and rapport [85]. "Translanguaging" is also

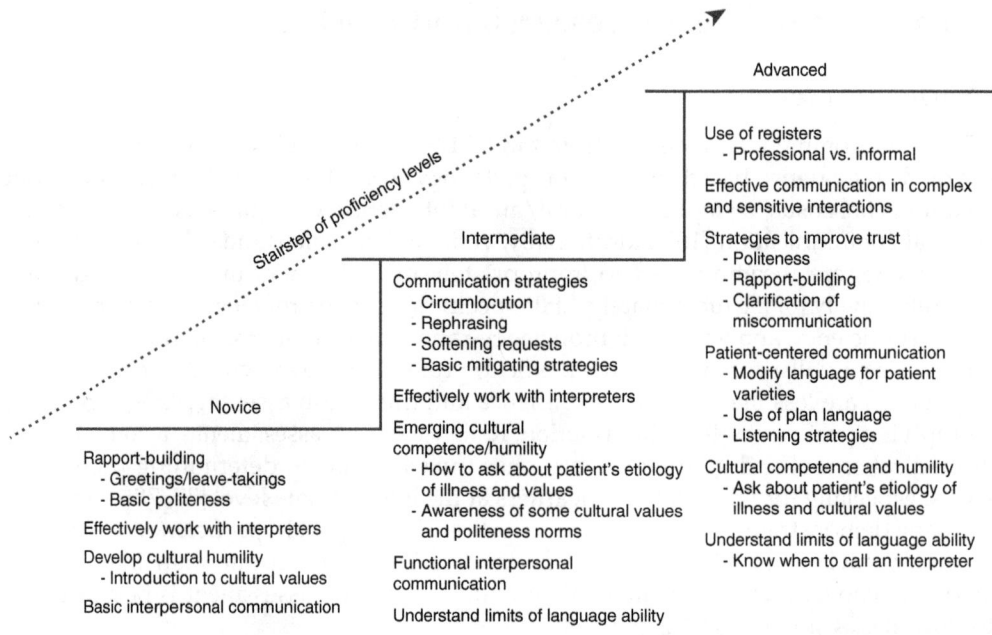

Figure 15.1 Proficiency levels and sample learner goals in language for healthcare purposes.

appropriate in clinical training to validate and support patient-centered language varieties sometimes considered nonstandard [89]. Translanguaging refers to what multilingual individuals do when moving back and forth between language systems as well as their movement beyond those systems to create new linguistic practices and meaning [90]. Conversations with patient focus groups and "ethical listening" may be starting points for learners to understand how their language impacts their listeners [68]. Ethical listening involves going beyond merely comprehending words or phrases to actively trying to understand the thoughts, experiences, and expectations of another person [16]. Figure 15.1 depicts sample proficiencies and goals.

Table 15.2 illustrates sample LHP pedagogy appropriate at the advanced level. Instruction at the intermediate level could use the same activities, adapting them for less complex and lower-stakes interaction. Rigorous methodological evaluation has yet to be determined, so this table is in no way comprehensive. Pedagogy should depend on needs-analysis results for the specific context and learners.

Educational levels

What are evidence-based teaching methods at the undergraduate, professional school, and career levels? Recall ACTFL's five goals for language learning: Communication, Cultures, Connections, Comparisons, and Communities. For LHP, *Context* and *Continuity* are additional goals tailored to the specific needs and purposes in healthcare [30]. Understanding the LHP context is crucial for a needs-based analysis, backward curricular design, and pedagogy to effectively teach healthcare-related content. Since language acquisition extends along an ongoing continuum, *Continuity* entails appropriately evaluating individual and programmatic language development

Table 15.2 Sample teaching methods in LHP targeting learners with advanced proficiency.

Communicative language goal	Sample activity
Interpersonal relationships: rapport with patients	• Clinical/on-the-job coaching [75] • Modeling rapport through authentic dialogues and videos [83–85] • Role-play and student-created dialogues • Supervised translation and interpreting [91]
Culture: humility and competence	• Written reflections and oral discussion of service-learning in healthcare contexts (e.g., assisting a nutrition or exercise class) • Reflections and oral discussion of language in clinical observation and shadowing experiences • Discuss and model best practices for working with an interpreter/when to call an interpreter [92] • Discuss patient-centered etiologies of illness • Social-dimension activities and cultural vignettes
Input: comprehensible content and ethical listening	• Problem- and task-based learning activities (system-based, communication task-based [58]) • Conversation with patient focus groups • Community service-learning [93]
Output: two-way interaction, negotiation, and co-construction of meaning	• Role-play/simulated patient interview [2] • Standardized patient interview/OSCE [87] • International clinical rotations [72] • LHP study abroad [94] • LHP internships
Metalinguistic awareness: translanguaging	• Role-play through authentic dialogues in different registers and language varieties [83] • Guest speakers on sociolinguistics • Interviews with focus groups of patients
Individual factors: student-directed learning	• Ongoing self-assessment and reflection [82]
Assessment and feedback	• Evaluate pre- and post-course proficiency through standardized patient interviews • Healthcare language coaching [75] • Independent validated assessment

as learners move through levels of language and healthcare instruction and longitudinal evaluations of programs [67]. Even as LHP has increased in demand, language education from early childhood through continuing education has yet to be well articulated in the United States, reflecting the need for more interprofessional collaboration [70, 91].

At the pre-health level, ongoing issues include traditional instruction focusing on reading and writing and emphases on formal presentations at the expense of spontaneous interpersonal conversations, authentic professional healthcare interaction, extended two-way communication, or patient language varieties. Classes tend to be student-centered, rather than relationship- or community-centered [16], and materials tend to focus on novice and intermediate proficiency levels [30]. Educators at this level could benefit from training on how to design and teach courses for specific purposes, experience in actual healthcare contexts, and collaboration with healthcare professionals in the community. Existing models propose targeting oral/aural communication through role-play [65], task-based learning [58], and community service learning [86, 93], while also emphasizing sociolinguistic awareness and culture [16]. Importantly, pre-health students tend to have much more time for language learning than later on in their training and practice.

At the medical/professional school level, LHP instruction has emphasized lectures, asynchronous online modules, and self-instruction, rather than active, student-centered, communicative methods [30]. Even the OSCE, which provides a standardized format, does not necessarily create contexts for small talk, rapport-building, or other types of spontaneous interaction. Because teaching methods for healthcare content differ from pedagogy for language content, instructors at this level could benefit from training on proficiency levels, communicative teaching methods, and methods of layering sociocultural awareness. The fact that many medical and health professional schools rely on volunteer students to teach healthcare language courses also remains problematic. Materials for this level are very limited, so instructors must cobble together resources [64]. Importantly, time constraints present challenges, so instructors should avoid shortcuts to language learning, such as focusing on memorized vocabulary or grammar exercises at the expense of spontaneous communication, rapport-building, and ethical listening to better understand the context for patient experiences.

Finally, graduate medical education (for resident physicians) and continuing career education (for practicing physicians) typically occur via on-the-job training, or learning by doing. There is very little time at this level to focus on language acquisition, so it is especially challenging to implement effective instruction. Few medical residencies have attempted bilingual tracks, but immersion experiences, language coaching, and international medical rotations seem to be effective [6, 95, 96]. One well-documented longitudinal program at this level provides a model for language development [6, 75]. Through standardized pre- and post-testing, preceptorship with a bilingual physician, on-the-job language coaching by interpreters, and an elective immersion, the program provides a unique language training for medical residents with intermediate language skills or higher. Materials targeting this educational level are virtually nonexistent due to the mode of learning while working [61, 65].

In summary, communicative LHP at the pre-health level (or earlier) provides an essential basis for attaining the highest level of proficiency possible during the undergraduate years before entering medical training and encountering stricter time constraints. Graduate and professional schools in healthcare are attempting to target higher levels of proficiency within an already intense curriculum, but it would be easier, more efficient, and more effective if more students already had an intermediate proficiency level or higher so that they could maximize benefits from LHP education. Some suggest that advanced language ability should already be in place by the time students are in residency programs [88]. Currently, the United States has no articulation between primary and secondary levels of language instruction and LSP/LHP. That is, language curricula are not geared toward actual use in career contexts. Instead, United States language programs tend toward a piecemeal approach in the early years (oriented to local school schedules and demand), followed by literature-oriented coursework in high school and college, variable language coursework in healthcare professional schools, and virtually no language training in residency. A sequenced plan for language instruction that emphasizes oral proficiency in the younger grades (e.g., dual immersion) and also includes LSPs in higher education could lead to more proficient speakers in the workplace. Finally, although on-the-job language training is beneficial, physicians are critically limited by time, career, and personal demands.

Future avenues for focus and research

Future avenues for research include evaluations of proprietary proficiency measures (e.g., the CCLA) as well as those used in hospital systems. Ideally, proficiency measures would be transparent and not for economic purposes; there is a need for validated LHP proficiency tests that are economical and appropriate to healthcare contexts. Additionally, study of the healthcare ILR self-assessment measure should continue in order to better understand its validity for LHP contexts and to gather additional data on intermediate-level self-assessment (previously shown to be less accurate than advanced or novice self-assessment). LHP program designers should keep in mind the limitations of proficiency measures since "[e]ven formal language assessments cannot guarantee proficiency for all situations" [29, p. 146], and standardized proficiency tests alone provide limited evidence regarding whether teaching has been effective [97].

There is a continuing need for textbooks and online resources targeting advanced proficiency levels with a communicative, socio-contextual approach. In particular, more effective language resources should be directed to practicing clinicians since audiovisual resources featuring actual healthcare interactions are limited. LHP should also develop and improve computer-assisted learning so that it reflects authentic two-way interaction.

Future training interventions should address the lack of pedagogical training for bilingual healthcare professionals who teach LHP and the lack of LSP and LHP training for language teachers who are designing and teaching courses. At the beginning and intermediate levels, there is an ongoing need for ethical implementation of curricula and realistic promises about what courses can help students achieve. This is especially true since studies suggest that students with some prior Spanish skills benefit most from LHP instruction. In high-stakes contexts, beginning and intermediate levels are inappropriate or even dangerous. Martinez highlights the need for more emphasis on understanding sociolinguistic context and ethical listening [16]. The goal for "complex conversations must be advanced proficiency, since overconfidence, time restraints, and reliance on inadequate language can result in unintended and adverse medical-legal consequences" [30, p. 654].

Conclusion

This chapter has identified significant gaps in literature applying SLA principles to LHP and a need for more evidence-based LHP pedagogy. First, we examined key terms, including proficiency. After an overview of SLA theories, we applied them to LHP. Next, applications and issues in training, curricular design, and resources were discussed. We also assessed pedagogy at each proficiency and educational level, offering suggestions based on model studies and areas for future focus.

In conclusion, the United States should acknowledge LHP work in other regions of the world as we establish best practices [98, 99]. Unfortunately, the United States faces the "intractable challenge" of increasing the number of practitioners with useful bilingual skills in the workplace [100, p. 377]. Despite years of language education, the proportion of students learning languages in formal educational contexts has remained stagnant for over 30 years and enrollment in higher education language classes has decreased [12, 97]. Language advocacy efforts and collaborative education across disciplines and public sectors are likely to most effectively impact the current situation; however, these efforts must be focused, needs-based, and articulated across educational levels.

Finally, we need to aim higher. We must maximize efforts to improve professional multilingualism by implementing best practices for instructor training, curricular design, and pedagogical methods that are rooted in language-acquisition research, patient-centered healthcare needs, and communicative language teaching. Ultimately, LHP pedagogical effectiveness will not be determined by research, instructors, or curricula, but by patient-provider relationships and health outcomes.

Highlights

- To effectively advance language for healthcare, we need textbooks and online resources targeting advanced learners, validated language for healthcare proficiency exams, instructor training, and objective longitudinal program evaluation.
- Teaching language is different from teaching healthcare content; at a minimum, instructors should be trained in language proficiency levels, effective communicative language teaching methods, and strategies for teaching sociocultural awareness.
- Language for healthcare courses should target intermediate proficiency or higher, focus on oral/aural interaction with patients and cross-cultural communication, and emphasize collaborative conversation over memorizing lists of vocabulary.

FURTHER READING

- This recent article provides well-documented information about a model longitudinal language program in a medical residency:

Cowden, J.D., Martínez, F.J., Dickmeyer, J.J., and Bratcher, D. (2022). Culture and language coaching for bilingual residents: The first 10 years of the CHiCoS model. *Teach. Learn. Med.* 1–12. https://doi.org/10.1080/10401334.2022.2092113.

- Grounded in theoretical and empirical studies, this comprehensive book offers information on most topics pertaining to Spanish and health care:

Martinez, G. (2020). *Spanish in Health Care: Policy, Practice and Pedagogy in Latino Health.* New York: Routledge.

- This reference book contains extensive information for language teachers that is grounded in SLA research:

Shrum, J.L. and Glisan, E.W. (2016). *Teacher's Handbook: Contextualized Language Instruction*, 5th ed. Boston: Cengage.

REFERENCES

1. Feuerherm, E.M., Showstack, R.E., Santos, M.G. et al. (2021). Language as a social determinant of health: partnerships for health equity. In: *Extending Applied Linguistics for Social Impact: Cross-Disciplinary Collaborations in Diverse Spaces of Public Inquiry* (ed. D.S. Wariner and E.R. Miller), 125–148. Bloomsbury Publishing.
2. Reuland, D.S., Frasier, P.Y., Slatt, L.M., and Alemán, M. (2008). A longitudinal medical Spanish program at one U.S. Medical School. *J. Gen. Intern. Med.* 23 (7): 1033–1037.
3. Diamond, L., Chung, S., Ferguson, W. et al. (2014). Relationship between self-assessed and tested non-English-language proficiency among primary care providers. *Med. Care* 52 (5): 435–438.
4. Diamond, L.C. and Jacobs, E.A. (2009). Let's not contribute to disparities: the best methods for teaching clinicians how to overcome language barriers to health care. *J. Gen. Intern. Med.* 25 (S2): 189–193.
5. Prince, D. and Nelson, M. (1995). Teaching Spanish to emergency medicine residents. *Acad. Emerg. Med.* 2 (1): 32–36.
6. Cowden, J.D., Thompson, D.A., Ellzey, J., and Artman, M. (2012). Getting past getting by: training culturally and linguistically competent bilingual physicians. *J. Pediatr.* 160 (6): 891–892.e1.
7. Richards, J.C. and Schmidt, D. (2002). *The Longman Dictionary of Language Teaching and Applied Linguistics*, 3ee. Harlow: Longman.
8. Ortega P, Francone NO, Santos MP, et al. Medical Spanish in US Medical Schools: a national survey to examine existing programs. *J. Gen. Intern. Med.* 2021;36(9):2724–2730. https://doi.org/10.1007/s11606-021-06735-3
9. Ellis, R. (1985). *Understanding Second Language Acquisition*. Oxford: Oxford University Press.
10. Valdés, G. (2001). Heritage language students: profiles and possibilities. In: *Heritage Languages in America: Preserving a National Resource* (ed. J.K. Peyton, D.A. Ranard, and S. McGinnis), 37–80. McHenry, IL: Center for Applied Linguistics.
11. Carreira, M. and Kagan, O. (2011). The results of the national heritage language survey: implications for teaching, curriculum design, and professional development. *Foreign Lang. Ann.* 44 (1): 40–64.
12. Rios-Font, W.C. (2017). Proficiency or exposure? Rethinking foreign language requirements within college curriculum reviews. *Hispania* 100 (1): 16–29.
13. American Council on the Teaching of Foreign Languages (2023). NCSSFL-ACTFL Can-Do Statements. ACTFL. https://www.actfl.org/resources/ncssfl-actfl-can-do-statements (accessed 26 February 2022).
14. American Council on the Teaching of Foreign Languages (2012).ACTFL Proficiency Guidelines 2012. ACTFL. https://www.actfl.org/resources/actfl-proficiency-guidelines-2012 (accessed 26 February 2022).
15. ACTFL Institutional Workshops. *ACTFL Language Connects*. https://www.actfl.org/learn/institutional-workshops (accessed 26 February 2022).
16. Martinez, G. (2020). *Spanish in Health Care: Policy, Practice and Pedagogy in Latino Health*. New York: Routledge.
17. Liskin-Gasparro, J.E. (2003). The ACTFL proficiency guidelines and the oral proficiency interview: a brief history and analysis of their survival. *Foreign Lang. Ann.* 36 (4): 483–490.
18. COERLL. *Teaching Methods*. University of Texas at Austin. https://oralproficiency.coerll.utexas.edu (accessed 26 February 2022).
19. Herzog, M. (n.d.). Interagency Language Roundtable. *History of the ILR Scale*. https://www.govtilr.org/Skills/IRL%20Scale%20History.htm (accessed 26 February 2022).
20. Common European Framework of Reference for Languages (CEFR) (2022). *The CEFR Descriptors*. Council of Europe.

https://www.coe.int/en/web/common-european-framework-reference-languages/the-cefr-descriptors (accessed 26 February 2022).
21. American Medical College Application Service *2022 AMCAS Application Guide* 2021. https://students-residents.aamc.org/media/11616/download (accessed 22 February 2022).
22. ACTFL Language Connects (2023). *Assigning CEFR Ratings to ACTFL Assessments*. https://www.actfl.org/resources/assigning-cefr-ratings-actfl-assessments (accessed 15 August 2023).
23. AAMC Electronic Residency Application Service. ERAS Applicant Worksheet. AAMC Electronic Residency Application Service. https://students-residents.aamc.org/media/9711/download (accessed 16 October 2022).
24. Vandergrift, L. (2006). *New Canadian Perspectives: Proposal for a Common Framework of Reference for Languages for Canada*. Ottawa: Department of Canadian Heritage.
25. Diamond, L., Toro Bejarano, M., Chung, S. et al. (2019). Factors associated with accuracy of self-assessment compared with tested non-English language proficiency among primary care providers. *Med. Care* 57 (5): 385–390.
26. Tang, G., Lanza, O., Rodriguez, F., and Chang, A. (2011). The Kaiser Permanente clinician cultural and linguistic assessment initiative: research and development in patient-provider language concordance. *Am. J. Public Health* 101: 205–208.
27. Truesdale D. Implementation of a Spanish Language Track at a Family Medicine Residency Program. Honors Thesis. Baylor University; 2018.
28. Reider B. Standardizing Proficiency: An Analysis of Linguistic and Cultural Indicators of Quality Care from Bilingual Physicians. Honors Thesis. Baylor University; 2022.
29. Regenstein, M., Andres, E., and Wynia, M.K. (2013). Appropriate use of non-English language skills in clinical care. *JAMA* 309 (2): 145–146.
30. Hardin, K. (2015). An overview of medical Spanish curricula in the United States. State-of-the-state feature article: medical Spanish in the United States. *Hispania* 98 (4): 640–661.
31. Fernández, A. and Pérez-Stable, E.J. (2015). ¿doctor, habla español? Increasing the supply and quality of language-concordant physicians for Spanish-speaking patients. *J. Gen. Intern. Med.* 30 (10): 1394–1396.
32. Rosenthal, A., Wang, F., Schillinger, D. et al. (2011). Accuracy of physician self-report of Spanish language proficiency. *J. Immigr. Minor. Health* 13: 239–243.
33. Shrum, J.L. and Glisan, E.W. (2016). *Teacher's Handbook: Contextualized Language Instruction*, 5ee. Boston: Cengage.
34. The Berlitz Method. Berlitz. www.berlitz.com (accessed 22 February 2022)
35. Vygotsky, L. (1962). *Thought and Language*. Cambridge, MA: MIT Press.
36. Pathan, H., Memon, R.A., Memon, S. et al. (2018). A critical review of Vygotsky's socio-cultural theory in second language acquisition. *Int. J. Engl. Linguist.* 8 (4): 232.
37. Chomsky, N. (1965). *Aspects of the Theory of Syntax*. Cambridge, MA: MIT Press.
38. Krashen, S.D. (1982). *Principles and Practice in Second Language Acquisition*. Oxford, UK: Pergamon.
39. VanPatten, B. and Williams, J. (ed.) (2015). *Theories in Second Language Acquisition: An Introduction*, 2ee. New York: Routledge.
40. Selinker, L. (1972). Interlanguage. *Int. Rev. Appl. Linguist. Lang. Teach.* 10: 209–231.
41. Anderson, R.W. (1984). The one to one principle of interlanguage construction. *Lang. Learn.* 34 (4): 77–95.
42. Isabelli-García, C., Brown, J., Plews, J.L., and Dewey, D.P. (2018). Language learning and study abroad. *Lang. Teach.* 51 (4): 439–484.
43. Savignon, S.J. (2001). *Communicative Language Teaching for the Twenty-First Century. Teaching English as a Second or Foreign Language*. Boston: Heinle & Heinle.
44. Long, M. (1981). Questions in foreigner talk discourse. *Lang. Learn.* 31: 135–158.
45. Pica, T. (1987). Second-language acquisition, social interaction, and the classroom. *Appl. Linguis.* 8 (1): 3–21.

46. Schmidt, R.W. (1990). The role of consciousness in second language learning. *Appl. Linguis.* 11 (2): 129–158.
47. Koike, D. (1994). Negation in Spanish and English suggestions and requests: mitigating effects? *J. Pragmat.* 21 (5): 513–526.
48. ACTFL (2023). *Facilitate Target Language Use.* ACTFL Language Connects. https://www.actfl.org/resources/guiding-principles-language-learning/target-language (acessed 15 August 2023).
49. Swain, M. (1985). Communicative competence: some roles of comprehensible input and comprehensible output in its development. In: *Input in Second Language Acquisition* (ed. S. Gass and C. Madden), 235–253. Rowley, MA: Newbury House.
50. American Council on the Teaching of Foreign Languages (2023). ACTFL Provide Effective Feedback. ACTFL Language Connects. https://www.actfl.org/resources/guiding-principles-language-learning/effective-feedback (accessed 15 August 2023).
51. American Council on the Teaching of Foreign Languages. ACTFL Standards Summary. ACTFL Language Connects. https://www.actfl.org/resources/world-readiness-standards-learning-languages/standards-summary (accessed 26 February 2022).
52. American Council on the Teaching of Foreign Languages. ACTFL Plan With Backward Design. ACTFL Language Connects. https://www.actfl.org/resources/guiding-principles-language-learning/backward-design (accessed 26 February 2022).
53. Lear, D. (2006). Spanish for medical professionals: implications for instructors. *Hispania* 89 (4): 927–936.
54. Wolfe, D.E. and Jones, G. (1982). Integrating total physical response strategy in a level I Spanish class. *Foreign Lang. Ann.* 15 (4): 273–280.
55. Mueller, R. (2017). Development and evaluation of an intermediate-level elective course on medical Spanish for pharmacy students. *Curr. Pharm. Teach. Learn.* 9 (2): 288–295.
56. Ray, B. and Seely, C. (2004). *Fluency through TPR Storytelling: Achieving Real Language Acquisition in School,* 4e. Blaine Ray Workshops: Command Performance Language Institute.
57. Rapstine, A.H. (2003). *Total Physical Response Storytelling (TPRS): A Practical and Theoretical Overview and Evaluation Within the Framework of the National Standards.* Michigan State University.
58. Coss MD. The case for a true task-based curriculum for medical Spanish courses. *Teach. Learn. Med.* 2022 35:224–239 https://doi.org/10.1080/10401334.2021.2020120
59. 2020 TESOL Electronic Village Online. Escape Rooms in ELT. https://escaperoomelt.wordpress.com (accessed 26 February 2022).
60. TalkAbroad. *Healthcare.* https://www.talkabroad.com/offering/healthcare (accessed 18 October 2022).
61. Ortega P, Hardin K, Pérez-Cordón C, Cox AO, Kim KC, Truesdale D, Chang R, Martínez GA, Miller de Rutté AM, Pérez-Muñoz C, Rolón L, Shin TM. An overview of online resources for physicians learning medical Spanish to improve healthcare for linguistic minorities. *Teach. Learn. Med.* 2021, 34:481–493 https://doi.org/10.1080/10401334.2021.1959335
62. Lafford, B.A. (2012). Languages for specific purposes in the United States in a global context: commentary on Grosse and Voght (1991) revisited. *Mod. Lang. J.* 96: 1–27.
63. Uber Grosse, C. and Voght, G.M. (2012). The continuing evolution of languages for specific purposes. *Mod. Lang. J.* 96: 190–202.
64. Shin, T., Hardin, K., Johnston, D. et al. (2021). Scoping review of textbooks for medical Spanish education in medical schools. *Med. Sci. Educ.* 13: 1519–1527.
65. Hardin K. Targeting oral and cultural proficiency for medical personnel: an examination of current medical Spanish textbooks. *Hispania* 2012;95(4):698–713. https://doi.org/10.1353/hpn.2012.0139.
66. Barahona, M. (2018). Trends in teacher development programs. In: *The TESOL Encyclopedia of English Language Teaching,* 1–14. Wiley Blackwell.

67. Hardin, K.J. and Hardin, D.M. Jr. (2013). Medical Spanish programs: a critical review of published studies and a proposal of best practices. *Teach. Learn. Med.* 25 (4): 306–311.
68. Martinez, G. (2016). Against medical Spanish: Spanish in the health professions yesterday, today, and tomorrow. *ADFL Bull.* 44 (1): 9–18.
69. King Ramirez, C. and Lafford, B. (ed.) (2018). *Transferable Skills for the 21st Century: Preparing Students for the Workplace Through World Languages for Specific Purposes*. Sabio Books.
70. Ortega, P., Diamond, L., Alemán, M.A. et al. (2020). Medical Spanish standardization in U.S. medical schools: consensus statement from a multidisciplinary expert panel. *Acad. Med.* 95 (1): 22–31.
71. Lie, D.A., Nodal, S., de la Torre, M. et al. (2020). Impact of a longitudinal medical Spanish curriculum on student communication skills. *J. Physician Assist. Educ.* 31 (1): 23–27.
72. Pechak, C., Diaz, D., and Dillon, L. (2014). Integrating Spanish language training across a doctor of physical therapy curriculum: a case report of one program's evolving model. *Phys. Ther.* 94 (12): 1807–1815.
73. Mospan, G.A. and Griffiths, C.L. (2016). Medical Spanish in US colleges and schools of pharmacy. *Innov. Pharm.* 7 (3). https://doi.org/10.24926/iip.v7i3.452.
74. Amerson, R. and Burgins, S. (2005). Hablamos Espanol: crossing communication barriers with the Latino population. *J. Nurs. Educ.* 44 (5): 241–242.
75. Cowden, J.D., Martínez, F.J., Dickmeyer, J.J., and Bratcher, D. (2022). Culture and language coaching for bilingual residents: the first 10 years of the CHiCoS model. *Teach. Learn. Med.* 1–12. https://doi.org/10.1080/10401334.2022.2092113.
76. Davidson, L. and Spaine Long, S. Medical Spanish for US medical students: a pilot case study. In: *Dimension 2013: World Language Learning Setting the Global Standard* (ed. P.B. Swanson and K. Hoyt), 9–22. Decatur, GA: Southern Conference on Language Teaching.
77. Tomoschuk, B., Ferreira, V.S., and Gollan, T.H. (2019). When a seven is not a seven: self-ratings of bilingual language proficiency differ between and within language populations. *Biling. Lang. Cogn.* 22 (3): 516–536.
78. Lion, K.C., Thompson, D.A., Cowden, J.D. et al. (2013). Clinical Spanish use and language proficiency testing among pediatric residents. *Acad. Med.* 88 (10): 1478–1484.
79. Wenyue, M. and Winke, P. (2019). Self-assessment: how reliable is it in assessing oral proficiency over time? *Foreign Lang. Ann.* 52 (1): 66–86.
80. Dejbord, S.P. (2019). *Beginning Medical Spanish Oral Proficiency and Cultural Humility*. New York: Routledge.
81. Maier, C. (1986). Fitting it all in one semester: an intensive introductory course in Spanish for healthcare personnel. *Hispania* 69 (3): 714–719.
82. Bloom, M., Timmerman, G.M., and Sands, D. (2006). Developing a course to teach Spanish for health care professionals. *J. Nurs. Educ.* 45 (7): 271–274.
83. Hardin, K. (2017). Exploring the relationship between authentic dialogue and Spanish for healthcare professionals. *J. Lang. Specif. Purp.* 4: 41–51.
84. Allison, A. and Hardin, K. (2020). Missed opportunities to build rapport: a pragmalinguistic analysis of interpreted medical interviews with Spanish-speaking patients. *Health Commun.* 35 (4): 494–501.
85. Magaña, D. (2022). *Building Confianza: Empowering Latinos/as Through Transcultural Health Care Communication*. Columbus, OH: Ohio State Press.
86. Sánchez-López, L. (2014). An analysis of the integration of service learning in undergraduate Spanish for specific purposes programs in higher education in the United States. *Cuadernos del ALDEEU* 28: 155–170.
87. Ortega, P., Park, Y.S., and Girotti, J.A. (2017). Evaluation of a medical Spanish elective for senior medical students: improving outcomes through OSCE assessments. *Med. Sci. Educ.* 27 (2): 329–337.

88. VanTyle, W.K., Kennedy, G., Vance, M.A., and Hancock, B. (2011). A Spanish language and culture initiative for a doctor of pharmacy curriculum. *Am. J. Pharm. Educ.* 75 (1): 1–8.
89. Ortega, P. and Prada, J. (2020). Words matter: translanguaging in medical skills training. *Perspect. Med. Educ.* 9 (4): 251–255.
90. García, O. and Li, W. (2018). Translanguaging. In: *Encyclopedia of Applied Linguistics* (ed. C. Chapelle), 1–7. Oxford: Wiley.
91. Showstack, R., Nicks, S., Woods, N.K., and Martínez, G. (2021). Interprofessional education for students of translation/interpreting and the health professions. *Hispania* 104 (3): 485–501.
92. Harrison AE, Mirza M. 2019 *Occupational Therapy Across Languages: Working with Interpreters to Ensure Effective and Ethical Practice*. https://www.aota.org/~/media/Corporate/Files/Publications/CE-Articles/CE_article_July_2019.pdf (accessed 18 October 2022).
93. Morin, R. (2010). Making connections: Spanish for medical purposes and service-learning. In: *Building Communications and Making Connections* (ed. S. Rivera-Mills and J.A. Trujillo), 16–39. Newcastle: Cambridge Scholars.
94. Reuland, D.S., Slatt, L.M., Alemán, M.A. et al. (2012). Effect of Spanish language immersion rotations on medical student Spanish fluency. *Fam. Med.* 44 (2): 110.
95. Valdini, A., Early, S., Augart, C. et al. (2009). Spanish language immersion and reinforcement during residency: a model for rapid acquisition of competency. *Teach. Learn. Med.* 21 (3): 261–266.
96. Chatterjee, A., Qin, L., García, M.P. et al. (2015). Improving linguistic and cultural competence in the health sector: a medical Spanish curriculum for resident physicians. *J. Span. Lang. Teach.* 2 (1): 36–50.
97. Norris, J.M. (2009). Understanding and improving language education through program evaluation. *Lang. Teach. Res.* 13: 1–13.
98. Staley, K., Allen, C., and Hamp, A. (2020). Case studies in ESP course development: medical English for Turkmen and Mexican medical specialists. *Eng. Teach. Forum* 58 (1): 2–9.
99. Bakić-Mirić, N. and Gaipov, D.E. (2015). The importance of teaching intercultural competence in English for specific purposes course in European medical schools. *Iperstoria* (5). https://doi.org/10.13136/2281-4582/2015.i5.267.
100. Rivers, W. and Robinson, J.P. (2012). The unchanging American capacity in languages other than English: speaking and learning languages other than English, 2000–2008. *Mod. Lang. J.* 96 (3): 369–379.

16 Centering Translanguaging for Inclusive Health Communication: Implications for Healthcare Professional Education

JOSH PRADA AND
ROBYN WOODWARD-KRON

Introduction

In this chapter, we approach healthcare encounters between health professionals and sociolinguistically diverse patients as spaces of conflict, marginalization and neglect, and thereby provide a framework for/in linguistically and culturally inclusive healthcare professional development as we pursue the articulation of more critical and equitable horizons for all. We engage with this issue from two perspectives and weave them together throughout the chapter. The first perspective is that of equitable multilingual education models driven by the communication practices, identities, and ways of knowing forged in language-minoritized, racialized communities. The other perspective is that of intercultural communication and the current education and practice of healthcare professionals. At the core of our proposal is the notion of translanguaging: the complex processes of meaning and sense-making engaged in by multilingual individuals during communication. Translanguaging focuses on the speaker and what they do with their linguistic and broader semiotic repertoires to make meaning. This emphasis on the language user's practices moves us away from understandings of languages as monolithic, static, and closed categories and orients us toward questioning the colonial nature of mainstream views of language and multilingualism. In line with this orientation, the perspective we present herein centers on the so-called heritage speaker as a linguistically and culturally appropriate expert in these contexts.

The chapter begins by laying out key foundations regarding the sociology and politics of language and multilingualism in today's world, with an emphasis on how grassroots ways of being, knowing, and doing are marginalized in these settings. We then move into healthcare encounters and the educational structures in place to support professional development in terms of language diversity as we recognize ways in which colonizer/settler/Eurocentric ideologies impinge on healthcare encounters with diverse patients. Moreover, these ideologies can further impinge on health professionals learning to communicate with linguistically diverse populations. We draw from this to move on to the nature of language practices in these contexts and continue by laying out a framework to guide renewal and just change. We, then, present practical recommendations for healthcare professional education.

The ordinariness of diversity and multilingualism

The last decades have seen increased activity concerning transnational mobility resulting in enhanced rates of migratory flows. This increase has been encouraged by conflict, war, and negative financial fluctuations, as well as more affordable international travel options. With these flows, new migrant communities have established themselves in areas that, quite often, were already home to previous waves of immigration, layering new characteristics as they bring with them their own linguistic and cultural practices, religious rituals, and ways of knowing and doing. This situation creates what Vertovec [1, 2] called superdiversity. Superdiverse communities are characterized by growing differences among people within ethnic, religious, and national categories as reflected in enhanced socioeconomic (and other) differences. While the complexity of recent contemporary superdiverse cosmopolitan spaces is worthy of attention, there is nothing new about linguistically and culturally diverse communities. The presence of First Nations and indigenous peoples, migrant peoples, the creation and changes in geopolitical borders through wars and land purchases, such as the Guadalupe Hidalgo Treaty, and the establishment of diasporic communities, all precede current understandings of linguistic diversity tied up to modernity. Moreover, in Asia and Africa, large multilingual communities where various languages cohabit and are mobilized flexibly with one another by locals in their daily interactions, are commonplace, and have never not been so. Similarly, at a smaller scale, these behaviors are relevant to the day-to-day lives of transnational, multilingual families across the world.

Multilingual practices, diverse cultural behaviors, and ways of being that cross monoglossic boundaries of appropriateness and national belonging are all part of the everyday lives of such minoritized communities, and increasingly, of so-called "monolingual" ones. These emergent multilingual practices are characterized by their flexibility and their fluidity, and despite their ordinariness, they are ideologized as subpar for certain contexts – particularly for contexts that reflect the values of Eurocentric and capitalist modernity – including healthcare encounters. The contextual inadequacy of these practices seems to violate the scientific/academic nature of healthcare work, an issue that, in what follows, we address in detail. This chapter calls for the centering of multilingual communities, their linguistic practices, and their ways of knowing and doing in healthcare encounters concerned with and committed to the well-being of their members. More concretely, we propose that the training of healthcare professionals, including doctors, nurses, technicians, and medical interpreters, among others, should be built on curricular approaches that question divides, and boundaries dictating who should say what to whom. To this end, we argue that "medical language" education (elaborated below) would benefit from a reformulation under the umbrella of "healthcare for local multilingual communities" that centers on the meaning- and sensemaking practices of diverse patients, including language (as practice), culture (as practice), and interaction as localized, bringing the healthcare encounter to bear on a spirit of care and respect for the person. Our understanding of language and culture as practice capitalizes on their practical nature, that is, how language and culture emerge through doing and flowing in real life, while emphasizing that attempts to cast them into monolithic patterns are reductive and faulty.

To accomplish this, the education and training of healthcare professionals should include pedagogical interventions to promote critical awareness of the linguistic and cultural aspects of communication that characterize "grassroots" multilingual communities, incorporating evidence showing the positive effects of language concordance and cultural alignment between clinician and patient, and equipping students/future healthcare professionals with the ideological tools for a more critical and humane consciousness in these contexts. In what follows, we chart out possibilities in different areas of pedagogy and practice to center translanguaging as a guiding element to stimulate new ways of thinking, knowing, and doing bi-/multilingualism in healthcare. To situate the reader, we begin by laying out the key foundations of translanguaging and poststructuralist views on language as a means to demystify bi-/multilingual practices.

Translanguaging: Approaching multilingualism from the multilingual's perspective

Structuralist language ideologies developed during colonial periods have remained dominant in our understanding of language. Such ideologies privilege Western European notions through a "one language, one people" conception of belonging, and reinforce the power of state-endorsed named languages [3]. These hierarchies and ideologies precipitated dominant models of bilingualism throughout the twentieth century, which characterized named languages (e.g., English, Spanish, and Chinese) as static, monolithic, and standardized skills one might "acquire." This view of named languages as static structures has great implications for how Western cultures conceive of multilingualism and of multilingual communities: a phenomenon identified as standard language cultures [4].

Our emphasis on "the West" is not without reason. The multilingual histories and practices of Asian and African contexts [e.g., 5, 6] and their potential to inform Western language scholars' views of multilingualism have only relatively recently been acknowledged in the "multilingual turn" [7]. The multilingual turn in language studies refers to a change in spirit, and consequently, in our approach to language, where multilingualism and the lives and practices of multilingual people are no longer relegated to a secondary role in our understanding of language. This multilingual turn has coincided with the aforementioned notion of superdiversity, somehow creating the illusion that multilingualism in modern, cosmopolitan, twenty-first century societies is a product of superdiversity [8–10].

In these conditions, where multilingual speakers from different backgrounds share spaces with one another, collaborate in different ways and shape the spaces which they inhabit, more fluid and organic understandings of bi-/multilingual communication are of the essence. Recognizing this issue, Garcia [11] proposed that bilingualism might be better described as dynamic, as bilinguals' language practices are learned in specific social contexts and are "multiple and ever adjusting to the multilingual multimodal terrain of the communicative act" [11 , p. 53] through a linguistic repertoire that is both individual to each person and always in flux [12]. This dynamic view of bi-/multilingual practices, which takes a first-person perspective using the multilingual individual's view as a point of departure [13] coupled with an understanding of named languages as products of imperialistic efforts are the foundational elements of translanguaging [14–16]. As reflected in Section "A framework for transformation: Guiding principles and concepts" (framework for change) below, we find the stance provided by translanguaging to hold great potential to reformulate some aspects of healthcare communications, and the language education of healthcare professionals, particularly as these pertain to intercultural contexts [17]. This perspective may serve as a means to move healthcare encounters with linguistically diverse patients toward a renewed understanding of the value of alignment beyond the superficiality of standard language ideologies and the practices they promote, and as we chart out strategic shifts in our view of the organizational structures at work in these settings.

Intercultural communication in healthcare

In healthcare, it is acknowledged that for communication to be effective and safe, it needs to be tailored to the needs, understandings, and socio-historical contexts of individuals and the communities that healthcare workers serve. This includes taking into consideration the languaging practices and preferences of culturally diverse communities in migrant destination countries and of First Nations peoples in settler environments. Despite these aspirations, language remains an enduring barrier in intercultural healthcare communication [18], for example, hindering the effective provision and exchange of health information [19]. Paternotte et al. [20] review of factors impacting intercultural communication found that language barriers (which we refer to as language discordance in this chapter) were frequently mentioned as contributing to miscommunication between patient and clinician, resulting in misunderstandings, frustrations, and tensions. Language discordance also impeded the healthcare provider from achieving shared decision-making about treatment [20]. There is considerable evidence of lasting and grave health outcomes resulting from miscommunication in intercultural healthcare, including poorer health outcomes for culturally diverse patients in both chronic and acute care [21, 22] and more adverse events [23], including patient death [24].

Much of the literature in medical and health sciences journals that reports on language discordance, framed as "language barriers" [e.g., 20], does not elaborate on the linguistic or socio-linguistic nature of the language barrier. The reader is left to interpret, for example, whether the barriers are due to complete or partial discordance of languages, or interference from one language to another due to lexicogrammar or phonological aspects. Further, Roberts [25] for example, points out that intercultural miscommunication may not be due to language aspects per se but to sociocultural factors that might impact interactions such as discourse styles or inferential processes. When the language discordance is attributed to a health professional who has undertaken their education in another linguistic or cultural setting, for example, an International Medical Graduate, the linguistic dimension of the health professional's communication has been investigated. The results of these explorations then inform educational interventions, for example, discursive patterns of patient-centered care [26, 27], and prosody [28].

Interpreter-mediated healthcare communication

Mediated health communication through interpreters is a major strategy adopted by both patients and health services to mitigate miscommunication arising from language discordance. Large hospitals in cities with culturally and linguistically diverse communities such as in Australia and the United States often have language service units from which both patients and healthcare professionals can request professional interpreters. Case studies of healthcare systems such as hospitals with in-house language services employing accredited, professional interpreters show decreased lengths of stay for their limited English proficiency patients and a decrease in their re-admission rates [29]. There is substantive, established evidence that patients have improved health outcomes when professional interpreters are involved compared to ad hoc interpreters such as family members [30]. Despite this evidence, numerous studies report healthcare professionals preferencing other forms of mediated communication, for example, reliance on automated interpreting or translation tools when professional interpreters are not readily available [31] and reliance on bilingual medical students undertaking clerkships [28].

Patients may sometimes opt to use family members as interpreters due to familiarity and trust, as well as privacy considerations since the professional interpreter may be part of the same community. Patients may also be unaware of their legal right to access a professional interpreter. A Dutch study of interpreter-mediated consultations in general practice [32], however, showed that trust in ad hoc interpreters could be misplaced. In this study, the ad hoc interpreters were found to take liberty with deciding what was interpreted and amplified their role. That is, ad hoc interpreters only interpreted about half of what was communicated. Further, the ad hoc interpreter asked their own questions and responded to the doctor's questions, thereby effectively silencing the patient. In a 2018, European symposium on mitigating language discordance in healthcare attended by practitioners and researcher working in intercultural communication system issues such as lack of professional interpreting services due to inadequate funding and resourcing also result in patients and clinicians utilizing ad hoc interpreters [33].

The professional interpreting model in healthcare is also not without criticism, particularly the notion that professional interpreters should remain neutral and act only as a conduit between interlocutors [34]. This is discussed in depth in Section II of this volume. Patients themselves may struggle to render emotions that they wish to convey; conversely, practitioners may need greater skills in expressing empathy and building rapport during a mediated encounter. Interpreters too may need enhanced skills in rendering these interpersonal aspects between languages [33]. The interpreter as a neutral conduit of information model also does not reflect the dynamic and interactional manner of medical encounters, in which participants signal their shared understandings and co-construct the encounter [34] through verbal and nonverbal feedback. Schouten et al. argue that instead of continuing the debate of whether to use professional or ad hoc interpreters in mediated communication, a combination of communication strategies is needed that resonate with interlocutor needs. For complex healthcare, this might include having both a professional interpreter present, as well as a family member/caregiver because, even though the family members should not be tasked with the role of ad hoc interpreting.

"...patients' family members can emotionally support the patient, advocate on their behalf and provide information about the patient that is relevant to their treatment, while professional interpreters have the skills for accurate interpretation and communication in a coordinated manner with each other, thereby enhancing the dynamic process of the co- construction of meaning between patients, interpreters and providers" [33, pp. 2605–2606].

Some medical encounters would benefit from having access to a professional interpreter, a family member present, and a bi-/multilingual clinician – particularly if this person is only partially bilingual and can use their skills to communicate some aspects independently and directly to the patient/family but may need help communicating other aspects through the interpreter.

There are established strategies and initiatives to support health professionals in mitigating some of the known issues to both professionally and informally-mediated language-discordant communication: for example, incorporating toolkits to assist with decision-making [35], the interpreter redesigning what was said by one speaker to the benefit of the other speaker [36], including the professional interpreter as part of the healthcare team [34], as well as professional development collaboratively delivered with language services staff, who may be interpreter educators, experienced interpreters or other communication experts [29].

The degree to which health professions students encounter education about working with interpreters specifically, and intercultural communication more generally, seems to vary considerably across health professions and programs. In the next section, we provide some snapshots from entry-to-practice medical education on interpreter-mediated communication, noting that our discussion does not address the sociocultural barriers and the cultural competency dimension of intercultural communication nor report on literature that addresses these significant aspects, for example [29, 37, 38].

Languaging in medical education

Intercultural communication in the medical curriculum

Throughout the last two decades, there have been sporadic calls in leading medical education journals for curriculum developers to pay greater attention to developing students' knowledge and skills for inclusive healthcare [e.g., 39, 40, 41]. Kachur and Altshuler's 2004 editorial advocates integrating cultural competence throughout the various clinical, ethical, bioscience, and medical domains, with bilingual interviewing mapped onto clinical skills during the clinical education component of the medical degree. Evidence of educating about cultural diversity, often framed as cultural competency, is increasingly required for accreditation of medical courses, and by organizations that set national standards for medical graduates, for example, in the United States [42–44]. National consensus statements for communication curricula in several countries make reference to culture and communication; for example, as a "specific issue" domain in the original 2008 United Kingdom consensus statement [45], and as an objective in Dutch medical curriculum documents [18]. However, there is little detail about pedagogy or evidence of the effectiveness or acceptability of these curriculum guidelines and requirements to the communities that these future doctors will serve. Recently qualified junior doctors from the United Kingdom, the United States, and Norway pointed out the gap between teaching approaches during medical school, and the communication skills they need for healthcare in the real world, including navigating language differences with patients in inner city hospitals [46]. To bridge this gap between education and reality of clinical practice, these doctors noted the need for opportunities to engage in authentic professional interpreter-mediated interactions, as well as more cultural competency/humility training. It seems reasonable to suggest that while there are admirable intentions to prepare medical students for healthcare for all, educating students for intercultural communication remains a siloed, and neglected area of the curriculum in many medical programs. Curriculum design mechanisms exist that can foster cultural awareness through community integration such as longitudinal clinical placements in community settings [47], and incorporating culturally diverse simulated patients [48] although the latter can be resource intensive, jeopardizing sustainability of the program when funding is an issue.

Interactional approach to teaching health professions students about interpreter-mediated communication

Fostering medical students' knowledge of and experiences with interpreted-mediated communication similarly appears to be a vulnerable area of the curriculum in terms of sustainability and status as core learning. There are concerns that accepted practices for teaching about interpret-mediated communication are simplistic, that is, guidelines widely used in medical education tend to focus on behavioral skills, (e.g., where the doctor should direct their gaze) logistical factors (e.g., booking the interpreter and briefings), and neglect the interactional dynamics that underpin patient-centered communication and foster patient understanding [48]. A consortium of international healthcare communication researchers and educators familiar with these guidelines have proposed an alternative model to the conduit model of interpreting in medical education: one that acknowledges the interpreter as a participant, contributing to co-constructing meanings, including intersubjective elements. Their alternative approach accommodates all participants continuously negotiating meanings, which would allow the doctor to monitor and adapt their speech and behavior accordingly to achieve shared goals. They also suggest that a more dynamic approach may help address doctors' reported reluctance to engage professional interpreters with the caveat that research is needed to monitor the efficacy and impact of an alternative pedagogy [48]. These suggestions also elide with developments in medical interpreting in which an empirical study found that there is a pressing need to include empathy training in medical interpreting training [49].

As with the placement, scope, and methodologies for teaching intercultural communication in medicine, there are curriculum initiatives reported in the literature that seek to improve medical students' attitudes toward and experiences of interpreter-mediated communication. For example, in Victoria, Australia, where the use of ad hoc interpreters is strongly discouraged in health services [50], one curriculum initiative has taken an interprofessional approach to teaching about mediated communication. Interprofessional education is widely used in prevocational as well as a vocational training as situated learning, adopting approaches such as simulation, in which two or more professions come together to learn with and from each other. In the Victorian study, volunteer medical students on their general practice rotation and Master of Interpreting and Translation students, for whom participation was compulsory, reported a high level of agreement about the value of learning about the other profession. The findings also showed a high level of agreement about the value of professional practices in interpreter-mediated communication such as pre- and post-briefings [51]. A United States medical school has implemented medical interpreter training for bilingual medical students with the aim of developing humanism [52]. The outcomes of this curriculum intervention included an increase in participating students' self-reported measures of empathy and humanism. Participating medical students also had the opportunity to gain certification as a qualified interpreter and train as a peer-mentor for future students participating in the study. Both curriculum innovations reflect a more general direction emerging in medical education redesign – known as *Value-Added* Medical Education (VAME), in which students learn in authentic settings as well as add capacity to health services by contributing to patient care [53]. VAME is seen to provide bidirectional benefits: to students in terms of their learning, for example, humanism and empathy, interprofessional learning; and to patients and the community by contributing to safe and high-quality healthcare that takes into account patients' languaging practices and preferences.

Student language practices within the clinical learning environment

The clinical component of medical education provides work-integrated learning so that students can transition to be work-ready. Supervisors must juggle facilitating student learning opportunities in a dynamic and unpredictable environment while ensuring safe and effective patient care. In culturally diverse societies, there will be opportunities to observe and participate in professional interpreter-mediated patient interactions; bilingual medical students are also likely to act as ad hoc interpreters in clinician-patient encounters. An Australian study investigating the prevalence of ad hoc interpreting while on clinical rotations found that more than one third of participants had reported acting as an ad hoc interpreter [31]. Students also reported interpreting for complex communication such as giving serious news and seeking informed consent despite students' variable linguistic competence and training/experience interpreting. Critically, in the Australian medical education setting, there is no formal acknowledgement of or engagement with the linguistic resources that multilingual students bring to medical education and how these resources might be safely and ethically deployed while on their clinical rotations. In some regards, this is quite different to the United States medical education and practice context. On the one hand, a similar study to Ryan et al.'s [31] study at two United States medical schools found that bilingual medical students reported being frequently asked to serve as ad hoc interpreters [54]. On the other hand, in the United States, medical language education has begun to spread in medical curricula as part of the languages for professional/specific purposes tradition [55].

Recent research has documented the rationales, demographics, and curricular structures characterizing these courses. Ongoing research [56] has surveyed over 300 medical students enrolled in a medical Spanish course simultaneously taught at 14 United States medical schools in 2021. The survey was completed prior to and after the course. This mixed-methods study revealed that current approaches to medical Spanish curricula and practice do not promote critical perspectives in and around language, and thus, recommendations were proposed to move toward "critical horizons" (as the authors termed this curricular journey). Moreover, and on a more positive note, the study revealed a general patient-oriented attitude toward language use among medical students, whereby students centered the needs of the patient beyond monolingual language ideologies that are typically promoted in foreign and second language teaching and learning. The authors took this to mean that medical Spanish students are rooted in patient-centeredness but lack the critical linguistic awareness and practical skills to bring their intuitions to practice.

Heritage speakers, heritage language education and their possibilities for medical language education

Some students enter into medical education with a pre-existing linguistic skillset in the target language developed throughout their lives, at home or in their communities, naturalistically (i.e., as opposed to through instruction), and with little (if any) educational support and representation in the school system. Importantly, this student profile's linguistic skill set is coupled with an expert cultural knowledge of the community(-ies) who use this language as they, themselves, are active members of these communities. Take, for example, United States Latinxs/Hispanics who grew up exposed to Spanish at home and who developed their bilingualism in Spanish (as a minoritized community language) and English (as the language of larger society and education) from an early age. Since the 1970s, in the United States and Canada, the term heritage speaker (HS) has been widely used to refer to this speaker profile [e.g., 57]. We find that this bilingual speaker profile, both as a language learner and as a healthcare professional, as well as current approaches to heritage language education hold tremendous potential for transforming multilingual healthcare encounters, presenting an opportunity for VAME that is largely untapped.

In short, heritage learner teaching/learning principles as endorsed by heritage language education professionals differ from L2 learners in a variety of ways (for a detailed account of L2 teaching and learning principles in relation to medical language we refer the reader to Chapter 15). Heritage language educators call for sociolinguistically oriented curricula, opportunities for experiential learning and bridges with the community, an emphasis on reflections on language, and a development of critical language/sociolinguistic awareness, alongside attention to the expansion of the linguistic and literacy skills HS bring into the heritage language classroom. Moreover, heritage language educators explore historical, political, and social aspects affecting the experiences of their HS student community, and center positive identity work in their discussions. Since the early 2000s, there has been increasing dialogue about the need for more criticality to be implemented in heritage language curricula [e.g., 58]. This approach to language education is more holistic and ecological, positions the multilingual speaker and their community in the center, and privileges a bottom-up understanding of multilingual practice that is often missing from L2/foreign language classrooms.

Considering the multilingual and culturally-diverse profiles HSs develop in their homes and communities, their knowledge of and experiences navigating elite monolingual spaces, and their personal connection with culturally-diverse patients, coupled with the ways heritage language education has evolved to recognize these and other issues and integrate them into curricular proposals, we find the field of heritage language studies, and the profile of HSs to be a key, if unexplored, pathway for growth in medical language education.

A framework for transformation: Guiding principles and concepts

Considering the above, we now present a conceptual framework for transformation of educational initiatives geared toward healthcare communication. For us, the education of healthcare professionals must incorporate spaces for critical reflection about the life histories, historical formations, and linguistic and cultural practices of the populations they serve. Specifically, we emphasize that such pedagogical modules must not only recognize the legitimacy of these practices (often deemed substandard), but they must socialize students and health professionals into ways of thinking and acting that embrace their possibilities for better healthcare provision. To that end, we must translanguage healthcare encounters, and in doing so, create pedagogical structures that reflect the complex interplay of linguistic, multimodal, emotional, and sociocultural dimensions that cut across meaning- and sense-making in real-life healthcare settings, and forgo current monolithic understandings of "medical languages." To accomplish this goal, as foreshadowed, we center translanguaging as a conceptual, organizational, and practical element.

Our proposal is based on four cornerstones, all of which bear on different aspects of translanguaging as a practical theory of language [59] and as pedagogy [60, 61]. We have revisited and restructured them to serve the purpose of our bringing healthcare communication to par with the realities of diverse local communities:

1. Re-epistemologizing "medical 'named languages'" through translanguaging
2. Trans-literacies in healthcare encounters
3. Understanding, assessing, and reformulating divides: trans-ing boundaries
4. The "heritage speaker" as a locally appropriate model: transgressing normativity

These cornerstones are collectively concerned with processes of re-epistemologizing, the inclusion of new models of literacy and appropriateness, and with the intentional exploration and undoing of specific boundaries and divides that structure healthcare encounters in ways that are detrimental to diverse, underserved patients. We provide an overview of our framework in Table 16.1 below.

Re-epistemologizing "medical 'named languages'" through translanguaging

Epistemologies are our theories about knowledge, particularly in terms of their validity, the methods we use to create such knowledge, and its scope. Through epistemological reasoning, we can differentiate what constitutes justified belief and what constitutes opinion. The emerging field of "medical language" teaching, with Spanish in the United States having become a stronghold of activity [55] may provide us with a model of what needs to be addressed in curricula to move toward more critical horizons in medical language education. The epistemologies of medical Spanish are the same as those undergirding other language courses for specific purposes, such as "English for tourism." This epistemological bedrock assumes stability (i.e., languages are static), countability (i.e., languages are countable, isolated, and independent from one another), and sufficiency (i.e., the target language will suffice). This view is inherently problematic because, among other things, it is not cognitively, socially, or historically true. The language of medicine as a social construct does not capture the complexity of intercultural interactions and may fall short in transparency in encounters with people whose education and socioeconomic levels are not on par with such discursive practices.

Linguistic shame, embarrassment, and insecurity play an important part in the social identity of migrants whose linguistic skills in the new language are still emerging, and it should not be surprising for these people to be overcome with fear and self-doubt in

Table 16.1 Cornerstones of Translanguaging as Applied to Medical Education and Practice.

Cornerstones of Translanguaging for change	Description	Strategies for Implementation
Re-epistemologizing "medical 'named languages'" through translanguaging	A focus on shifting the foundational bedrock of what constitutes language(s) through a bottom-up approach, and its implications for understanding, teaching/learning, and using language for medical purposes	Students become familiar with how multilingual community members deploy their language resources in their day-to-day lives. Students reflect on these data-sets, and are guided to understand their organic, fluid, purposeful nature. They make connections between these emerging understandings and theoretical concepts, such as translanguaging, standard language, and native speakers.
Trans-literacies in healthcare encounters	Going beyond the idea of using language and knowledge that is contextually appropriate to navigating meaning- and sense-making as socioculturally relevant.	Students interview community members to co-explore their experiences in healthcare settings. Attention is placed on how formal approaches to "literacy" often fail to satisfy and meet patients' needs. Students and patients design alternative routes of communication, thinking about meaning and sense-making in ways that transcend academic, medical language. These are shared in their peers and instructor.
Understanding, assessing, and reformulating divides: trans-ing boundaries	Investigating the philosophical foundations of specific roles and elements characteristic of healthcare encounters and their dichotomic relationships.	Students develop skills to utilize technology and intercultural communication tools in ways that give patients autonomy in situations where interpreters are not available.

(Continued)

Table 16.1 (Continued)

Cornerstones of Translanguaging for change	Description	Strategies for Implementation
The "heritage speaker" as a locally appropriate model: transgressing normativity	Creating spaces that center HSs in curricula and in practice.	Instructors and curriculum designers include HSs in conversations around material development, turning to their expertise to reflect vernacular realities. HSs serve as teaching assistants, hold internships and/or guide discussions to educate L2 speakers around community issues.

situations where an elite form of monolingualism in the new language is expected. We must, first, recognize this as a social justice problem stemming from institutionalized neglect of racialized and minoritized bodies, and second, acknowledge that such ideology guides professional language curricula and translates into healthcare encounters.

This type of curricular politization (even when unconsciously done) serves the purpose of upholding the social hierarchies that marginalize communities of color, peoples of lower socioeconomic backgrounds, and linguistically and culturally diverse populations. It is, therefore, of the essence to unsettle these foundations through epistemological renewal, as called for in other language-related fields, such as language education [61] and in media and communications [62]. Regardless, efforts to dismantle and restructure this ideological and practical meshwork in curricula and in practice are scarce. The power differentials shaping these situations must be included in educational proposals concerned with the well-being of linguistically diverse communities, including medical interpreting courses, medical translation courses, medical language courses for clinicians, and any other educational proposals that focus on the imagined language abstractions that, supposedly, are used in particular spaces.

A translanguaging view asks us to center the patient, the healthcare professional, and the means and media available to them for meaning- and sense-making during their encounters. Importantly, these means, media, and resources are never just "the target language" – a fundamental, yet critically overlooked issue. A translingual orientation around the healthcare professional's linguistic knowledge is key, but so is their cultural sensitivity, their dexterousness in navigating technological tools, as well as their ability to actively and accurately include multimodal resources, such as pictures, sounds, and videos. These must be coupled with skills to utilize the required technologies, and the individual's openness to navigate these ecologically complex contexts meaningfully and compassionately, as they center each patient's needs, lives, and well-being, rather than what is told, or how it is told. This orientation must guide renewal efforts to re-epistemologize this area of practice through the notion that language is something we do as we engage with our entire repertoires (linguistic, semiotic, spatial) in ways that bring to the fore our personhood in context, our emotions, our identities, and our life trajectories.

Trans-literacies in healthcare encounters

While folk understandings of literacy are connected to our ability to read and write, and to other traditional ways of engaging with and producing knowledge; from an educational perspective, literacy is the ability to mobilize knowledge for specific purposes. Being literate is always on a grayscale: as knowledge and its nature change, so do the ways in which that knowledge is accessed, operationalized, and brought into dialogue through practices. By contrast, the idea of multiliteracies [63], questions the assumptions of literacy and situates learning and meaning-making in a more realistic plane. Multiliteracies is the concept of understanding information and the design of meaning through the manipulation of individual modes, these being: linguistic meaning, visual meaning, audio meaning, and gestural/tactile/spatial meaning. Alternatively, yet closely related, the ability to fluidly move among these and other resources, means, media, and platforms is referred to as transliteracy. A model of translitearcies encompasses information creation and consumption capabilities, information and communication technologies, communication and collaboration, creativity, and critical thinking [e.g., 64].

In our context, the development of multiliteracies and transliteracies is geared toward developing practices, knowledges, and spaces that draw on the cultural, linguistic, and cognitive dimensions that all bring into healthcare encounters while centering on patients' needs and histories. An existing gap that requires attention resides in current approaches to the notion of health literacy. According to the United States Health Resources and Services Administration, health literacy is "the degree to which individuals have the capacity to obtain, process, and understand basic health information needed to make appropriate health decisions" [65]. HRSA also reports that low health literacy is more prevalent among older adults. Minority populations, people with low socioeconomic status, and medically underserved people. As we see it, trans-perspectives have great potential to advance this notion. A trans-perspective on health literacy capitalizes on understanding the different abilities, skills, and mindsets with which individuals from specific cultural and linguistic communities' approach and navigate health knowledge and decisions. The nature of a trans-approach to health literacy is critical and interdisciplinary, and its application brings to how language-minoritized people engage with health knowledge and practices. Our lens proposes to incorporate this focus on emergent ways of grassroots ways of knowing and acting as a key element of the cultural foundation of healthcare education and provision. We direct the reader to Chapter 9 in this volume for more on health literacy in culturally and linguistically diverse populations.

Understanding, assessing, and reformulating divides: Trans-ing boundaries

Fields like anthropology have a tradition of adopting post-structuralist perspectives. These post-structuralist perspectives help us deconstruct our knowledge and the platforms they shape, as we approach its different components as mobile, dynamic, and complex. As we see it, this perspective has great possibilities to unsettle the divides and dichotomies that lay out the roadmap for the linguistic and sociocultural practices of healthcare encounters with minoritized and racialized multilingual patients. These divides and dichotomies include, but are not limited to, the sharp distinction between interpreters versus bilingual healthcare professionals, professional versus nonprofessional interpreters, technology-mediated versus in-person interpretation, family versus nonfamily members, languages such as Spanish versus English, or formal versus informal registers. Preconceived ideas of who must take what role in these contexts may play against the objectives of healthcare, and a more dynamic approach to meaning- and sense-making where teams are reassembled to address specific encounters seems to be more appropriate.

Let us take for example the activities engaged during translating and interpreting, whereby the speaker navigates contextual needs and pressures by carefully deploying different features of their semiotic repertoires in order to meet communication needs. A translanguaging view, also introduced that this is naturally done across named languages, language varieties, registers, and discourses, and in a diverse range of contexts: everyday multilingual settings involving community interpreting and cultural brokering, embodied interaction, and text-based commodities. Following Baynham and Lee [66], we must focus on developing a practice-based account of translation (which we expand to interpreting).

We envision collaborations between bilingual health professionals, medical interpreters, community members and patient relatives, through linguistically and socioculturally appropriate materials and practices aligned with the patient's needs. We also envision readily available team members who will be able to bridge the culture of the clinic/hospital, the mainstream culture, and the patient's culture, in ways that incorporate a clear and solid grasp on institutional protocols while engaging in culturally sensitive practices that privilege the patient's profile. To accomplish this, new appropriateness models must be developed, and to that end, we turn our attention to the so-called "heritage speaker."

The "heritage speaker" as a locally appropriate model: Transgressing normativity

Research shows a preference for individuals to choose others who are similar to themselves as partners. Such trends also take place in healthcare encounters and apply to constructs such as language and race/ethnicity. The notion of language concordance is particularly useful in this regard. Language concordance refers to the linguistic alignment between health professionals and patients, positively affects the relationship between them [67], enhances the quality of care and patient satisfaction [68, 69], and improves health outcomes [70, 71] and better understanding medication and dosage [72]. Additionally, alignment of racio-linguistic profiles between patients and health professionals also leads to positive outcomes as encounters are developed through more culturally appropriate practices, such as the use of specific discourse and genre elements, the flow into the nondominant language practices for small talk, and the disclosure of personal information on part of the clinician for exemplification and rapport building [73–76]. In pursuing the centering of language, racio-ethnic profiles, and knowledge concordance, we turn to the expertise of local knowers whose experiential repertoires have been developed in translingual, transnational, and diverse spaces: the HS.

As foreshadowed, HSs are multilingual people who grew up speaking a minoritized language at home or in the community, while acquiring a majority language through education and through everyday interactions in the majority culture. HSs have been described in the literature as "incomplete acquirers," [77] and "semilinguals" [78] given their proneness to engage in nonstandard language practices. They are socially positioned as not from here nor from there [79] and often internalize deficit discourses regarding their value as multilingual speakers and cultural experts. As Prada describes [16], the HS label fails to integrate the expertise and complexity of their personhood, their nuanced understanding of emergent practices, and their full meaning- and sense-making abilities as it focuses on one element of the individual's linguistic repertoire. Importantly, this label assumes a monolithic understanding of languages, leaving no room for conceptualizing their practical abilities as translanguaging and transcultural emergent behaviors.

If we seek to serve the diverse community members with whom this chapter is concerned, pathways for education, interaction, and policy in healthcare encounters must shift in ways modeled after the community members themselves. To set up baselines of what is communicatively and interactionally best for these patients, their own offspring (i.e., HSs) and other community members hold the key for renewal. Their linguistic practices align with those of their patients, granting them a particularly advantageous position to provide information in understandable ways. Importantly, this alignment is key for relationship building as they undo boundaries stemming from linguistic hierarchies, allowing for relatability. As we mentioned earlier, this often translates into trustworthiness and clarity, which positively impacts the outcomes of healthcare encounters on the whole.

To materialize this vision, some key action points are in order. First, racialized and minoritized multilinguals from local communities must find appropriate support as they complete their educational journeys, or as they continue developing professionally once in the field. This type of support must tap into a variety of social, historical, and sociocultural areas through readings, reflections, and guided conversations with critical language professionals. The goal of these support structures is to help them reposition themselves as rightful multilinguals in the workplace and beyond. As they develop more empowered profiles, they will be able to identify how organizational structures and policies produce important divides that deepen marginalization. As these roadblocks are identified, allies and stakeholders must partner to open spaces to transgress normativity and move toward justice, service and representation. We wonder, what would healthcare education and practice look like when modeled after the practices, realities, and values of historically marginalized communities? We find the concepts of VAME and translanguaging, presented earlier, to be helpful in helping us shift to placing appropriate value on what HSs and other racialized, minoritized community members bring to the table.

Conclusions

This chapter has laid out key tenets to stimulate shifts in how professional healthcare providers approach encounters with linguistically and culturally-diverse community members. Our emphasis is on the intersection between ideologies, language, and cultural practice at its interfaces with education, and how this interplay bears great possibilities to move multilingualism in healthcare encounters toward more humane, realistic, and socially-oriented realizations. To achieve that, we draw heavily from translanguaging, a practical theory of language developed through the lens afforded by the embodied, historically, socially, and politically situated multilingual experiences of grassroots communities. Translanguaging conceives of language and culture as practice: that is, something people do in their meaning- and sense-making, blurring the lines between dichotomic boundaries and divides. Because of the transformative nature of translanguaging, we call for centering it in professional discourse rhetoric in general, and in healthcare encounters and the education of healthcare professionals in particular.

The chapter has also highlighted the tenuous and marginalized space education for intercultural communication holds in many medical curricula. The overview of innovative practices in this space suggests that there are opportunities to harness and embed interprofessional education with translation and interpreting students, explore interpreting for bilingual medical students, as well as medical language education through a critical lens in ways that transform all, reformulating healthcare encounters through emergent understandings of language and culture as inherently interwoven also in these contexts. An important step forward is to reimagine multilingual and culturally diverse health encounters through the experiences of the communities being served. This perspective helps us reconsider "languages for medical purposes" or "medical [named] languages" as healthcare provision [for minoritized communities].

REFERENCES

1. Vertovec, S. (2007). Super-diversity and its implications. *Ethn. Racial Stud.* 30 (6): 1024–1054.
2. Eguren, J. and Vertovec, S. (ed.) (2013). *Anthropology of Migration and Multiculturalism*, vol. 33, 208–212. Migraciones: Publicación del Instituto Universitario de Estudios sobre Migraciones.
3. Makoni, S. and Pennycook, A. (2012). Disinventing multilingualism: from monological multilingualism to multilingua francas. In: *The Routledge Handbook of Multilingualism* (ed. M. Martin-Jones, A. Blackledge, and A. Creese), 451–465. Routledge.
4. Milroy, J. (2001). Language ideologies and the consequences of standardization. *J. Socioling.* 5 (4): 530–555.
5. Canagarajah, S. and Liyanage, I. (2012). Lessons from pre-colonial multilingualism. In: *The Routledge Handbook of Multilingualism* (ed. M. Martin-Jones, A. Blackledge, and A. Creese), 67–83. Routledge.
6. Khubchandani, L.M. (1997). Language policy and education in the Indian subcontinent. In: *Encyclopedia of Language and Education: Language Policy and Political Issues in Education* (ed. R. Wodak and P. Corson), 179–187. Lan, N., & Leung, E. 2022. Empathy as embodied in medical interpreting: A case study of medical-interpreter trainees' turn-taking management.
7. May, S. (ed.) (2013). *The Multilingual Turn: Implications for SLA, TESOL, and Bilingual Education*. Routledge.
8. Arnaut, K., Blommaert, J., Rampton, B., and Spotti, M. (ed.) (2015). *Language and Superdiversity*. Routledge.
9. Blommaert, J. (2010). *The Sociolinguistics of Globalization*. Cambridge University Press.
10. Jørgensen, J.N. (2008). Polylingual languaging around and among children and adolescents. *Int. J. Multiling.* 5 (3): 161–176.
11. Garcia, O. (2009). *Bilingual Education in the 21st Century: A Global Perspective*. Wiley-Blackwell.
12. Otheguy, R., García, O., and Reid, W. (2015). Clarifying translanguaging and

deconstructing named languages: a perspective from linguistics. *Appl. Linguist. Rev.* 6 (3): 281–307.
13. Kalaja, P. and Melo-Pfeifer, S. (ed.) (2019). *Visualising Multilingual Lives: More than Words*. Multilingual Matters.
14. García, O. and Wei, L. (2014). Language, bilingualism and education. In: *Translanguaging: Language, Bilingualism and Education* (ed. O. García and A.M.Y. Lin), 46–62. London: Palgrave Pivot.
15. Vogel, S. and García, O. (2017). Translanguaging. In: *Oxford Research Encyclopedia of Education* (ed. G. Noblit and L. Moll). Oxford University Press.
16. Prada, J. (2021). Translanguaging awareness in heritage language education. In: *Heritage Language Teaching: Critical Language Awareness Perspectives for Research and Pedagogy* (ed. S. Loza and S.M. Beaudrie), 101–118. Routledge.
17. Ortega, P. and Prada, J. (2020). Words matter: translanguaging in medical communication skills training. *Perspect. Med. Educ.* 9: 251–255.
18. Paternotte, E., Fokkema, J.P., Van Loon, K.A. et al. (2014). Cultural diversity: blind spot in medical curriculum documents, a document analysis. *BMC Med. Educ.* 14: 1–6.
19. Suurmond, J., Uiters, E., de Bruijne, M.C. et al. (2011). Negative health care experiences of immigrant patients: a qualitative study. *BMC Health Serv. Res.* 11: 1–8.
20. Paternotte, E., van Dulmen, S., van der Lee, N., Scherpbier, A. J., & Scheele, F. (2015). Factors influencing intercultural doctor-patient communication: a realist review. *Patient Educ. Couns.*, 98(4), 420–445. https://doi.org/10.1016/j.pec.2014.11.018
21. Parker, M.M., Fernández, A., Moffet, H.H. et al. (2017). Association of patient-physician language concordance and glycemic control for limited–English proficiency Latinos with type 2 diabetes. *JAMA Intern. Med.* 177 (3): 380–387.
22. Woodward-Kron, R., Fraser, C., Rashid, H. et al. (2016). Perspectives of junior doctor intercultural clinical communication: lessons for medical education. *Focus Health Prof. Educ. Multidiscip. J.* 17 (3): 82–95.
23. Divi C, Koss RG, Schmaltz SP, Loeb JM. Language proficiency and adverse events in US hospitals: a pilot study. *Int. J. Qual. Health Care* 2007; 19(2): 60–67. https://doi.org/10.1093/intqhc/mzl069.
24. Woodward-Kron, R. and Story, D. (2020). Intercultural communication and safe, effective healthcare for all. *Future Lead. Commun.* 5 (3): 11–13.
25. Roberts, C. (2008). 12. Intercultural Communication in Healthcare Settings. De Gruyter Mouton.
26. Dahm, M.R. (2011). Patient centred care: are international medical graduates' expert novices'? *Aust. Fam. Physician* 40 (11): 895–900.
27. Woodward-Kron, R. (2016). International medical graduates and the discursive patterns of patient-centred communication. *Language Learning in Higher Education* 6 (1): 253–273.
28. Woodward-Kron, R., Stevens, M., and Flynn, E. (2011). The medical educator, the discourse analyst, and the phonetician: a collaborative feedback methodology for clinical communication. *Acad. Med.* 86 (5): 565–570.
29. Hlavac J, Beagley J, Zucchi E. Applications of policy and the advancement of patients' health outcomes through interpreting services: data and viewpoints from a major public healthcare provider. *J. Transl. Interpreting* 2018; 10(1): 111–136. https://doi.org/10.12807/ti.110201.2018.a07.
30. Karliner, L., Marks, A., and Mutha, S. (2016). Reducing health care disparities for minority women in the era of the affordable care act: opportunities within primary care. *J. Health Care Poor Underserved* 27 (2): 392–415.
31. Ryan, A.T., Fisher, C., and Chiavaroli, N. (2019). Medical students as interpreters in health care situations: "... it's a grey area". *Med. J. Aust.* 211 (4): 170–174.
32. Zendedel, R., Schouten, B.C., van Weert, J.C., and van den Putte, B. (2018). Informal interpreting in general practice: are interpreters' roles related to perceived control, trust, and satisfaction? *Patient Educ. Couns.* 101 (6): 1058–1065.

33. Schouten, B.C., Cox, A., Duran, G. et al. (2020). Mitigating language and cultural barriers in healthcare communication: toward a holistic approach. *Patient Educ. Couns.* 103 (12): 2604–2608.
34. Li S, Gerwing J, Krystallidou D, Rowlands A, Cox A, Pype P. Interaction-a missing piece of the jigsaw in interpreter-mediated medical consultation models. *Patient Educ. Couns.* 2017; 100(9): 1769–71. https://doi.org/10.1016/j.pec.2017.04.021
35. Gray, B., Hilder, J., and Stubbe, M. (2015). How to use interpreters in general practice: the development of a New Zealand toolkit. *J. Prim. Health Care* 4: 52–61.
36. Baraldi, C. and Gavioli, L. (2014). Are close renditions the golden standard? Some thoughts on translating accurately in healthcare interpreter-mediated interaction. *Interpret. Transl. Train.* 8 (3): 336–353.
37. Roberts, C. (2007). Intercultural communication in healthcare settings. In: *Handbook of Intercultural Communication* (ed. K. Knapp, G. Antos, H. Kotthoff, and H. Spencer-Oatey), 243–262. Berlin: Mouton de Gruyter.
38. Skelton, J.R., Kai, J., and Loudon, R.F. (2001). Cross-cultural communication in medicine: questions for educators. *Med. Educ.* 35 (3): 257–261.
39. Kachur, E.K. and Altshuler, L. (2004). Cultural competence is everyone's responsibility! *Med. Teach.* 26 (2): 101–105.
40. Prideaux, D. and Edmondson, W. (2001). Cultural identity and representing culture in medical education. Who does it? *Med. Educ.* 35 (3): 186–187.
41. Sorensen, J., Norredam, M., Dogra, N. et al. (2017). Enhancing cultural competence in medical education. *Int. J. Med. Educ.* 8: 28.
42. Ortega P. Spanish language concordance in U.S. medical care: a multifaceted challenge and call to action. *Acad. Med.* 2018; 93(9): 1276–1280. https://doi.org/10.1097/ACM.0000000000002307
43. Accreditation Council for Graduate Medical Education. *ACGME Core Competencies*. https://www.ecfmg.org/echo/acgme-core-competencies.html. Updated 2007. (accessed 15 May 2018).
44. Liaison Committee on Medical Education (2018). *Functions and Structure of a Medical School: Standards for Accreditation of Medical Education Programs Leading to the MD Degree. Effective Academic Year: 2019–20.* Association of American Medical Colleges and American Medical Association http://lcme.org/publications (accessed 15 May 2018).
45. Von Fragstein, M., Silverman, J., Cushing, A. et al. (2008). UK consensus statement on the content of communication curricula in undergraduate medical education. *Med. Educ.* 42 (11): 1100–1107.
46. Malhotra, A., Gregory, I., Darvill, E. et al. (2009). Mind the gap: learners' perspectives on what they learn in communication compared to how they and others behave in the real world. *Patient Educ. Couns.* 76 (3): 385–390.
47. Roberts, C., Daly, M., Held, F., and Lyle, D. (2017). Social learning in a longitudinal integrated clinical placement. *Adv. Health Sci. Educ.* 22: 1011–1029.
48. Min-Yu Lau, P., Woodward-Kron, R., Livesay, K. et al. (2016). Cultural respect encompassing simulation training: being heard about health through broadband. *J. Public Health Res.* 5 (1): 657. jphr-2016.
49. Lan N, Leung E. Empathy as embodied in medical interpreting: a case study of medical-interpreter trainees' turn-taking management. In: Moratto R, Li D, eds. *Global Insights into Public Service Interpreting*. London: Taylor and Francis; 2021. https://doi.org/10.4324/9781003197027
50. Department of Health and Human Services, Victoria (2017). *Language Services Policy and Guidelines*. Melbourne: Victorian Government https://www.dhhs.vic.gov.au/publications/language-services-policy-and-guidelines.
51. Hlavac J, Harrison C. Interpreter-mediated doctor-patient interactions: interprofessional education in the training of future interpreters and doctors. *Perspectives* 2021; 29(4): 572–590. https://doi.org/10.1080/0907676X.2021.1873397.
52. Vargas Pelaez, A.F., Ramirez, S.I., Valdes Sanchez, C. et al. (2018). Implementing a

medical student interpreter training program as a strategy to developing humanism. *BMC Med. Educ.* 18 (1): 1.
53. Gonzalo, J.D., Lucey, C., Wolpaw, T., and Chang, A. (2017). Value-added clinical systems learning roles for medical students that transform education and health: a guide for building partnerships between medical schools and health systems. *Acad. Med.* 92 (5): 602–607.
54. Vela, M.B., Fritz, C., Press, V.G., and Girotti, J. (2016). Medical students' experiences and perspectives on interpreting for LEP patients at two US medical schools. *J. Racial Ethn. Health Disparities* 3: 245–249.
55. Ortega P, Diamond L, Alemán MA, et al. Medical Spanish standardization in U.S. Medical schools: consensus statement from a multidisciplinary expert panel. *Acad. Med.* 2020; 95(1): 22–31. https://doi.org/10.1097/ACM.0000000000002917
56. Prada, J., Tan, K., and Ortega P. Medical Student Linguistic Perspectives and Their Implications for Teaching Spanish for the Health Professions: Towards Critical Horizons. Unpublished Manuscript.
57. Pascual y Cabo, D. and Prada, J. (2015). Understanding the Spanish heritage language speaker/learner. *EuroAmerican J. Appl. Linguist. Lang.* 2 (2): 1–10.
58. Leeman, J. and Martínez, G. (2007). From identity to commodity: ideologies of Spanish in heritage language textbooks. *Crit. Inq. Lang. Stud.* 4 (1): 35–65.
59. Wei, L. (2018). Translanguaging as a practical theory of language. *Appl. Linguis.* 39 (1): 9–30.
60. Seltzer, K., Ascenzi-Moreno, L., and Aponte, G.Y. (2020). Translanguaging and early childhood education in the USA: insights from the CUNY-NYSIEB project. In: *Inclusion, Education and Translanguaging: How to Promote Social Justice in (Teacher) Education?* (ed. J.A. Panagiotopoulou, L. Rosen, and J. Strzykala), 23–39. Springer Nature.
61. Prada, J. and Turnbull, B. (2018). The role of translanguaging in the multilingual turn: driving philosophical and conceptual renewal in language education. *EuroAmerican J. Appl. Linguist. Lang.* 5: 8–23.
62. Prada, J. Forgoing multilingualism as a collection of elite monolingualisms through trans-rhetoric. In: *Communicative Spaces in Bilingual Contexts: Discourses, Synergies and Counterflows in Spanish and English* (ed. A. Sánchez-Muñoz and J. Retis), 13–31. Taylor & Francis.
63. Cazden, C., Cope, B., Fairclough, N. et al. (1996). A pedagogy of multiliteracies: designing social futures. *Harv. Educ. Rev.* 66 (1): 60–92.
64. Stornaiuolo, A., Smith, A., and Phillips, N.C. (2017). Developing a transliteracies framework for a connected world. *J. Lit. Res.* 49 (1): 68–91.
65. Health Resources and Services Administration. *Health* Literacy. https://www.hrsa.gov/about/organization/bureaus/ohe/health-literacy.
66. Baynham, M. and Lee, T.K. (2019). *Translation and Translanguaging*. Routledge.
67. Menon, U., Szalacha, L.A., Martinez, G.A. et al. (2022). Efficacy of a language-concordant health coaching intervention for latinx with diabetes. *Patient Educ. Couns.* 105 (7): 2174–2182.
68. González, H.M., Vega, W.A., and Tarraf, W. (2010). Health care quality perceptions among foreign-born Latinos and the importance of speaking the same language. *J. Am. Board Fam. Med.* 23 (6): 745–752.
69. Eskes, C., Salisbury, H., Johannsson, M., and Chene, Y. (2013). Patient satisfaction with language-concordant care. *J. Physician Assist. Educ.* 24 (3): 14–22.
70. Traylor, A.H., Schmittdiel, J.A., Uratsu, C.S. et al. (2010). Adherence to cardiovascular disease medications: does patient-provider race/ethnicity and language concordance matter? *J. Gen. Intern. Med.* 25: 1172–1177.
71. Diamond L, Izquierdo K, Canfield D, Matsoukas K, Gany F. A systematic review of the impact of patient-physician non-English language concordance on quality of care and outcomes. *J. Gen. Intern. Med.* 2019; 34(8): 1591–1606. https://doi.org/10.1007/s11606-019-04847-5.
72. Bailey, S.C., Sarkar, U., Chen, A.H. et al. (2012). Evaluation of language concordant, patient-centered drug label instructions. *J. Gen. Intern. Med.* 27: 1707–1713.

73. Fuchsel, C.M. (2017). *Yes I Can, (Sí, Yo Puedo): An Empowerment Program for Immigrant Latina Women in Group Settings*. Oxford University Press.
74. Magaña, S., Lopez, K., Aguinaga, A., and Morton, H. (2013). Access to diagnosis and treatment services among Latino children with autism spectrum disorders. *Intellect. Dev. Disabil.* 51 (3): 141–153.
75. Plough, A., Fielding, J.E., Chandra, A. et al. (2013). Building community disaster resilience: perspectives from a large urban county department of public health. *Am. J. Public Health* 103 (7): 1190–1197.
76. Vickers, C. and Goble, R. (2011). Well, now, okey dokey: english discourse markers in Spanish-language medical consultations. *Can. Mod. Lang. Rev.* 67 (4): 536–567.
77. Montrul, S. (2010). Current issues in heritage language acquisition. *Annu. Rev. Appl. Linguist.* 30: 3–23.
78. Hansegård, N.E. (1962). Tomedalen—en svensk bygd utan sprak. *Samtid och Framtid* 4: 215–219.
79. Urciuoli, B. (2008). Whose Spanish?: the tension between linguistic correctness. In: *Bilingualism and Identity: Spanish at the Crossroads with Other Languages*, vol. vol. 37 (ed. M. Niño-Murcia and J. Rothman), 257. John Benjamins Publishing.

17 Dedicated Medical Spanish Courses and Crosslinguistic Healthcare Communication Skills

MARCO A. ALEMÁN
AND ALEJANDRA ZAPIÉN-HIDALGO

Introduction

Hispanic/Latinx populations are a fast-growing and highly heterogeneous ethnic group from various countries of origin, social, and cultural backgrounds. According to the 2020 United States Census [1], Hispanics (an official term created for the Census) comprised 18.5% of the total population in 2022, and it is estimated that by the year 2050, 26% of the country's population will be Hispanic [2]. There are 41 million people in the United States who speak Spanish at home and 16.2 million Spanish speakers who have limited English proficiency (LEP), defined as, speaking English less than "very well," accounting for 64% of all persons with LEP in the nation [3]. Individuals with non-English language preference have more challenges than those with English preference when they engage with the healthcare system. Miscommunication due to lack of or ineffective use of the patient's preferred language can lead to medical errors and poor health outcomes [4], increase the cost of medical care [5], and have potential adverse clinical consequences [6]. At a population level, federal law through Title VI mandates that any healthcare entity that receives federal funds use interpreters or other methods to bridge this language gap [7]. Offering medical interpretation services is an opportunity to provide equitable and high-quality healthcare to populations with non-English language preferences (NELP) [8]. The inclusion of professional medical interpreters is associated with better prevention screening, better outcomes, and improved utilization of services [6]. While many medical institutions contract medical interpreters to meet this goal, these efforts are affected by the availability of trained interpreters and variability in the use of interpreters by healthcare staff [9]. In addition, in one study, the use of professional interpreters, when compared to language-concordant clinicians, did not

---

The Handbook of Language in Public Health and Healthcare, First Edition.
Edited by Pilar Ortega, Glenn Martínez, Maichou Lor, and A. Susana Ramírez.
© 2024 John Wiley & Sons, Inc. Published 2024 by John Wiley & Sons, Inc.

mitigate and may have worsened patients' negative perceptions of the care provided by their language-discordant clinicians [10]. Interpreters also act as "cultural brokers" and co-constructors of meaning (joint understanding) in medical interactions [11]. However, dual-role interpreters (who are generally ad hoc interpreters who are hired in an administrative or clinical position as their primary role but use their bilingual language skills to serve as interpreters in a secondary role), have been documented to omit, reduce, or revise the majority of physician attempts to establish rapport with a patient [12]. This may influence findings that Spanish-speaking patients in the emergency department who had an interpreter during their visit rated their physician as less friendly, respectful, or concerned compared to patients who did not have an interpreter [13].

Language-concordant care is the ability of the patient and clinician to directly communicate with one another in the patient's preferred language. Data show that patients with NELP who have language-concordant clinicians had better recall of health information and asked more questions of a clinical encounter [14]. Furthermore, patients in another study reported being more satisfied or receiving better care from language-concordant clinicians [9].

Patients with Spanish-language preference are often not able to receive care from Spanish-speaking clinicians due to a shortage of clinicians trained and proficient in medical Spanish [15–17]. Medical Spanish education in the United States arose from a need to bridge a communication gap and improve the care provided to Spanish-speaking people. Currently, some medical Spanish education programs in United States medical schools aim to increase the number of trained Spanish-speaking clinicians who can directly communicate with their patients [18, 19]. However, there is no federal or medical school requirement for the teaching of medical Spanish nor its curriculum. In a 2021 national survey, 78% of United States medical schools reported offering some form of medical Spanish training for their students [20]. However, medical schools varied in the instruction of medical Spanish, from structured programs with dedicated language and/or physician faculty-led programs to medical student-run programs, online programs, or a combination of all of these [20]. The content, length, and evaluation [21] of medical Spanish programs vary [18, 21–23].

Teaching clinicians to communicate with linguistically diverse patients: Historical development

Crosslinguistic healthcare communication skills

In the medical literature, the term "global linguistic competence" has been used to refer to the communication skillset needed by a clinician to effectively communicate with patients across languages. Given multiple meanings of "global linguistic skills" in the language literature, we will use the term "crosslinguistic communication skills" to refer to the skillset required for healthcare communication with linguistically diverse patient populations. Ortega et al. have proposed that all medical students should be instructed on crosslinguistic competence within a longitudinal communication skills curriculum that includes: (1) understanding the diversity and the impact of language and population health; (2) embracing self-awareness of language proficiency in any nondominant languages and limitations for using those languages in medical settings; (3) achieving competency in the use of a professional medical interpreter; and (4) understanding cultural issues in health that may confound successful medical communication with linguistically diverse populations [24].

Understanding the diversity and the impact of language and population health

Educators have proposed training medical students and clinicians to serve the growing diverse population [24]. In response, medical schools are updating their interpersonal and communication skills training to meet competencies as outlined by the Liaison Committee of Medical Education (LCME) [25], which sets standards for medical education in the United States. The LCME competencies also require that medical schools address structural competence, cultural competence, and health inequities, which are important for the future physician when caring for the diverse U.S. population. This includes a better understanding of the diverse ways people perceive their illness, the presence of health disparities and their impact on the targeted population, and how to recognize and address health inequities, among others. In addition, healthcare professionals are seeking information and training to recognize and answer to the cultural and linguistic needs of the patient or community [26].

Self-awareness of language proficiency in any nondominant languages and limitations for using those languages in medical settings

Linguistic competence is the operational knowledge of a language that allows a person to match sounds and meanings to communicate with others [27] Healthcare professionals who can communicate successfully and effectively respond to the patients and their community achieve linguistic competence. This includes considering the needs of people with NELP (or nondominant language preferences), low health literacy skills, or other communication challenges, including individuals with disabilities, to identify the best communication strategy [28].

Improving communication with linguistically diverse populations includes incorporating individuals and systems of health with knowledge of the targeted population, being aware of the different languages spoken, and finding opportunities to provide training to patient-facing staff and healthcare professionals. Training in cultural and linguistic skills should occur before trainees' clinical experiences with patients and should continue throughout their undergraduate, graduate medical education, and afterward through continuing medical education [29]. Communication problems due to language discordance and lack of use of qualified medical interpreters are the leading cause of patient safety events and healthcare expenditures in people who have LEP [8].

In the United States, there are healthcare professionals who are bilingual and bicultural and are eager to provide care to populations with NELP. The Joint Commission is the nation's oldest and largest standards-setting and accrediting body in health care. This independent and not-for-profit organization does not prevent healthcare professionals from directly communicating with their patients in their preferred language without the presence of a medical interpreter. However, it does recommend that clinics and hospitals have an action plan, such as proficiency assessments, to assure that bilingual clinicians can effectively communicate with and fulfill the needs of the patients. Individuals who are considered "qualified bilingual providers" are able to communicate directly with patients in their preferred language, and, in some cases, support colleagues to bridge the communication gap as dual-role interpreters [30]. However, the proficiency level at which a clinician is considered a "qualified bilingual provider" is ill-defined, leaving the decision largely up to individual hospitals/medical centers and oftentimes up to individual clinicians. Thus, there is a need for trainees and clinicians to learn to appropriately self-assess their language skills as well as recognize their limitations in the non-English languages they speak. It is recommended for clinicians to learn to use standardized language assessments, when they are available, before communicating with their patients without a professional interpreter [31]. For example, clinicians can use the Clinician Cultural Linguistic Assessment (CCLA), which is commercially available in a variety of languages [32].

Competency in the use of a professional medical interpreter

Given the lack of clarity or standardization in defining what it takes or what it means to be a "qualified bilingual provider," it is particularly essential for all healthcare professionals to receive training in how to best work with professional medical interpreters. They should also understand the need to reduce ad hoc, untrained, interpreters in order to reduce medical errors [33]. Training should include pre- and post-encounter debriefing with the interpreter to maximize the communication with the patient and the clinician's self-improvement. Using the presession to discuss the patient's clinical situation and any specific goal with the interpreter will benefit all parties and ensure a successful clinical interaction [34].

Cultural issues in health that may confound successful medical communication with linguistically diverse populations

Social and cultural constructs and beliefs are intertwined with language. Cultural training interventions can improve medical students' and resident physicians' understanding of racial/ethnic differences in disease burdens, traditional cultural practices, influences of patient culture on clinicians' behaviors, best practices for working with interpreters, as well as immigration and other legal issues that intersect with language [33]. In addition, patient mistrust with the clinician may occur due to lack of language concordance, prior inadequate interactions with the health system, variations of patient's health literacy, or the clinician's lack of cultural humility.

Medical Spanish education

Medical Spanish education in the United States began for public education purposes. In the early 1920s, the League of Latin American Citizens (LULAC) organization was founded in Texas. Through their *Movimiento Pro Salud* program, LULAC provided health promotion and prevention education to Mexican communities in Texas to address public health disparities in collaboration with local and state public health partners [35]. One important collaborator was Ruben C. Ortega, a Methodist minister who, for his presentations, adapted his Spanish language and incorporated cultural nuances to meet the needs of his audience [35]. Later, in the early 1970s, medical Spanish began to be taught at the college level and several textbooks were published to meet this need [35].

In 1987, Gonzalez-Lee and Simon published their innovative teaching of medical Spanish to second-year medical students, integrating language seminars and "cross-cultural" clinical experiences with Spanish-speaking patients and physicians [36]. In 2008, the curriculum guiding principles by Reuland et al. [18] informed medical Spanish educators in medical schools. In 2015, a national survey of medical Spanish courses taught in U.S. medical schools, created and administered by the Latino Medical Student Association (LMSA), identified a heterogeneity of instruction and student evaluation in the 66% of medical schools that responded to the survey [37]. An updated survey showed an increase (78%) in medical Spanish education in United States medical schools, but only 21% provided a formal curriculum, a faculty educator, learner assessment, and institutional credit [20]. To offer guidance, an interdisciplinary group met in 2018 and provided a model for the standardization of instruction, evaluation, and research in medical Spanish [19]. This group evolved into the Medical Spanish Taskforce and in 2020 became the National Association of Medical Spanish (NAMS) [38].

Based on expert recommendations in the peer-reviewed literature, medical Spanish programs should target students who have been assessed as having intermediate or greater proficiency in Spanish [18, 19], as they represent the cohort who are more likely to reach the goal of being successful in conducting a medical encounter in Spanish without the need of an interpreter. Educators starting a medical Spanish program should use a standardized process to assess learner suitability to enroll in a medical Spanish course or program [18, 23]. One option is the Interagency Language Roundtable (ILR), a tool developed by the United States Government in collaboration with nongovernment agencies to assess language fluency. The ILR has undergone several revisions [39] and a modified version, sometimes referred to as the ILR scale for healthcare (ILR-H) has been validated for self-assessment by physicians. The ILR-H uses proficiency categories related to conversational healthcare skills rated as "poor," "fair," "good," "very good" and "excellent" [40, 41]. While the ILR-H is comparably accurate to validated oral interviews at the lower or higher end of the scale, it is less accurate for those self-assessing in the intermediate range [41] and this needs to be considered in the selection of learners for the program. An alternate option is the ALTA Spanish Speaking and Listening Assessment (SLA) [18], which is a validated and recorded telephone interview test that requires students to respond to 12 prompts regarding general and health-related concerns from a large pool of questions. The SLA is scored on a scale of 1 (beginner) to 12 (native speaker) and has been mapped to the ILR [42]. A panel of medical and language experts [19] has recommended that students enrolling in a medical Spanish course should have a minimum self-assessed score of "fair" on the ILR-H while others recommend a minimum score of 6 (intermediate) on the ALTA SLA [18] that corresponds to level 2 on the ILR scale [42]. Chapter 15 provides additional information about medical Spanish proficiency level and scales for its evaluation. In this chapter, we focus our attention on medical Spanish courses in the medical school level in the United States context and on medical student learners. However, other health disciplines and schools, such as physician assistant [43], nursing [44, 45], and pharmacy [46, 47] schools have a similar need to train their learners in medical Spanish and have started programs to meet those needs.

Medical Spanish curricula should begin with a needs assessment, and be developed with a standardized framework such as Kern's Six Steps [48], after first identifying the end goal for the intended learner.

An expert consensus recommends that medical Spanish curricula be standardized and include core competencies and learner skill assessment that include the use of standardized patient (SP) encounters [19]. The curriculum should include training and evaluation of medical Spanish knowledge of organ systems and interviewing; medical Spanish knowledge of common illnesses and associated cultural colloquialisms that may be used by the patient; patient-centered explanation of the diagnoses, their evaluation and treatment plan, and self-assessment of learners' language skills and need to work with an interpreter in selected situations. The recommended language structures by language experts include vocabulary in health contexts, grammar as relevant to health contexts, integrated cultural and sociolinguistic content, and communicative activities [21]. That is, the course material needs to be applicable to the end goal and needs of the learner [49] when interfacing with Spanish-speaking patients in their student or professional healthcare roles.

The structure of medical Spanish programs can vary, according to the medical school's curriculum, educator availability, and student interest. Programs may be time-limited such as two or four weeks of intense instruction, semester-long, longitudinal [18, 19] either in person, online, or a hybrid [20, 49]. Currently, there is a lack of evidence that one particular structure to teach medical Spanish is better. Medical Spanish educators in the United States are heterogeneous [21] and can vary from bilingual and bicultural native speakers or non-native speakers and from physicians to nonphysicians such as medical students [50, 51], language educators, second-language acquisition (SLA) experts, and preferably a combination of these [18–20, 22, 52]. Since medical content experts who teach medical Spanish (mostly physicians) are not usually trained to teach languages while SLA experts such as Spanish educators or linguists are experts in language instruction but not medical content, it is recommended that a hybrid collaboration of these educators would provide a more robust curricula and assessment of the program [22]. Courses taught by students were less likely to have an assessment or provide feedback to the learner [20], limiting interpretation of its curricular benefit to learners and increasing the potential for incomplete training and risk for false fluency [9, 17, 53] that can negatively affect their future interactions with patients. Identifying the best-trained educators knowledgeable in curriculum design and assessment and providing them with institutional support, including dedicated funding, is imperative to the program's success. However, currently there is a lack of standardization regarding the prerequisites and training needed for medical Spanish educators [54]. Collaborators who can co-teach can add to the program's success and include interpreters, community health outreach workers, or others who bring expertise and lived experience in language, communication, culture, real-world expectations, and use of Spanish by the patient population.

Critical issues and topics in medical Spanish education

In this section, we will discuss the targeting of the type of learners, learning objectives, instructional methods, and assessment of a medical Spanish program.

Guiding principles for medical Spanish education

Currently, standardized medical Spanish curriculum, pedagogy, and evaluation processes do not exist.

Several training programs have incorporated Reuland et al. guiding principles [18] when creating a medical Spanish curriculum. These principles include the following:

- The program should be longitudinal and provide multiple learning modalities.
- The program should focus on learners with an intermediate or advanced level of Spanish proficiency.

- The program should have an official status within the medical school and students should receive credit.
- Encourage integration of the program into the preexisting medical school curriculum.
- The primary focus should be on language and communication skills. Culture is an important and secondary focus.
- Use validated and reliable measurements of language proficiency for student assessments and program evaluation.

The guiding principles can be modified as needed to fit the program's curricular design and end goals. For example, course credit hours provided vary according to the length of the program and the individual medical school's criteria for course credit. Providing credit encourages a commitment to complete the program as greater attrition of students occurs in non-credit courses. The use of standardized assessment tools of linguistic skills provides a more exact appraisal of a student meeting these goals [18, 23].

The focus of medical Spanish training should be on oral bidirectional communication with the patient [18, 22] and therefore, it is recommended that educators group learners based on oral proficiency [22]. While there is also a need to provide written instructions in Spanish to the patient, this should not be the focus of the course. The course methodology can be modified to fit the learner's needs, preexisting medical knowledge, and clinical experiences. For example, preclinical medical students (students who have not yet begun their clinical experiences) may benefit from an interview-based course structure focusing on learning how to conduct a general interview for an acute complaint and other elements of the history, physical exam, assessment, and plan. An organ system-based approach (e.g., cardiovascular and respiratory) can be used for students with prior knowledge of the general interview and exam or those with more clinical experiences. Learners, especially as they progress in their clinical learning, in medical school, residency training, or beyond, will need programs that meet their real-life patient encounter needs. The instructor should consider applying Task-Based Language Teaching (TBLT) [52], Content Based Instruction (CBI) or Project-based Learning (PBL) SLA methodologies. CBI "allows for explicit language instruction, integrated with content instruction, in a relevant and purposeful context" [55]. To enhance contextual learning, it is best to couple the medical Spanish course with the general medical school curricula [18], with topics occurring shortly after each is taught in English, to enhance the learning of the new material in Spanish using the prior knowledge in English, reinforcing and facilitating learning [51].

Targeting resident and practicing physicians

The Accreditation Council for Graduate Medical Education (ACGME) [56] establishes the competencies for physicians in graduate medical training programs, known as house staff or resident physicians. One of the six ACGME competencies is interpersonal and communication skills. Compared to teaching medical students, teaching resident physicians includes different challenges including their busy clinical workweek, limited time for structured teaching sessions [57], and variable clinical opportunities to practice medical Spanish. Benefits of medical Spanish training for resident physicians may include personal satisfaction, increased knowledge and confidence, potential savings to the hospital with the need for less utilization of medical interpreters [58, 59], and an increase in patient and family satisfaction [59].

Resident physicians underestimate their language proficiency even in written case scenarios, yet many provide care to patients in Spanish [60]. Resident physicians wishing to learn medical Spanish may be motivated by the immediate applicability of the new knowledge, often in complex and time-limited encounters, to provide high-quality care to their patients. That is, the stakes are higher for resident physicians versus medical students who are not yet legally responsible for the care of their assigned patients. Educational programs for resident physicians should be tailored to fit their busy schedules and greater access to patients to provide real-world experience and feedback. A good example is the CHiCos (Clínica Hispana de Cuidados de Salud, or Hispanic Health Care Clinic), a three-year program for pediatric residents based in their required continuity outpatient clinic that includes Spanish-English bilingual training, ongoing language evaluation and collaboration between bilingual supervisory physicians and medical interpreters [61, 62]. While online modules and self-paced learning seem alluring for the busy resident, they may not meet all of the medical Spanish learner competencies [63] and should not be the sole method of instruction. Additionally, time-limited programs may not always yield the desired results since brief-intervention medical Spanish programs may decrease interpreter use, despite the learner's limited language proficiency at the conclusion of the course [59, 64]. In contrast, one longitudinal resident physician program for family medicine residents identified an improvement in oral proficiency using the CCLA [58]. Another longitudinal study on emergency medicine residents showed improvement in oral and listening comprehension assessments performed by the same trained evaluator using the ILR scale and the Oral Proficiency Interview (OPI) that is based on the American Council of Teaching of Foreign Languages (ACTFL) guidelines [65].

Medical Spanish programs for residents ought to focus on the end goal for the resident physician learner that varies according to medical specialty. For example, a resident in orthopedics would need to learn how to describe the indication for a total knee replacement, the procedure and its risks and benefits to the patient and how to answer the patient's questions regarding the procedure and obtain the signed consent for the surgery. A resident in ophthalmology would need to explain what macular degeneration is to a patient, using the related medical vocabulary and explain how it can affect the patient's eyes, including the natural progression of the disease if left untreated and inform the patient regarding useful therapies ranging from oral medications to those medications that are injected directly into the eye.

Compared to the resident physician, the practicing clinician has similar time limitations yet more clinical experience, from which to draw upon for contextual learning. The published medical Spanish training programs for practicing clinicians is limited and its outcomes were not well-evaluated [66] and are insufficient to guide the educator regarding creating medical Spanish programs for this group. In a recent study of a heterogeneous population of practicing physicians, including residents, nurses, and other clinicians taking an interprofessional education (IPE) course consisting of two eight-week sessions of medical Spanish, "Spanish-speaking patients reported a lower-quality communication from clinicians learning Spanish than do English-speaking patients" [67]. More research is needed in medical Spanish education for practicing clinicians.

We recommend that students prepare for class using appropriate resources and use the class time to integrate information such as medical Spanish vocabulary in real-world role-play cases [49] as skills practiced and acquired in classroom role-plays transfer to real world medical tasks [52, 68]. A recent review of medical Spanish textbooks performed by a combination of medical Spanish professionals and language experts identified a difference in their evaluations of the same textbooks, with language experts assigning lower scores for vocabulary and grammar, culture, and communicative abilities [69]. The study found that many published medical Spanish textbooks [69] and online resources [63] are not designed for the intended audience of medical Spanish courses (i.e., learners with intermediate Spanish level and above); rather, most resources target beginner learners. Additionally, few are appropriate as stand-alone resources for medical students or physician learners [69]. For example, educators can use a textbook [70] or other resources that provide an interview-based format for an interview-based course. Educators may need to adopt a variety of learning resources, such as including more than one textbook to meet learners' educational goals, core competencies, and language structures. Non-clinician educators and even clinicians without the time, resources, or knowledge to create role-play cases can utilize compiled or published cases [71]. According to a published scoping review, online resources are also varied in quality, emphasizing interactive virtual activities, listening exercises, and vocabulary review that may enhance classroom learning and activities, and allow for independent study [69]. However, no online resources were found to meet the criteria for medical Spanish learner competencies, while only one online resource was found to be suitable for the self-assessment competency [63].

Targeting medical Spanish competencies

In this section, we present content and pedagogy useful in the teaching of the various components of the clinical encounter. We also address how to best assess the medical Spanish skills of the learner.

Teaching students to conduct the medical interview

Up to 80% of diagnoses in medicine can be obtained by a good interview [72, 73] thus making the instruction of medical interviewing in Spanish a crucial and foundational element of medical Spanish training [74]. Building rapport with the patient, including recognizing a patient's cultural preferences and applying cultural humility [75] that "emphasizes curiosity and self-reflection over mastery" [76], will maximize the interview and its yield. To prevent creating generalizations and stereotypes, learners should be taught how to inquire about what name the patient gives to his or her illness and their interpretation of such as well as the expectations or goals for the visit [77]. This strategy helps eliminate implicit bias and can help address health disparities. In addition, communicating diagnoses, their meaning, evaluation and therapeutic options along with their risks and benefits to the individual is critical.

Educators should emphasize the need to recognize cultural and linguistic nuances that help the clinician build rapport with Spanish-speaking patients and the skills needed to modify interviewing techniques accordingly. These include affiliative humor ("intended to elicit laughter and/or other forms of amusement in targets"), mitigation of directives (softening of suggestions, recommendations, requests, commands, and acts), and inclusive pronouns for solidarity (using "us" or "we" to protect alignment and positive face), words of empathy, apologies, and compliments [12]. Educators may use audio or video recordings of authentic [78] or simulated dialogue [71] between the clinician and patient and ask learners to reflect on the interactions. Hispanic/Latinx patients typically expect their physician to relate to them at a personal level, a concept called *personalismo,* and this should be incorporated in the teaching of the interview [79]. Learners can practice how to use pleasantries such as asking about the patient's general well-being or family before starting the actual interview and this will allow for a better physician-patient connection and interaction [80].

Learners need to acquire knowledge in Spanish of all the major anatomical parts of the body that can be achieved via vocabulary lists in textbooks [70], online resources [63] or created by the educators. Selected vocabulary list unit(s) can be assigned as homework and incorporated by educators, along with a Spanish grammar unit, as they relate to a segment of the medical history or performing part of the physical exam. This will help them build a foundation for learning basic and advanced questions and expressions useful when interviewing with a Spanish-speaking patient. Teaching strategies include using a mnemonic strategy called total physical response [81], such as the game, "Simon Says." The instructor provides a command to learners asking them to touch a part of their body, demonstrating its location and students perform the task, reciting the anatomical part in the target language. This helps to teach the major parts of the body using physical and oral student participation and responses. Educators can use oral corrective feedback [82, 83] to ensure proper pronunciation or identification of the body part. Showing pictures of people with normal or abnormal specific body parts (for example a person with a sunburn or a red eye) can be used in class to trigger recall of the name of the anatomical part in Spanish and the learner who responds is asked to use that newly learned word in a question or statement directed to the patient. [In a conversation with M. Alemán, MD (July 2022)]. Educators should also focus on teaching basic illness scripts [84] in the target language, by using case-based methodology. This allows a contextual use of new medical Spanish vocabulary and application of prior medical knowledge [81] to create plausible questions for the patient and her condition. Strategies can include using large group participation or small groups of 2–4 students in which the educator provides the class with a short statement of the patient's illness (e.g., left acute knee pain and redness) and asks the learners to create the questions, in Spanish, to be used when interviewing the patient with this complaint [In a conversation with Marco Alemán, MD (July 2022)]. Educators provide oral corrective feedback to learners regarding the language and clinical accuracy of their responses. Educators can select common conditions such as someone with a sore throat or abdominal pain to more complex medical conditions with usual and unusual presentations, increasing their complexity as determined by the learners' needs and readiness by Spanish language or clinical knowledge. In addition, emphasis should also be placed on phrases used in transitions between segments of the interview. A useful technique can be to assign learner groups in pairs, provide them with a skeleton text from an actual conversation, [78] and ask them to use role-play to complete the sentence(s) and communicate the transition sentence(s) or request(s). Another option is to ask the student pairs to create, in Spanish, these transitions that occur during the interview or provide the students with sample transition phrases in English and request that they translate them to Spanish. Students then use these answers in role-plays and the instructor provides oral corrective feedback [82, 83].

Building interactive classroom methods for student application of learned medical Spanish vocabulary should be paramount. This can include using individual or small group work using case-based methods for contextual learning. For example, students create questions or phrases that are useful during the medical interview or as responses to patients' replies and utilize their answers during in-classroom role-plays, where they play the role of the physician as well as the patient, improving on their oral and aural communication [85]. Afterwards the instructor provides corrective feedback [82, 83] to facilitate the appropriate use of grammar, vocabulary and pronunciation to enhance and assess comprehension. Another method is to use trigger tapes/videos of prerecorded student encounters with an SP and ask learners to write down their follow up questions for a segment of the interview and use these questions later in a role-play in class using small groups or with an SP, playing the role of the clinician. These exercises are targeted, task-directed skills that are realistic and applicable in the future in simulated or real-life patient encounters, anchored in TBLT [52].

The instruction should also include recognizing and preventing potential misunderstandings related to words or slang used by their Spanish-speaking patients to describe common objects or conditions that are unknown to the interviewer. Educators can use role-play, as an information gap activity, using a brief exchange of information between two learners that includes some of the various words used to mean cheeks, calves, or eyeglasses used by people from various Spanish-speaking countries. Students are asked to voice clarifying questions of their role-play partner to identify their knowledge gap. Educators may also use modeling, open-ended questions or show pictures of these objects to elicit learners' responses. Some Spanish-speakers may also mix use of two languages, such as Spanish and English (sometimes referred to as *Spanglish*). Recognizing this concept and other ways in which multilingual people incorporate hybrid use of multiple languages is called translanguaging, and serves to inform that our patients may incorporate *non-standard* features (by monolingual language standards), regionalisms, and influences from multiple languages [86–88]. Additionally, training should include recognizing when patients may not understand the clinician's questions or information and practicing how to address this issue by rephrasing the same question or concept in Spanish. This can include asking learners in role-play to use the teach back technique [89], using phrasings requesting that the patient voice back what they have understood from what was said to them by the learner. The instructor provides the learner with oral corrective feedback, including prompts for self-repair, to clarify and improve language acquisition [82, 83].

Additionally, educators should address how and when to selectively inquire about immigration status in a sensitive manner, especially when it affects healthcare or access to healthcare services. Directly asking patients about their immigration status risks losing trust with the patient and negatively affecting the communication and encounter. Clinicians may instead consider focusing on an indirect approach to obtain needed medical information, such as asking "When was the last time you had the opportunity to return to your home country?" Learners should be exposed, via didactic or interactive methods, to issues that affect health and health disparities in Hispanic/Latinx patients. For example, these can include the diverse immigrant experience that can be more traumatic for some, relocation challenges, adjusting to a new language and country, access to healthcare [90, 91] due to lack of finances, immigration status [92], racism, and discrimination. Educators can incorporate one or more of these elements in cases for in-classroom role-play with provision of oral corrective feedback or in SP encounters. Alternatively, use of audio or video recordings of real or simulated patient encounters can help in triggering reflection and in-class discussion regarding these important themes.

One of the medical Spanish course learning objectives should be how to recognize one's language and cultural limitations and know when to request and work with a professional interpreter [33, 34]. This applies to all medical Spanish learners, regardless of their proficiency level. For example, intermediate and advanced-level learners may need to use professional interpreters to explain complex medical information or treatment plans, including information beyond the clinician's scope of practice, deliver bad news, or simply to validate the history obtained from the patient. Furthermore, to fulfill crosslinguistic competencies, all learners and clinicians, not just those in medical Spanish programs, need to learn to work with interpreters since all students will encounter patients with whom they have a language discordance. This training should encompass how to recognize trained interpreters and how to access, work with and collaborate with interpreters to ensure a successful interpreted encounter that includes bidirectional feedback between interpreter and clinician that promotes learning about language and cultural issues that affect the care of the patient [33]. The learner of crosslinguistic communication skills needs to learn how to recognize problems with the interpreted encounter and how to resolve the issue [33]. This training should include how to recognize when the interpreter is not interpreting all of the patient's words, paraphrasing or adding words that can change the meaning and negatively affect the encounter [12]. Meanwhile, the medical Spanish learner who works with interpreters may have an advantage in recognizing this mismatch between what the patient says and what is interpreted. Useful techniques can include the use of video clips of simulated interpreted encounters or role-play by educators demonstrating improper interpretation in Spanish followed by debriefing by the instructor. In addition, educators can provide groups of two students with scripts of correct and incorrect dialogue of an interpreted encounter for use in role-plays followed by oral correction and in-class debriefing.

Teaching students to conduct the physical examination

Training should teach how to communicate effectively during the physical exam, a sensitive portion of the medical encounter. Additionally, training should include expressions used to obtain the patient's consent to proceed to the exam as well as phrasings for each element of the exam, including sensitive body areas (genitalia, rectal exam, and others). Educators can obtain physical exam vocabulary from textbooks [70], online resources [63], or create their own. This training should include the concepts of common Hispanic/Latinx values such as *personalismo* ("personalism"), *simpatía* ("harmony/warmth in a relationship"), *respeto*, ("respect") and *confianza* ("trust") in class, didactic or interactive method [93, 94]. For example, students can review recorded simulated video encounters in pairs identifying if the above concepts are present and/or appropriately addressed by the clinician and orally communicate this to their partner. Most importantly, the learner needs to practice communicating these concepts with appropriate feedback, either in the classroom through role-play exercises or structured practice with SPs. This aligns with focusing the learning with end-goals in mind, per Kern's principles and TBLT [48, 52]. Educators may also use simulated encounters or provide model dialogues that represent communication during the physical examination. Additionally, educators can provide tasks, in English, related to specific exam components and instruct the learner to use the appropriate Spanish-language and culturally appropriate phrasing in a role-play.

Teaching students how to discuss the diagnosis and assessment with patients

One of the most important elements of the medical Spanish training program is instruction in providing a plausible explanation of the patient's problem, synthesizing the clinical information, and proving a potential evaluation and therapeutic plan. This advanced training should be sequenced after learners' mastery of basic interviewing skills and in line with the learners' stage of medical knowledge. Scheduling it beforehand would risk misunderstandings by both learner and patient and risk adherence to the plan and potentially the quality of care provided. For example, a learner who does not know how to recognize, evaluate, or treat gallbladder stones or appendicitis would have a more difficult time conveying this information accurately and answering the patient's concerns let alone explaining the risk and benefits to the testing, treatment and plan of therapy in Spanish. We recommend using interactive class activities that encourage learners to practice providing disease-specific explanations and needed testing and therapeutic plans to the patient. Classroom methods can include providing students with a written summary of a task to be used in role-play in pairs; for example, (1) inform a healthy 35-year-old woman that she has low back pain and not a bladder infection that she was worried about, addressing her fears and questions; (2) inform a young woman that she has an ectopic pregnancy and explain its risks and the need for an emergent consultation with an obstetrician/gynecologist; or (3) inform the father of a six-year-old that he has COVID-19, its severity and therapeutic plan as well as isolation recommendations. Educators can then provide real-time feedback to the learner to ensure learning of correct phrases and addressing the learner's questions. Creating condition or disease-specific phrasings to be learned ensure that this task-based goal is mastered and transferred to real world situations [51].

Integrating sociocultural context in medical Spanish education

Culture is integral to understanding a community and communicating with its members. Therefore, we encourage the inclusion of cultural topics relevant to the Spanish-speaking population in interactive classroom activities, student presentations, role-play cases, and testing scenarios with SPs.

The Hispanic/Latinx population is heterogeneous and educators should avoid promoting cultural stereotypes [23]. Integrating and training our students on cultural humility is crucial. Students must learn that culture is complex and dynamic, affects all people, does not determine behavior and cannot be distilled into a body of traits that is used as a checklist, implied by the term cultural competence [95]. Therefore, it is not possible to assume the patient's perception of health or behaviors based on their race, ethnicity, or country of origin [96]. We need to encourage and train learners and clinicians to become culturally humble and to create respectful partnerships with their patients [95]. Cultural humility invites healthcare providers to practice self-reflection, self-awareness, and commit to a lifelong learning about their patients and the community they serve. This approach makes them more open and humble to each patient's perspectives and goals, leaving behind the false sense of security that stereotyping gives and promoting a collaborative approach when establishing the treatment plan [75].

The inclusion of service-learning opportunities [18, 97, 98] and international immersion [18] are high-value elements that can promote cultural exposure and reflection to maximize cultural humility proficiency. Participation in required service-learning opportunities that involve direct patient care has been associated with higher cultural scores in nursing students [97] and should be part of the program when feasible.

Intentionally incorporating cultural nuances when creating realistic role-play cases is one of the most used methods to expose medical Spanish learners to cultural issues affecting Spanish-speaking populations. They can include cultural preferences for communication such as recognizing the benefit of using the more formal Spanish *usted* ("you") when addressing older people, of higher social status (e.g., professionals and clergy), or unknown to the interviewer to create an atmosphere of respect and avoid creating a cultural transgression that may limit communication. Incorporating *familismo* [93, 99], the concept of the value of the extended family unit, in cases can assist learners in exploring its potential role in decision-making to the Hispanic/Latinx patient. Other cultural aspects to incorporate in role-play cases include use of two last names and potential for name errors in the chart, use of alternative or complementary medicine, sharing of medications, procurement and use of medications from their home country [100], nutrition and food choices [101], cultural health beliefs, and death and dying preferences. Educators need to be cognizant of the danger of creating stereotypes of the Hispanic/Latinx population by only presenting a subset of their cultural aspects to the learners [102] and inform their learners of such.

Assessment of learner medical Spanish skills

The best method of evaluating competency in medical Spanish is through oral assessment [22]. The evaluation tools utilized to assess competency after this training need to reflect the real-world goal and the assessment is best accomplished by use of high-quality case scenarios utilizing trained SPs. SPs are trained actors who play the role of a patient with a specific medical problem, and SP encounters are a routine part of clinical skills training and assessment in U.S. medical education. Creating SP encounters consisting of simple to complex medical care scenarios aligned to assess course objectives in a safe environment, helps provide the learner with formative and summative evaluations of their medical Spanish. How learners' skills are assessed during these encounters is variable and the subject of ongoing research. According to some educators, students' use of language during medical encounters is assessed on pronunciation, grammar accuracy, grammar sophistication, vocabulary, formality (e.g., correct and consistent use of tú/usted), pace and fluency, comprehensibility and comprehension, and feedback is provided [Conversation between Marco Alemán, MD and Carmen Pérez-Muñoz, PhD (July 2022)]. In addition, this feedback may reduce any learner overconfidence that would otherwise lead to overestimation of their medical Spanish skills in clinical encounters without recognizing their errors, known as false-fluency [9, 17] and that has been associated with medical errors [4].

The cases should strive to assess all aspects of the medical encounter in Spanish, including the medical interview, exam commands, and the explanation of an assessment/diagnosis, evaluation, and management plan to the patient. The SPs selected should reflect the regional and linguistic background of the patient in the case to make it realistic (e.g., an SP whose variety of Spanish is aligned with the nationality of the patient being portrayed, such as an actor with a Caribbean accent to represent a patient from Cuba or the Dominican Republic) and should undergo training to improve the reliability of case representation and reduce variability [103]. The encounter checklists should represent the specific goals of the encounter such as specific history items that allow for higher complex history and decision-making, provision of commands for instructions of a sensitive or invasive exam (e.g., pelvic and rectal), provision of serious news, or discussion of goals of care, among others. Provision of specific feedback to the learner allows the targeting of tailored and goal-oriented areas for improvement as the learner progresses in medical Spanish training. The Comunicación y Habilidades Interpersonales (CAI), a Spanish Communication and Interpersonal Skills (CIS) scale, is a validated tool adapted for cultural and linguistic elements for use by SPs and that can serve to provide learners with feedback about their interpersonal skills in standardized medical Spanish encounters [104].

Recommendations for medical language education and research

Recommendations for research in medical Spanish education

Standardizing medical Spanish education teaching and learner assessment will help meet linguistic, medical, and ethical standards. To achieve this, robust and structured research methodology and evaluation metrics are needed. The professional non-profit organization NAMS [38] has been working to meet this goal. The NAMS consists of physicians, Spanish language professors, linguists, medical interpreters, and students who are committed to identify, conduct research on, and disseminate the best medical Spanish education teaching and evaluation practices. NAMS aims to create and administer a national medical Spanish certifying exam [105]; similar to the now discontinued United States Medical Licensing Examination (USMLE) Step 2 Clinical Skills (CS) [106] to assess learners' clinical skills proficiency in medical Spanish. We encourage medical Spanish educators to join or collaborate with NAMS.

Future research should focus on the best methodologies for training learners in medical Spanish. For example, what classroom techniques yield the highest benefit for learning and applying the new medical Spanish training in direct patient care? Research should continue to explore the best learning resources and this includes creating training resources suitable to the advanced learner. We should explore the benefits of using TBLT, as has been recently proposed [52], CBI and PBL SLA methodologies to teach medical Spanish. We recognize the value of combining language and clinical experts to optimize best training practices. NAMS is currently studying the standardization of curriculum and assessment used by medical Spanish educators. More research is also needed on how we can assist those institutions with limited resources of trained personnel or evaluation resources. The COVID-19 pandemic begat an expansion of virtual learning that has provided educators with new opportunities to collaborate virtually, including in medical Spanish education [54], allowing various educators to share their expertise across what were once geographic limitations. More research on virtual medical Spanish education is needed.

The benefit of ongoing contact with Spanish-speaking individuals and their communities during the training is critical for learning and applying medical Spanish lessons but also allows for contextual learning and exploration of the target populations' culture.

Research should continue to explore the benefits and limitations of various approaches to accomplish this, including service learning and immersion.

As we expand medical Spanish programs, research should continue to explore the benefit of using SPs for formative and summative evaluations. Research should help identify a standardized method for evaluating these SP encounters for programmatic needs and, eventually, for a national standardized exam.

Another area rich for research is teaching medical Spanish to resident physicians who are in graduate medical education training programs. Alignment with ACGME standards [107] that programs must adhere to is crucial. Currently, some of this work has started by individuals and selected training programs that are part of NAMS.

Recommendations for education

Recommendations for teaching crosslinguistic communication skills

All health professional learners should undergo training in crosslinguistic skills to engage with their non-English-speaking patients. This includes recognizing and understanding the linguistic diversity and the impact of language on population health. Similarly, medical Spanish learners should receive and build on that knowledge, expanding it as it relates to the heterogeneous Spanish-speaking population. Medical Spanish learners benefit from exploring the heterogeneity of Spanish and how it affects their communication with their patients. In addition, medical Spanish learners should examine how their patients' lack of English language proficiency affects their access to healthcare, understanding of medical information, and knowledge that contributes to health disparities in the Hispanic/Latinx population.

Cross-cultural medicine has a variety of approaches that healthcare professionals can utilize to elicit patients' health beliefs without stereotyping [76]. Researchers have identified the value of adapting the motivational interviewing principles to include cultural aspects. Integrating cultural values and beliefs in motivational interviewing has helped establish confidence and improve treatment adherence among patients in global settings [108].

All clinicians, including medical Spanish learners, need training in how their patient's culture affects communication and their patient's interpretation of their illness and goals of care. However, the medical Spanish learners would behoove themselves to be even more attentive to the specific cultural norms of the Hispanic/Latinx patient. For example, knowing the most common types of foods consumed by specific Hispanic/Latinx subgroups can help identify how to guide the nutrition history and provide specific modifications that are suitable to that person. One would recommend eating less tortillas to their Mexican patients with diabetes and less arepas to those who are from Venezuela, but not vice-versa.

All clinicians need to recognize and be self-aware of their non-English language proficiency to identify when they need to request an interpreter. Even intermediate and advanced non-English language speakers benefit if they have not undergone training in medical vocabulary and other aspects in the target language. Lastly, all health professions students and clinicians need to be educated on how to identify and work with professional medical interpreters [33]. This helps improve communication with the patient, reduce costs of care, encourage more patient questions, improve patient satisfaction with the encounter, and reduce health disparities.

Recommendations for medical Spanish education

Educators should adhere to Reuland's principles [18] in creating a medical Spanish curriculum including selecting and grouping intermediate to advanced learners according to their proficiency level. When possible, we highly recommend combining a clinician with a second language acquisition (SLA) specialist [22], each providing their expertise, intertwining their knowledge, and enriching the experience for the learner. Interactive sessions, maximizing oral communication by learners to create, modify and utilize medical Spanish vocabulary and phrasing useful in the patient interaction is preferred [22]. Intertwining medical Spanish course material with the learners' usual medical school curricula will enhance their learning by contextualizing the experience [109]. The inclusion of the importance and exploration of culture in the Hispanic/Latinx population in-class activities, reflection, and service learning is paramount. Educators and researchers should collaborate to create, expand, and investigate new print and online resources for use in medical Spanish education given the limited scope of online resources [63] and print materials for intermediate to advanced learners of medical Spanish [69] currently available. The curriculum should include methods for the learner to self-assess regarding their language skills [69], self-correct in real time during encounters and identify their limitations and the need to include an interpreter. Self-assessment is crucial, as the learner may not have external feedback on their performance in the future after the training is completed.

Educators should advocate for a standardized process for certification of bilingual Spanish-speaking healthcare students and clinicians at their home institutions and teaching hospitals [34, 60]. The Clinician Cultural and Linguistic Assessment-Spanish (CCLA-S) [32] is an available standardized assessment to ascertain if a clinician is qualified to practice as a bilingual provider. Additional research is needed to develop other methods for establishing that clinicians are qualified to use a nondominant language in patient care. Employers should incentivize the bilingual clinician certification process by allocating additional pay, as has been done in some entities [17]. This recognizes and rewards participation in a medical language training programs, incentivizes future learners, and helps increase the pool of available Spanish-speaking clinicians. Lessons learned in medical Spanish education may be modified for use when teaching other non-English medical languages in medicine or other health professions.

Conclusion

All health professions students, including medical students, should be trained in crosslinguistic healthcare communication skills to engage with patients of diverse linguistic and cultural backgrounds and needs. In the United States context, the LCME advocates and lists communication skills as foundation skills to be taught in medical schools while leaving the methods to the discretion of the individual medical schools [25]. This training enhances communication with patients and their families to improve health and reduce health disparities. Educators outside the United States should consider developing crosslinguistic healthcare communication skills training as appropriate for their learners and the needs of their respective communities.

The United States, like other countries, has a plurality of immigrants and languages used by their respective communities. Many individuals from linguistically diverse communities are unable to communicate with their clinicians without an interpreter, yet professional interpreters may not be easily available to them. Furthermore, language-concordant care is superior to interpreter-mediated care and has been identified as a goal for better communication of clinicians with their NELP patients [10]. Depending on the population served, healthcare systems need to not only hire professional interpreters but must also train and recruit bilingual and bicultural clinicians to adequately meet the language needs of the local population.

The Hispanic/Latinx population in the United States is the largest segment of the population with many being Spanish speaking and accounting for the majority of the United States population with non-English language preference. Medical Spanish training programs can increase the number of language-concordant clinicians and be pivotal in bridging the communication gap between the Spanish-speaking populations and their clinicians. Such medical Spanish programs have a high degree of variability in their goals, methods of instruction, and evaluation. This variation is both a limitation as well as an opportunity to contribute valuable research and methodology to the field. There is a growing list of resources, individuals, and academic and non-profit institutions seeking to enhance and standardize medical Spanish training and evaluation. Through collaboration, invested educators and researchers can help identify and secure the needed funding that will allow for evidence-based growth of both crosslinguistic communication training and medical language education for clinicians caring for linguistically diverse populations.

Highlights

- More research is needed to continually evaluate evidence-based methods to assess bilingual Spanish-speaking clinicians and ensure appropriate qualification to independently communicate with Spanish-speaking patients.
- Educators should select intermediate and advanced learners for medical Spanish training and group them by proficiency level for their training.
- Individuals who teach and assess medical Spanish skills should emphasize oral communication in clinician training, clinician skills assessment, and evaluation of program effectiveness.
- All health professional learners should undergo training in crosslinguistic skills to engage with their non-English-speaking patients.
- Healthcare systems should actively recruit, train, and compensate the language skills of bilingual and bicultural clinicians.
- Unless determined to be qualified by a validated assessment method for medical language proficiency, clinicians should work with professional interpreters in clinical encounters with patients who prefer non-English languages for health communication.

REFERENCES

1. U.S. Census Bureau Quick Facts: United States (2022). https://www.census.gov/quickfacts/fact/table/US/RHI725219 (accessed 15 August 2023).

2. U.S. Census Bureau: Hispanic Population to Reach 111 Million by 2060. U.S. Census Bureau. 2018. https://www.census.gov/library/visualizations/2018/comm/

hispanic-projected-pop.html (accessed 30 July 2022).
3. Zhong, J. and Batalova, J. (2015). *The Limited English Proficient Population in the United States in 2013*. Migration Policy Institute. https://www.migrationpolicy.org/article/limited-english-proficient-population-united-states-2013 (accessed 30 July 2022).
4. Divi, C., Koss, R.G., Schmaltz, S.P., and Loeb, J.M. (2007). Language proficiency and adverse events in US hospitals: a pilot study. *Int. J. Qual. Health Care* 19 (2): 60–67.
5. Hampers, L.C., Cha, S., Gutglass, D.J. et al. (1999). Language barriers and resource utilization in a pediatric emergency department. *Pediatrics* 103 (6 Pt 1): 1253–1256.
6. Flores, G. (2005). The impact of medical interpreter services on the quality of health care: a systematic review. *Med. Care Res. Rev.* 62 (3): 255–299.
7. The U.S. Department of Health and Human Services (2013). *Guidance to Federal Financial Assistance Recipients Regarding Title VI and the Prohibition Against National Origin Discrimination Affecting Limited English Proficient Persons - Summary*. The Office for Civil Rights. https://www.hhs.gov/civil-rights/for-providers/laws-regulations-guidance/guidance-federal-financial-assistance-title-vi/index.html (accessed 31 July 2022).
8. Karliner, L.S., Pérez-Stable, E.J., and Gregorich, S.E. (2017). Convenient access to professional interpreters in the hospital decreases readmission rates and estimated hospital expenditures for patients with limited English proficiency. *Med. Care* 55 (3): 199–206.
9. Diamond, L.C., Schenker, Y., Curry, L. et al. (2009). Getting by: underuse of interpreters by resident physicians. *J. Gen. Intern. Med.* 24 (2): 256–262.
10. Ngo-Metzger, Q., Sorkin, D.H., Phillips, R.S. et al. (2007). Providing high-quality care for limited English proficient patients: the importance of language concordance and interpreter use. *J. Gen. Intern. Med.* 22 (Suppl 2): 324–330.
11. Aranguri, C., Davidson, B., and Ramirez, R. (2006). Patterns of communication through interpreters: a detailed sociolinguistic analysis. *J. Gen. Intern. Med.* 21 (6): 623–629.
12. Allison, A. and Hardin, K. (2020). Missed opportunities to build rapport: a pragmalinguistic analysis of interpreted medical conversations with Spanish-speaking patients. *Health Commun.* 35 (4): 494–501.
13. Rivadeneyra, R., Elderkin-Thompson, V., Silver, R.C., and Waitzkin, H. (2000). Patient centeredness in medical encounters requiring an interpreter. *Am. J. Med.* 108 (6): 470–474.
14. Seijo, R., Gomez, H., and Freidenberg, J. (1991). Language as a communication barrier in medical care for Hispanic patients. *Hisp. J. Behav. Sci.* 13 (4): 363–376.
15. Association of American Medical Colleges (2023). *Table B-4: Total U.S. Medical School Graduates by Race/Ethnicity and Sex, 2018–2019 through 2022–2023*. https://www.aamc.org/download/321536/data/factstableb4.pdf.
16. Garcia, M.E., Bindman, A.B., and Coffman, J. (2019). Language-concordant primary care physicians for a diverse population: the view from California. *Health Equity* 3 (1): 343–349.
17. Fernández, A. and Pérez-Stable, E.J. (2015). Doctor, habla español? Increasing the supply and quality of language-concordant physicians for Spanish-speaking patients. *J. Gen. Intern. Med.* 30 (10): 1394–1396.
18. Reuland, D.S., Frasier, P.Y., Slatt, L.M., and Alemán, M.A. (2008). A longitudinal medical Spanish program at one US medical school. *J. Gen. Intern. Med.* 23 (7): 1033.
19. Ortega, P., Diamond, L., Alemán, M.A. et al. (2020). Medical Spanish standardization in US medical schools: consensus statement from a multidisciplinary expert panel. *Acad. Med.* 95 (1): 22–31.
20. Ortega, P., Francone, N.O., Santos, M.P. et al. (2021). Medical Spanish in US medical schools: a national survey to examine existing programs. *J. Gen. Intern. Med.* 36 (9): 2724–2730.

21. Hardin, K. (2012). Targeting oral and cultural proficiency for medical personnel: an examination of current medical Spanish textbooks. *Hispania* 95 (4): 698–713.
22. Ortega, K.J. and Hardin, D.M. (2013). Medical Spanish programs in the United States: a critical review of published studies and a proposal of best practices. *Teach. Learn. Med.* 25 (4): 306–311.
23. Ortega, P., Park, Y.S., and Girotti, J.A. (2017). Evaluation of a medical Spanish elective for senior medical students: improving outcomes through OSCE assessments. *Med. Sci. Educ.* 27 (2): 329–337.
24. Ortega, P., Pérez, N., Robles, B. et al. (2019). Strategies for teaching linguistic preparedness for physicians: medical Spanish and global linguistic competence in undergraduate medical education. *Health Equity* 3 (1): 312–318.
25. (2023). Liaison Committee on Medical Education https://lcme.org/ (accessed 15 August 2023).
26. Puebla Fortier, J., Shaw Taylor, Y., Convissor, R., and Pacheco, G. (1999). *Assuring Cultural Competence in Health Care: Recommendations for National Standards and an Outcomes-Focused Research Agenda (1999)*. Washington, DC: US Department of Health and Human Services Office of Minority Health.
27. Chomsky, N. (1980). *Rules and Representations*. Columbia University Press.
28. Georgetown University NC for CC *What is Linguistic Competency?* New Jersey Statewide Network for Cultural Competence https://www.nj.gov/njsncc/resources/what-is/ (accessed 31 July 2022).
29. O'Toole, J.K., Alvarado-Little, W., and Ledford, C.J. (2019). Communication with diverse patients: addressing culture and language. *Pediatr. Clin.* 66 (4): 791–804.
30. The Joint Commission (2017). *Language Access and Interpreters Services- Understanding the Requirements. Manual: Hospital and Hospital Clinics Chapter: Rights and Responsibilities of the Individual*. The Joint Commission https://www.jointcommission.org/standards/standard-faqs/hospital-and-hospital-clinics/rights-and-responsibilities-of-the-individual-ri/000002120/ (accessed 31 July 2022).
31. Diamond, L.C., Tuot, D.S., and Karliner, L.S. (2012). The use of Spanish language skills by physicians and nurses: policy implications for teaching and testing. *J. Gen. Intern. Med.* 27 (1): 117–123. https://doi.org/10.1007/s11606-011-1779-5.
32. Clinician Cultural and Linguistic Assessment (CCLA) ALTA Language Services. https://www.altalang.com/language-testing/ccla/ (accessed 31 July 2022).
33. Diamond, L.C. and Jacobs, E.A. (2010). Let's not contribute to disparities: the best methods for teaching clinicians how to overcome language barriers to health care. *J. Gen. Intern. Med.* 25 (2): 189–193.
34. Hadziabdic, E. and Hjelm, K. (2013). Working with interpreters: practical advice for use of an interpreter in healthcare. *Int. J. Evid. Based Healthc.* 11 (1): 69–76.
35. Martínez, G.A. (2020). *Spanish in Health Care*. New York: Taylor & Francis.
36. Gonzalez-Lee, T. and Simon, H.J. (1987). Teaching Spanish and cross-cultural sensitivity to medical students. *West. J. Med.* 146 (4): 502–504.
37. Morales, R., Rodriguez, L., Singh, A. et al. (2015). National survey of medical Spanish curriculum in U.S. medical schools. *J. Gen. Intern. Med.* 30 (10): 1434–1439.
38. National Association of Medical Spanish *Working Together for Healthier Communication*. National Association of Medical Spanish. https://www.namspanish.org/ (accessed 31 July 2022).
39. Interagency Language Roundtable. *Interagency Language Roundtable*. 2011. https://www.govtilr.org/ (accessed 30 July 2022).
40. Diamond, L.C., Luft, H.S., Chung, S., and Jacobs, E.A. (2012). "Does this doctor speak my language?" Improving the characterization of physician non-English language skills. *Health Serv. Res.* 47 (1 Pt 2): 556–569.
41. Diamond, L., Chung, S., Ferguson, W. et al. (2014). Relationship between self-assessed and tested non-English-language proficiency among primary care providers. *Med. Care* 52 (5): 435–438.

42. Reuland, D.S., Frasier, P.Y., Olson, M.D. et al. (2009). Accuracy of self-assessed Spanish fluency in medical students. *Teach. Learn. Med.* 21 (4): 305–309.
43. Lie, D.A., Nodal, S., de la Torre, M. et al. (2020). Impact of a longitudinal medical Spanish curriculum on student communication skills. *J. Physician Assist. Educ.* 31 (1): 23–27.
44. Bloom, M., Timmerman, G.M., and Sands, D. (2006). Developing a course to teach Spanish for health care professionals. *J. Nurs. Educ.* 45 (7): 271–274.
45. Martinez, G.A., Parés-Avila, J.A., Graham, M. et al. (2021). Communicating and coaching in Spanish for chronic care. *J. Nurs. Educ.* 60 (1): 34–37.
46. Garavalia, L.S., Chan, L., Ortiz, M. et al. (2017). Student-led co-curricular medical Spanish training in a pharmacy professional program. *Curr. Pharm. Teach. Learn.* 9 (4): 644–651.
47. Mueller, R. (2017). Development and evaluation of an intermediate-level elective course on medical Spanish for pharmacy students. *Curr. Pharm. Teach. Learn.* 9 (2): 288–295.
48. Thomas, P.A., Kern, D.E., Hughes, M.T. et al. (ed.) (2022). *Curriculum Development for Medical Education: A Six-Step Approach*. JHU Press.
49. Long, M. (2014). *Second Language Acquisition and Task-Based Language Teaching*. John Wiley & Sons.
50. O'Rourke, K., Gruener, G., Quinones, D. et al. (2013). Spanish bilingual medical student certification. *MedEdPORTAL Publications*. (accessed 5 February, 2022). https://www.mededportal.org/doi/10.15766/mep_2374-8265.9400.
51. Vega, T.A., Contag, A.G., Urbanowicz, E. et al. (2021). Introductory medical Spanish elective: creating and evaluating a case-based course compatible with an 18-month pre-clinical medical curriculum. *Med. Sci. Educ.* 31 (2): 495–502.
52. Coss, M.D. (2022). The case for a true task-based curriculum for medical Spanish courses. *Teach. Learn. Med.* 35: 1–16.
53. Flores, G. and Mendoza, F.S. (2002). ¿Dolor aquí? ¿Fiebre?: a little knowledge requires caution. *Arch. Pediatr. Adolesc. Med.* 156 (7): 638–640.
54. Ortega, P., Shin, T.M., Francone, N.O. et al. (2021). Student and faculty diversity is insufficient to ensure high-quality medical Spanish education in US medical schools. *J. Immigr. Minor. Health* 23 (5): 1105–1109.
55. Content Based Instruction (2011). *Teaching and Researching Reading* (ed. W. Grabe and F.L. Stoller). Harlow, England: Longman/Pearson Print.
56. Accreditation Council for Graduate Medical Education. *ACGME Core Competencies*. https://www.acgme.org/what-we-do/accreditation/common-program-requirements/.
57. Chatterjee, A. and Talwalkar, J.S. (2012). An innovative medical Spanish curriculum for resident doctors. *Med. Educ.* 46 (5): 521–522.
58. Barr, W.B., Valdini, A., Louis, J.S. et al. (2018). Sí, tu puedes: an integrated Spanish language acquisition in residency utilizing personal instruction. *J. Grad. Med. Educ.* 10 (3): 343–344.
59. Mazor, S.S., Hampers, L.C., Chande, V.T., and Krug, S.E. (2002). Teaching Spanish to pediatric emergency physicians: effects on patient satisfaction. *Arch. Pediatr. Adolesc. Med.* 156 (7): 693–695.
60. Lion, K.C., Thompson, D.A., Cowden, J.D. et al. (2013). Clinical Spanish use and language proficiency testing among pediatric residents. *Acad. Med.* 88 (10): 1478–1484.
61. Cowden, J.D., Thompson, D.A., Ellzey, J., and Artman, M. (2012). Getting past getting by: training culturally and linguistically competent bilingual physicians. *J. Pediatr.* 160 (6): 891–892.e1.
62. Cowden, J.D., Martinez, F.J., Dickmeyer, J.J., and Bratcher, D. (2022). Culture and language coaching for bilingual residents: the first 10 years of the CHiCoS model. *Teach. Learn. Med.* 1–12. https://doi.org/10.1080/10401334.2022.2092113.
63. Ortega, P., Hardin, K., Pérez-Cordón, C. et al. (2021). An overview of online resources for medical Spanish education for effective communication with Spanish-speaking patients. *Teach. Learn. Med.* 34: 1–13.

64. Prince, D. and Nelson, M. (1995). Teaching Spanish to emergency medicine residents. *Acad. Emerg. Med.* 2 (1): 32–36. discussion 36.
65. Grall, K.H., Panchal, A.R., Chuffe, E., and Stoneking, L.R. (2016). Feasibility of Spanish-language acquisition for acute medical care providers: novel curriculum for emergency medicine residencies. *Adv. Med. Educ. Pract.* 7: 81–86.
66. Hardin, K. (2015). An overview of medical Spanish curricula in the United States. *Hispania* 98: 640–661.
67. Ortega, P., Avila, S., and Park, Y.S. (2022). Patient-reported quality of communication skills in the clinical workplace for clinicians learning medical Spanish. *Cureus* 14 (2): e22222.
68. Nguyen, H.T. (2016). Interactional practices across settings: from classroom role-plays to workplace patient consultations. *Appl. Linguis.* 39 (2): 213–235.
69. Shin, T.M., Hardin, K., Johnston, D. et al. (2021). Scoping review of textbooks for medical Spanish education. *Med. Sci. Educ.* 31 (4): 1519–1527.
70. Ortega, P. (2016). *Spanish and the Medical Interview: A Textbook for Clinically Relevant Medical Spanish*, 2ee. Philadelphia, PA: Elsevier.
71. Ortega, P. and Alemán, M.A. (2022). *Spanish and the Medical Interview: Clinical Cases and Exam Review*, 1ee. Philadelphia, PA: Elsevier.
72. Peterson, M.C., Holbrook, J.H., Von Hales, D. et al. (1992). Contributions of the history, physical examination, and laboratory investigation in making medical diagnoses. *West. J. Med.* 156 (2): 163–165. 2. Lown B. The lost art of healing: practicing compassion in medicine. New York Ballantine Books: 1999.
73. Hampton, J.R., Harrison, M.J., Mitchell, J.R. et al. (1975). Relative contributions of history-taking, physical examination, and laboratory investigation to diagnosis and management of medical outpatients. *Br. Med. J.* 2 (5969): 486–489.
74. Ortega, P., Pérez, N., Robles, B. et al. (2019). Teaching medical Spanish to improve population health: evidence for incorporating language education and assessment in U.S. medical schools. *Health Equity* 3 (1): 557–566.
75. Tervalon, M. and Murray-García, J. (1998). Cultural humility versus cultural competence: a critical distinction in defining physician training outcomes in multicultural education. *J. Health Care Poor Underserved* 9 (2): 117–125.
76. Solchanyk, D., Ekeh, O., Saffran, L. et al. (2021). Integrating cultural humility into the medical education curriculum: strategies for educators. *Teach. Learn. Med.* 33: 1–7.
77. Kleinman, A., Eisenberg, L., and Good, B. (1978). Culture, illness, and care: clinical lessons from anthropologic and cross-cultural research. *Ann. Intern. Med.* 88 (2): 251–258.
78. Koester, A.J. (2002). The performance of speech acts in workplace conversations and the teaching of communicative functions. *System* 30 (2): 167–184.
79. Davis, R.E., Lee, S., Johnson, T.P., and Rothschild, S.K. (2019). Measuring the elusive construct of personalismo among mexican american, puerto rican, and cuban american adults. *Hisp. J. Behav. Sci.* 41 (1): 103–121.
80. Platt, F.W. and McMath, J.C. (1979). Clinical hypocompetence: the interview. *Ann. Intern. Med.* 91 (6): 898–902.
81. Oxford, R.L. (2001). Language learning strategies. In: *The Cambridge Guide to Teaching English to Speakers of Other Languages* (ed. R. Carter and D. Nunan), 166–172. Cambridge: Cambridge University Press (The Cambridge Guides).
82. Hellman, A.B., Wilbur, A., Harris, K.A., and Short, D. (2019). *The 6 Principles for Exemplary Teaching of English Learners®: Adult Education and Workforce Development*. Chicago: TESOL Press.
83. Tedick, D. and Gortari, B. (1998). *Research on Error Correction and Implications for Classroom Teaching*, vol. vol 1. The Bridge, ACIE Newsletter. Center for Advanced Research on Language Acquisition, University of Minnesota http://www.carla.umn.edu/immersion/acie/vol1/May1998.pd.

84. Keemink, Y., Custers, E.J.F.M., van Dijk, S., and Ten Cate, O. (2018). Illness script development in pre-clinical education through case-based clinical reasoning training. *Int. J. Med. Educ.* 9: 35–41.
85. Davidson, Lauren, and Sheri Spaine Long. (2013). "Medical Spanish for US Medical Students: A Pilot Case Study." Dimension 2013: World Language Learning Setting the Global Standard. Ed. Peter B. Swanson and Kristin Hoyt. Decatur. Southern Conference on Language Teaching. 9–22. https://eric.ed.gov/?id=EJ1211308.
86. García, O. and Wei, L. (2012). Translanguaging. In: *The Encyclopedia of Applied Linguistics* (ed. C.A. Chapelle), 1–7. Wiley.
87. Ortega, P. and Prada, J. (2020). Words matter: Translanguaging in medical communication skills training. *Perspect. Med. Educ.* 9 (4): 251–255.
88. Arteaga, D. and Llorente, L. (2009). Spanish as an international language: implications for teachers and learners. In: *Multilingual Matters*. ProQuest Ebook Central. https://ebookcentral-proquest-com.libproxy.lib.unc.edu/lib/unc/detail.action?docID=449884.
89. Anderson, K.M., Leister, S., and De Rego, R. (2020). The 5Ts for teach back: an operational definition for teach-back training. *Health Lit. Res. Pract.* 4 (2): e94–e103.
90. Ackert, E., Hong, S.H., Martinez, J. et al. (2021). Understanding the health landscapes where latinx immigrants establish residence in the US. *Health Aff. (Millwood)* 40 (7): 1108–1116.
91. Friedman, A.S. and Venkataramani, A.S. (2021). Chilling effects: US immigration enforcement and health care seeking among Hispanic adults. *Health Aff. (Millwood)* 40 (7): 1056–1065.
92. Philbin, M.M., Flake, M., Hatzenbuehler, M.L., and Hirsch, J.S. (2018). State-level immigration and immigrant-focused policies as drivers of Latino health disparities in the United States. *Soc. Sci. Med.* 199: 29–38.
93. Dingfelder, S.F. (2005). Cultural considerations. *Monit. Psychol.* 36 (1): 59. http://www.apa.org/monitor/jan05/considerations.
94. Magaña, D. (2021). *Building Confianza: Empowering Latinos/as through Transcultural Health Care Communication*. The Ohio State University Press.
95. Hunt, L.M. (2019). Beyond cultural competence: Applying humility to clinical settings. In: *The Social Medicine Reader, Volume II, Third Edition*, 127–131. Duke University Press.
96. O'Connor, B.B. (1996). Promoting cultural competence in HIV/AIDS care. *J. Assoc. Nurses AIDS Care* 7: 41–53.
97. Abrams, M.P., Chalise, S., Peralta, H., and Simms-Cendan, J. (2021). Social, demographic, Spanish language, and experiential factors influencing nursing students' cultural competence. *J. Nurs. Educ.* 60 (1): 29–33.
98. Gazsi, C.C. and Oriel, K.N. (2010). The impact of a service learning experience to enhance curricular integration in a physical therapist education program. *J. Allied Health* 39 (2): 61E–67E.
99. Smith-Morris, C., Morales-Campos, D., Alvarez, E.A.C., and Turner, M. (2013). An anthropology of familismo. *Hisp. J. Behav. Sci.* 35 (1): 35–60.
100. Vissman, A.T., Bloom, F.R., Leichliter, J.S. et al. (2011). Exploring the use of nonmedical sources of prescription drugs among immigrant Latinos in the rural southeastern USA. *J. Rural Health* 27 (2): 159–167.
101. Mattei, J., Sotres-Alvarez, D., Daviglus, M.L. et al. (2016). Diet quality and its association with cardiometabolic risk factors vary by Hispanic and Latino ethnic background in the Hispanic Community Health Study/Study of Latinos. *J. Nutr.* 146 (10): 2035–2044.
102. Ortega, P., Martínez, G., Alemán, M.A. et al. (2022). Recognizing and dismantling raciolinguistic hierarchies in latinx health. *AMA J. Ethics* 24 (4): E296–E304.
103. Cleland, J.A., Abe, K., and Rethans, J.-J. (2009). The use of simulated patients in medical education: AMEE Guide No 42. *Med. Teach.* 31 (6): 477–486.

104. Ortega, P., Moxon, N.R., Chokshi, A.K. et al. (2021). Validity evidence supporting the comunicación y habilidades interpersonales (CAI) scale for medical Spanish communication and interpersonal skills assessment. *Acad. Med.* 96 (11S): S93–S102.
105. Ortega, P. (2018). Spanish language concordance in U.S. medical care: a multifaceted challenge and call to action. *Acad. Med.* 93 (9): 1276–1280.
106. USMLE Step 2 Clinical Skills Wikipedia, the free encyclopedia. https://en.wikipedia.org/wiki/USMLE_Step_2_Clinical_Skills (accessed 1 August 2022).
107. Accreditation Council of Graduate Medical Education. Accreditation Council of Graduate Medical Education. https://www.acgme.org/ (accessed 1 August 2022).
108. Oh, H. and Lee, C. (2016). Culture and motivational interviewing. *Patient Educ. Couns.* 99 (11): 1914–1919.
109. Shrum, J. and Glisan, E. (2010). *Teacher's Handbook: Contextualized Language Instruction*, 4ee. Boston, MA: Heinle.

18 Medical Language Programs to Enhance Engagement with Diverse Communities in the United States and Around the World

ROSE L. MOLINA AND JENNIFER KASPER

Introduction

We live in a richly diverse linguistic biome: more than 7000 languages are spoken among the 7.9 billion people (and counting) who inhabit our planet [1]. While the five most spoken languages are English (1.13 billion speakers), Mandarin (1.12 billion), Hindi (615 million), Spanish (534 million), and French (280 million speakers), each continent has an astounding linguistic variety within their borders. For example, there are more than 1500 languages in Sub-Saharan Africa alone [2].

Languages infuse every aspect of our globalized world and are critical to communication in health-related clinical care, research, teaching, and advocacy in all countries. A plethora of data demonstrates the power of the spoken word to enhance the therapeutic alliance and patient experience [3–5]; reduce medical errors and enrich patient care [6, 7]; and diminish health inequities and improve health outcomes [8–11]. With increasingly diverse student bodies and patient populations everywhere, undergraduate and preprofessional training are optimal times to expand language proficiency to improve patient outcomes, promote authentic collaboration, reduce burden on local staff and communities, enhance equity, and begin to mitigate centuries of racism and colonialism and their impacts on health.

Language learning is just as critical in the United States, as it is around the world, because of the number of individuals, including both immigrants and United States-born persons, who prefer to communicate in non-English languages. More than 350 languages are spoken in the United States, resulting in broad linguistic diversity of the patient populations seen at many medical institutions throughout the country. In the United States,

---

The Handbook of Language in Public Health and Healthcare, First Edition.
Edited by Pilar Ortega, Glenn Martínez, Maichou Lor, and A. Susana Ramírez.
© 2024 John Wiley & Sons, Inc. Published 2024 by John Wiley & Sons, Inc.

approximately 10% of the population aged 16–64 years old reports having limited English proficiency (defined as speaking English less than very well), with approximately one-third speaking Spanish as their preferred language [12]. The population with limited English proficiency has lower education and earns less than the population with English proficiency [12]. Importantly, approximately 13% of the population with limited English proficiency are born in the United States [12]. Language prevalence varies by metropolitan area and may not always reflect the prevalence at the state level [13].

There is a growing need for medical and other health professionals to develop language skills in the most common non-English languages spoken in their geographic area in order to communicate directly and effectively with patients of different linguistic preferences. Linguistic minorities face additional access and communication barriers when there are less available interpreters and language-concordant clinicians [14]. While many medical schools offer courses for students to improve skills in Spanish [15], the most common non-English language spoken in the United States, much less information is available about providing medical language education in other non-English languages. While Mandarin is far more commonly spoken than Spanish on a global scale [1], there are very few medical Mandarin courses published in the peer-reviewed literature [16]. Offering medical language education in multiple languages is critical to build an inclusive healthcare workforce that can provide language-concordant care and better meet the needs of the diverse patient populations throughout the United States [17].

In this chapter, we present a case study of the Medical Language Program and opportunities for students to apply their language skills in global health electives at Harvard Medical School (HMS). The HMS Medical Language Program includes courses in Spanish, Portuguese, and Mandarin, with recent pilot courses based on student demand in Arabic and French. We also explore the relevance of language acquisition for global health engagement among medical students and other health professional students. We end with recommendations for building a robust medical language program based on our decades of experience in offering a variety of language courses.

Case study of the medical language program at Harvard Medical School

Background and history

HMS has been a national leader in offering a variety of medical language courses for decades (Figure 18.1). In the early 1970s, Dr. Guillermo Herrera, an internal medicine physician at Brigham and Women's Hospital who worked at both HMS and Harvard Chan School of Public Health, created the first credit-bearing HMS medical Spanish course and linked it with a primary care clinical elective in Colombia. Since the 1990s, the medical Spanish courses have expanded to include both longitudinal semester-long courses and intensive one-month courses at a variety of language proficiency levels. Additional longitudinal medical language courses in Mandarin, Portuguese, Haitian-Kreyol, French, and Arabic have been offered based on funding, student interest, and local language demographics. Matriculating students fill out a survey about their interest in enrolling in medical language courses, which is used to identify the number

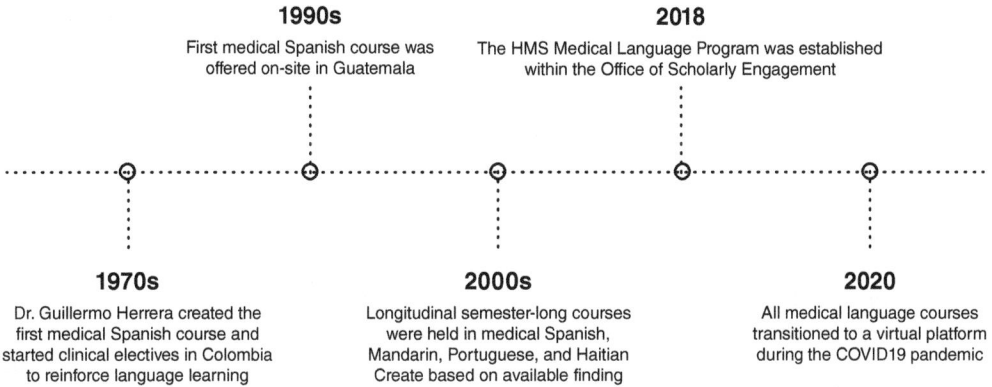

Figure 18.1 Timeline of the Harvard Medical School Medical Language Program.

and type of language courses offered each academic year. There is a required minimum of six enrolled students to hold a course. To date, student demand has mirrored language prevalence in Massachusetts [18], with the highest student demand for Spanish, Portuguese, and Mandarin. However, language prevalence varies by neighborhood within the Boston Metro Area [19], where HMS is located. All medical language courses are electives and are given for credit. Since the 1990s, medical students have also had the opportunity to pursue clinical electives with partner sites abroad to continue applying their language skills in clinical training. More than 1000 HMS students have taken a medical language course since the first medical Spanish course was offered in the 1970s.

In 2018, the Medical Language Program was formally established within the Office of Scholarly Engagement at HMS. This milestone created a sustainable home for the longitudinal medical language courses that were previously organized by medical students and dependent on external funding. A faculty director, administrative support staff, and a budget within the Office of Scholarly Engagement ensured that the Medical Language Program had the administrative oversight to provide continuity and growth opportunities for the students enrolled in the elective courses. Additionally, the Office of Scholarly Engagement is exploring how to incorporate language assessments prior to participation in global health electives and scholarly projects to ensure that students have the appropriate language skills and resources to participate in experiences in countries where the predominant language is not English. One study showed the lack of standardization across medical Spanish curricula in the United States, including study abroad initiatives and language assessment and preparation prior to global health experiences that require additional language skills [15].

Current medical language program scope

The goal of the HMS Medical Language Program is to advance equitable care by training medical students to provide language-concordant and culturally humble care for diverse patient populations. To that end, the Medical Language Program currently offers the following longitudinal medical language courses, which are designed for first-year Harvard medical students but open to any Harvard student, including those from other Harvard schools.

- Intermediate Medical Spanish (Fall and Spring semesters)
- Advanced Medical Spanish (Fall and Spring semesters)
- Intermediate Medical Portuguese (Fall semester only)
- Intermediate Medical Mandarin (Fall and Spring semesters)

Auditors from other area medical schools and affiliated hospitals are welcome to join if space permits. The average enrollment varies from 5 to 15 students per course, with a maximum of 15 students per instructor. The courses meet weekly for 1.5 hours for a total of 13 weeks each semester. In 2018–2019, approximately one-quarter of HMS students enrolled in at least one semester of a longitudinal medical language course or the intensive language elective course.

These courses are designed for at least intermediate-level students because students need a foundation in the language before learning additional medical terminology and their application in clinical care [20]. The medical language courses focus on developing oral proficiency with less emphasis on reading and writing proficiency. To facilitate oral proficiency in the Mandarin course for students who may lack reading and writing proficiency, the instructor uses both Chinese characters and pinyin pronunciation in the classroom.

The medical language instructors are clinicians experienced in medical training, teaching, and the language being taught. Most instructors are native speakers and have received university-level education in the target language. Only a few instructors are heritage speakers. None of the instructors trained in linguistics or language instruction, specifically. The instructors have been recruited through job postings in the HMS Program in Medical Education job board and through professional networks of faculty who have participated as guest speakers in the language courses in prior years and/or had listed language skills on their hospital websites. Applicants must have a HMS appointment or affiliation with a HMS clinical site. We require a cover letter with a statement about motivation for teaching a medical language course, updated CV, and an interview with our Office of Scholarly Engagement staff. We prioritize selecting faculty who have done at least some of their medical training in the target language and who have had prior experience with teaching HMS students. Of our current language instructors, all are physicians except for one clinical psychologist. In the past, we have extended teaching positions to allied health professionals for specific languages for which it was more difficult to recruit faculty. For example, the pilot course in medical Arabic was led by a professional medical interpreter at a clinical affiliate of HMS who had extensive experience in teaching Arabic in other adult learning settings. The professional Arabic interpreter was able to recruit faculty guest speakers to cover specific medical material that he felt less comfortable teaching.

A separate long-standing, credit-bearing intensive four-week medical Spanish course is designed for fourth-year medical students at the beginner, intermediate, or low-advanced levels. This course is currently taught by instructors from the International Health Central American Institute (IHCAI) in Costa Rica who can teach at various proficiency levels. HMS has maintained a long-standing institutional relationship with IHCAI Institute in the clinical exchange program through which medical students from HMS and from Costa Rica participate. Prior to the COVID-19 pandemic, IHCAI Institute instructors traveled to Boston to teach the course. During the COVID-19 pandemic, the instructors have taught remotely from Costa Rica. Instructors with expertise in Spanish grammar partner with physicians and medical students who also serve as language teachers to build proficiency through discussing medical cases from the beginner level. In our experience at HMS, intensive language learning is the fastest way to bring students with little experience in the language up to the level where they can collect pertinent medical information from a patient and present it in the target language by the time they finish the course. The IHCAI instructors have developed a simple history and physical exam case assessment to demonstrate student proficiency in obtaining basic medical information, which all students in the intensive course have passed.

Curriculum development and innovation

One aim of the Medical Language Program is to standardize the curricula for the medical language courses across the languages taught. In the mid-late 2000s, the continuity of curricular content and instructors of the medical language courses varied according to student interest, available instructors, and available funding. Once the Medical Language Program was incorporated into the Office of Scholarly Engagement, the Director began a process of aligning both the various medical language course curricula with each other and with the Practice of Medicine course, which is the foundational clinical course for first-year students that covers the comprehensive medical history and physical exam. This alignment was important for the following purposes: (1) to ensure that students learn clinical content first in English before being expected to learn it in a secondary language, (2) to ensure that the content in the secondary language reinforces the content taught in Practice of Medicine, and (3) to harmonize the experiences of students who take any medical language course such that the content is consistent if students choose to take more than one medical language course.

The first step to align the curricula and pedagogy across language courses was to obtain instructor buy-in on this idea across the courses. We co-led a two-hour workshop with the Director of the Office of Educational Quality Improvement in which all language instructors learned about methods for curricular development and alignment. Instructors shared what worked in their classrooms and collaborated to find solutions to common challenges, such as scheduling the sessions far enough in advance to accommodate the availability of guest speakers and interpreters. Additionally, we realized that the medical language schedule should follow the Practice of Medicine course by one to two weeks given the different days of the week students are assigned to each course. They also discussed the transition to teaching in the virtual platform in the context of the COVID-19 pandemic. The complete Practice of Medicine teaching materials were shared with medical language instructors as a reference for the content students learned in their core English-language course. As a result of the workshop, the instructors redesigned their curricula and pedagogy and shared their revised syllabi to ensure alignment with each other and with the Practice of Medicine course. The Office of Scholarly Engagement staff reviewed the syllabi of all medical language courses to ensure the topics followed the order of the Practice of Medicine course.

In addition to aligning the curricular content around the history and physical exam, the Director also sought to integrate sessions that aligned with the HMS societal themes of health equity and interprofessional training that were established in 2019. Each language course instructor dedicated at least one session to cultural humility, cultural context for addressing health issues, and overcoming inequities experienced by specific linguistic minority populations. For example, the medical Mandarin course included a session on culturally sensitive ways of approaching discussions regarding end-of-life care in East Asian cultures. Additionally, each course included a session on working with interpreters in the target language, which was led by an interpreter from an affiliated hospital. In their course evaluations, students consistently raved about the interpreter session because they learned relevant, actionable best practices for collaborating with an interpreter to bridge linguistic and cultural differences. Prior to the COVID-19 pandemic, the Medical Language Program provided students with opportunities to shadow interpreters in the target language for a morning or afternoon at the affiliated clinical sites to enhance their clinical language learning experiences. Students always reported the experience as a meaningful one and sought it out when it was available.

The pedagogy of the medical language courses deploys a variety of methods, including didactic sessions, case-based discussion, role play in small and large groups, and 1:1 practice with primary language speakers, including practicing bilingual physicians, bilingual researchers, and bilingual graduate students. Guest speakers join the class from affiliated hospitals in-person (or virtually during the COVID-19 pandemic), and guests from other countries join via the virtual platform. Prior to the formation of the Medical Language Program, many course instructors made small improvements to their curricula over time based on student feedback, but there was limited interaction among language instructors to learn from each other regarding effective pedagogical approaches. Most of the language instructors are trained as clinicians, not teachers, so there was an opportunity for faculty development in curricular innovation across the language courses. Since the establishment of the Medical Language Program, language instructors meet regularly with the Office of Scholarly Engagement leadership to share lessons learned and opportunities for improvement. For example, consistent comments from students across language courses center on the importance of interactions with bilingual individuals for improving their oral language skills. Students also appreciated learning about regional variations in language, when applicable. All medical language courses have now developed networks of bilingual health professionals and students who serve as teaching assistants and language practice partners for students taking the courses. During the COVID-19 pandemic, these interactions were facilitated across countries through the virtual platform.

Transition to virtual platforms

In response to the COVID-19 pandemic, we transitioned our Medical Language Program to online courses via the Zoom platform. At first, there were administrative and technological issues that required attention, such as gaining familiarity with the technical capacities. Additionally, learning how to build a sense of community in the virtual classroom required additional attention, especially when pandemic fatigue ran high, and students craved in-person interactions. However, students and faculty were quick to adapt to the virtual environment, which had been required of other courses and work-related responsibilities. We maintained student enrollment in our medical language courses despite the pandemic. Furthermore, there were several silver linings of the transition to virtual learning. First, the virtual platform allowed for schedule flexibility in maximizing student and faculty attendance. Prior to the COVID-19 pandemic, some students and faculty had schedule limitations in commuting across town from their clinical sites to be able to teach and learn in person. The virtual environment allowed students and faculty to log in from anywhere, which maximized opportunities to engage in language learning. Second, the virtual platform enabled bidirectional learning across geographic boundaries and even across countries. Language instructors arranged for

HMS students to meet other students and faculty from collaborating institutions in other countries, such as China, Brazil, and Colombia. These opportunities may not have surfaced prior to the transition to remote learning and have only strengthened our relationships with partner sites for our clinical exchange program. Third, virtual classrooms enabled the Medical Language Program to hold the intensive medical Spanish course in two separate months each year during the pandemic, which doubled student enrollment. Lastly, the virtual environment allowed for easy small group or 1:1 language practice with primary speakers via breakout rooms. Recruiting sufficient primary speakers and physical space to make this happen in the in-person classroom would have been challenging.

Language assessment

Benchmarking language proficiency is an ongoing area of work in the HMS Medical Language Program. To triage students into the appropriate language level course, we ask students to report their language skills based on the Interagency Language Roundtable scale [21]. The medical Spanish instructors have also developed a three to five minutes video quiz for students to self-assess their understanding of spoken Spanish, which allows the instructors to differentiate students into the intermediate and advanced Spanish courses. For students who desired to enroll in Intermediate Spanish, they watched a video of the instructor presenting a patient scenario and were asked how much of the video they understood on a scale of 0–100. For the students who desired to enroll in Advanced Spanish, they watched a video of the instructor presenting a patient scenario and were asked several factual questions about the encounter that they needed to respond to in written Spanish. Most students thought this exercise was somewhat to very useful in identifying which level course matched their language skills.

As part of the curricular and pedagogy alignment, all longitudinal language courses end with a formative assessment using the Objective Structured Clinical Examination (OSCE). The instructors recruit bilingual speakers (typically physicians known through their professional networks or through the Office of Scholarly Engagement) to act as standardized patients. They discuss the case in advance, review the grading rubric, and answer any questions. Students perform a history and physical exam of the standardized patients in clinical scenarios (e.g., primary care visit for a patient with chest pain with interview in the Fall and added physical exam in the Spring). Students also take quizzes and give oral presentations throughout the course and receive feedback to enhance their language skills. The courses are given for credit as pass/fail, so there is no letter grade or numerical rank to determine proficiency level. Rather, at the end of the course, written results of a formative assessment are given to each student to enhance their individualized language learning. The rubric for the assessment included respectful greetings and closing, accurate history gathering, building rapport with the patient, and identifying personal/cultural context relevant to the medical encounter.

There is growing demand from physicians and students for a standardized proficiency benchmark to ensure quality and safety in patient encounters [22–24]. Students and faculty are sensitive to the risks of miscommunication when language skills between clinicians and patients are not concordant. For this reason, the session on working with interpreters is included in all longitudinal medical language courses. The Medical Language Program does not set the expectation that students who take the language courses will attain the level of proficiency to hold clinical sessions without an interpreter in the secondary language. The goal is to gain medical vocabulary and a communication approach (including building rapport and understanding cultural context) needed to gather a basic history and conduct a physical exam. To measure their language skills at a moment in time, students have the opportunity to take the Clinician Cultural and Linguistic Assessment (CCLA) from ALTA Language Services [25], which has been used in affiliated hospitals as a benchmark for clinician language proficiency. Since 2019, only four students out of 103 in the semester-long courses opted in to take the CCLA ALTA assessment at the beginning of their courses. Only one of the four took the assessment at the end of the semester course. None of the four students passed the proficiency benchmark of 80 at the beginning of the course. Five students who took the intensive medical Spanish course took the CCLA ALTA assessment at the beginning and at the end of the course. All five students demonstrated improvement in their scores, and two of them met the cut off of at least 80 for professional proficiency.

Longitudinal learning and maintenance of language skills

Medical students who participate in the Medical Language Program often seek additional opportunities to apply their language skills in clinical settings with appropriate supervision. Several clerkships and core curriculum courses match students to clinical sites based on their language preference for the patient population and/or faculty member. Students also have the opportunity to participate in electives in community health centers that serve large numbers of linguistic minority populations. In 2020–2022, there were nine students who enrolled in a longitudinal medical language course or the intensive medical Spanish course and elected to take one of the community health electives. Additionally, approximately one-quarter of post-clerkship HMS students travel abroad for a clinical rotation, an independent study/scholarly research project, or as part of the HMS clinical elective exchange program. Fourth-year students can enroll in clinical electives in Brazil, Chile, China, Colombia, Costa Rica, France, Guatemala, Israel/Palestine, Spain, and Taiwan with affiliated sites where HMS has clinical elective exchange programs. In the clinical elective exchange program, students engage in medical training, cross-cultural learning, and strengthen their language skills in clinical encounters. Among 130 students who took the intensive medical Spanish course between 2012 and 2019, 63 (48%) also participated in a clinical elective abroad in Latin America or Spain. In their reports on their experiences, students who took both the language course and the clinical training said they either improved their language skills or felt more at ease speaking in Spanish after the abroad experience.

In a survey we conducted of HMS alumni who participated in a medical language course, we found that 3% reported full proficiency before taking the language course and 16% reported full proficiency at the time of the survey (years after they completed the language course), suggesting that the courses may equip physicians to practice language-concordant care in their careers and catalyze long-term language learning [26]. More than half of alumni reported taking the medical language courses to use the language in their future careers, recognizing the value of being able to provide language-concordant care to patients both in the United States and in other countries [26].

Path forward

Since the first medical Spanish course in the early 1970s, the student-led efforts in the mid-2000s in other medical language courses, and the formalization of the HMS Medical Language Program in 2018, student demand for language training has continually increased. Students are vocal about the need for second language skills in both local community health settings and in their global health engagements. We continue to adapt the curricula on an ongoing basis to ensure alignment with longitudinal themes and Practice of Medicine content. New pedagogical approaches are applied, particularly as we have adapted to the virtual learning environment during the COVID-19 pandemic. We continue to build long-term language learning opportunities, including community engagement through community-based organizations and global health electives. Benchmarking language proficiency remains an ongoing area of focus for our teachers and learners. We plan to continue to build collaborations with language directors at other medical schools across the United States and other countries to share best practices and resources to assess language learning in the context of the clinical encounter.

Application of language learning to global health engagement

While there is an ever-growing sensitivity to caring for linguistically diverse patient populations in the United States, there is a more nascent recognition of the importance of language concordance in global health work. The tenets of humanistic medical professionalism exhort us to communicate authentically and holistically (e.g., by using spoken language, body language, facial expression, and demeanor); this is a prerequisite to establishing trusting relationships with patients [27, 28]. The onus of responsibility is on the global health worker to name, understand, and respect with "absolute integrity" local culture, which includes complying with what language the host country team decides is appropriate in different types of interactions (e.g., research and patient care) [29]. For example, in any clinical setting, failure to adequately communicate a treatment plan and medication use can have adverse health consequences [30]. In addition, the healthcare worker who lacks proficiency in speaking and understanding the local language creates an added burden on the local staff who in many cases are called upon to interpret and accommodate visiting clinicians and other types of volunteers.

The global health field consists of a mix of 10 of 1000 of nongovernmental organizations; national (e.g., the United States Agency for International Development) and supra-national [e.g., World Health Organization (WHO)] agencies; religious, missionary organizations (e.g., World Vision); academic institutions; and financial institutions (e.g., World Bank, International Monetary Fund) that engage in health, humanitarian relief, policy, research, education, and advocacy [31]. This mix of diverse actors from wealthy and less wealthy countries is at risk of perpetuating colonialism, the persistence of power relations that subjugate a former colony that is now a sovereign nation. Richardson defined "coloniality" as "attempts to capture the racial, political-economic, social, epistemological, linguistic, and gendered hierarchical orders imposed by European colonialism that have transcended 'decolonization' and continue to oppress.... [p. 103]" [32]. Students may be engaged in global health interventions at risk of perpetuating coloniality in multiple realms [33–35].

Even though the practice of global health has colonial roots, there is a growing commitment to mitigate and eliminate current and future neocolonial interventions. Language infuses global health clinical care, humanitarian relief, policy, research, education, and advocacy. As such, it is a key dimension to counter coloniality. One key strategy involves local language knowledge production, use, and circulation in languages other than English. Another strategy includes translating publications written in other languages to English or other official languages of the WHO. Visiting global health workers need to elevate the credibility of non-English-speaking local colleagues so the local colleagues are the leading protagonists in describing their reality in their chosen language, prioritizing problems, and initiating solutions.

Numerous articles on global health research state unequivocally that the researcher is obligated to seek written or verbal consent from a potential research participant [36–38]. This can be challenging and fraught with pitfalls if language discordance is not addressed. In addition, collaboration throughout the research process and assigning appropriate authorship is necessary to counter "extractive research" [39] and the disproportionate advantage given to some researchers due to many factors, including language ability [40]. English is the dominant language of scientific research, yet only approximately 5% of the world's population speaks English as its first language [41]. Those who are not proficient in reading and writing English are less able to engage in English language scientific discourse. Efforts from organizations such as the Healthcare Information for All [42] expert working group on multilingualism are advocating to change the status quo [33]. Dissemination of research findings into local languages of the populations most impacted by the research is critical [43].

Language proficiency is warranted in health education and health advocacy arenas as well. Authors of a commentary on the Ebola epidemic state how it is incumbent on workers from wealthier countries (the global North) to listen and create space for local teams to lead advocacy and education in their local languages to counter stigma, build community trust, and improve care [44].

Global health workers, including medical students, who work in countries outside their home country need heightened sensitivity to how language can exacerbate or mitigate the ethical complexity of their work. For example, power dynamics between ex-pats and in-country personnel can develop for many reasons. There are inherent geopolitical inequities in who can and cannot cross borders that heightens the privilege of trainees and full-fledged professionals from other countries. The length of time they spend in a country (typically short, intermittent, at the convenience of the global health worker's professional and personal commitments, and infrequently longitudinal) constrains the development of meaningful relationships and the creation of authentic partnerships with local teams. A global health trainee's awareness of their linguistic limitations is, in many cases, different from trainees in-country. However, the global health trainees are given more attention and credence by patients or local staff and can undermine the local practice, even for senior professionals. It is crucial that all global health workers appreciate and view their learning as an ever-evolving endeavor. Language fluency and proficiency can mitigate misunderstanding and lessen power imbalances [45]. They are key components of respectful, collaborative, community-centered, and community-driven initiatives.

Global health opportunities presented to medical trainees continue to grow at a rapid rate. One in four medical students in the United States who completed the Association of American Medical Colleges 2019 Graduation questionnaire reported participating in a global health experience [46]. During the last decade, 68 HMS students traveled to 33 countries for clinical electives; 103 traveled to 9 countries as part of the HMS global clinical electives exchange program; and 158 participated in one- or two-month clinical electives with HMS exchange partner medical schools in 7 Latin American countries (Figure 18.2). Since 2017, 76 students conducted their scholarly project graduation requirement in 33 different countries.

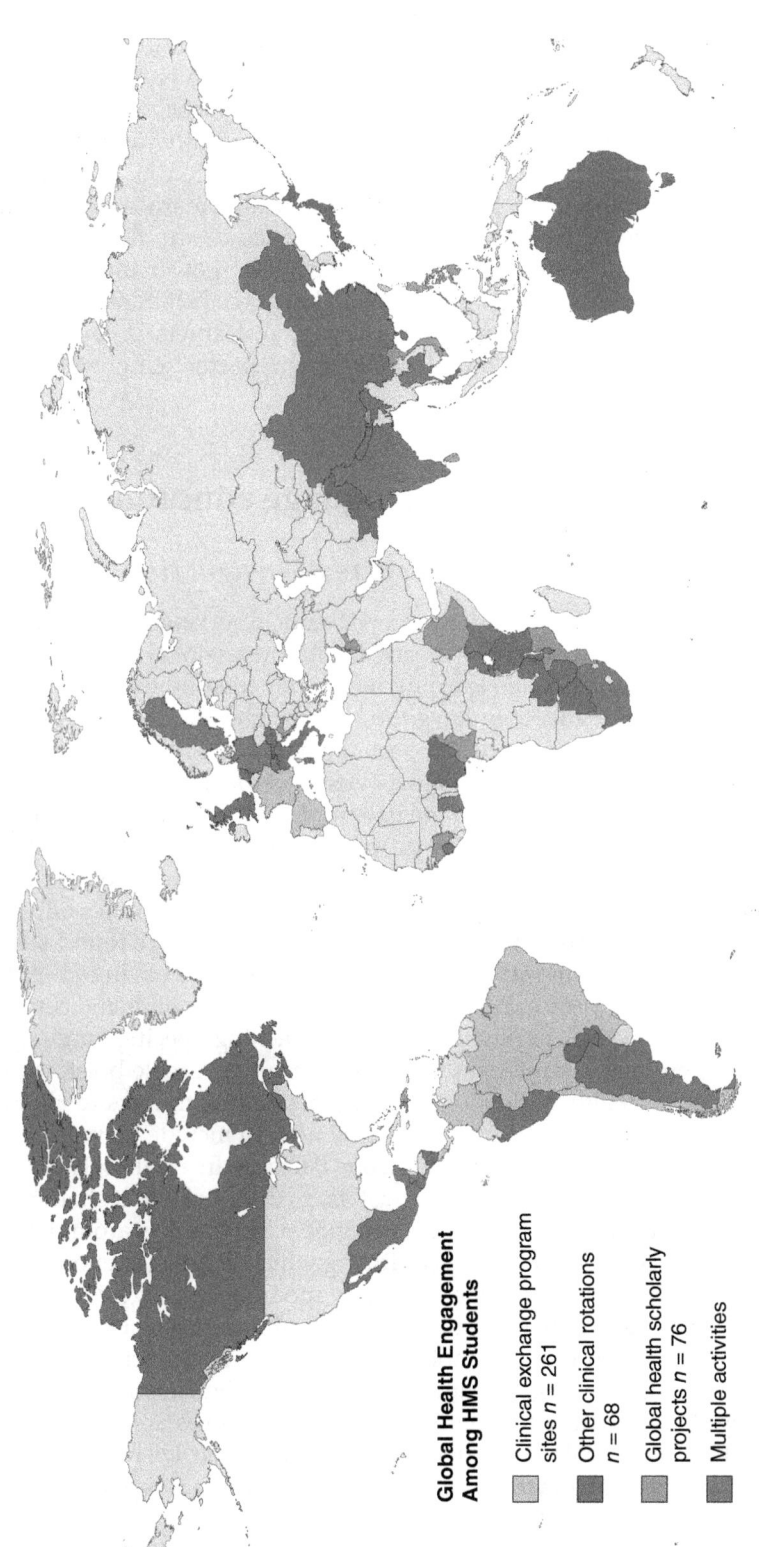

Figure 18.2 Map of Global Health Engagement among Harvard Medical School Students. *Source:* Created by the authors with https://mapchart.net (Creative Commons Attribution-ShareAlike 4.0 International License).

To prepare students for engaging in ethical global health work, numerous schools provide predeparture training; HMS is no exception, but there is a lack of focus on language [47, 48]. In a study of medical and nursing student participants, 77% thought that language was an important topic to cover during predeparture training [49]. In the ethics literature, articles stress that trainees need to be instructed in "language capability" as part of formal training [50, 51]. Yet it is unclear how many schools with predeparture training include a discussion of language concordance; the importance of communication in the local language; and how to address power imbalances, colonialism, and inequities as they relate to differences in language [52]. A recent systematic review of predeparture training programs for a variety of learners in undergraduate, graduate, and residency programs found only 25% reported language as a key competency [48].

Recommendations for medical language education

Selecting languages and language levels of instruction

We recommend attending to both student interest and local language prevalence in deciding which language courses to offer during health professional training. Students are often most committed to language learning when they identify their own language interests and needs. Additionally, they have the best insight into their long-term language goals and integration into their health professional careers. At the same time, it is also important to maintain focus on the linguistic needs of the local population. We recognize that not all students will remain in the geographic area of their medical training and may want to learn a language that may be more prevalent in their next career destination, so balancing these needs is important. Additionally, finding language instructors in less commonly spoken languages may be a challenge that precludes offering any language course based on student demand alone. However, we have found success in posting job positions first within our HMS community and then having HMS faculty circulate the posting in other professional networks. Lastly, we recommend considering local, institutional, and societal imperatives around teaching specific languages. For example, at HMS, there was a large demand to learn Haitian Creole bolstered by the work led by Partners In Health, a global health organization with links to HMS. HMS offered Haitian Creole courses and expanded enrollment to include Harvard students from other schools as well as staff members from Partners In Health. There was an increase in demand around the time of the devastating earthquake that shattered Haiti in 2010. Attending to such local, institutional, and global imperatives around language learning should also be considered when prioritizing which languages to offer.

While some experts have recommended teaching medical language courses at least at the intermediate level [20], there may still be value in offering intensive courses at the beginner level. We have seen demonstrable improvements in proficiency among the students taking the intensive medical Spanish course, even when taught at the beginner level. Additionally, it is important to identify additional resources in the community to boost language skills at the beginning level for students who wish to enroll in the intermediate-level medical language course but require additional support.

Instructor recruitment and qualifications

Recruitment of medical language instructors should include an official job posting with desired qualifications, scope of teaching, expected time commitment, and any available teaching stipend or compensation. Criteria for selecting candidates should include an assessment of the instructor's language proficiency, their medical knowledge for teaching the appropriate course content for medical or other health professional students, and their understanding of cultural issues relevant to the language of instruction and clinical care. Maintaining a database of multilingual clinicians is a valuable investment for recruiting instructors, teaching assistants, or guest speakers.

Aligning curricula across languages

Standardizing medical language curricula to reflect the learning objectives and course content of what students learn as part of their health professional training (e.g., history and physical exam, explanation of diagnosis and management plans) is critical to meet the goal of building a healthcare workforce able to provide language-concordant care. To achieve this, creating buy-in among language instructors is an important first step. Additionally, providing the administrative support to make the curricular changes as easy as possible is critical to overcome barriers. For example, providing all the curricular material that is taught in English and a simplified calendar for language instructors to follow several months in advance of the courses has been helpful in our experience. Having a dedicated director and staff with expertise in the history of the Medical Language Program to review course materials across language courses has been particularly helpful in identifying opportunities to streamline and learn best practices across courses. We hold biannual faculty meetings of our Medical Language Program, which allows instructors from all language courses to interact with and learn from each other. These meetings are important for alignment and community building. Lastly, for medical language courses other than Spanish, there are far fewer articles in the published literature about medical language curricula to adapt and expand. Our Mandarin and Portuguese instructors have offered online videos, podcasts, and written materials to provide extra practice for students.

Optimizing the virtual learning environment for language learning

The COVID-19 pandemic pushed learners and teachers to adapt to virtual environments. We recommend leveraging the advantages of virtual learning and mitigating the disadvantages. Virtual environments afford the most scheduling flexibility for both teachers and learners, which includes opening opportunities to engage with people across geographies and time zones in other countries. Additionally, large group, small group, and 1:1 conversations can happen relatively seamlessly. However, community building in the virtual classroom presents a distinct set of challenges, especially as many learners may be prone to multitasking and less able to engage with each other while on the virtual platform, especially if internet access and bandwidth are limited.

As the COVID-19 pandemic continues to undulate, we have planned to have several in-person sessions (one at the beginning of the course, and one at the end of the course) with the remaining sessions being virtual. We recommend attending to both student and instructor preferences, as well as institutional policies, regarding the division of in-person vs. online classes. Lastly, additional research is needed to evaluate different types of online resources for learning (e.g., podcasts and videos).

Assessing language proficiency and its application to clinical care

To optimize placement of students into the most appropriate language level, we recommend requiring students to report their language skills based on the Interagency Language Roundtable scale. Language instructors may also want to create videos that students interact with to appraise their spoken language proficiency. A variety of pedagogical tools (e.g., quizzes and oral presentations) can be implemented to evaluate student progress during a language course. At course completion, we recommend each student undergo a formative assessment of their ability to engage effectively in a clinical encounter using standardized patients in the Objective Structured Clinical Examination (OSCE). Finally, another useful tool that can be used prior to and at course end is the CCLA from ALTA Language Services or other validated assessment tool. Implementing robust, objective assessment tools will help students to understand their strengths and areas for improvement in clinical encounters and engagement in local and international contexts. Such assessments will also assist instructors in evaluating aspects of their course that work well and aspects that need improvement.

Enhancing opportunities to connect language learning to health equity locally and around the world

Medical language learning does not end in the classroom. Putting language skills into practice with appropriate supervision is critical for developing and maintaining proficiency. We recommend identifying opportunities for students to apply their language skills in clinical and community-based settings that are acceptable to community members.

Any comprehensive, equitable, collaborative global health partnership requires an equally comprehensive predeparture training that includes language [53]. Medical and other students are "voting with their feet" in learning languages to relate to diverse patients both in the United States and abroad [54]. In addition, a robust curriculum for medical students and other trainees should include a discussion of language concordance; communication in local languages; power imbalances, colonialism, and inequities as they relate to differences in language; the role and limitations of language courses; and language proficiency assessments. Teaching faculty ought to involve participants from countries where the target language is used, discuss problems that arise from language discordance between the students and the local partners, and explore how to ameliorate these language barriers to enhance communication, understanding, and outcomes [55]. Finally, students should be sensitive to and operate within their language limitations and seek ongoing language support to minimize barriers to optimal, equitable global health outcomes.

Conclusion

In this chapter, we described a case study of the Medical Language Program at HMS that showcases the variety of languages offered and teaching models at our institution. We also highlight language learning as a gateway to approaching the understanding of culture with humility. Language concordance is critical–but not always possible–for clinical care, research, education, and advocacy, especially in a multilingual society and world. Language concordance can reduce power imbalances, enhance true collaboration and partnerships, and be a key driver of health equity, community, and country sovereignty. Nurturing curiosity about language and supporting language acquisition align with elevating human dignity and the human rights of patients everywhere.

Highlights

- We describe the history of the Medical Language Program at HMS as a demonstration project of how to formalize, strengthen, and expand language learning for medical students.
- There are curricular opportunities to align language learning longitudinally across courses and clerkships in undergraduate medical education.
- Standardized assessment of language skills is critical to ensure appropriate use of the language and collaboration with interpreters in clinical care and research.
- Greater investment is needed to create and enhance language training, assessment, and impact as a fundamental part of global health engagement.

Acknowledgments

We would like to dedicate this chapter to Dr. Guillermo Herrera (1932–2022) for being the vanguard in developing medical language courses for medical students at HMS. We are grateful to Kari Hannibal for her many years of managing the HMS Medical Language Program and her assistance in critically reviewing the chapter. We would also like to acknowledge Marcie Naumowicz who has provided administrative support to the HMS Medical Language Program since 2021 and has contributed to this chapter.

REFERENCES

1. Berlitz. *The Most Spoken Languages in the World*. 2021. https://www.berlitz.com/en-uy/blog/most-spoken-languages-world (accessed 25 January 2022).
2. The World Bank. *Teaching Young Children in the Language they Speak at Home is Essential to Eliminate Learning Poverty*. 2021. The World Bank Press Release 2021/005/HD. https://www.worldbank.org/en/news/press-release/2021/07/14/teaching-young-children-in-the-language-they-speak-at-home-is-essential-to-eliminate-learning-poverty (accessed 25 January 2022).
3. Flores, G., Abreu, M., Olivar, M.A., and Kastner, B. (1998). Access barriers to health

care for Latino children. *Arch. Pediatr. Adolesc. Med.* 152 (11): 1119–1125.
4. Carrasquillo, O., Orav, E.J., Brennan, T.A., and Burstin, H.R. (1999). Impact of language barriers on patient satisfaction in an emergency department. *J. Gen. Intern. Med.* 14 (2): 82–87.
5. Yeheskel, A. and Rawal, S. (2019). Exploring the "patient experience" of individuals with limited English proficiency: a scoping review. *J. Immigr. Minor. Health* 21 (4): 853–878.
6. Divi, C., Koss, R.G., Schmaltz, S.P., and Loeb, J.M. (2007). Language proficiency and adverse events in US hospitals: a pilot study. *Int. J. Qual. Health Care* 19 (2): 60–67.
7. Schyve, P.M. (2007). Language differences as a barrier to quality and safety in health care: the joint commission perspective. *J. Gen. Intern. Med.* 22 (Suppl 2): 360–361.
8. Ngo-Metzger, Q., Sorkin, D.H., Phillips, R.S. et al. (2007). Providing high-quality care for limited English proficient patients: the importance of language concordance and interpreter use. *J. Gen. Intern. Med.* 22 (Suppl 2): 324–330.
9. Institute of Medicine (2012). *How Far have we come in Reducing Health Disparities? Progress since 2000: Workshop Summary*. Washington, DC: National Academies Press.
10. Smedley, B.D., Stith, A.Y., and Nelson, A.R. (2003). *Unequal Treatment: Confronting Racial and Ethnic Disparities in Health Care*. Washington, DC: National Academies Press.
11. Lor, M. and Martinez, G.A. (2020). Scoping review: definitions and outcomes of patient-provider language concordance in healthcare. *Patient Educ. Couns.* 103 (10): 1883–1901.
12. Wilson, J.H. (2014). *Investing in English Skills: The Limited English Proficient Workforce in U.S. Metropolitan Areas*. Washington, DC: The Brookings Institute. https://www.brookings.edu/research/investing-in-english-skills-the-limited-english-proficient-workforce-in-u-s-metropolitan-areas/ (accessed 25 January 2022).
13. Rumbaut, R.G. and Massey, D.S. (2013). Immigration and language diversity in the United States. *Daedalus* 142 (3): 141–154.
14. Espinoza, J. and Derrington, S. (2021). How should clinicians respond to language barriers that exacerbate health inequity? *AMA J. Ethics* 23 (2): E109–E116.
15. Ortega, P., Francone, N.O., Santos, M.P. et al. (2021). Medical spanish in US medical schools: a national survey to examine existing programs. *J. Gen. Intern. Med.* 36 (9): 2724–2730.
16. Zhang, C., Sangarlangkarn, A., Luo, D. et al. (2009). *Essential Medical Mandarin for Health Care Providers*. MedEdPORTAL.
17. Molina, R.L. and Kasper, J. (2019). The power of language-concordant care: a call to action for medical schools. *BMC Med. Educ.* 19 (1): 378.
18. Migration Policy Institute (2022). *State Demographics Data*. Massachusetts: Migration Policy Institute. https://www.migrationpolicy.org/data/state-profiles/state/language/MA# (accessed 6 July 2022).
19. City of Boston (2018). *Language and Communications Access*. https://www.boston.gov/sites/default/files/document-file-11-2018/demographic_data_report_-_neighborhood_depth_lep_with_accom_notice_2.pdf (accessed 6 July 2022).
20. Ortega, P., Diamond, L., Alemán, M.A. et al. (2020). Medical spanish standardization in U.S. medical schools: consensus statement from a multidisciplinary expert panel. *Acad. Med.* 95 (1): 22–31.
21. Interagency Language Roundtable. *Interagency Language Roundtable*. 2011. https://www.govtilr.org/Skills/ILRscale1.htm (accessed 25 May 2020).
22. Diamond, L.C., Luft, H.S., Chung, S., and Jacobs, E.A. (2012). "Does this doctor speak my language?" improving the characterization of physician non-English language skills. *Health Serv. Res.* 47 (1 Pt 2): 556–569.
23. Diamond, L., Chung, S., Ferguson, W. et al. (2014). Relationship between self-assessed and tested non-English-language proficiency among primary care providers. *Med. Care* 52 (5): 435–438.
24. Diamond, L., Toro Bejarano, M., Chung, S. et al. (2019). Factors associated with

accuracy of self-assessment compared with tested non-English language proficiency among primary care providers. *Med. Care* 57 (5): 385–390.
25. ALTA Language Services, Inc (2023). *Clinician Cultural and Linguistic Assessment*. https://www.altalang.com/language-testing/ccla/ (accessed 15 August 2023).
26. Pereira, J.A., Hannibal, K., Stecker, J. et al. (2020). Professional language use by alumni of the Harvard Medical School Medical Language Program. *BMC Med. Educ.* 20 (1): 407.
27. Benatar, S. and Upshur, R. (2014). Virtues and values in medicine revisited: individual and global health. *Clin. Med.* 14 (5): 495–499.
28. Astle, B., Faerron Guzmán, C.A., Landry, A. et al. (2018). *Global Health Education Competencies Toolkit*, 2ee. Washington, DC: Consortium of Universities for Global Health https://www.cugh.org/wp-content/uploads/sites/95/2020/05/CUGH-Global-Health-Toolkit-Web-Version.pdf.
29. White, M. and Evert, J. (2014). Developing ethical awareness in global health: four cases for medical educators. *Dev. World Bioeth.* 14 (3): 111–116.
30. Romo, M.L. and DeCamp, M. (2015). Ethics in global health outreach: three key considerations for pharmacists. *Int. J. Pharm. Pract.* 23 (1): 86–89.
31. Bush, S.S. and Hadden, J. (2019). Density and decline in the founding of international NGOs in the United States. *Int. Stud. Q.* 63 (4): 1133–1146.
32. Richardson, E.T. (2019). On the coloniality of global public health. *MAT* 6 (4): 101–118.
33. Whitehead, C., Wondimagegn, D., Baheretibeb, Y., and Hodges, B. (2018). The international partner as invited guest: beyond colonial and import-export models of medical education. *Acad. Med.* 93 (12): 1760–1763.
34. Spiegel, J.M., Breilh, J., and Yassi, A. (2015). Why language matters: insights and challenges in applying a social determination of health approach in a North-South collaborative research program. *Glob. Health* 11: 9.
35. Bhakuni, H. and Abimbola, S. (2021). Epistemic injustice in academic global health. *Lancet Glob. Health* 9 (10): e1465–e1470.
36. Emanuel, E.J., Wendler, D., Killen, J., and Grady, C. (2004). What makes clinical research in developing countries ethical? The benchmarks of ethical research. *J. Infect. Dis.* 189 (5): 930–937.
37. Ruiz-Casares, M. (2014). Research ethics in global mental health: advancing culturally responsive mental health research. *Transcult. Psychiatry* 51 (6): 790–805.
38. Stapleton, G., Schröder-Bäck, P., Laaser, U. et al. (2014). Global health ethics: an introduction to prominent theories and relevant topics. *Glob. Health Action* 7: 23569.
39. Chu, K.M., Jayaraman, S., Kyamanywa, P., and Ntakiyiruta, G. (2014). Building research capacity in Africa: equity and global health collaborations. *PLoS Med.* 11 (3): e1001612.
40. Smith, E., Hunt, M., and Master, Z. (2014). Authorship ethics in global health research partnerships between researchers from low or middle income countries and high income countries. *BMC Med. Ethics* 15 (1): 42.
41. Pakenham-Walsh, N. and Healthcare Information For All working group on multilingualism (2018). Improving the availability of health research in languages other than English. *Lancet Glob. Health* 6 (12): e1282.
42. Health Information for All (2006–2017). *Health Information for All*. Global Healthcare Information Network. https://hifa.org (accessed 24 January 2022).
43. Binagwaho, A., Allotey, P., Sangano, E. et al. (2021). A call to action to reform academic global health partnerships. *BMJ* 375: n2658.
44. Myser, C. (2015). Defining "global health ethics": offering a research agenda for more bioethics and multidisciplinary contributions-from the global south and beyond the health sciences-to enrich global health and global health ethics initiatives. *J. Bioeth. Inq.* 12 (1): 5–10.
45. Lahey, T. (2012). Perspective: a proposed medical school curriculum to help

students recognize and resolve ethical issues of global health outreach work. *Acad. Med.* 87 (2): 210–215.
46. Association of American Medical Colleges *Medical Education*. Graduation Questionnaire (GQ). https://www.aamc.org/data-reports/students-residents/report/graduation-questionnaire-gq (accessed 25 January 2022).
47. Kasper, J., Mulye, A., Doobay-Persaud, A. et al. (2020). Perspectives and solutions from clinical trainees and mentors regarding ethical challenges during global health experiences. *Ann. Glob. Health* 86 (1): 34.
48. Kalbarczyk, A., Nagourney, E., Martin, N.A. et al. (2019). Are you ready? A systematic review of pre-departure resources for global health electives. *BMC Med. Educ.* 19 (1): 166.
49. Kironji, A.G., Cox, J.T., Edwardson, J. et al. (2018). Pre-departure training for healthcare students going abroad: impact on preparedness. *Ann. Glob. Health* 84 (4): 683–691.
50. Crump, J.A., Sugarman, J., and Working Group on Ethics Guidelines for Global Health Training (WEIGHT) (2010). Ethics and best practice guidelines for training experiences in global health. *Am. J. Trop. Med. Hyg.* 83 (6): 1178–1182.
51. Pinto, A.D. and Upshur, R.E.G. (2009). Global health ethics for students. *Dev. World Bioeth.* 9 (1): 1–10.
52. Peluso, M.J., Forrestel, A.K., Hafler, J.P., and Rohrbaugh, R.M. (2013). Structured global health programs in U.S. medical schools: a web-based review of certificates, tracks, and concentrations. *Acad. Med.* 88 (1): 124–130.
53. Provenzano, A.M., Graber, L.K., Elansary, M. et al. (2010). Short-term global health research projects by US medical students: ethical challenges for partnerships. *Am. J. Trop. Med. Hyg.* 83 (2): 211–214.
54. Schmuter, G. (2020). Learning a second language: diversifying medical school from within. *Acad. Med.* 95 (2): 172.
55. Peluso, M.J., van Schalkwyk, S., Kellett, A. et al. (2017). Reframing undergraduate medical education in global health: rationale and key principles from the Bellagio Global Health Education Initiative. *Med. Teach.* 39 (6): 639–645.

19 Clinical Communication Skills Training in Minoritized Languages

CARMEN PÉREZ-MUÑOZ
AND TIFFANY M. SHIN

Introduction

With strong interest and demand from professionals and educational institutions alike, the field of medical language education continues to grow rapidly. Its speedy development, though, has led some to question its ability to maintain sound pedagogical methods. This chapter analyzes the underpinnings of medical language education and offers ways in which instructors can ensure healthy growth in this valuable discipline. A better understanding of its place in language education, including a look at the broader field of languages for specific purposes (LSP), will help in developing best practices and successful educational programs. The push-and-pull between medicine and language pedagogy experts and the necessity for cross-dialogue make medical language education particularly fascinating, where successful interdisciplinary collaboration can result in positive progress that is multiplicative rather than summative alone. The following pages are targeted to both language and medical professionals interested in maximizing the learning experience of their medical language students to ensure they receive the best possible training and contribute to building a better and more equitable health system.

This chapter focuses on the different aspects related to medical language teaching, including diving into its context, challenges, and critical issues to be considered, offering practical recommendations, and providing suggestions for further development. Medical language education pertinent to clinical skills is addressed here, referring to the ability to gather patient information through effective verbal and nonverbal communication and the ability to synthesize, and apply patient information in the clinical setting.

The chapter is meant to provide guidance both to those already in the field of medical language teaching and who are interested in continuing to explore venues to maximize

---

The Handbook of Language in Public Health and Healthcare, First Edition.
Edited by Pilar Ortega, Glenn Martínez, Maichou Lor, and A. Susana Ramírez.
© 2024 John Wiley & Sons, Inc. Published 2024 by John Wiley & Sons, Inc.

the success of their programs, and to those who are new to it, offering background and tools to create a successful and sustainable course. Given the background and experience of the authors, special emphasis is given to undergraduate college medical language courses and medical school courses.

Historical development

Historical development of medical language education

In recent years, scholarly work on medical languages has thrived, ranging from descriptive pieces about the current state of medical language teaching [1], to analyses of benefits [2], to pedagogical methodologies [3] and evaluation tools [4]. Medical languages are a subcategory of the field of LSP, which focuses on language acquisition with an emphasis on a particular field for its application. In 1977, Peter Strevens wrote, "Among current developments in the learning and teaching of languages, the change which appears to be moving at the fastest rate and which brings in its train the greatest consequences for learners and teachers alike, is the trend towards the learning of languages for specific rather than for general purposes" [5], foreseeing the impact that LSP would have on the field of language teaching and learning. Despite not being a novel field, the lack of formal literature about LSP left it without the same recognition as other branches of language teaching for decades, but recent years have brought new scholarship and focus on LSP, conforming a network of resources and tools to formally establish this field.

One of the interesting things about the particular case of medical languages is that this newfound interest comes from both of the involved fields: language and medical education. However, articles like Hardin's "Overview of Medical Spanish Curricula in the United States" highlights the dangers of the trend of offering medical language courses, stating that quantity does not necessarily imply quality [6]. As a language instructor, Hardin was one of the first to advise caution and signal the critical importance of sound curriculum design and other pedagogical factors that affect the efficacy and outcomes of medical language courses. Hardin points out the aforementioned lack of literature, finding only 35 scholarly works on medical Spanish education in 38 years in her systematic review. Adding to what Hardin had already stated, Matthew D. Coss criticizes the way in which many medical language courses and programs in medical schools have been developed "without significant input from experts in the fields of applied linguistics and second language acquisition" [7], contributing to the lack of consistency among these courses and programs.

Nevertheless, identifying problems is the first step toward finding solutions. In recent years, experts from both the medical and language teaching fields have been collaborating in a more structured and official way to promote and implement a standardized approach to the teaching of medical languages. In 2018, a panel of medical Spanish experts organized a forum where they "outlined national [United States] standards for the teaching and application of medical Spanish skills in patient-physician communication, establish curricular and competency guidelines for courses in medical schools, propose best practices for skill assessment and certification, and identify next steps needed for the implementation of the proposed national standards" [8]. This assembly was one of the first steps in the creation of the National Association of Medical Spanish (NAMS), which is in itself a step toward achieving more uniformity in medical language education in medical schools and undergraduate programs. The association is comprised of professionals in the fields of linguistics, pedagogy, medicine, interpreting, and others, who are working to create a standardized, evidence-based approach to teaching medical Spanish. Although NAMS focuses on medical Spanish, its progress and contributions may serve as a model for professionals working with other minoritized languages.

The need for standardized curricula and best practices in medical language education is not simply a pedagogically sound practice, but also an act of responsibility. The ultimate goals of medical language teaching are to address health equity, break down structural barriers that prevent linguistically minoritized groups from accessing care, and ensure quality of care. The lack of standardization in clinician training in medical languages to serve minoritized populations may translate into not only a failure to achieve these goals but also promote a false sense of accomplishment of equity in the healthcare system. Offering medical language programs should not only be a checkbox that is marked and make us feel that just trying is enough; in order to create real and long-lasting changes in the health system, this training needs to follow the same rigorous process as any other area in medical education.

There is a significant void in valuable pedagogical methodology in LSP. A substantial amount of the theories and practices used in the LSP classroom are simply adaptations from English for Specific Purposes (ESP), as already noted by Trace, Hudson, and Brown [9]. ESP is a well-established field, likely related to the global position of English as a bridge language (i.e., a language used as a way to communicate by groups who do not share a common native language). However, the simple translation of ESP for LSP pedagogy presents significant challenges and disadvantages. When English is regularly used by non-native speakers to communicate with other non-native speakers (i.e., two individuals from non-English-speaking countries communicate in English), it can lead to mistakes and misunderstandings, as Grandin noted, "Global English is a risky and limited form of communication. Aside from its purely linguistic limitations, and resulting potential for misunderstanding, it bars us from cultural nuances and isolates us from the inner language of our conversational partners. It keeps us at the surface level and never lets us into the other person's world" [10]. Grandin's words highlight the crucial nature of the cultural component in LSP course development. In the clinical setting in particular, nuances can be extremely relevant both when patients share their stories and when providers make decisions about their diagnosis and plan of care. Simplifying content to the surface level just so that basic communication can happen is a dangerous practice that leads to a lesser quality of care for these patients by, for instance, asking less questions or assuming information. LSP courses must thwart the danger of becoming glorified vocabulary lessons or focusing on teaching learners to merely do a direct translation of what they would say in their dominant language. LSP courses should foster language accuracy as much as effective communication skills within the specific cultural context. For these same reasons, LSP instructors need to establish formal methodologies beyond ESP and particular to the target language and cultures they cover. In other words, LSP is not a one-size-fits-all field, but a sewing pattern that requires tailoring to fit the specific needs of each particular language and each specific field in which said language is used.

LSP within fields like medicine, business, engineering, and diplomacy is growing quickly, as professionals see the advantages of communicating directly with speakers in their preferred languages and eliminating the need for an interpreter. In healthcare, medical language education finds its place amidst communication skills training, cultural humility training, and health equity and justice, though unfortunately it is often offered as extracurricular rather than a required part of curricula. In the United States, having limited English proficiency (LEP) is associated with a higher likelihood of suffering medical errors. One recent study at seven hospitals across the United States demonstrated that families of hospitalized children who reported LEP were twice as likely to experience medical errors [11]. Medical language educators have the potential to improve healthcare safety as they train professionals to care for patients in their preferred languages.

Specific recommendations for medical language courses are offered in more detail later in this chapter. From curriculum design to teaching tools and methods of evaluation, LSP courses must be intentional in content, learning objectives, teaching methodologies, and student assessments.

Conceptual framework for clinical skills education

Medical language education pertinent to clinical skills refers to the ability to gather patient information through effective verbal and nonverbal communication and the ability to interpret and apply this patient information in the clinical setting. These skills typically are assessed in a variety of manners, often with observed encounters with patients or patient actors, which is often referred to as simulation training or working with standardized patients (SPs). Evaluation of clinical skills often includes assessing a learner's action, performance, competence, and knowledge when interacting in the clinical setting. The educational assessment of skills relates to the clinical tasks of the particular healthcare professional, whether it is for medicine, nursing, pharmacy, physical therapy, or others. Each healthcare field typically has a standard set of core clinical competencies required of students upon graduation. These core competencies within each field should be used as a framework for medical language courses in order for learners to achieve clinical competency in nondominant languages.

Critical issues and topics in clinical skills training

Two main pillars in course design are course objectives –referring to what learners need to acquire during the class– and learner profile –pertaining to who the students are and what their skill level is. In the case of LSP courses, the focus on the practical application of language skills tends to result in the favorable intersection of instructors' learning objectives and individual learners' goals. By developing clear objectives, faculty can ensure proper instruction and fair assessment.

Traditionally, beginner and intermediate language courses place a strong emphasis on written communication, making students feel more confident reading and writing than listening and speaking. On the other hand, LSP courses often focus on those last two skills of listening and speaking alone, as they gear toward in-person communication contexts. However, this is not to say that skills based on written formats – reading and writing – do not have a place in medical language learning. Given the nature of these courses, a strong emphasis should be put on oral proficiency, but instructors may also incorporate written components, such as through authentic healthcare-related readings and written assignments, to approach language learning in a well-rounded manner. Readings offer students the possibility to increase exposure to new vocabulary and frequency of encountering it [12], which helps in the acquisition process (studies show that words need to be encountered between 6 and 20 times before being learned [13, 14]). Subsequently, there is evidence that improvement in vocabulary knowledge facilitates speaking skills [15], highlighting the direct connection between reading and speaking.

Occasionally, oral communication may be inappropriately associated with less formally correct language, one where "making oneself understood" is enough, or just conveying the main ideas without the necessity for completely accurate grammar or vocabulary. To avoid this problem, objectives should state clearly that accuracy is relevant in every form of communication, particularly in the clinical setting. For that same reason, acquisition of specialized medical vocabulary is as important as the ability to simplify language and explain technical terms to patients. This is where written assignments can become a useful tool. Concision and clarity are two of the most important skills in effective communication and are particularly relevant in the often fast-paced clinical setting (and even more so in potentially intercultural communication). Offering students short written assignments where they have a limited space to explain a diagnosis, give instructions, etc., can be a useful way to practice those skills. Written assignments give students the opportunity to spend more time actively thinking about how to say something without the threat of immediacy that oral assignments carry, fostering critical thinking, and analytical processes that they can later apply to their oral skills.

The hybrid nature of LSP courses, where language learning is connected to specific areas of application, presents a particular challenge for instructors, who must evaluate and determine the progression of specific skills framed within a field that may not necessarily be their specialty. For example, in languages for medical purposes, the instructor needs to gauge what kind of health-related knowledge students should have at any given point during their training when designing the course. The interdisciplinary nature of medical language teaching makes collaboration one of the best tools to achieve effective results [16, 17]. Developing clinical communication skills in a different language, as well as acquiring the ability to use them effectively, may be better accomplished through the guidance of both medical and language experts, particularly at a graduate level. Language instructors can help students develop proficiency in language and cultural skills; clinical instructors can guide them in best practices to communicate with patients effectively and with compassion. Both types of instructors together can demonstrate the ways in which the complementary skills enable the clinician to provide patients with quality care and a positive experience. Cultural content needs to be included organically throughout course objectives, in combination with the rest of the material, rather than as a side note or addendum to the curriculum [18]. Instructors should emphasize the need to increase understanding of and sensitivity toward the different cultures (particularly within the United States) with respect to healthcare-related beliefs, practices, and social interactions. Instructors may have difficulties selecting cultural content while avoiding stereotyping patients given the many cultures, traditions, and perspectives that often reside within a single language. For that reason, teaching cultural humility and strategies to develop it is an approach that can help mitigate the impossibility of teaching all cultural aspects related to a specific language. At the same time, developing cultural humility addresses potential unconscious biases that students may have since it "incorporates a lifelong commitment to self-evaluation and self-critique, to redressing the power imbalances in the patient-physician dynamic, and to developing mutually beneficial and nonpaternalistic clinical and advocacy partnerships with communities on behalf of individuals and defined populations" [19].

When discussing course design in detail, it is best to approach the topic by the level and context in which these courses take place to address specific components and factors to be considered in the process.

Undergraduate programs

In the United States, students interested in pursuing a career in healthcare start by completing a four-year undergraduate college degree. These students show a diverse range of interests in their degree preferences, from pre-med, to biology, to psychology, and more. This diversity can pose challenges for instructors when designing medical language courses. In course design, it is important to remember that the focus of LSP courses is successful communication within a particular context. Language instructors should always prioritize teaching effective communication skills and not context-based content (in this case medical), as that is not their area of expertise. Just like students are learning the language to be used as a tool within that particular context, the context should be simply a vehicle for the LSP instructor when teaching effective communication skills in any particular language. This means that the clinical setting should simply be the background for learning activities. In this sense, backward design is a useful instrument when creating an LSP course: "one starts with the end—the desired results [. . .]– and then derives the curriculum from the evidence of learning (performances) called for by the standard and the teaching needed to equip students to perform" [20]. In other words, starting with the final stage that students should achieve after course completion, educators can build back a curriculum that would achieve the course objectives and goals in a scaffolded and realistic way.

Undergraduate medical language courses are often mostly made up of premedical students planning to apply to medical school. Other students include those pursuing careers in nursing, social work, or public health. Depending on the timing of the undergraduate language course, many students have not yet received formal professional career training in their area of interest. Thus, undergraduate medical language courses should be designed to provide students with a contextualized but general overview of the patients they want to serve and instill a sense of the need to tackle health disparities. A public health approach is one form of introducing topics related to said disparities and issues affecting racially, ethnically, and linguistically minoritized groups in healthcare: "The public health approach involves defining and measuring the problem, determining the cause or risk factors for the problem, determining how to prevent or ameliorate the problem, and implementing effective strategies on a larger scale and evaluating the impact" [21]. In an undergraduate medical language course, this approach framed within the target language and cultures may offer a great basis for students interested in developing clinical skills in that particular language.

Language instruction for undergraduate students should focus on significantly advancing proficiency and relevant cultural humility in order to establish the basis for good communication skills. Language proficiency development should include acquiring context-specific vocabulary, mastering grammar, developing fluency, and improving pronunciation. Deepening students' understanding of the background, strengths, and challenges of the population is a vital piece that should be prioritized in course design. Cultural content may include, though is not limited to: demographics of the specific minoritized language group, racism in healthcare, lack of access and structural barriers experienced by the patient population, culturally relevant practices that affect health, and the effects of migration [22, 23].

Using field-specific content, instructors should build their course to connect vocabulary topics, create activities to allow them to review and practice specific grammar skills, and include opportunities for oral practice in a realistic setting. If these are achieved successfully, students will have an excellent basis to continue their medical language training at a postbaccalaureate level if given the opportunity.

Graduate programs in healthcare

Students who complete undergraduate language studies will ideally continue their training at the graduate level to acquire language skills for professional application. The primary difference between undergraduate and graduate medical language courses resides in the core material that is emphasized. Both should include linguistic and cultural content and provide students with an accurate view of the population groups. While undergraduate courses should lay the basis for students to develop their language proficiency, upon which they will build field-specific skills, graduate courses benefit from following the core curriculum's objectives in specialty-specific communication skills (such as the medical interview in medical school) [24]. Graduate medical language courses ultimately provide students with a more specialized communication skillset for professional use compared to undergraduate courses. The main objective of graduate medical language courses is the acquisition of the skills, knowledge, and attitudes necessary for effective patient communication. As in every stage of training, the objectives of graduate medical language courses must appropriately parallel the roles and responsibilities of these learners.

Limited flexible time in a graduate curriculum can be a challenge for medical language training. A variety of approaches can be taken, including offering medical language courses as an opportunity to receive course credit for graduation requirements or providing supplementary offerings such as certificate programs. Because language learning takes time and the overall goal is the retention of language skills upon graduation, longitudinal medical language programs that follow students throughout their years of training seem like a logical best option, but also a more logistically challenging one. For institutions that do not have the necessary resources to provide longitudinal training, including faculty support, a possible alternative can be short intensive programs. Traditionally, short-term programs last for eight weeks or less, although there are no established parameters in terms of number of meetings per week or the duration of these meetings. These shorter programs would particularly benefit from collaborations with language pedagogy experts [3, 17], as they may provide guidance in ways to use time more efficiently to maximize language development.

Medical school programs

Clinical communication skills training begins in the first year of medical school, typically starting with learning how to greet a patient and set the stage for a medical encounter. Students gradually learn how to ask questions to obtain the patient's medical history, which includes asking about their current and past medical issues, information about their family's health, and their social situation. More advanced clinical communication skills training may occur during the second year of medical school, such as learning to break bad news, address difficult emotions, obtain informed consent, give motivational counseling, and discuss medical errors in an appropriate and considerate way. As medical students enter their clinical years of training and spend time working in hospitals or clinics, they benefit from learning communication skills applicable to specific clinical specialties [25]. Students are required to rotate in a variety of specialties for at least one month or more at a time. These specialties typically include, but are not limited to, internal medicine, pediatrics, obstetrics and gynecology, surgery, neurology, psychiatry, and ambulatory medicine. Students interact directly with patients and work collaboratively with healthcare teams to provide patient care, particularly during real-life encounters with patients, students benefit from direct observations and feedback from instructors [26].

Clinical communication skills training in minoritized languages for medical students focuses on the roles and responsibilities of clinicians-in-training. As a medical school's core curriculum involves clinical communication skills for all students, medical language education would benefit from paralleling this core material and teaching students the same skills in a specific language. By using existing schemata, i.e., the content of their courses in English, the process of language learning is facilitated for students [27], and the material is positively reinforced in both languages. Ideally, students acquire new clinical communication skills first in the dominant language and then learn it in the target language.

Given the variation in programs' duration, curricula, and expected outcomes, there is no consensus about the base language level that students should have prior to starting them. However, in general terms, it seems safe to state that intermediate levels (B1 to B2 in the Common European Framework of Reference for Languages or CEFR system) are a good starting point for most current medical school language programs. Nevertheless, instructors need to ensure that students are realistically able to achieve effective patient-centered clinical communication skills by the end of their training. Still, it is not possible to guarantee that a single course will result in sustainable language skills without the need for any further intervention or assessment. Thus, medical language programs should teach continual self-assessment by providing students with tools to objectively evaluate their abilities to communicate effectively without an interpreter; these tools should include both practice opportunities and self-reflection rubrics or forms to foster this analytical process [28, 29]. This aspect is a key element in achieving the goals of medical language programs to genuinely address health inequities and improve healthcare access for speakers of minoritized languages.

Medical instructors should collaborate with language pedagogy experts in order to develop effective courses from the perspective of both fields. There is more to language courses than curriculum design: teaching methods, evaluation tools, and language pedagogy knowledge (techniques for language correction, scaffolding material, learning strategies, etc.) are only some of the aspects with which language instructors can contribute and become valuable additions to these programs. An interdisciplinary approach to clinical skills training combines language instructor expertise with that of medical instructors so that programs can offer students a well-rounded experience tailored to their specific needs and goals.

Some students without sufficient language proficiency who wish to join medical language programs have a genuine interest in communicating, even if partially, with patients who speak minoritized languages. Courses at the beginner level can be offered so that these learners may obtain the basis to at least greet and say goodbye to their patients, carry out some informal conversation, and have some other low-stakes exchanges that would not pose a threat to patients if there are errors; at the same time, this helps build rapport and trust when patients observe a clinician making an effort to help them feel welcomed and comfortable. A recent systematic review points out that "LEP patients with language-concordant physicians report receiving more education about their care, have fewer unasked questions, and have better medication adherence and fewer emergency room visits" [30] and, although these very basic exchanges do not equate true doctor-patient language concordance, they may still have a positive impact on patients with non-English language preference.

Given the dynamic context of clinical encounters, students likewise should learn best practices when working with interpreters. They must recognize that their ability to communicate in a target language often will vary depending on the context and content of the clinical encounter. Upon completion of a medical language program, students must understand that calling on an interpreter should not be viewed as a failure. Rather, certified medical interpreters may enhance patient care in many ways beyond language, including advocating for patients and acting as cultural brokers.

Resident physician training programs

To become a board-certified physician in the United States, individuals graduate from medical school and then proceed to residency training programs in their specialty of choice. Here, they gain the specific skills necessary to practice medicine and pass board certification exams. Residency training programs vary in length, ranging from three years to six years or more depending on the specialty. To subspecialize in a particular field, a doctor may graduate from residency and enter into what is known as a fellowship program, which can last one to three or more years.

Given their expanded professional role and responsibilities, resident physicians need a much greater depth of clinical communication skills compared to medical students. Here, their training in language-specific skills may be deepened by acquiring medical specialty-specific vocabulary and phrases as well as strategies to address cultural factors of particular relevance to a specialty. For example, a pediatric resident physician may benefit from learning how to ask a parent about a child's developmental milestones, such as cooing, babbling, and speech. A psychiatric resident physician needs to know how to ask about mental health, symptoms of psychosis, and suicidality in a professional and culturally sensitive manner. This is a natural continuation of the skillset they developed during their medical school years but with a much more specific focus. In terms of assessment, self-evaluation using validated tools has some benefits, but there are other creative ways involving collaboration that can prove useful for students to get detailed feedback about their performance and progress. An innovative example is the use of the culture and language coach (CLC), a figure that provides mentoring as well as additional opportunities for practice and evaluation of students' skills for three years [31].

Programs for physicians-in-practice

Clinical communication skills courses and objectives for physicians-in-practice are often similar to those for resident physicians. Physicians-in-practice need language learning to be specific to their medical field. Educational programs should teach them to accurately self-assess and understand their strengths, limitations, and abilities to use the target language in the medical setting. Often, the roles and responsibilities of a practicing physician change over time. As physicians are required to complete maintenance of certification and continuing education requirements to maintain their medical licensing, they should also seek to maintain and regularly update medical language skills.

Programs for non-physician healthcare professionals

Accordingly, all healthcare professional programs should develop clinical communication skills training in minoritized languages to target the specific roles and responsibilities of specific healthcare fields. Course objectives should account for variations in practical skills, roles, and responsibilities within a specific medical field. For instance, pharmacy school students may focus on communication skills centered on medication plans and counseling, nursing school students may focus on language related to their specific patient care tasks, and social workers should likewise acquire communication skills to discuss social determinants of health and mental health terminology in a culturally sensitive manner.

Medical languages and advocacy

Healthcare workers who have been trained in a minoritized language are in a good position to become strong advocates for that population. Medical language programs should instill and foster a sense of responsibility during their training that remains with them once they become professionals. Instructors can help students gain the understanding, ability, and responsibility to become agents of change for a more inclusive and accessible healthcare system. Instructors can provide examples of professionals advocating for patients who speak minoritized languages. In public health, for instance, public health workers can promote research on issues that particularly affect a population with a minoritized language/culture. Other professionals, like pharmacists, can ensure that detailed translations of instructions and information about drugs are available and accurate. In clinics, nurses and doctors can advocate for pamphlets, charts, and signage to be available in the common language(s) of minoritized populations in their geographic area. Healthcare professionals can apply their skills and position beyond communication with patients for advocacy and system change.

Recommendations for medical language education and research

The scarcity of formal literature in medical languages is one of the aspects that, although improving, still demands further development. Research should be approached from both the language pedagogy and the medical education fields and delve into successful and innovative teaching methodologies, strategies for assessment, and accomplishment of program objectives, among other topics. Data gathering is a useful tool in the process of measuring and analyzing student success, skills development, and other components in the medical language arena. Instructors are recommended to obtain regular feedback from students that will provide information about practices that entail improvements in their communication skills. However, a constant flow of forms and surveys about every detail of their course or program should be avoided to not overwhelm students.

Gathered data can be used for future course improvement and may have different approaches. The examples that follow are suggestions to improve/modify courses based on specific factors, including the type of student, previous medical language training, perception of skills, teaching tools, and evaluation tools.

Type of student

Offering an analysis of the student population that makes up their programs helps instructors and their peers in similar institutions design the tools to tailor their teaching for better success rates. At a college undergraduate level, for instance, knowing whether students are mostly in a pre-med track, interested in nursing, public health, or other areas, allows instructors to focus on particular topics when designing class activities, evaluation tools, and assignments in order to better train them for their future career. More tailored courses would likely keep fostering their motivation, encouraging them to continue with medical language programs as graduate students if given the opportunity.

Previous medical language training and connection to language development

This kind of study can be most useful for graduate courses and programs. Obtaining data about potential past participation in medical language courses and linking it to their progress and development in their current program can provide useful information. Students should be assessed regularly, starting with preprogram data and adding systematic checkpoints. Both instructor evaluations and self-assessment (ideally both) can be used for this type of research. Collaboration between language and medical professionals is an encouraged practice in medical language teaching, as previously noted, but it does not necessarily have to be limited to instruction in the same course. This type of study can help design a more seamless continuity between undergraduate and graduate programs in medical languages and ensure student success and maximum development of skills.

Perception of skills (self-evaluation)

Linked to the previous area, instructors can focus more deeply on students' own perception of their skills and progress. It has been mentioned how developing awareness and an accurate sense of language limitations among students is a key factor in medical language programs that contributes to ensuring accountability once they are graduated and unsupervised. Having students complete regular self-assessments and see how they match with those provided by instructors or SPs will offer that information. The side-by-side comparison of scores will be a useful aid for students in calibrating their own perspectives, and publication of these results will help set up models and standards across institutions and programs.

Teaching tools

There is a wealth of possibilities within this area. Reliance on techniques and strategies from other fields, such as ESL, can only be overcome by increasing and developing language-specific tools and activities. These should be designed to promote language development at the same time that they are framed in a culturally relevant way that fosters awareness and deepening of knowledge. Creating a corpus of best practices, sample assignments, and class activities that appear to be pedagogically resounding tools for instructors will solidify the framework of medical language teaching.

Evaluation tools

Similarly, there is still much to be done in regard to how students are evaluated. Both undergraduate and graduate courses would benefit from more research on ways in which we can successfully assess students in their language, cultural, and clinical skills within these programs. Given the amount of variation within programs in length and other particular characteristics, it would be ideal to have a variety of assessment tools available to choose from and adapt to the particular needs of a program or course. Ideally, these tools would evaluate distinct skills (intercultural competence, language fluency, and accuracy, ability to connect with patients, and more) and do it in different manners (from more objective quiz-like formats to more subjective role-play activities, for instance).

These are just a few general topics to be considered when approaching the area of scholarly work within the medical language field, but there is certainly a longer list of avenues that can be taken in developing it. The main point here is to demonstrate through all of these possibilities that medical languages are indeed an established field; for now, it is more so in practice, but there is plenty of room to make it so from a theoretical standpoint as well. The future of medical language instruction relies on facilitating and fostering collaborative relationships between clinical and language professionals. Important steps have been taken in recent years in solidifying the discipline. It is now time to take the next step and move toward a true interdisciplinary approach to teaching and researching medical languages. In the pages that follow, we provide recommendations for best practices regarding key components of medical language education, with a particular focus on those that use real-life scenarios to offer students the most effective training for their future careers.

Clinical skills and interpersonal communication training and assessment

Language learning is a long process, and it normally takes years to achieve a level of proficiency good enough to allow learners to confidently communicate orally. Instructors should take a well-rounded approach to clinical skills training, including authentic speaking and listening practice for students, as well as opportunities to engage in reading and writing of medical languages. Assigning articles in the target language about relevant topics in the healthcare field exposes students to the vocabulary, solidifies sentence construction, and allows them to gauge recommended levels of formality in these contexts, among other benefits [12]. Written assignments are a valuable opportunity to let students take the time to put together their ideas, exercise critical thinking, and practice their language skills without the threat of immediacy that oral communication poses. In the words of linguist Alister Cumming, "writing elicits an attention to form-meaning relations that may prompt learners to refine their linguistic expression" [32].

Even so, aural and oral skills remain the most valuable in medical languages, as the ultimate objective is often direct communication with native speakers in an oral conversation setting. As a first-stage type of training for this situation, role-play activities in class are a useful tool. Instructors can create scenarios for a patient-doctor situation that needs to be role-played by students, who would then practice both their language and communication skills. However, there are other ways to help students acquire additional practice speaking in a realistic health setting. Students benefit from organized, practical opportunities to use these skills, such as simulation training with SPs, community service, or immersion experiences (i.e., study abroad programs) that may involve living with a host family, taking language courses, and completing an internship in a foreign country. Whether locally or abroad, course content fostering direct contact with target language speakers can and should be included in medical language courses, but it is important that it reflects roles and responsibilities within reach for a student at that level.

Because it affects all aspects of communication, cultural learning needs to be interwoven throughout the curriculum, objectives, practice, and assessments, rather than relegated to a topic to be covered in a finite number of sessions. Students should learn to recognize their limits of cultural understanding and the existence of potential unconscious and conscious biases [4, 19]. Along with cultural humility, students must learn appropriate self-awareness and self-assessment of medical language skills [4]. Because language skills naturally vary with use (or lack thereof), it is important for them to continually use them as they progress through training and their careers. All physicians should be able to self-assess whether or not working with an interpreter is necessary for ensuring quality of care and patient safety, but particularly those who have not worked with patients in the target language for an extended amount of time.

Assessments should focus on practical skills within a real-life or simulated patient care setting. Every assessment that instructors choose to include in their course should have a grading rubric that accompanies it and accurately reflects the specific skills that are been tested. The lack of standardization in medical language courses is particularly noticeable in the area of assessment with regard to rubrics, as there are no formal guidelines [33]. In general terms, it can be stated that, just like medical language courses are a hybrid field, rubrics should not focus solely on language or clinical skills, but combine both. Language and medical instructors should clearly detail the expectations from students for each assessment, and grading rubrics should reflect those same expectations regarding both language and clinical communication skills. Needless to say, grading must be fair. For example, students should not be penalized for not demonstrating knowledge of technical terms in an SP encounter, as they may be trying to avoid those words in that specific context in order to be more accessible to the patient. In that sense, if instructors want to test knowledge of medical jargon, they can create a separate assignment or request a more formal written summary of the encounter in Spanish after it has taken place. Feedback is most effective when both medical and language faculty provide formative, individual comments, as students benefit from their complementary but unique expertise and experiences. Students should also be asked to self-assess their performance regularly, fostering self-awareness of strengths, limitations, and areas for growth. They should compare their self-evaluation with the feedback they get from their instructors to learn how to calibrate their perception of their skills.

Case-based learning and simulation training

Understanding the core tasks and clinical communication skills expected of the learner in the dominant language helps provide a framework for medical language programs.

Faculty must design these programs to accomplish the clinical communication objectives necessary for the specific learner's level of training and responsibilities. Accordingly, clinical cases help students contextualize medical language content and seem to be also their preferred learning method according to a recent study [34]. Case-based learning can occur in class in large groups, in pairs, or with faculty, native language speakers, or SPs. Cases can be used asynchronously before or after class, but they should always be written specifically for the target language, reflecting the heterogeneity of speakers from varying nationalities, educational levels, and socioeconomic status reflective of real-life encounters. The intention is for students to learn cultural humility, not to burden them with the unreasonable expectation to learn every possible cultural practice or regional variation of words.

SP encounters are common in medical professional training, and they are particularly useful in language training as an opportunity to practice and evaluate students' practical communication skills. Educators can work with medical school administrators overseeing clinical simulation programs to use the clinical simulation center, if one is available, as well as to identify and select SPs for a language program. An ideal pool of SPs will have native proficiency in the target language and reflect the diversity among language speakers within the community, including age, socioeconomic status, and national heritage. If SPs are not available, alternative options include role-playing with faculty or fellow students. SPs, as well as faculty or students who play the role of "patient" in simulation activities, should be trained on specific cases and be prompted to intentionally present cultural aspects or nuances while taking care not to present unintentional stereotypes [35]. Learners should learn to identify and ask for clarification readily and quickly, rather than assuming or assigning meaning. For example, when a patient uses a regional word or cultural reference that is unclear or uncertain, a student should identify this and ask for clarification. SP cases can also present students with potential miscommunications or communication challenges, such as giving bad news or explaining a plan of care, in the simulated low-risk environment. Students likewise benefit from simulations on working with interpreters in a variety of medical contexts, including learning how to recognize signs of poor interpretation. Case-writing is an excellent opportunity for instructors to benefit from interdisciplinary collaborations by ensuring cases include relevant linguistic, cultural, and clinical aspects for student practice.

Service learning in clinical settings

According to the National Service-Learning Clearinghouse, "Service-learning is a teaching and learning strategy that integrates meaningful community service with instruction and reflection to enrich the learning experience, teach civic responsibility, and strengthen communities" [36]. Service learning is a key component of multidimensional language learning that enables students to integrate clinical communication skills. Students can contextualize language learning within population health and public advocacy. Service learning may include volunteering at a community clinic or involvement with a local nongovernmental association serving the target population. Caring for patients appropriately involves understanding the many factors influencing public health and individual well-being. Students should learn to thoughtfully observe, listen, engage with compassion and humility, and dialogue with faculty and fellow learners. Through community engagement, students can begin to understand points of strength, resilience, and need. They can become familiar with organizations and businesses that provide fellowship opportunities and foster an appreciation for culture, history, and arts. Faculty can facilitate community tours and introductions to community physicians and key community members to inform students' learning and engagement. With appropriate supervision and guidance, learners who dedicate time to service-learning activities where they are speaking the target language rapidly improve and integrate their medical language skills beyond their peers.

By definition, it is clear that service learning perfectly matches some of the main goals inherent to medical language training. Nonetheless, there are many different ways to approach service learning in medical language courses. For instance, Dr. Lourdes Sánchez-López offered a review of the background and some of the models that have been used throughout the years and proposed an adaptation and expansion of the Comprehensive Integration Model. According to Sánchez-López, in order to achieve a "meaningful and successful service-learning course," four elements must be present: The service-learning opportunity must be (1) built into the course to link integrated theory and practice, (2) designed by the instructor, service-learning professional, and community partner, (3) fully integrated into class discussions, projects, and assessments, and (4) required of all students participating in the program [37].

In addition to these pillars that can help medical language instructors shape their courses, instructors can add a number of guidelines that can increase the success and effectiveness of the service-learning component in medical language teaching. To begin with, programs must emphasize that the target-speaking community is not a learning tool. Students must be aware that the concept of "service" relies on mutually beneficial relationships, not solely for the experiential benefit of the person offering service. Community voices should lead and guide needs assessments, and the community service opportunities provided for students must be sustainable and ethical. Instructors should instill a sense of respect and compassion for these communities; being able to develop a deeper awareness of their reality and practice, language skills are simply collateral benefits. Additionally, opportunities should be curated by instructors. Although this can be a time and energy-consuming activity, it is necessary to ensure that the community project in which students will be collaborating is suited for their level and that the experience lines up with the learning goals of their medical language course.

Oftentimes, free clinics frequented by speakers of minoritized languages may not have the resources to have language-concordant clinicians or certified medical interpreters. For that reason, volunteers are often asked to act as interpreters, which is rarely something that they are trained for. There are ways in which programs can help ensure appropriate volunteer involvement: first, instructors should guarantee language assessment protocols are in place, and that the protocols match the responsibilities of volunteers; if said protocols are not in place, instructors should make sure not to send students who are not proficient enough to interpret. Accordingly, instructors can potentially look for other options for these students to engage in real-world conversations in a low-stakes environment with the target population, such as helping them fill out basic forms or accompanying patients who are alone in the hospital.

The benefits of service learning are many and well-known, but the real impact this activity has on communities must guide the process of creating these opportunities.

Study abroad programs

Learners often seek study abroad programs in regions where the target language is spoken. For example, undergraduate students frequently spend a semester or more abroad honing their language skills and benefiting from direct contact with the language and culture. In some cases, students can carry out internships during their time abroad, gaining an extra perspective on the approach to a specific field, such as medicine, in that particular region or culture. Medical students and residents often have the ability to spend an elective abroad too, learning in a medical setting in another country often for a month at a time. While there are many benefits to language immersion and host family stays, significant limitations include students' lack of time or financial limitations. Other concerns include ethical considerations such as a lack of supervision and the dangers of medical tourism [38]. Learners should seek opportunities that involve community-based, sustainable healthcare and provide appropriate faculty supervision and interpreter support. Learners should receive training before studying abroad to ensure that they know their abilities and limitations.

On their part, instructors should actively participate in selecting (or sometimes even creating) recommended programs that will offer quality training for these students and help them achieve their learning goals, both linguistic and clinical. Faculty can help guide learners to explore regional and national service opportunities.

Nevertheless, it is not necessary to travel to a different country to become a good clinician for linguistically marginalized populations. Local medical language programs should strive to include opportunities for local community engagement. As of 2018, the Center for Immigration Studies reported that more than 67 million people in the United States speak languages other than English at home [39]. Although groups and numbers vary significantly in different areas, learners can likely find opportunities within their own communities to immerse themselves and learn from those experiences without having to leave the country. Virtual opportunities for language immersion are rapidly increasing and are also viable options given less financial and time commitments, such as virtual one-on-one tutoring or conversation sessions with teachers based at a language school where the target language is the dominant language.

Virtual education

The lack of resources (funding, trained instructors, and more) is one of the main reasons why many institutions do not offer medical language courses. Virtual medical language education could offer increased accessibility for learners if thoughtfully developed to meet the same language competencies required by in-person courses. When developing programs, institutions may explore virtual instruction delivery, which would facilitate hiring experts on the field when none are available locally, for instance. However, adopting preexisting online courses over which they do not have any input regarding curriculum or assessment may not be a recommendable option. In the case of medical Spanish, Ortega et al. found that, overall, existing online courses did not meet the criteria to adequately fulfill learner competencies or cultural elements, and all but one failed to achieve competency in self-assessment [40].

The COVID-19 pandemic forced a significant development in the area of online learning. If approached with best practices in mind, virtual educational methodologies can help address health disparities in a way that is in reach to all students, rather than dependent on the specific institution's ability to provide quality medical language education. In that sense, preexisting online courses can be used as supplemental tools but should not be considered as comprehensive alternatives to quality medical language programs.

Conclusion

Clinical communication skills training in minoritized languages is an often-overlooked opportunity to improve health equity. A thoughtfully developed training program provides learners with the skills to improve healthcare access, quality, and safety for patients who speak nondominant languages. By offering a health equity-focused approach to education, teaching faculty will equip clinicians with the perspective, knowledge, and abilities to be agents of change within their communities and improve the health and well-being of target populations.

Highlights

- There is not a "one size fits all" approach to medical language education; courses and programs must be tailored to the specific level, institution, and context in which they take place.
- When creating or reviewing a medical language course or program, instructors need to assess their student population, resources, and intended objectives before designing the details of the class.
- Objectives should align with assessment or, in other words, the evaluation tools need to address specific goals that the course/program has outlined for students.
- Instructors need to be realistic about what can be accomplished through their course/program and avoid unreasonable expectations.
- Whenever possible, language and medical educators should establish collaborations to improve and enhance medical language courses and programs based on their individual strengths and expertise.
- Data gathering is an essential tool to produce more literature on medical language education (regarding teaching methodologies, assessment, etc.) that will help solidify and standardize the field.

REFERENCES

1. Morales, R., Rodriguez, L., Singh, A. et al. (2015). National survey of medical Spanish curriculum in U.S. medical schools. *J. Gen. Intern. Med.* 30 (10): 1434–1439. https://doi.org/10.1007/s11606-015-3309-3.
2. Mazor, S.S., Hampers, L.C., Chande, V.T., and Krug, S.E. (2002). Teaching Spanish to pediatric emergency physicians: effects on patient satisfaction. *Arch. Pediatr. Adolesc. Med.* 156 (7): 693. https://jamanetwork.com/journals/jamapediatrics/article-abstract/203643 (accessed 2 February 2023).
3. Ortega, P., Pérez, N., Robles, B. et al. (2019). Strategies for teaching linguistic preparedness for physicians: medical Spanish and global linguistic competence in undergraduate medical education. *Health Equity* 3 (1): 312–318. https://doi.org/10.1089/heq.2019.0029.

4. Lie, D.A., Forest, C.P., and Richter-Lagha, R. (2018). Evaluating medical Spanish proficiency: a comparison of physician assistant student self-assessment to standardized patient and expert faculty member ratings: a comparison of physician assistant student self-assessment to standardized patient and expert faculty member ratings. *J. Physician Assist. Educ.* 29 (3): 162–166. https://journals.lww.com/jpae/FullText/2018/09000/Evaluating_Medical_Spanish_Proficiency__A.7.aspx (accessed 2 February 2023).
5. Strevens, P. (1977). Special-purpose language learning: a perspective. *Lang. Teach. Linguist. Abstr.* Cambridge University Press 10 (3): 145–163.
6. Hardin, K. (2015). An overview of medical Spanish curricula in the United States. *Hispania* 98 (4): 640–661.
7. Coss, M.D. (2022). The case for a true task-based curriculum for medical Spanish courses. *Teach. Learn. Med.* 35: 1–16.
8. Ortega, P., Diamond, L., Alemán, M.A. et al. (2020). Medical Spanish standardization in U.S. Medical Schools. *Acad. Med.* 95 (1): 22–31.
9. Trace, J., Hudson, T., and Brown, J.D. (2015). *Developing Courses in Languages for Specific Purposes*. ScholarSpace at University of Hawaii at Manoa: Home. https://scholarspace.manoa.hawaii.edu/handle/10125/14573 (accessed 1 March 2022).
10. Grandin, J.M. (2005). Globalization and its implications for the profession. In: *ACTFL 2005–2015: Realizing Our Vision of Languages for All* (ed. A.L. Heining-Boynton), 175–198. Upper Saddle River, NJ: Prentice Hall.
11. Khan, A., Yin, H.S., Brach, C. et al. (2020). Association between parent comfort with English and adverse events among hospitalized children. *JAMA Pediatr.* 174 (12): e203215.
12. Zahar, R., Cobb, T., and Spada, N. (2001). Acquiring vocabulary through reading: effects of frequency and contextual richness. *Can. Mod. Lang. Rev.* 57 (4): 541–572. https://doi.org/10.3138/cmlr.57.4.541.
13. Saragi, T., Nation, I.S.P., and Meister, G.F. (1978). Vocabulary learning and reading. *System* 6 (2): 72–78. https://www.sciencedirect.com/science/article/pii/0346251X78900271.
14. Herman, P.A., Anderson, R.C., Pearson, P.D., and Nagy, W.E. (1987). Incidental acquisition of word meaning from expositions with varied text features. *Read. Res. Q.* 22 (3): 263. https://psycnet.apa.org/fulltext/1988-02742-001.pdf.
15. Mart, C.T. (2012). Developing speaking skills through reading. *Int. J. Engl. Linguist.* 2 (6): 91. https://doi.org/10.5539/ijel.v2n6p91.
16. Riejos, R. and María, A. (1999). Applications of cognitive theory to interdisciplinary work in languages for specific purposes. *Ibérica* 1: 29–37. https://www.redalyc.org/pdf/2870/287026296002.pdf.
17. Pérez Muñoz, C. and Shin, T.M. (2021). Collaboration and evaluation in medical Spanish teaching [Innovation and digital technologies in Languages for Specific Purposes]. In: *Multilingual academic and professional communication in a networked world Proceedings of AELFE-TAPP 2021 (19th AELFE Conference, 2nd TAPP Conference) Vilanova i la Geltrú (Barcelona), 7–9 July 2021*, 978–984. Universitat Politècnica de Catalunya.
18. Lavrenteva, E. and Orland-Barak, L. (2015). The treatment of culture in the foreign language curriculum: an analysis of national curriculum documents. *J. Curric. Stud.* 47 (5): 653–684. https://doi.org/10.1080/00220272.2015.1056233.
19. Tervalon, M. and Murray-García, J. (1998). Cultural humility versus cultural competence: a critical distinction in defining physician training outcomes in multicultural education. *J. Health Care Poor Underserved* 9 (2): 117–125. https://doi.org/10.1353/hpu.2010.0233.
20. Wiggins, G.P. and McTighe, J. (2008). *Understanding by Design*. Alexandria, VA: Association for Supervision and Curriculum Development.
21. Satcher, D. and Higginbotham, E.J. (2008). The public health approach to eliminating disparities in health. *Am. J. Public Health* 98 (9 Suppl): S8–S11. https://doi.org/10.2105/ajph.98.supplement_1.s8.

22. Oliver, M., Fernberg, T., Lyons, P. et al. (2022). Addressing health disparities in Hispanic communities through an innovative team-based medical Spanish program at the medical school level—a single-institution study. *BMC Med. Educ.* 22 (1): 98. https://doi.org/10.1186/s12909-022-03151-x.
23. Braun, R., Nevels, M., and Frey, M.C. (2020). Teaching a health equity course at a Midwestern private university—a pilot study. *Int. Q. Community Health Educ.* 40 (3): 201–207. https://doi.org/10.1177/0272684X19874974.
24. Ortega, P., Diamond, L., Alemán, M.A. et al. (2020). Medical Spanish standardization in U.S. medical schools: consensus statement from a multidisciplinary expert panel. *Acad. Med.* 95 (1): 22–31. https://doi.org/10.1097/ACM.0000000000002917.
25. Blood, A.D., Farnan, J.M., and Fitz-William, W. (2020). Curriculum changes and trends 2010-2020: a focused national review using the AAMC Curriculum Inventory and the LCME Annual Medical School Questionnaire Part II. *Acad. Med.* 95 (9S A Snapshot of Medical Student Education in the United States and Canada: Reports From 145 Schools): S5–S14. https://journals.lww.com/academicmedicine/fulltext/2020/09001/curriculum_changes_and_trends_2010_2020__a_focused.3.aspx (accessed 2 February 2023).
26. Kandiah, D.A. (2017). Perception of educational value in clinical rotations by medical students. *Adv. Med. Educ. Pract.* 8: 149–162. https://doi.org/10.2147/AMEP.S129183.
27. Alptekin, C. (1993). Target-language culture in EFL materials. *ELT J.* 47 (2): 136–143. https://academic.oup.com/eltj/article-abstract/47/2/136/365896 (accessed 2 February 2023).
28. Kissling, E.M. and O'Donnell, M.E. (2015). Increasing language awareness and self-efficacy of FL students using self-assessment and the ACTFL proficiency guidelines. *Lang. Aware.* 24 (4): 283–302. https://doi.org/10.1080/09658416.2015.1099659.
29. Symons, A.B., Swanson, A., McGuigan, D. et al. (2009). A tool for self-assessment of communication skills and professionalism in residents. *BMC Med. Educ.* 9 (1): 1. https://doi.org/10.1186/1472-6920-9-1.
30. Diamond, L., Izquierdo, K., Canfield, D. et al. (2019). A systematic review of the impact of patient–physician non-English language concordance on quality of care and outcomes. *J. Gen. Intern. Med.* 34 (8): 1591–1606.
31. Cowden, J.D., Martinez, F.J., Dickmeyer, J.J., and Bratcher, D. (2022). Culture and language coaching for bilingual residents: the first 10 years of the CHiCoS model. *Teach. Learn. Med.* 1–12. https://doi.org/10.1080/10401334.2022.2092113.
32. Cumming, A. (1990). Expertise in evaluating second language compositions. *Lang. Test.* 7 (1): 31–51. https://doi.org/10.1177/026553229000700104.
33. Ortega, P., Francone, N.O., Santos, M.P. et al. (2021). Medical Spanish in US Medical Schools: a national survey to examine existing programs. *J. Gen. Intern. Med.* 36 (9): 2724–2730. https://doi.org/10.1007/s11606-021-06735-3.
34. George, T., Carey, R.A.B., Abraham, O.C. et al. (2020). Trainee doctors in medicine prefer case-based learning compared to didactic teaching. *J. Family Med. Prim. Care* 9 (2): 580–584. https://doi.org/10.4103/jfmpc.jfmpc_1093_19.
35. Ortega, P., Martínez, G., Alemán, M.A. et al. (2022). Recognizing and dismantling raciolinguistic hierarchies in latinx health. *AMA J. Ethics* 24 (4): E296–E304.
36. Seifer, S.D. and Connors, K. (ed.) (2007). *Faculty Toolkit for Service-Learning in Higher Education*. Scotts Valley, CA: Learn & Serve America, National Service-Learning Clearinghouse.
37. Sánchez-López, L. (2013). Service-learning course design for languages for specific purposes programs. *Hispania* 96 (2): 383–396.
38. Caldwell, P. and Purtzer, M.A. (2015). Long-term learning in a short-term study abroad program: "are we really truly helping the community?". *Public Health Nurs.* 32 (5): 577–583. https://doi.org/10.1111/phn.12168.

39. McHugh, P. (2019). *67.3 Million in the United States Spoke a Foreign Language at Home in 2018*. Center for Immigration Studies. https://cis.org/Report/673-Million-United-States-Spoke-Foreign-Language-Home-2018 (accessed 1 March 2022).

40. Ortega, P., Hardin, K., Pérez-Cordón, C. et al. (2021). An overview of online resources for medical Spanish education for effective communication with Spanish-speaking patients. *Teach. Learn. Med.* 34: 1–13.

20 Faculty Development in Medical Language Education

MÓNICA B. VELA AND
ADRIANA C. BLACK MOROCOIMA

Introduction

Countries with large non-English speaking patient populations, like the United States, struggle to provide language-concordant healthcare. In the United States, Title VI of the Civil Rights Act of 1964 requires institutions receiving federal funding to make a reasonable effort to provide language-concordant care [1]. However, this law is rarely enacted, enforced, or used to seek legal recourse [2]. The impact of this deficit in language-concordant care is dire, as patients with limited English proficiency (LEP) are more likely to face poor health outcomes and are unable (due to poor communication) to establish trust in healthcare workers (HCW); furthermore, healthcare systems experience a greater number of medical errors and are less likely to seek care due to fear of untoward consequences [2]. Patients with LEP are likely to belong to populations with other marginalized identities (e.g., immigrant populations and communities with lower socioeconomic status) and face social determinants (e.g., poor housing quality and food insecurity) that predispose them to poorer health [3].

HCWs are complicit in creating health disparities for patients who speak non-English languages, inclusive of American Sign Language (ASL), due to a healthcare culture that ignores basic communication needs. HCWs are incentivized to move quickly, see a high volume of patients, and are often compensated for acquiring a patient base with high-quality metrics (e.g., well-controlled chronic diseases like hypertension and diabetes, as well as up-to-date cancer screenings). These incentives often lead to cherry-picking patients with significant means and concordant communication styles, leaving patients with LEP with poorer access to quality care. Moreover, HCWs and organizations are not reimbursed for interpreter services by insurance entities such as Medicare or Medicaid [4, 5].

Linguistic marginalization occurs early in the process of seeking healthcare and the default language in United States healthcare systems is English in person, on websites, and in even telehealth [6]. Healthcare systems also do not punish hospitals and clinics for failure to provide language-concordant care. The Joint Commission, formerly known as the Joint Commission on Accreditation of Healthcare Organizations, or JCAHO,

---

The Handbook of Language in Public Health and Healthcare, First Edition.
Edited by Pilar Ortega, Glenn Martínez, Maichou Lor, and A. Susana Ramírez.
© 2024 John Wiley & Sons, Inc. Published 2024 by John Wiley & Sons, Inc.

responsible for accrediting hospitals, has had standards for providing translation and interpreter services since the 1990s [7]. It was not until 2010 that the Joint Commission introduced the word "qualified" to describe those services, but the Joint Commission still does not require the use of "certified interpreters." These nebulous standards provide little protection for linguistically diverse populations.

The culture allowing for poorer standards of care for linguistically diverse populations is established early. Undergraduate and graduate medical education do little to address healthcare worker bias against linguistically diverse patients. Medical school and residency applicants are not assessed for linguistic diversity, are not advantaged for speaking multiple languages in standard admissions practices, and are not screened for bias of any number of marginalized patient populations. Similarly, clinical and teaching faculty are not recognized in any way for their linguistic diversity and capital, despite the clear advantages of providing inclusive medical education and clinical care. Linguistic capital, as defined by Tara Yosso, is "the scholarly and social skills that are captured when communicating in multiple languages or styles" [8]. We apply Yosso's definition of linguistic capital in healthcare to refer to an individual's capacity to: (1) appropriately identify patients who would benefit from interpreter services, (2) communicate effectively in a nondominant language, (3) deploy language tools to improve the accessibility and utilization of high-quality care services to patients who communicate most effectively in a nondominant language, and (4) educate others on the critical need for language-concordant care. Admissions and recruitment officers for all allied health schools would do well to screen for varying levels of linguistic capital among their applicants.

Furthermore, there is no standardized instruction provided in United States medical education on providing language-concordant care, the use of interpreter services, or language law. Leaders in medical education have noted several obstacles to incorporating language-specific coursework or even coursework related to language equity, citing little time in the curriculum for additional topics, a concern that the issues would only be of interest to a small number of students, and few faculty qualified to lead this instruction. Two national surveys of medical education coursework related to medical Spanish noted that, when offered, there was often little to no course credit assigned to enrolled students, little to no monetary incentive or administrative support to the faculty instructors, and there was often a lack of curricular standards or certification upon completion of the coursework [9, 10]. These mechanistic obstacles have served to diminish the value and importance of this education and to disincentivize faculty from developing this field of study. The concern that there are very few faculty available to lead this instruction must be addressed through greater efforts to address a lack of diversity among academic faculty [11, 12].

The lack of racial and ethnic diversity among academic faculty in the medical profession has been documented repeatedly. As an example, the Association of American Medical Colleges notes that 5.5% of medical school faculty are Hispanic, Latinx, or of Spanish origin; 3.6% are Black or African American; and only 0.2% are Native American or Alaskan Native [13]. Linguistic diversity is also an issue. In the United States, the language spoken most frequently among LEP populations is Spanish (over 37 million people) followed by Chinese and Tagalog [14]. Lisa Diamond et al. have demonstrated that 37% of resident physicians in training spoke at least one non-English language, although the languages they spoke were not those in greatest need for the population. Spanish, for example, had the lowest national resident physician to patient ratio [15, 16]. As a result, the lack of faculty development to support and incentivize language-concordant care in medical education has significantly affected the United States Latinx community and has allowed for raciolinguistic hierarchies within Latinx health [17]. Other non-English speaking populations have likely been similarly impacted. Medical education should promote the development of academic faculty with linguistic capital in order to change a healthcare culture that allows a differential quality of care for linguistically diverse patients who do not speak English.

In this chapter, we will: (1) explore frameworks for conceptualizing faculty development to improve language-concordant healthcare delivery with an ultimate focus on health equity, (2) identify areas for growth, and (3) propose recommendations.

Terminology for faculty development

The following terms (Table 20.1) will be utilized throughout this chapter to help present strategies that will improve the clinical and academic faculty development and support needed to promote language-concordant care. From here forward, we propose the use of the term, "Clinical Language Equity Education" (CLEE). This term will be defined as that education designed to expand communication between HCWs and patients to be inclusive of linguistically diverse populations for the purpose of improving HCW-patient trust, accessibility of healthcare services, healthcare outcomes, and ultimately health equity. It is also important to center these efforts on multilingual faculty, who often have intersecting, minoritized identities, as they have often been the LEP group in professional settings and exposed to oppressive practices and behaviors. The work of promoting health equity is the work of all allied HCWs and academicians. The development of medical language education curriculum should be led by those with authentic, shared lived experiences with those speaking nondominant languages, and those with a personal drive to effect change regardless of their identities [28]. An educator or trainer's personal experience with discrimination often impacts their effectiveness as perceived by trainees [29].

With the assistance of this terminology, we also hope to provide readers with a framework that they can utilize to discuss critical issues and potential recommendations that will support faculty in teaching, researching, and providing language-concordant care. We will address challenges and provide potential action steps that faculty can implement within their respective professional settings. In sum, we hope that patients and HCW can partner and advocate for quality, language-concordant, and equitable care.

Theoretical framework

In order to best address the power imbalances that infiltrate systems and institutions that communities interact with daily, Yosso presents a framework that helps shift existing power dynamics and centers the cultural capital that faculty could bring into medical schools, hospitals, and clinics [8]. This framework, the Community Cultural Wealth model, comprises six different forms of cultural capital: linguistic, navigational, familial, social, resistance, and aspirational.

Linguistic capital is a term for the communication and intellectual skills cultivated through the experiences of speaking in more than one language or style. Navigational capital refers to the skills needed to move through unjust, institutional systems. Familial capital refers to the cultural knowledge that an individual gains from relatives

Table 20.1 Terminology Related to Faculty Development in Clinical Language Equity Education.

Term	Definition	Example(s)
Clinical Language Equity Education (CLEE)	Education that serves to broaden communication between healthcare workers (HCW) and patients to be inclusive of linguistically diverse populations for the purpose of improving HCW-patient trust, accessibility of healthcare services, healthcare outcomes, and ultimately health equity.	1. HCWs learn to work effectively with interpreter services 2. HCWs learn to recognize the need for non-English concordant care in the clinical setting
Cultural Humility	A lifelong process and commitment to self-reflection and analysis, to repair power imbalances in the HCW-patient relationship, and to developing mutually beneficial, non-paternalistic advocacy partnerships with individuals and communities [18].	Clinical educators broaden and enrich learners' understanding of the heterogenous, linguistically diverse populations. The stereotype that patients who speak languages other than English are uneducated or health illiterate is false and promotes bias and differential care.
Faculty Development (FD)	An organized, goal-directed process to achieve career progression and growth. Inherent in this process is the acquisition of skills that enable one to contribute in a meaningful way to the advancement of a field of interest, whether educational, operational, or scientific. The process requires attention to technical skills, personal attributes, and explicit goals. Supportive mentorship is optimal [19]	FD in CLEE includes: 1. HCWs track quality metrics for patients who speak a language other than English. 2. HCWs engage in cultural humility training that includes linguistic diversity and promotion of linguistic capital. 3. Students engage in language certification and advance their linguistic skills to achieve the level of competency needed to care for patients without interpreter services. 4. Trainees are taught about language-concordant care and to recognize when and how to access certified interpreters in person, virtually, or through telephonic means. 5. HCWs promote healthcare accessibility and promote the use of languages other than English on websites, in public service announcements, hospital and clinic signage, availability of interpreter services, use of electronic record alerts, written patient materials, etc.

Term	Definition	Example
Flourish	The presence of both mental health and social well-being with positive feeling and positive functioning [20].	HCWs promote health and well-being of their patients and are trained to focus on assets and salubrious outcomes. Patients deserve the opportunity to experience the healthcare system as a positive entity that promotes both health and well-being rather than an entity that only diminishes illness.
Health Equity	Achieved when every individual has the opportunity to reach their full potential and no individual is disadvantaged from achieving this potential because of social position or other socially determined circumstances [21].	HCWs address the impact of social determinants of health to mitigate the inequities that marginalized populations experience in health and healthcare. These social determinants include, but are not limited to: insurance status, housing, wealth and income, educational status, and interactions with racism, and discrimination.
Language-Concordant Care	A healthcare experience where the HCW and patient communicate in the same language [22–24].	Language-concordant care can be achieved through multiple means: 1. HCWs and patients speak the same language. 2. Highly trained and certified interpreters are available in person to facilitate communication. 3. Highly trained and certified interpreters are available via electronic or other assistive devices.
Language Equity	A component of Health Equity that is achieved when a patient is able to communicate using their preferred language [25].	1. A hospital trains patient intake staff to ask patients about language preference, and non-English language preference, when applicable, becomes incorporated into the patient's care plans. 2. A hospital institute's a care plan for patients with non-English language preference that coordinates language services and clinical services, preferentially matching patients with language-concordant clinicians whenever possible. 3. Medical students with multilingual skills are granted the opportunity to professionalize their non-English language skills in healthcare contexts.

(Continued)

Table 20.1 (Continued)

Term	Definition	Example(s)
Limited English Proficiency (LEP)	Individuals who do not speak English as their primary language and who have a limited ability to read, speak, write, or understand English [26]. Potential questions to ask to identify LEP in clinical care include [27]: 1. How well do you speak English? 2. In what language do you prefer to receive your medical care?	HCWs learn to identify language needs and share appropriate options and resources with their patients through various trainings. Patients' knowledge, opportunities, and access to quality care should not be hindered due to healthcare workers' lack of thoroughly understanding the health assessments, options, or resources available when language discordance occurs.
Linguistic Capital	The scholarly and social skills that are captured when communicating in multiple languages or styles [8].	The ability for HCW to: 1. Identify patients who would benefit from interpreter services. 2. Communicate effectively in nondominant languages. 3. Deploy a shared language or language tools to improve the accessibility and utilization of high-quality care services to patients who communicate most effectively in a nondominant language. 4. Promote a culture of advocacy for language equity in clinical settings.
Linguistic Marginalization	Also referred to as linguistic minoritization, is commonly recognized as a major barrier to access to health services and health information [6].	Healthcare workers eliminate the bias that exists around English being the default language in the United States healthcare system and therefore other language speakers being marginalized or minoritized. This demonstrates a monolingual bias for English speakers and mitigating this bias will be important for HCWs who seek to provide equitable care.

about community interactions, resources, and cultural intuition. Social capital consists of the crucial network composed of both people and resources within a community that can help to navigate institutions. Resistance capital is critical as it addresses the knowledge and behavior necessary to challenge inequities. Finally, aspirational capital is the ability to remain hopeful despite all the injustices present in one's environment [8].

Community cultural wealth in linguistically diverse populations

All of these forms of capital come together to form cultural capital. This cultural capital can assist linguistically minoritized communities in explicitly maneuvering around the systemic challenges in place that are upheld by a lack of access to trained, quality interpreters, accessibility to language-concordant hospitals, administrators to setup appointments, and bilingual or multilingual HCW, among other barriers [2]. Without providing more language options – both oral and written – healthcare systems and HCWs are failing to protect LEP patients and in turn, causing harm.

Having family present during healthcare appointments is one potential way in which linguistically diverse communities' cultural capital can be utilized. Using family members as ad hoc interpreters is illegal, unethical (diminishes patient autonomy and confidentiality) and has been proven to diminish the quality of care being delivered when compared to a trained interpreter. However, family members can successfully partner with HCW in being advocates for the best quality care for the patient by requesting language-concordant care and being familiar with patients' rights, and when permitted by the patient, asking for clarification on complex issues. This strategy raises familial, social, and navigational capitals, helps to reduce potential bias with HCWs, patients, and families working in tandem with one common goal, and ultimately places value on the patient's experience in the clinical setting. Researchers have recommended establishing the LEP Patient Family Advocate role, allowing for a family member to be part of the healthcare team and serve as a bridge between all healthcare staff and the patient's family [30]. The LEP Patient Family Advocate may be a cultural resource by identifying and addressing topics related to access, quality, literacy, and safety. Researchers noted that incorporating this team member had a positive effect on communication, trust, and partnership among the patient and team members, while also improving continuity of care and safety of the patient. Additionally, families reported lower levels of stress related to their family member's care.

Community cultural wealth among faculty

Faculty who develop and teach medical language courses must apply an assets-based approach, such as the Community Cultural Wealth model, to their work. Too often, intersecting, minoritized identities are viewed as "disadvantaged" or as a burden to the healthcare system. The lack of faculty who identify as having intersecting minoritized identities in medical education settings is an extension of the same problem. This is despite emerging data demonstrating, for example, that racial concordance between patient and HCW are associated with improved patient outcomes [31, 32]. Yosso's model allows for a macro-level approach that centers on the skillset and assets that linguistically diverse groups bring to educational spaces [8]. In order for faculty to utilize their social capital, they must first acknowledge the power, privilege, and positionality they hold within academia and medicine. Marjorie Rosenthal proposes that HCWs and academicians reconsider academic hierarchies by engaging and partnering meaningfully with the local communities and bringing knowledge gained from interacting with local communities into teaching, clinical practice, and research [33]. Ultimately, promoting a culture of advocacy for language equity in educational, research, and clinical settings will assist in establishing a community where faculty are trained, become experts in disseminating CLEE, and can then mentor incoming trainees to do the same.

Critical issues and topics

The currency of published scholarship depends highly upon the sociopolitical climate of healthcare, as well as that of the country in which it is housed. For decades, research related to care of poor, "vulnerable," "indigent," or immigrant populations, as well as other literature related to health services, was not as highly valued in academic circles when compared to basic science, clinical, or translational science [34]. In fact, scholarship related to the impact of racism and discrimination on health and healthcare was unlikely to be published in high-impact journals [35, 36]. In the last two decades, the mounting literature on racial and ethnic health and healthcare disparities [37], the rise of the Affordable Care Act [38], the impact of the COVID-19 pandemic on minoritized communities [39], and racialized violence [40] have all contributed to a renewed focus on health equity. Within health equity, language equity has only recently been defined and has risen as a recognized field of attention-worthy scholarship [6].

Teaching health equity in medical education

It has only been in the last 15 years that there has been a demand within medical education for coursework on health equity [41]. In July 2022, the Association of American Medical Colleges published a report titled, "Diversity, Equity and Inclusion Competencies Across the Learning Continuum," with guidelines designed to, "develop physicians who are more fully equipped to address inequities in healthcare and who value diversity in all its forms" [42]. Unfortunately, issues related to language-concordant care were not included in their report. Some clinical educators have begun to incorporate guidelines on language-concordant care as part of health equity promotion [43].

Recommendations for research, education, and clinical practice

In order to comprehensively address language-concordant care and mitigate health and language inequities, sustainable structures must be put in place at multiple levels across the educational continuum and within healthcare delivery systems. In this section, we focus on recommendations related to medical language faculty development. Faculty must be actively engaged in improving language equity in the various settings in which they work. This will require implementing processes and policies within student curricula, in clinical settings, and also in research practice. Additionally, it is imperative to continuously collect data and evaluate the progress that is made as these programs are established. These qualitative and quantitative measures will dictate what future adjustments are required and will support the overall sustainability of the programs. Finally, it is the goal that these recommendations, listed below in four categories – curricular, clinical, research, and evaluation – will be able to be duplicated in many medical schools and healthcare systems.

1. **Curricular Recommendations**. Clinical Language Equity Education expertise (CLEE) must be incorporated into academic medicine, such as through the following strategies:

a. Focus on equity measures and incorporating CLEE in the curriculum (across four years), admissions (recognizing language as an asset), financial aid (rewarding students with multilingual capacity), and through awards and promotions.
b. Develop coursework with educational credits for learners and continuing medical education credits for practicing physicians. Institutional approval and course credit serve as markers for quality and provide incentives for participation. This could be approached similarly to recent Title IX learning requirements which are standard at most United States medical institutions and teach faculty how to prevent and report sexual discrimination and harassment.
c. Establish regularly scheduled trainings on CLEE. Completing these trainings would be incentivized with ties to promotion and salary adjustments.
2. **Clinical Recommendations**. Clinical practices must be guided by CLEE through measures such as the following:
   a. Add Language Equity Specialists to planning and policy committees. Their participation may help address appropriate signage and signal inclusion at multiple entry points (e.g., online, phone communications, written communications, telehealth, public service announcements, and in-person clinical settings).
   b. Create electronic record notations alerting faculty and staff that a patient has a non-English language preference.
   c. Require clinical documentation of how language-appropriate care was provided, such as language-concordant care being provided by a qualified clinician or interpreter services being offered at check-in and in the clinical encounter.
3. **Research Recommendations.** Institutions and funding agencies, such as the National Institutes of Health, should consider the following:
   a. Create new research opportunities for the study of Clinical Language Equity Education and language outcomes for the health populations.
   b. Engage CLEE Specialists to review calls for clinical research studies and grants requesting that they incorporate the following key language equity strategies:
      i. Add language equity consultants to projects.
      ii. Require cultural humility trainings for Principal Investigators and other key members of research teams.
      iii. Promote CLEE specialist positions on research teams and/or require CLEE training for research teams.
      iv. Incorporate a CLEE specialist on Institutional Review Boards to safeguard protections for research participants from linguistically diverse communities and ensure the inclusion of linguistically representative groups in clinical trials.
4. **Evaluation Recommendations.** Create Language Equity Report Card to provide metrics with respect to recommendations 1–3.
   a. **Metric.** Is language capability viewed as a valuable asset in holistic review of student, staff, and faculty recruitment and evaluations?
   b. **Metric.** Are patients adequately screened for language preferences and subsequently provided with either a language-concordant HCW or a professional interpreter to achieve language-appropriate care?
   c. **Metric.** Are study populations linguistically diverse?
   d. **Metric.** Are faculty and staff trained in language equity and cultural humility?

In addition to the four main categories listed above, the following recommendations are centered on the forms of capital posited in the Community Cultural Wealth Framework. Below, in Table 20.2, recommendations are listed in alignment with the form

Table 20.2 Faculty Development in Clinical Language Equity Education Recommendations for Academic Leaders.

Recommendation for Clinical Language Equity Faculty	Meaning	Form of capital [8]	Challenge	Action steps
Encourage all medical students, trainees, and faculty to experience working with linguistically diverse patients and utilize interpreter services [44].	Provides a climate where steps are taken to ensure that language equity is achieved.	Linguistic	Shifting existing narratives and the current status quo in healthcare services where English is the default language and those who do not speak English are forced to assimilate and are frequently seen as a problem or a burden.	Establish policies, processes, trainings, and procedures that can be standardized, duplicated, and measured for quality of care outcomes across medical schools and healthcare systems in a sustainable way.
Add CLEE Specialists to planning and policy committees in order to ensure all new clinical endeavors are language inclusive.	Creates a space that is easier for LEP patients to maneuver; thus, providing a more welcoming environment of belonging.	Navigational	Creating new job descriptions that fully detail the expertise and depth needed to address these language gaps.	Partner with Human Resources, external linguistic consultants, and the Office of Equal Opportunity to create job descriptions, search committees, and interview processes that are just and evidence-based.
Support well-defined family roles on clinical teams as assets to health promotion [44].	Builds a foundation for family engagement playing a role in supporting high-quality outcomes [45]. Future research may demonstrate that in clinical settings, shared linguistic capital may be a mechanism to promote family engagement.	Familial	Leveraging family and culture as assets and not as "ad hoc" interpreters.	Engage family on language equity rights and how to be an advocate for themselves as patients.

Protect patients and students from medical and legal consequences of language-discordant care and role model appropriate use of interpreters [44]. Partner with certified interpreters when providing care for patients with LEP instead of using students and staff as ad hoc interpreters.	Cultivates an environment of trust, justice, and unity between patients, their families, and HCW. Creates opportunities for interpreters to utilize their skills in-person or via telephone, and/or video. In turn, patients feel more comfortable during their visit and students engage in interprofessional education.	Social	Learning and becoming knowledgeable about legal policies and resources about providing language-concordant care.	Teach both patients and students that LEP patients have a legal right to professional interpretation services and/or competent language-concordant care [44, 46, 47].
		Resistance	Changing the culture of academic medicine that is the legal, moral, and ethical mandate required to promote an equitable and safe clinical environment for all patients.	1. Teach staff to ask about patient language preferences and how to effectively work with medical interpreters [48]. 2. Highlight patients' rights to request an interpreter. 3. Provide multilingual marketing materials (e.g., signage, pamphlets, websites, and public services announcements).
Recognize the value of providing language-concordant care, treating LEP patients with dignity and respect, and aspire to deliver the highest quality care and outcomes possible for all patients –regardless of shared or unshared linguistic capital.	Creates a culturally humble environment where power structures are recognized and balanced.	Aspirational	Allocating time to engage in self-reflective and introspective practices where all HCWs are able to self-assess their own power, privilege, and positionality in professional spaces related to linguistic capital.	1. Provide regular trainings about language-concordant care to faculty and HCW, in addition to trainings that discuss how to implement culturally humble practices in classroom and clinical settings. 2. Provide language certification for proficient trainees competent to care for patients without interpreter services present.

of capital that is being utilized. As these efforts are never simple or straightforward, we transparently share challenges that these recommendations bring and what action steps are required to achieve them.

Conclusion

Despite legal and financial incentives to provide language-concordant care and incorporate language equity policies into systems of care, a language equity culture has not yet been adopted by leadership, researchers, HCWs, and medical educators in the United States healthcare context. A culture shift can only take place through a process that incorporates self-reflection, self-education, and, finally, action steps. This culture shift will also require significant resourced and enforced policies throughout systems of care, education, and scholarship. It is incumbent upon those interested in addressing health disparities and creating an equitable world where everyone can flourish that language equity be promoted, supported, and sustained in all mechanistic delivery systems. In turn, this will help generate health equity for all patients.

Highlights

- Institutions and funders can create new research opportunities for the study of Clinical Language Equity Education and language-related health outcomes. They should also engage language equity experts to review calls for clinical research studies and grants.
- Clinical Language Equity Education (CLEE) expertise must be incorporated into academic medicine by focusing on equity measures and longitudinally incorporating CLEE in the curriculum, admissions process (recognizing language as an asset), financial aid (rewarding students with multilingual skills), and through awards and promotions.
- A more inclusive healthcare system will also improve a sense of belonging for HCWs from linguistically diverse communities and will fuel an avenue of research scholarship and faculty development centered on providing language-concordant care with health equity as the ultimate goal.

REFERENCES

1. Office of the Assistant Secretary for Administration & Management *Title VI, Civil Rights Act of 1964*. U.S. Department of Labor. https://www.dol.gov/agencies/oasam/regulatory/statutes/title-vi-civil-rights-act-of-1964 (accessed 29 April 2022).
2. Steinberg, E.M., Valenzuela-Araujo, D., Zickafoose, J.S. et al. (2016). The "Battle" of Managing Language Barriers in Health Care. *Clin. Pediatr. (Phila)* 55 (14): 1318–1327.
3. Fischer, A., Conigliaro, J., Allicock, S., and Kim, E.J. (2021). Examination of social determinants of health among patients with

limited English proficiency. *BMC. Res. Notes* 14 (1): 299.
4. Jacobs, B., Ryan, A.M., Henrichs, K.S., and Weiss, B.D. (2018). Medical interpreters in outpatient practice. *Ann. Fam. Med.* 16 (1): 70–76.
5. Translation and Interpretation Services *Medicaid*. Centers for Medicare & Medicaid Services. https://www.medicaid.gov/medicaid/financial-management/medicaid-administrative-claiming/translation-and-interpretation-services/index.html. http://Medicaid.gov/ (accessed 29 April 2022).
6. Showstack R, Santos M, Feuerherm E, Jacobson H, Martinez G. *Language as a Social Determinant of Health: An Applied Linguistics Perspective on Health Equity*. 2018. AAALetter.
7. The Joint Commission (2017). *Language Access and Interpreter Services – Understanding The Requirements. Behavioral Health. Rights and Responsibilities of the Individual*. Joint Commission Enterprise. https://www.jointcommission.org/standards/standard-faqs/behavioral-health/rights-and-responsibilities-of-the-individual-ri/000002120 (accessed 29 April 2022).
8. Yosso, T.J. (2005). Whose culture has capital? A critical race theory discussion of community cultural wealth. *Race Ethn. Educ.* 8 (1): 69–91.
9. Morales, R., Rodriguez, L., Singh, A. et al. (2015). National Survey of medical Spanish curriculum in U.S. medical schools. *J. Gen. Intern. Med.* 30 (10): 1434–1439.
10. Ortega, P., Francone, N.O., Santos, M.P. et al. (2021). Medical Spanish in US medical schools: a National Survey to examine existing programs. *J. Gen. Intern. Med.* 36 (9): 2724–2730.
11. Ortega, P., Shin, T.M., Francone, N.O. et al. (2021). Student and faculty diversity is insufficient to ensure high-quality medical Spanish education in US medical schools. *J. Immigr. Minor. Health* 23 (5): 1105–1109.
12. Kamran, S.C., Winkfield, K.M., Reede, J.Y., and Vapiwala, N. (2022). Intersectional analysis of U.S. medical faculty diversity over four decades. *N. Engl. J. Med.* 386 (14): 1363–1371.
13. (2019). *Diversity in Medicine: Facts and Figures*. Washington, DC: Association of American Medical Colleges. https://www.aamc.org/data-reports/workforce/report/diversity-medicine-facts-and-figures-2019.
14. Migration Policy Institute. *Top 10 Languages Spoken by Limited English Proficient U.S. Residents and LEP Share*. 2013. https://www.migrationpolicy.org/programs/data-hub/charts/top-10-languages-spoken-limited-english-proficient-us-residents-and-lep.
15. Diamond, L.C., Mujawar, I., Vickstrom, E. et al. (2020). Supply and demand: association between non-English language-speaking first year resident physicians and areas of need in the USA. *J. Gen. Intern. Med.* 35 (8): 2289–2295.
16. Diamond, L., Grbic, D., Genoff, M. et al. (2014). Non-English-language proficiency of applicants to US residency programs. *JAMA* 312 (22): 2405–2407.
17. Ortega, P., Martínez, G., Alemán, M.A. et al. (2022). Recognizing and dismantling raciolinguistic hierarchies in Latinx health. *AMA J. Ethics* 24 (4): E296–E304.
18. Danso, R. (2018). Cultural competence and cultural humility: a critical reflection on key cultural diversity concepts. *J. Soc. Work.* 18 (4): 410–430.
19. Hamilton, G.C. and Brown, J.E. (2003). Faculty development: what is faculty development? *Acad. Emerg. Med.* 10 (12): 1334–1336.
20. Levin, J. (2020). Human flourishing and population health: meaning, measurement, and implications. *Perspect. Biol. Med.* 63: 401–419.
21. Centers for Disease Control and Prevention. *Health Equity*. 2022. https://www.cdc.gov/chronicdisease/healthequity/index.htm (accessed 29 April 2022).
22. Ngo-Metzger, Q., Sorkin, D.H., Phillips, R.S. et al. (2007). Providing high-quality care for limited English proficient patients: the importance of language concordance and interpreter use. *J. Gen. Intern. Med.* 22 (Suppl 2): 324–330.
23. Molina, R.L. and Kasper, J. (2019). The power of language-concordant care: a call to action for medical schools. *BMC Med.*

Educ. 19 (1): https://doi.org/10.1186/S12909-019-1807-4.
24. Ortega, P. (2018). Spanish language concordance in U.S. medical care: a multifaceted challenge and call to action. *Acad. Med.* 93: 1.
25. Ortega P. *Language Equity Definition*. 2022.
26. US Department of Justice. *Limited English Proficiency*. https://www.lep.gov.
27. Karliner, L.S., Jacobs, E.A., Chen, A.H., and Mutha, S. (2007). Do professional interpreters improve clinical care for patients with limited English proficiency? A systematic review of the literature. *Health Serv. Res.* 42 (2): 727–754.
28. Vela, M.B., Chin, M.H., and Peek, M.E. (2021). Keeping our promise - supporting trainees from groups that are underrepresented in medicine. *N. Engl. J. Med.* 385 (6): 487–489.
29. Liberman, B.E., Block, C.J., and Koch, S.M. (2011). Diversity trainer preconceptions: the effects of trainer race and gender on perceptions of diversity trainer effectiveness. *Basic Appl. Soc. Psychol.* 33 (3): 279–293.
30. Gil, S., Hooke, M.C., and Niess, D. (2016). The limited English proficiency patient family advocate role: fostering respectful and effective care across language and culture in a pediatric oncology setting. *J. Pediatr. Oncol. Nurs.* 33 (3): 190–198.
31. Greenwood, B.N., Hardeman, R.R., Huang, L., and Sojourner, A. (2020). Physician–patient racial concordance and disparities in birthing mortality for newborns. *Proc. Natl. Acad. Sci.* 117 (35): 21194–21200.
32. Alsan, M., Garrick, O., and Graziani, G. (2019). Does diversity matter for health? Experimental evidence from Oakland. *Am. Econ. Rev.* 109 (12): 4071–4111.
33. Rosenthal, M.S. (2015). What we might accomplish by engaging in our local communities. *Prev. Med. Rep.* 2: 13–14.
34. Lett, E., Adekunle, D., McMurray, P. et al. (2022). Health equity tourism: ravaging the justice landscape. *J. Med. Syst.* 46 (3): 17.
35. Hardeman, R.R., Murphy, K.A., Karbeah, J., and Kozhimannil, K.B. (2018). Naming institutionalized racism in the public health literature: a systematic literature review. *Public Health Rep.* 133 (3): 240–249.
36. Krieger, N., Boyd, R.W., Maio, F.D., and Maybank, A. (2021). *Medicine's Privileged Gatekeepers: Producing Harmful Ignorance About Racism And Health*. Health Aff Blog https://www.healthaffairs.org/do/10.1377/forefront.20210415.305480/full.
37. Betancourt, J.R. and Maina, A.W. (2004). The Institute of Medicine report "unequal treatment": implications for academic health centers. *Mt. Sinai J. Med.* 71 (5): 314–321.
38. Buchmueller, T.C. and Levy, H.G. (2020). The ACA's impact on racial and ethnic disparities in health insurance coverage and access to care. *Health Aff.* 39 (3): 395–402.
39. Tai, D.B.G., Shah, A., Doubeni, C.A. et al. (2021). The disproportionate impact of COVID-19 on racial and ethnic minorities in the United States. *Clin. Infect. Dis. Off. Publ. Infect. Dis. Soc. Am.* 72 (4): 703–706.
40. Sharif, M.Z., García, J.J., Mitchell, U. et al. (2022). Racism and structural violence: interconnected threats to health equity. *Front. Public Health* 9: 676783. https://www.frontiersin.org/articles/10.3389/fpubh.2021.676783.
41. Gonzalez, C.M. and Bussey-Jones, J. (2010). Disparities education: what do students want? *J. Gen. Intern. Med.* 25 (Suppl 2): S102–S107.
42. American Association of Medical Colleges. *American Association of Medical Colleges Diversity, Equity and Inclusion Competencies across the Learning Continuum Report*. 2022. https://www.aamc.org/data-reports/report/diversity-equity-and-inclusion-competencies-across-learning-continuum.
43. Pincavage, A.T., Osman, N.Y., Alexandraki, I. et al. (2022). AAIM recommendations to promote equity in the clerkship clinical learning environment. *Am. J. Med.* 135 (8): 1021–1028.
44. Vela, M. (2022). *Use of Certified Interpreters in Clinical Clerkships*. Alliance for Academic Internal Medicine p. Appendix. https://www.im.org/resources/ume-gme-program-resources/resources-equity-clerkship-cle.

45. Cené, C.W., Johnson, B.H., Wells, N. et al. (2016). A Narrative Review of Patient and Family Engagement: The "Foundation" of the Medical "Home". *Med. Care* 54 (7): 697–705.
46. Vela, M., Fritz, C., Press, V., and Girotti, J. (2016). Medical students' experiences and perspectives on interpreting for LEP patients at two US medical schools. *J. Racial Ethn. Health Disparities* 3 (2): 245–249. https://doi.org/10.1007/s40615-015-0134-7.
47. Vela, M., Fritz, C., and Jacobs, E. (2015). Establishing medical Students' cultural and linguistic competence for the Care of Spanish-Speaking Limited English Proficient Patients. *J. Racial Ethn. Health Disparities* 3: 484–488.
48. Ortega, P. and Shin, T.M. (2021). *Language Is Not A Barrier—It Is An Opportunity To Improve Health Equity Through Education*. Health Aff Blog. https://www.healthaffairs.org/content/forefront/language-not-barrier-opportunity-improve-health-equity-through-education.

Part V Mass Communication and Health: Theory, Research, and Application with and for Linguistically Diverse Populations

Introduction to Part V

A. Susana Ramírez

In this section, we move beyond clinical settings to examine the global health information environment and to consider the role played by the mass media in communicating health information – and misinformation – about, for, and to linguistically diverse populations. The goal of the section is to demonstrate how information disseminated through mass media technologies (i.e., to mass audiences) influences population health and the extent to which linguistically diverse populations are considered in this literature.

We begin this section with a historical perspective on research in mass communication and health, including an overview of the predominant theories of mass communication. Mass media is defined as a diverse set of technologies that can reach mass audiences, such as television, radio, magazines, and increasingly, digital media. In Chapter 21, Katharine Head and Katherine Ridley-Merriweather trace the development of mediated interventions for public health in the context of communicable disease prevention, the shift to considering the influence of the information environment on patients' knowledge and behaviors, through the current focus on information seeking behaviors and misinformation effects. Advances in mass media technologies, including the introduction and rise of social media, are discussed, along with areas for future research and practice considerations relevant to linguistically diverse populations.

The Handbook of Language in Public Health and Healthcare, First Edition.
Edited by Pilar Ortega, Glenn Martínez, Maichou Lor, and A. Susana Ramírez.
© 2024 John Wiley & Sons, Inc. Published 2024 by John Wiley & Sons, Inc.

In Chapter 22, the focus turns to the information environment and the research on information seeking. Beginning from the twin premises that health information seeking has significant consequences on patient health, even as the efficacy of seeking is limited by linguistic and other barriers, Christine Swoboda, Priti Singh, Susana Ramírez, and Naleef Fareed present a conceptual framework to examine critical issues in health information seeking behaviors and outcomes among linguistically diverse populations. Focusing on the United States context, the goals of this chapter are to: Synthesize what is known about health-information-seeking behaviors and outcomes, including disparities; analyze critical issues in health-information seeking as they relate to linguistic minority populations; and present recommendations for research, education, and practice.

In Chapter 23, Suruchi Sood and Rachael HaileSelasse explore the dynamic relationship between linguistic diversity and entertainment-education strategies that promote social and behavioral change. They briefly review the modern histories and definitions of both linguistic diversity and entertainment-education, describing the organic cross-influence between the two disciplines. Linguistic diversity is more broadly the use of different languages but includes language variation within culture and cultural variation within language. As a communication strategy, entertainment-education inherently influences language via a wide variety of media channels including audio, video, and visual arts. Sood and HaileSelasse articulate a compelling argument for the bidirectional relationship between language and entertainment-education, illustrated by intervention examples from the field: Entertainment-education impacts linguistic diversity by providing new ways to describe relationships, experiences, and actions, using abbreviations, shortcuts, mnemonics, and the introduction of new terminology. Principles from applied linguistics are utilized in entertainment-education through its careful attention to formative research and audience segmentation, as well as its reliance on culture-centric messaging and the use of narratives to enhance program reach and engagement.

Chapter 24 specifically explores the use of graphic medicine (comics) as a strategy for communicating with linguistically diverse populations. MK Czerwiec, Jane Zhao, Isa Álvarez, and Pilar Ortega situate the emergence of graphic medicine within the context of narrative medicine, sharing examples of comics developed for health education and then proposing graphic medicine as a tool to improve public health messaging, patient–clinician communication, and clinician wellness among healthcare students and professionals from linguistically diverse backgrounds.

Chapter 25 examines the health implications of social media use. Despite a vast and growing scholarship on the relationship between social media use and health, much of this work has focused on English language content and on platforms popular within Western countries. Anna Gaysynsky, Katherine Heley, and Sylvia Chou discuss the importance of studying social media use in linguistically diverse populations, highlight the potential benefits and harms of social media use for these populations, and outline future directions for research and practice.

This section concludes with a sobering review of the role of communication during public health crises. In this chapter, Victoria Ledford, Susana Ramírez, and Xiaoli Nan argue that public health crises—whether localized, such as wildfires, or global, such as infectious disease pandemics—are a unique context for health communication: During public health crises, clear, accurate, and actionable information must be disseminated to multiple audiences swiftly, even as the science and context may be evolving quickly. The challenges for effectively reaching linguistically diverse audiences are multiplied in public health crises. This chapter contextualizes and theorizes understanding potential pitfalls in communicating during public health emergencies and reviews relevant theoretical frameworks and the research evidence to guide effective communication efforts to mitigate disparities in access to health information and resultant disparities in health outcomes. Using the COVID-19 pandemic as a primary example, in this chapter, the authors describe the challenges and strategies that health actors (e.g., medical personnel, health agencies, policymakers, and individuals) may face and use when communicating urgent information in public health crises.

Together, these six chapters lay out key theoretical traditions and the existing evidence for the ways in which mass media influence population health. These chapters present an overarching argument for the need to expand media and health theorizing to consider the ways in which linguistic minority audiences experience and are influenced by health information from the media. That is, despite the long traditions of mass media for health promotion, the theoretical mechanisms and empirical evidence for the effectiveness of such approaches, and the ways in which modern media contexts contribute to poor health outcomes, a significant limitation in this scholarship is (lack of) attention to the growing linguistic diversity of modern societies. In this section, scholarly readers will appreciate this overview of the field and find suggestions for much-needed scholarship. Optimistic and practice-oriented readers will appreciate the suggestions for how mass media can be leveraged in the context of linguistically diverse populations in support of health equity.

21 Mass Media and Health Research in, with, and for Linguistically Diverse Populations

KATHARINE J. HEAD AND
KATHERINE E. RIDLEY-MERRIWEATHER

Introduction

In 1896, movie-goers in Paris viewed a 50-second-long silent film called L'Arrivée d'un train en gare de La Ciotat ("The Arrival of a Train at La Ciotat Station") in which a train is pulling into a train station. The film's directors, Auguste and Louis Lumière, positioned the shot such that the train seemingly rushed straight toward the camera, and thus, straight toward the audience (Figure 21.1). Rumored accounts say that audience members were astonished by the illusion of this moving image, with some reports claiming that individuals ran to the back of the theater because they were overwhelmed with fear and panic that the train was coming directly at them [1]. This early account of media effects persists to this day as an example of the proposed naïveté of audience members in believing information fed to them from the mass media. Luckily, society—and our understanding of media effects and the use of media—has evolved to recognize that we have a more nuanced relationship with mass media than is depicted in this folklore story.

Mass media, in the most basic sense, are simply the technologies used to deliver content to a wide audience. (Note: media is plural for "medium.") However, from a pragmatic and scholarly perspective, the term mass media has evolved to incorporate the production, distribution, and consumption of content across a variety of mass media platforms, such as radio, television, and, increasingly, digital media such as social media platforms [2]. Health and mass media have always been intertwined, with the ability for health-related messages to reach large portions of the general

---

The Handbook of Language in Public Health and Healthcare, First Edition.
Edited by Pilar Ortega, Glenn Martínez, Maichou Lor, and A. Susana Ramírez.
© 2024 John Wiley & Sons, Inc. Published 2024 by John Wiley & Sons, Inc.

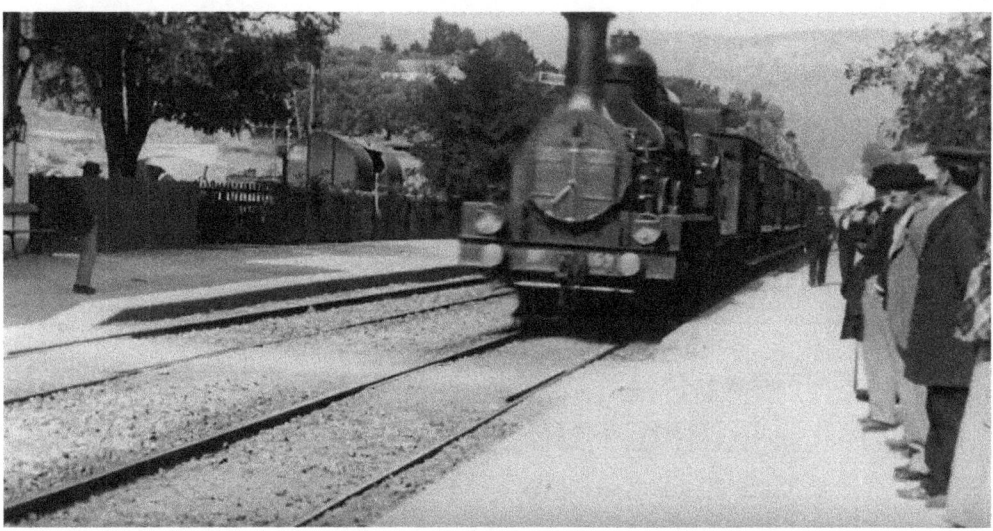

Figure 21.1 Still image from L'Arrivée d'un train en gare de La Ciotat ("The Arrival of a Train at La Ciotat Station") film. *Source:* Shim Harno / Alamy Stock Photo.

public through the mass media's reach. In the early 1900s, for instance, New York-based NBC broadcast health-related radio programs to its affiliates featuring experts speaking on topics such as baby's health and preventing cancer [3]. On the other hand, much of the health information that the general public encounters in the mass media is not always accurate, and may even be downright quackery [4]. Fraudulent medical advertisements promoting "cures" like the one shown below were common in the twentieth century and could be found in magazines and mass mailings (Figure 21.2).

And, while it may be easy for us to look at such messages and be puzzled about how anyone could believe the information, we know that health misinformation in the mass media today represents perhaps an even bigger threat than it did back then.

In this chapter, we first provide a broad historical overview of the major areas of mass media and health research. This includes mass media effects theories, mediated health interventions, and individual's health information seeking through the use of mass media. We then review several critical issues in the study of mass media on health. Finally, we conclude with directions for future research and practice. The purpose of this chapter is to provide a broad overview of the traditions of mass media research as pertaining to health and well-being; other chapters in this section elaborate on specific topical areas and the issues and opportunities for understanding how mass media is used within, and for, linguistically diverse populations. Through it all, we hope the reader will come to recognize that though the mass media are not an all-powerful force (nor does it have the ability to leap off the screen and hurt us!), individuals' lives and their well-being are nonetheless affected by the cumulative and overarching power of the mass media.

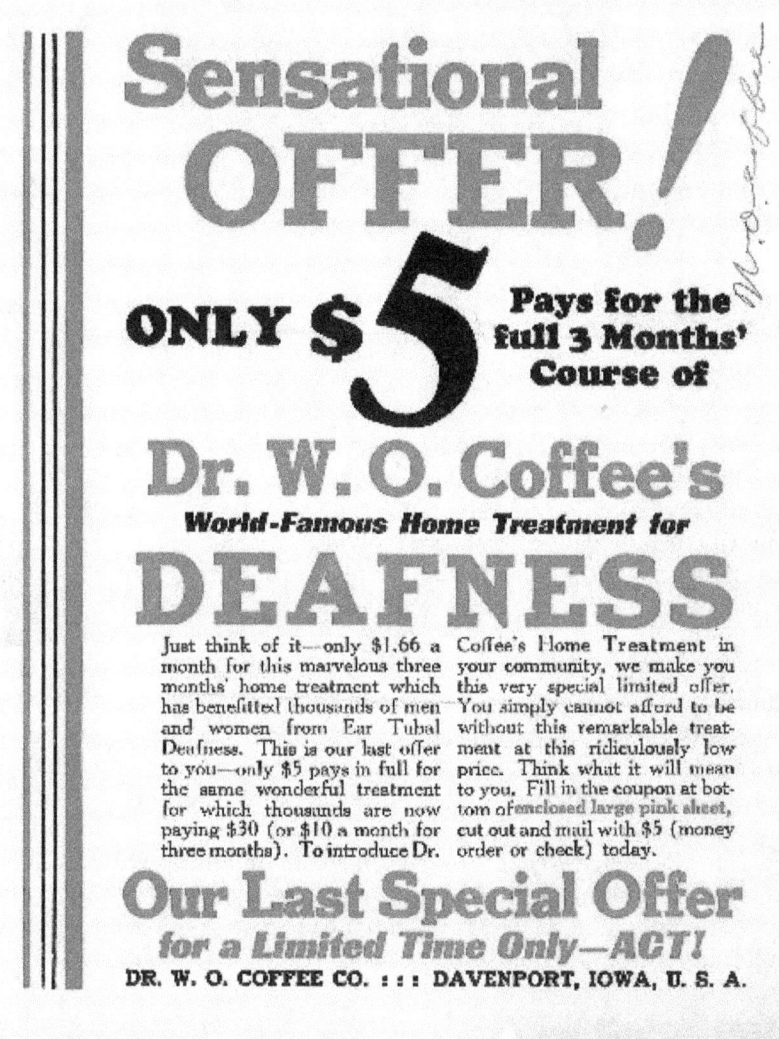

Figure 21.2 Quackery medical advertisement. *Source:* Coffee [5], American Medical Association Archives.

Historical and theoretical overview of mass media and health

Mass media effects

Since their birth, the mass media have played an important role in influencing health beliefs, attitudes, behaviors, and outcomes. While early conceptualizations of the mass media as having a "magic bullet" or "hypodermic needle" effect on audiences through simply shooting information into the minds of passive audiences [6], scholars have since developed much more nuanced theoretical frameworks for explaining and predicting the effects of mass media. Much of the development of these theories took place in the 1950s, 1960s, and 1970s during the growth of mass communication research as a discipline distinct from its sociological and psychological parentage. In this section, we will review four of the major theoretical traditions for studying mass media effects—agenda-setting theory, framing, social cognitive theory (SCT), and cultivation analysis—and provide examples of studies that have examined these theories in the context of health within linguistically diverse populations.

Agenda-setting theory

In late 2019 and early 2020, before the COVID-19 pandemic had reached most people's doorsteps, news media coverage of a novel coronavirus was increasing. In December 2019, the AP News reported that China was investigating a new respiratory illness that had already killed more than 20 people [7]; by February 2020, the BBC reported that the World Health Organization (WHO) had named the disease "COVID-19" [8]; by the time the WHO officially declared the outbreak a pandemic, in March 2020, news coverage about COVID-19 had grown to a near-constant level and it seemed that the pandemic was all that anyone could talk about. Importantly, *before most of us had any personal experience with the virus*, it was already an important topic in our minds. This is an example of the agenda-setting role of the media, which is a theoretical model that helps to explicate the ability of the mass media to influence the salience of topics on the public agenda [9].

McCombs and Shaw conducted the seminal study elucidating the agenda-setting role of the media [10]. They collected two sources of data during the 1968 presidential election: interviews with 100 undecided voters in North Carolina in which they asked participants to describe the major campaign issues, and a collection of major mass media news stories, which were content-analyzed to determine what topics were being reported on. By comparing the two data sources, they concluded that "the evidence in this study that voters tend to share the media's *composite* definition of what is important strongly suggests an agenda-setting function of the mass media." (p. 184, emphasis original).

Agenda-setting research has evolved as the nature of the mass media itself has evolved. For example, a basic assumption of agenda-setting theory is that the public is habitually exposed to homogenous content, yet today's media-rich environment – which now includes hundreds of television channels, online websites, and user-generated content such as podcasts and blogs – contains much more heterogeneous content [11]. Additionally, research has shown that the media not only influences the salience of certain topics, but that the agenda-setting function can also lead to other observable effects, such as influencing the public's opinions, attitudes, and even behaviors.

Agenda-setting media effects are well-studied in the health context. For example, an examination of newspaper stories in Japan from 1945 to 1990 showed that the coverage had influenced national smoking control policies [12]. The findings revealed that coverage about smoking grew over time, showed periodic changes in content (e.g., hazards of smoking, nonsmokers' rights, smoking control in other countries), and that as media coverage grew, so too did policy actions to curb smoking behaviors. The author argued that agenda-setting can be understood as "issue building" to help support policy change, and that "mass media creates a 'space' for bureaucratic action." (p. 35) There are important demographic differences to consider when studying agenda-setting in health. For example, in one study of college-aged women and their mothers, scholars found that on the topic of breast cancer screening, the older mothers were more influenced by mass media sources, and the younger daughters were more influenced by interpersonal sources of information [13]. This study reminds us that the media does not set the agenda equally for all audiences, especially in today's complex media world.

When considering agenda-setting effects among linguistically diverse and minority populations, it is important to note that people from these groups may not be consuming mainstream, English-language media; as such, the "agenda" of the media they do consume may be different than those of populations monolingual in the dominant language. Ethnic and linguistic minority media may cover different information, in different ways. For example, in one study comparing Spanish-language newspapers with English-language newspapers in the United States, health news coverage was significantly higher in the English-language outlets [14]. They also found that the topics of stories differed, with English-language newspapers covering health policy and politics more than Spanish-language newspapers. On the other hand, there may be some geographic areas with linguistic minorities, which are severely lacking in language-matching local mass media, suggesting there is room for improvement in reaching these audiences with appropriate, targeted media [15]. In any case, more work is needed to assess potentially differential agenda-setting effects across linguistically diverse and minority populations, including for populations who are multilingual and may be consuming different media with differing, and potentially competing agendas.

Framing

If the mass media has the power to set the agenda, they also have the power to frame the ways that topics and stories are presented. The metaphor of a "frame" was originally proposed by sociologist Erving Goffman in 1974, who believed that individuals rely on interpretive schema as a way to understand a given event or idea [16]. Building on this idea, and with influences from psychology and communication disciplines, scholars began to study how news and mass media framed issues [17]. A comprehensive definition of framing is offered by Entman [18], who said:

> To frame is to *select some aspects of a perceived reality and make them more salient in a communicating text, in such a way as to promote a particular problem definition, causal interpretation, moral evaluation, and/or treatment recommendation* for the item described. (p. 52, emphasis original)

Frames can take many forms and can be generic or issue-specific [19]. Beyond that, there are certain elements within a news story that can affect the frame; Tankard [20] offered a list of 11 potential framing mechanisms that serve as a useful guide:

1. Headlines
2. Subheadings
3. Photos
4. Photo captions
5. Leads
6. Source selection

7. Quotes selection
8. Pull quotes
9. Logos
10. Statistics and charts
11. Concluding statements and paragraphs

Mass media coverage of health topics contains multitudinous examples of framing. For example, in a quantitative content analysis of media coverage of three different mass shootings in the United States (occurring in 1991, 2007, and 2015), researchers found that source selection by the news media relied more on internal and informal sources for the earlier shootings, while the 2015 news coverage relied more heavily on politician sources [21]. The frames used to explain the shootings also shifted; the earlier shooting used individual character and workplace bullying to set up the story, while the 2007 shooting focused on mental health, and the most common frame used in the 2015 media coverage focused on gun control policy. Despite the very real danger that mass shootings pose to the public, especially in the United States, the authors noted that none of the news coverage analyzed in this study used public health as a major explanatory frame. Ramírez and colleagues also noted the conspicuous absence of public health frames in English-language compared with a Latino-targeted bilingual (English–Spanish) newspapers [15].

Beyond traditional mass media sources, social media provides an exciting medium for studying framing because it allows for an examination of how media producers and media consumers simultaneously understand and frame an issue. For example, Tian found strong correlations between producer and consumer framings in a comparison of YouTube videos about organ donation and associated audience comments—positively valenced frames were overwhelmingly present in both, and the top two frames ("donors are good people" and "it is important to donate organs because of organ shortage") were the same in both [22]. Interestingly, the author noted that coverage of this health topic on YouTube differs from the frames used in other media, such as more negative framing of organ donation in entertainment television, suggesting the need to examine frames across a variety of channels, and, in the context of linguistically diverse media, across languages. See Chapter 25 in this book for a more thorough look at social media and health.

Finally, investigating the potentially different framing effects taking place depending on the source and audience is important to consider, especially among linguistically diverse audiences. For example, some research suggests that US Latinos trust Spanish-language news outlets when delivered by Spanish-language journalists, compared to English-language mainstream news [23]. A recent study of Spanish-language Twitter COVID-19 vaccine messages found that 31% of tweets were anti-vaccine, with 63% of those anti-vaccine tweets falling within the "safety" (i.e., side effects) frame [24]. This differs from a study of English-language Twitter COVID-19 vaccine messages conducted around the same time, which found that only 23.8% were anti-vaccine, and of those, the specific "safety" frame was only present in 18.1% tweets [25]. And, in an acknowledgment of the ever-increasing global power of social media and the user-generated content which comes from it, one recent study found that popular Chinese migrant YouTube vloggers living across the globe constructed narrative frames around their COVID-19 experiences which strongly incorporated their Chinese culture (e.g., pre-pandemic Chinese cultural norms of mask-wearing, references to Chinese historical figures and media) and language (i.e., Mandarin) [26]. A novel study like this pushes us to consider the transnational and trans-language power of social media to reach audiences where they are, and with frames which may reflect the geographic origin of their cultural and linguistic identities.

Social cognitive theory

The SCT of mass communication focuses on the psychosocial mechanisms through which individuals learn about the world and alter their behaviors [27]. The social psychologist Albert Bandura first posited that human learning occurs through observation and imitation of others. In Bandura's most famous experiment, the 1961 "Bobo Doll Experiment," children were shown either (a) a researcher aggressively playing with a blow-up clown Bobo doll (e.g., punching it, throwing it, verbal aggression, etc.) or (b) a researcher ignoring the Bobo doll, and then left in the playroom with the Bobo doll. Children in the aggressive condition showed significantly higher tendency to aggressively interact with the Bobo doll after the researcher left, including, and especially, imitating the aggressive acts performed by the researcher [28].

Building on this work, the SCT focuses on the process of reciprocal determinism, in that human behavior can be best understood as the interplay and transaction between personal, behavioral, and environmental factors. SCT is a complex theory with many intertwining concepts, but as it relates to mass media, this theory has helped us identify the ways in which audiences learn about and form perceptions about health and health behaviors from what they observe in the mass media [27]. The concepts of vicarious learning and outcome expectations (e.g., beliefs about the likely outcomes of performing a behavior), for instance, are well-studied concepts within this theoretical tradition. In an experimental study of adults in Austria, exposure to a television show featuring various portrayals of alcohol consumption behaviors and consequences led to differential outcome expectations, which were also influenced by the participants' personal alcohol consumption levels [29]. Self-efficacy, or an individual's belief that they can engage in a behavior, is another important aspect of SCT. In a survey study in Hong Kong, researchers showed that exposure to different news media channels and content about the Ebola epidemic was associated with higher self-efficacy in performing protective behaviors [30]. And, while SCT can be thought of as a media effects theory, it is also frequently used as a guide for designing mediated health interventions across different languages, races, and countries, as well [31]. In sum, the SCT tradition of scholarship helps researchers and practitioners to understand the position that the mass media plays in teaching the world about health and health behaviors. In the context of communicating with linguistically diverse audiences, SCT has been foundational for the development of entertainment education programs (refer to Chapters 3 and 23 in this volume).

Cultivation analysis

In 1967, George Gerbner and colleagues started the longitudinal Cultural Indicators Project, aiming to investigate how exposure to television content over time can affect audiences' perceptions of reality [32]. In his seminal essay, Gerbner notes that television creates a "common culture through which communities cultivate shared and public notions about facts, values, and contingencies of human existence." [33] (p. 138). Then and now, this focus on long-term "cultivation" rather than more immediate "effects" has set this scope of research apart from other mass media work [32].

The most well-known findings from the first few decades of the Cultural Indicators Project had to do with measuring repeated exposure to violent content on television and its association with audiences' perceptions of the levels of real-world violence. Pivotal to this work is the consistent finding that heavy viewers of television which contains violent content will significantly overestimate the prevalence of violence in the real world—something dubbed the "mean world syndrome" [34]. Importantly, the television landscape of the 1960s and 1970s, when the study was conducted, is vastly different from the landscape today. Rather than a relatively small and homogenous choice of content, "television" today could mean audiences are watching cable, satellite, streaming services, and more. As television has diversified, so has cultivation analysis, including more nuanced ways to measure exposure and a focus on genre-specific content [35]. Cultivation work has shown that heavy viewers of health-related dramas, for example, are more likely to believe doctors are courageous and superhuman, something that could affect how people interact with healthcare providers when receiving care [36]. Fatalism, or the belief that (health) events are inevitable and individuals have little power to change the outcome, is a concept with an interesting and complicated relationship with media exposure and health behavior research. While some research shows, for example, that heavy viewers of health-related dramas are more likely to adopt more fatalistic views about cancer and underestimate its impact on society [37], other work has argued that there is scant evidence of causal direction, owing to the different ways in which fatalism has been conceptualized and operationalized – it may be that fatalism itself, as a personality trait or cultural belief, affects individuals' media exposure [38]. Other recent research has argued that information overload, the result of access to information in multiple languages among ethnic minorities, may be responsible for health behavior effects mistakenly attributed to fatalistic attitudes [39]. As research on this topic evolves, practitioners and providers would be wise to acknowledge that exposure to health-related mass media is strongly associated with important concepts like fatalism that are in turn associated with health behaviors and outcomes.

With the popularity of health-related dramas and the news' ever-present focus on health-related content, scholars and practitioners alike will need to stay vigilant about assessing the long-term cultivation of health beliefs and perceptions. International research even shows that the more audience members consume medical news and entertainment media, the more likely they are to genderize diseases, such as believing that women are more likely to have certain diseases which do not align with real-life incidence rates [40]. Perhaps most important, a recent meta-analysis provides evidence that cultivation varies not only depending on the type of media an audience is consuming but also varies by key subgroups such as political affiliation, educational attainment, and income level [41]. These types of studies are relevant for public health practitioners and healthcare providers because they help shed light on why individuals from certain demographic groups may hold certain, persisting health beliefs. While research is scant on the topic, there may be linguistic differences in cultivation effects as well.

These four theoretical traditions—agenda-setting, framing, SCT, and cultivation analysis—represent some of the more well-known approaches to studying media effects and give a good primer on the types of work happening in this area and its relevance for understanding potential consequences of mass media on the health of linguistically diverse populations. However, it should be noted that there are other theoretical and conceptual approaches that were not discussed here. For a more comprehensive look at the major theories and research in mass media effects, we suggest the fourth edition of "Media Effects: Advances in Theory and Research" [42].

Mass media health interventions

History and context

Contextualized within the study of mass media effects, scholars and practitioners have also long recognized the intentional use of mass media to influence health beliefs, attitudes, and behaviors. Mediated communication campaigns and interventions possess a rich history and are defined as mass media driven, organized communication activities targeted toward a particular audience, usually for a particular period of time, and focused on achieving a particular goal [43].

A 2006 10-year retrospective of research on mass media health communication campaigns identified and elucidated the effects on health knowledge, beliefs, and attitudes—as well as behaviors—attributable to mass media and translatable to major public health impacts [31]. This review named different historical eras of health campaigns and pointed out that the period of minimal effects (1940s/1950s), in which evidence related to both campaign planning and evaluation were still being developed, was succeeded by some hope-generating campaign successes in the 1960s and 1970s as scholars developed more nuanced understandings designing effective health campaigns. Eventually, during the 1980s and 1990s, as scholars gained and applied more knowledge about campaigns, and therefore, experienced more success, we entered a "moderate effects era." Finally, as communication theory and science developed and more rigorous campaign planning, execution, and evaluation efforts were formalized, we are now in the "conditional effects era."

In the current campaign climate, it is important to note turning points that assisted health communication scholars in creating more successful campaigns. For example, many health communication scholars consider the successful collaboration of a physician with a communication expert that resulted in the Stanford Heart Disease Prevention Program (SHDPP), to be integral to the rise and validation of the health communication field [44]. The SHDPP messaging was targeted to high-risk individuals through the mass media and emphasized exercise, smoking cessation, dietary attention, and stress reduction. The campaign successfully helped reduce heart disease in two California communities, designating a third, similar community as a control. This "proof of concept" interdisciplinary approach energized the fields of medicine, public health, and health communication to recognize the power of the mass media to effect real health changes.

Mass-mediated health campaign efforts

Working successfully in mass media health promotion requires acknowledgment of certain considerations well known in health campaign work, regardless of the targeted population. In this section, we review some examples of mass media health campaign design and execution, raising attention to issues of linguistic diversity.

Formative research and audience analysis
Researchers focused on creating appropriate and effective health campaigns must seek community involvement and partnership in better understanding audience characteristics, assessing media use and preferences, and gaining input and feedback on designing messages [45]. In the 1990s, for example, researchers from communication and psychology discovered the importance of developing and targeting antidrug messaging in the mass media based on the audience characteristic of "sensation-seeking" [46].

This involved the development and testing of messages that had high stimulating potential for an audience which responded best to mediated messages like this [47]. The importance of formative research has been made particularly clear during the time since the dawn of the COVID-19 pandemic. In Australia, for example, behavioral scholars employed participatory research practices and partnered with community leaders in culturally diverse areas to address the challenges of successfully communicating COVID-19 protocols and achieving better outcomes [48]. The community groups were able to successfully identify several recommendations for health officials, including not only creating messages and translating them but also ensuring the messages were delivered by trusted messengers through appropriate channels and identifying a need for a national advisory group focused on addressing linguistically diverse populations in that country. Rigorous formative research and audience awareness like this can determine the difference between creating a mediocre mediated campaign and a very successful one.

Global mass media campaigns
In 1967, Miguel Sabido devised a method of designing the content of supermarket magazines to both entertain and educate inner-city customers in Mexico about their health [49]. Through these magazines, Sabido was successful at greatly increasing community members' attendance at local community health clinics. Over the course of the next 20 years, Sabido transferred these approaches and ideas to fictional television shows, known as telenovelas in Mexico, and the field of "edutainment" – entertainment education – was born. This strategic mix of entertainment and education diffused from Mexico through other countries [50] and is still a popular form of mass media health promotion today. See Chapter 23 in this book for a more thorough examination of entertainment education and Chapter 3 for critical interrogation of "illness narratives."

Entertainment education is just one kind of, or one use of, mass media in health campaigns. Before beginning any kind of mass media campaign or program, scholars should possess full understanding of the limits of mass media in the context of health. For example, diffusion of innovations theory (DoI) allows that mass media's role may be good for awareness and/or knowledge, but it is through the combination of mass media coverage and public dialogue with opinion leaders and interpersonal influences within the community that really drive adoption of new health behaviors [51, 52]. The "Clean India" health campaign presents an important example of the use of DoI principles for understanding and guiding a health campaign with a mass media component. In 2014, Narendra Modi was swept into office as prime minister of India on a flurry of tweets, winning the first election in India to be determined by a candidate's social media presence [53]. After the election, the new prime minister continuously communicated with his followers through many social media platforms, informing them about his "Clean India" campaign and entreating them to promote cleanliness to help stop open defecation in the streets by the time of Mahatma Ghandi's 150th birthday in 2019 [54]. In 2014, only about 40% of rural Indian households owned a toilet; however, by 2019 that number had risen to 95%. Through increased government funding to support the building of toilets in homes and villages, enlisting dozens of social and political influencers (including opposition leaders and celebrities) who served as opinion leaders within their regional, ethnic, and linguistic communities to help him spread the word about the importance of this campaign, and linking the campaign to an emotionally positive goal date, Modi successfully led a health campaign that encouraged adoption of increased sanitation.

Health campaigns in linguistically diverse US populations

Within the United States, there is ample opportunity to consider the diverse language needs of the public. Over 8% of people over the age of five living in the United States do not speak English very well, according to the United States Census Bureau [55]. Since members of these populations are likely to live closely grouped together, mediated health campaigns launched in those areas must be mindful of executing linguistically appropriate channels. In our own work, we work with clinical and community organizations to design and disseminate health communication materials that are sensitive to language needs. For example, the Komen Tissue Bank (KTB), a unique breast tissue biobank in Indianapolis, Indiana, considers the regional language diversity when designing recruitment outreach materials: KTB information booklets, flyers, and website pages are translated into Spanish, Vietnamese, and traditional and simplified Chinese. Importantly, the content of the materials for each group also incorporates the cultural norms of the KTB intended audiences, making a true interpretation rather than a simpler translation [56]. Similarly, the Indiana Region of the American Red Cross collaborated with a coalition of over 65 community organizations to help facilitate conversations between individuals and groups about COVID-19 vaccinations and also launched a multimedia health campaign to promote vaccination [57]. This campaign, which created a website containing videos, social media content, and graphics to be used freely by any organization wanting to facilitate critical vaccination conversations, included content translated into the seven most prominent languages besides English used in Indiana: Spanish, Arabic, French, Burmese, Hakha Chin, Chinese, and Polish. Well-done interpretations and placement of campaign messages in linguistically and culturally appropriate channels are essential conditions to ensure the campaigns reach the target audience and stand a chance to achieve the intended effects.

Future of mass media health campaigns

Harnessing the use of mass media to effect health change is not new, and the evidence base for successful mass media health campaigns grows each day. The United States Centers for Disease Control and Prevention (CDC) features a number of mass media campaigns on their website, ranging in topics from awareness about pregnancy-related complications, to antismoking campaigns, to colorectal cancer screening efforts [58]. Many of these campaigns contain extensive information about how the campaigns are used within diverse and linguistic minority populations, including targeted messaging examples. Mediated campaigns have shown real successes yet need to continue to evolve with the changing media landscape. One of the most important foci of campaign research in the next decade will be further enhancing and refining the use of social media [59].

Health information seeking in the global village

Canadian philosopher and media scholar Marshall McCluhan is often cited for his well-known observation that "the medium is the message" [60]. Although somewhat antithetical to the thesis of this book, with its focus on the diversity of language and messages, this famous adage has helped shaped the way that media scholars and practitioners think about the importance of, and focus on, the media or channel through which messages are delivered. However, McCluhan also wrote extensively about the influence of mass media on our society and coined the term "global village" to describe the power of media to both shrink and expand our cultures simultaneously. McCluhan has been criticized for this oversimplistic view of media effects on society, but perhaps at the heart of his observation is that mass media can increase our access to the world in previously unimaginable ways. In other words, in addition to studying mass media effects on health and designing mass media health interventions, it is also paramount that scholars and practitioners recognize and understand individuals' use of media to access health information and health-related stories.

Health information seeking is defined as "...an active effort to obtain information about a specific topic, using any source(s) to obtain desired information, that occurs outside of routine patterns of interpersonal communication or general media use" [61] (p. 400). Health Information Seeking (HIS) is a robust field of study that relies on various theories, methods, and measures to assess the health contexts/topics, populations, and channels people use to obtain their desired information. As with most human behavior, we see patterns in how different audiences seek out health information. For example, women are more likely to engage in HIS than men, while variables like education, family situation, and race influence the different sources of health information that individuals may seek out [62]. The Internet, in particular, has revolutionized the capacity for individuals to seek information beyond their own social networks [63]. In addition to the role that HIS can play in leading to potential increases in health knowledge and health literacy, practitioners would do well to recognize that HIS is important as it relates to concepts like patient participation, shared decision-making, and patient involvement in care [64, 65]. For more detailed information on HIS in linguistically diverse populations, we recommend Chapter 22 in this volume.

It is important to acknowledge that just seeking out health information does not mean that individuals find credible information or that they have the ability to process that information. Beyond just considering the role of individuals' health literacy when designing health materials (see also Chapters 1 and 9 in this book), researchers and practitioners must also consider how an individual's health literacy affects their ability to find, make sense of, and act on digital and mass media content they come across, which is part of the idea of ehealth literacy [66]. Common sense is a nonprofit organization devoted to helping young people navigate the complex news media world in which we live, and they have ample resources on their website directed at improving individual's news and media literacy skills [67].

As mass media continues to expand and evolve, and individuals have increasing access to global content, scholars and practitioners must continue to monitor and study how individuals seek out certain health-related media and what they believe are the benefits of each kind of media.

Critical issues in mass media and health

As the field of mass media has developed more nuanced understandings of media use and media effects, so too has the field recognized assumptions and limitations of how this scholarship has been approached. In this section, we briefly review three critical issues about this field of inquiry: the overreliance on quantitative methodologies, the pressing concerns about mass media access and the digital divide, and the growing problem of health misinformation.

First, much of the research on mass media has relied on post-positivist and quantitative methodologies. Given the scope of "mass" audiences, a quantitative approach that relies on, for example, survey methodologies, is understandable because it allows researchers to capture large amounts of data across many participants. Additionally, the use of experimental methodologies for assessing media effects and engaging in mediated health campaign evaluation is also necessary for showing movement in certain metrics (e.g., a change in attitudes or behavior). However, as the mass media continue to evolve, a stronger reliance on qualitative, critical, and mixed-methods approaches is essential to understanding the effects of that evolution. For example, mental healthcare providers may be particularly interested in a mixed-methods study in which researchers found that the surveys yielded important statistics about the number of students experiencing significant mental health challenges and the types of social media platforms they used for support [68]. However, it was during the follow-up, qualitative interviews with students that revealed more in-depth and nuanced findings about the different life stressors that were leading to the mental health challenges, and how each social media platform afforded different kinds of help.

Second, inherent in any discussion of mass media and health must be the acknowledgment that significant communication inequalities exist in terms of access to and ability to make sense of information and resources. The digital divide continues to persist in the United States, where rural residents are less likely than their suburban and urban counterparts to have home broadband Internet access [69]. The divide is even more pronounced globally, where almost half of the world's population does not have access to Internet – most of those people living in developing countries [70]. Beyond geographic access to the technology, as the digital divide was originally conceptualized, a further divide for linguistic minority populations is linguistically available access [71]. There are many challenges that exist to providing clear and effective linguistically appropriate health information to different communities, and those working in health and media need to be prepared to tackle this challenge and to devote resources to ensuring good access to health messages [72].

Third, anyone working in health promotion and healthcare today must acknowledge the very real threat of health misinformation. Health misinformation abounds, particularly on social media platforms and other media that rely heavily on user-generated content (e.g., podcasts), and these types of information present significant challenges for public health [73]. In fact, given the increasing amount and reach of health misinformation in recent years, the United States Surgeon General has declared that one of his office's priorities is to tackle this issue and has even developed a toolkit for addressing misinformation in everyday life [74]. Additionally, mass-mediated health campaigns need to acknowledge that some of their efforts may need to be devoted to "battling" misinformation about the same topics. The COVID-19 pandemic was hounded by such unparalleled volumes of misinformation that the public, particularly those in minority linguistic communities, could not determine whom to trust or where to turn for good information [75]. The CDC, presumably the predominant source of national health information and guidance in the United States, found itself in the unfortunate position of being forced by misinformation campaigns to play catch-up about COVID-19 vaccination messaging [76]. Going forward, a variety of evidence-based techniques will need to be employed to address this very real public health threat of misinformation [77].

Directions for future research and practice

The many ways in which mass media and health intersect, especially as new media emerge and our understandings of health evolve, means that there is fertile ground for new work and new ways of thinking in this area. We offer three areas for future research and practice relevant to mass media and health: the adoption of the paradigm represented in the Masspersonal Model of Communication (MMoC), the application of critical theory of multiliteracies, and the consideration of the intersection of diverse consumption patterns and different mass media in our society. Each of these suggestions is geared less toward adopting new specific practices or pointing to specific gaps in the research literature and is instead more focused on helping readers and practitioners shift their understandings of how humans and mass media interact.

First, we encourage researchers and practitioners to adopt the MMoC as a way of conceptualizing how we communicate in today's world (MMoC, shown below, Figure 21.3). The MMoC reconceptualizes our understanding of the traditional categories, or levels, of communication which were traditionally based on the number of people – senders and receivers – involved in the interaction (e.g., interpersonal, group, organizational, and mass.) This represented a useful, but simple, way of defining and categorizing human communication. Instead, the MMoC model asks us to consider how the accessibility and personalization of the *message* should define our understanding of a communication context and can help us better identify how and why that message may have certain effects [78].

Since its publication in 2018, the MMoC has been highly cited and adopted. For example, in a qualitative study assessing citizen's perspectives of Vietnamese government messaging during the first 5 months of the COVID-19 pandemic, researchers found that citizens believed that the government's reliance on and coordination of messages across multiple interpersonal and mass media channels (i.e., intersecting contexts in the masspersonal space) led to high perceptions of the government's effective management of the pandemic [79]. Other countries' governments, large public health agencies, and healthcare organizations can learn from this that their communication plans with their stakeholders (e.g., citizens and patients) may best be designed in a multimedia, message-centered way.

Application of the MMoC also has important implications for those audiences who immersively utilize social media for health purposes. Because the MMoC has moved away from thinking about communication within strict categories, it allows us to better examine how something like health communication on social media platforms can be *simultaneously* public (i.e., mass) and personalized, something that other media has historically been unable to accomplish well [80]. Consider the current (at the time of this writing) decision of the Supreme Court to overturn Roe vs. Wade on June 24, 2022, effectively banning abortions in many states [81]. Immediately upon the release of this information, social media was buzzing with the news about the decision and everyone from political leaders to celebrities to everyday individuals were expressing their perspectives. In other words, according to the MMoC, this information was highly public and accessible. Couched within many of those public social media posts, however, were also highly personalized messages about the very real and very personal fall-out of this decision for individual women's autonomy and wellbeing. Consider, for example, the tweet posted by singer–songwriter Taylor Swift on June 24th (Figure 21.4).

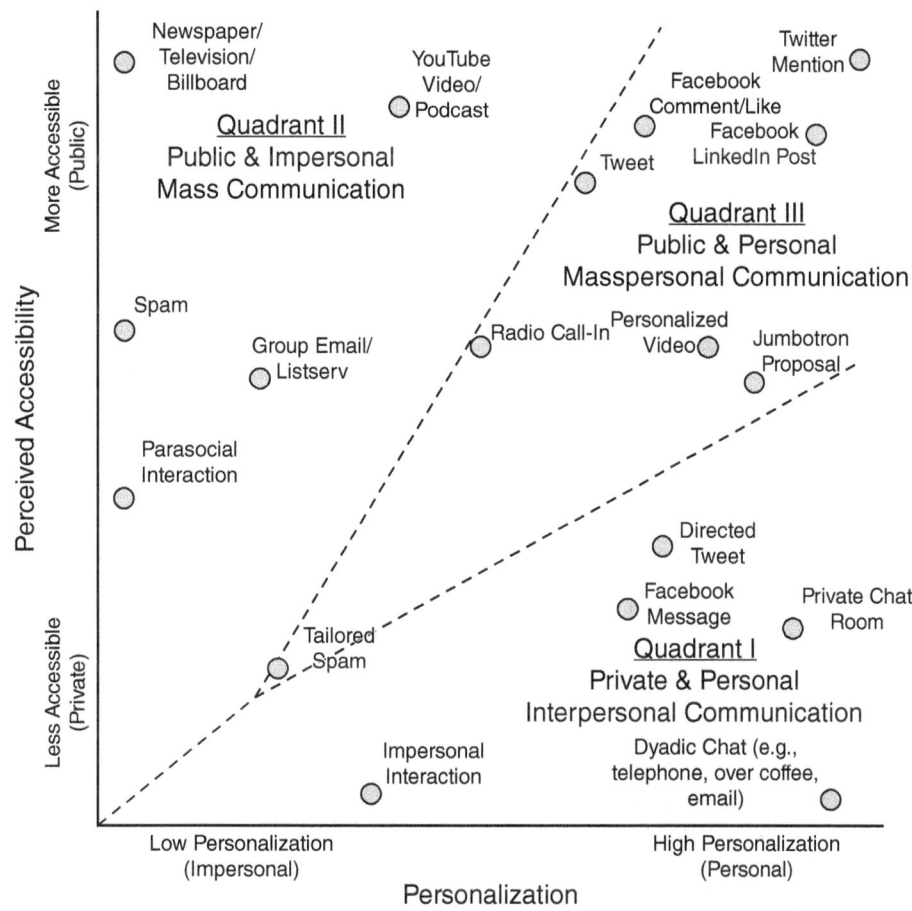

Figure 21.3 Masspersonal Model of Communication. *Source:* O'Sullivan and Carr [78]. Reproduced with permission of SAGE publications.

Ms. Swift not only shared (i.e., "re-tweeted") a formal statement written by former First Lady Michele Obama about the Supreme Court's decision and the implications it will have for women's reproductive healthcare—amplifying Ms. Obama's message among a potentially different demographic (i.e., their follower networks)—and also included her own personal thoughts, including her personal fear about what this decision means for hers and other women's bodies. Because of the interactive, two-way nature of social media, Ms. Swift's post was liked more than 800,000 times, retweeted more than 150,000 times, and more than 10,000 users responded to her tweet. A post like this, from someone with a global reach of 91 million followers, includes both public and personal communicative elements – and therefore, this message may have a particularly large impact on how her followers and fans think about the topic of women's reproductive rights.

Second, we must continue to move the field from a consumption model (i.e., audiences as passive consumers of media) to what Mirra and colleagues call a critical theory of multiliteracies [83]. Building on previous theoretical and practical assumptions about how individuals interact with media (including especially uses and gratifications theory,

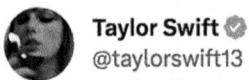

Figure 21.4 Singer–songwriter Taylor Swift's retweet of Former First Lady Michelle Obama's tweet on June 24, 2022 regarding the overturning of Roe vs. Wade by the US Supreme Court. *Source:* Swift [82].

which was not discussed in this chapter), this multiliteracies approach firmly places media consumers—and thus, patients—in an active role. Conceptualizing the role of consumers as not only consuming, but also producing, distributing, and even inventing new digital content across diverse platforms can open our eyes to a wider understanding of how media and the public interact. For example, "Breast Cancer Pink" is a song and music video, created by an academic diagnosed with breast cancer, that subverts and rejects the traditional media narratives around breast cancer (e.g., the dominating "pinkness" and heteronormative femininity of these narratives in the United States) and instead focuses the content on queer experimentation, alienation, and frustration inherent in this person's unique cancer experience [84]. Young people, in particular, reject the notion of industry-regulated power in controlling the media and its content and being cast as passive consumers, and instead demand a role in the creation and distribution of media content about health, particularly in digital spaces [85]. From an intervention and behavior change perspective, the multiliteracies model may help us better engage with our target audiences by working *with* them to create focused, targeted health-oriented content.

Third, we challenge researchers and practitioners to consider the diversity of health information consumption patterns and, in building on the MMoC presented above, the intersection of different forms of mass media in our society in how health information is distributed and consumed. Consider, for example, recent statistics about news consumption in the United States. In an ongoing study of news consumption over the past several years, here are some of the findings from the Pew Research Center [86]:

- 23% of United States adults sometimes or often get their news from podcasts
- 69% percent of Twitter users say they get news from the site (and 70% of those have turned to Twitter for breaking news, in particular)
- 50% of United States adults report that they prefer to consume their news from a smartphone, computer, or tablet vs. only 5% who prefer print publications
- Circulation for Hispanic newspapers in the United States has dropped in recent years, but viewership for the evening news on Univision and Telemundo local affiliates is rising
- 60% of Black Americans report preferring to get their news from television, compared to 43% of White Americans

What drives these differing and intersecting consumption patterns? By acknowledging the diversity and intersection of different types of media use and why some individuals may rely on different sources for health information, we can, for example, better approach how we design health interventions for reaching different audiences. In addition, through acknowledgment of the possibilities of these intersecting media, healthcare providers and health communication scholars can consider the different ways our patient populations learn about health in their day-to-day lives.

Conclusion

This chapter provided a broad historical, theoretical, and practical overview of the role of mass media in health. Mass media serves as an important source of health information, whether through consumption of news, actively searching for health information, or the design of health communication campaigns designed to reach specific audiences.

The ever-changing nature of this field is greatly affected by the growing mass media options available to individuals across the globe and the acknowledgment that linguistic diversity does and should play an important role in how health media is consumed, understood, and acted upon. Importantly, we must reconcile this complex mass media landscape with the also ever-changing nature of health and health risks. As noted by renowned health communication scholar Gary Kreps:

> Responding effectively to health problems is complex, with the need to address many different health risks, each with unique symptoms, causes, and treatments. We live in a rapidly changing health information environment, where new advances expand health knowledge, such as the need to keep abreast of new strategies for disease prevention, screening, diagnosis, and treatment. There are significant barriers to disseminating complex and changing health information to diverse audiences, especially for at-risk populations, who may suffer from limited levels of information access, health literacy, education, and social capital [87].

With this in mind, health communication researchers, public health practitioners, and healthcare providers must be ready and willing to grow and adapt in order to remain effective in their work. This is particularly important as we acknowledge the salience of performing and promoting masspersonal and multiliterate frameworks to better guide and explore evolving health information consumption patterns in our diverse public and patient populations.

Highlights

- The study of mass media and health has a long and rich history.
- Several theoretical frameworks provide guidance on studying and understanding the effects of mass media on health.
- Mass-mediated campaigns can be designed to influence health beliefs, attitudes, and behaviors across a variety of audiences.
- Individuals have increasing access to global health content through a variety of media channels, and health information seeking is an important area for scholars and practitioners to monitor.
- The future of media and health will incorporate more critical/cultural and nuanced understandings of how individuals consume and create mediated content.

REFERENCES

1. Loiperdinger, M. and Elzer, B. (2004). Lumiere's arrival of the train: cinema's founding myth. *Mov. Image* 4 (1): 89–118.
2. Grossberg, L., Wartella, E., Whitney, D.C., and Wise, J.M. (2006). *MediaMaking: Mass Media in a Popular Culture*, 524. SAGE.
3. Holland, C. (2015). Next on your radio dial, 15 minutes of healthy talk. In: *National Museum of American History*. Smithsonian (O Say Can You See? Stories from the Museum). https://americanhistory.si.edu/blog/next-your-radio-dial-15-minutes-healthy-talk (accessed 6 July 2022).

4. Dushman, A. (2018). Ads and labels from early 20th-century health fraud promotions. *AMA J. Ethics* 20 (11): 1082–1093.
5. Coffee, W.O. (n.d.). *Dr W.O. Coffee's World-Famous Home Treatment for Deafness*. American Medical Association Acrhives: Historical Health Fraud and Alternative Medicine Collection.
6. Bineham, J.L. (1988). A historical account of the hypodermic model in mass communication. *Commun. Monogr.* 55 (3): 230–246.
7. China Investigates Respiratory Illness Outbreak Sickening 27. AP NEWS. https://apnews.com/article/wuhan-health-international-news-china-severe-acute-respiratory-syndrome-00c78d1974410d96fe031f67edbd86ec (accessed 19 April 2022).
8. (2020). *Coronavirus Disease Named Covid-19*. BBC News. https://www.bbc.com/news/world-asia-china-51466362 (accessed 19 April 2022).
9. McCombs, M. and Reynolds, A. (2002). News influence on our pictures of the world. In: *Media Effects: Advances in Theory and Research*, 2ee, 11–28. Routledge.
10. McCombs, M.E. and Shaw, D.L. (1972). The agenda-setting function of mass media. *Public Opin. Q.* 36 (2): 176–187.
11. McCombs, M. (2005). A look at agenda-setting: past, present and future. *J. Stud.* 6 (4): 543–557.
12. Sato, H. (2003). Agenda setting for smoking control in Japan, 1945–1990: influence of the mass media on National Health Policy making. *J. Health Commun.* 8 (1): 23–40.
13. Ogata Jones, K., Denham, B.E., and Springston, J.K. (2006). Effects of mass and interpersonal communication on breast cancer screening: advancing agenda-setting theory in health contexts. *J. Appl. Commun. Res.* 34 (1): 94–113.
14. Villar, M.E. and Olson, Y.B. (2013). Differences in English- and Spanish-language health news: a comparison of newspapers in two cities. *Howard J. Commun.* 24 (1): 57–70.
15. Ramírez, A.S., Estrada, E., and Ruiz, A. (2017). Mapping the health information landscape in a rural, culturally diverse region: implications for interventions to reduce information inequality. *J. Prim. Prev.* 38 (4): 345–362.
16. Goffman, E. (1974). *Frame Analysis: An Essay on the Organization of Experience*, vol. vol. IX, 586. Cambridge, MA: Harvard University Press (Frame analysis: An essay on the organization of experience).
17. Tewksbury, D. and Scheufele, D.A. (2019). News framing theory and research. In: *Media Effects: Advances in Theory and Research*, 3ee, 51–68. Routledge.
18. Entman, R.M. (1993). Framing: toward clarification of a fractured paradigm. *J. Commun.* 43 (4): 51–58.
19. Vreese, C.H. (2005). News framing: theory and typology. *Inf. Des. J.* 13 (1): 51–62.
20. Tankard, J.W. Jr. (2001). The empirical approach to the study of media framing. In: *Framing Public Life*, 1ee (ed. S.D. Reese, O.H. Gandy Jr., and A.E. Grant), 95–106. Routledge.
21. DeFoster, R. and Swalve, N. (2018). Guns, culture or mental health? Framing mass shootings as a public health crisis. *Health Commun.* 33 (10): 1211–1222.
22. Tian, Y. (2010). Organ donation on web 2.0: content and audience analysis of organ donation videos on YouTube. *Health Commun.* 25 (3): 238–246.
23. Gomez-Aguinaga, B., Oaxaca, A.L., Barreto, M.A., and Sanchez, G.R. (2021). Spanish-language news consumption and Latino reactions to COVID-19. *Int. J. Environ. Res. Public Health* 18 (18): 9629.
24. Herrera-Peco, I., Jiménez-Gómez, B., Romero Magdalena, C.S. et al. (2021). Antivaccine movement and COVID-19 negationism: a content analysis of Spanish-written messages on twitter. *Vaccines* 9 (6): 656.
25. Huangfu, L., Mo, Y., Zhang, P. et al. (2022). COVID-19 vaccine tweets after vaccine rollout: sentiment–based topic modeling. *J. Med. Internet Res.* 24 (2): e31726.
26. Zhang, L.T. and Zhao, S. (2020). Diaspora micro-influencers and COVID-19 communication on social media: the case of Chinese-speaking YouTube vloggers. *Multilingua* 39 (5): 553–563.

27. McAlister, A.L., Perry, C.L., and Parcel, G.S. (2008). How individuals, environments, and health behaviors interact. In: *Health Behavior and Health Education: Theory, Research, and Practice*, 4ee (ed. K. Glanz, B.K. Rimer, and K. Viswanath), 169–188. Jossey-Bass.
28. Bandura, A., Ross, D., and Ross, S.A. (1961). Transmission of aggression through imitation of aggressive models. *J. Abnorm. Soc. Psychol.* 63 (3): 575–582.
29. Mayrhofer, M. and Naderer, B. (2019). Mass media as alcohol educator for everyone? Effects of portrayed alcohol consequences and the influence of viewers' characteristics. *Media Psychol.* 22 (2): 217–243.
30. Li, X. (2018). Media exposure, perceived efficacy, and protective behaviors in a public health emergency. *Int. J. Commun.* 19328036 12: 2641–2660.
31. Noar, S.M. (2006). A 10-year retrospective of research in health mass media campaigns: where do we go from here? *J. Health Commun.* 11 (1): 21–42.
32. Gerbner, G., Gross, L., Morgan, M. et al. (2002). Growing up with television: cultivation processes. In: *Media Effects: Advances in Theory and Research*, LEA's Communication Series, 2ee (ed. J. Bryant and D. Zillmann), 43–67. Mahwah, NJ: Lawrence Erlbaum Associates Publishers.
33. Gerbner, G. (1969). Toward "cultural indicators": the analysis of mass mediated public message systems. *AV Commun. Rev.* 17 (2): 137–148.
34. Gerbner, G., Gross, L., Eleey, M.F. et al. (1977). TV violence profile no. 8: the highlights. *J. Commun.* 27 (2): 171–180.
35. Record, R.A. (2018). Genre-specific television viewing: state of the literature. *Ann. Int. Commun. Assoc.* 42 (3): 155–180.
36. Quick, B.L. (2009). The effects of viewing Grey's Anatomy on perceptions of doctors and patient satisfaction. *J. Broadcast. Electron. Media* 53 (1): 38–55.
37. Chung, J.E. (2014). Medical dramas and viewer perception of health: testing cultivation effects. *Hum. Commun. Res.* 40 (3): 333–349.
38. Ramondt, S. and Ramírez, A.S. (2017). Fatalism and exposure to health information from the media: examining the evidence for causal influence. *Ann. Int. Commun. Assoc.* 41 (3–4): 298–320.
39. Ramírez, A.S. and Arellano-Carmona, K. (2018). Beyond fatalism: information overload as a mechanism to understand health disparities. *Soc. Sci. Med.* 219: 11–18.
40. van Driel, I., Myrick, J.G., Pavelko, R. et al. (2018). The role of media use in the genderization of disease: the interplay of sex, culture, and cultivation. *Int. J. Commun. Health* 13: 1–10.
41. Hermann, E., Morgan, M., and Shanahan, J. (2021). Television, continuity, and change: a meta-analysis of five decades of cultivation research. *J. Commun.* 71 (4): 515–544.
42. Oliver, M.B., Raney, A.A., and Bryant, J. (ed.) (2019). *Media Effects: Advances in Theory and Research*, 4ee, 454. Taylor & Francis https://www.routledge.com/Media-Effects-Advances-in-Theory-and-Research/Oliver-Raney-Bryant/p/book/9781138590229 (accessed 26 April 2022).
43. Snyder, L.B. (2007). Meta-analyses of mediated health campaigns. In: *Mass Media Effects Research: Advances Through Meta-Analysis* (ed. R.W. Preiss, B.M. Gayle, N. Burrell, et al.), 327–344. Earlbaum.
44. Rogers, E.M. (1996). Up-to-date report. *J. Health Commun.* 1 (1): 15–24.
45. Atkin, C.K. and Freimuth, V. (2013). Guidelines for formative evaluation research in campaign design. In: *Public Communication Campaigns* (ed. R.E. Rice and C.K. Atkin), 53–68. Sage.
46. Donohew, L., Palmgreen, P., and Lorch, E.P. (1994). Attention, need for sensation, and health communication campaigns. *Am. Behav. Sci.* 38 (2): 310–322.
47. Stephenson, M.T. and Southwell, B.G. (2006). Sensation seeking, the activation model, and mass media health campaigns: current findings and future directions for cancer communication. *J. Commun.* 56 (suppl_1): S38–S56.
48. Wild, A., Kunstler, B., Goodwin, D. et al. (2021). Communicating COVID-19 health information to culturally and linguistically diverse communities: insights from a participatory research collaboration. *Public Health Res. Pract.* 31 (1): 1–5.

49. Sabido, M. (2021). Miguel Sabido's entertainment-education. In: *Entertainment-Education Behind the Scenes* (ed. L.B. Frank and P. Falzone), 15–21. Cham: Palgrave Macmillan.
50. Singhal, A., Rogers, E.M., and Brown, W.J. (1993). Harnessing the potential of entertainment-education telenovelas. *Gaz. Leiden. Neth.* 51 (1): 1–18.
51. Moseley, S.F. (2004). Everett Rogers' diffusion of innovations theory: its utility and value in public health. *J. Health Commun.* 9 (Suppl 1): 149–151.
52. Rogers, E.M. (2003). *Diffusion of Innnovations*, 5ee. Free Press.
53. Rodrigues, U.M. and Niemann, M. (2017). Social media as a platform for incessant political communication: a case study of Modi's "Clean India" campaign. *Int. J. Commun.* 11: 23.
54. Curtis, V. (2019). Explaining the outcomes of the "Clean India" campaign: institutional behaviour and sanitation transformation in India. *BMJ Glob. Health* 4 (5): e001892.
55. U. S. Census Bureau (2022). *Selected Social Characteristics in the United States*. US Department of Commerce.
56. Ridley-Merriweather, K.E., Head, K.J., Younker, S.M. et al. (2022). A novel qualitative approach for identifying effective communication for recruitment of minority women to a breast cancer prevention study. *Contemp. Clin. Trials Commun.* 27: 1–9.
57. American Red Cross IR. *The COVID-19 "Have the Talk" Campaign.* 2022.
58. Media Campaigns | CDC. 2022 https://www.cdc.gov/chronicdisease/programs-impact/campaigns/index.htm (accessed 3 May 2022).
59. Merchant, R.M., South, E.C., and Lurie, N. (2021). Public health messaging in an era of social media. *JAMA* 325 (3): 223–224.
60. McLuhan, M. (1964). *Understanding Media: The Extensions of Man*. McGraw-Hill.
61. Lewis, N., Shekter-Porat, N., and Nasir, H. (2021). Health information seeking. In: *The Routledge Handbook of Health Communication*, 3ee (ed. T. Thompson and N.G. Harrington), 399–411. Routledge.
62. Percheski, C. and Hargittai, E. (2011). Health information-seeking in the digital age. *J. Am. Coll. Health* 59 (5): 379–386.
63. Jacobs, W., Amuta, A.O., and Jeon, K.C. (2017). Health information seeking in the digital age: an analysis of health information seeking behavior among US adults. Alvares C, editor. *Cogent Soc. Sci.* 3 (1): 1302785.
64. Anker, A.E., Reinhart, A.M., and Feeley, T.H. (2011). Health information seeking: a review of measures and methods. *Patient Educ. Couns.* 82 (3): 346–354.
65. Wong, D.K.K. and Cheung, M.K. (2019). Online health information seeking and eHealth literacy among patients attending a primary care clinic in Hong Kong: a cross-sectional survey. *J. Med. Internet Res.* 21 (3): e10831.
66. Norman, C.D. and Skinner, H.A. (2006). eHEALS: the eHealth literacy scale. *J. Med. Internet Res.* 8 (4): e507.
67. News and Media Literacy Resource Center. *Common Sense Education*. 2019. https://www.commonsense.org/education/news-media-literacy-resource-center (accessed 30 April 2022).
68. Vornholt, P. and Choudhury, M.D. (2021). Understanding the role of social media–based mental health support among college students: survey and semistructured interviews. *JMIR Ment. Health* 8 (7): e24512.
69. Vogels, E.A. (2021). *Some Digital Divides Persist Between Rural, Urban and Suburban America*. Pew Research Center. https://www.pewresearch.org/fact-tank/2021/08/19/some-digital-divides-persist-between-rural-urban-and-suburban-america (accessed 3 May 2022).
70. With Almost Half of World's Population Still Offline, Digital Divide Risks Becoming 'New Face of Inequality', Deputy Secretary-General Warns General Assembly | Meetings Coverage and Press Releases. (2021). https://www.un.org/press/en/2021/dsgsm1579.doc.htm (accessed 3 May 2022).
71. (2021). *The Importance of Language Services in Public Health Campaigns*. Telelanguage. https://telelanguage.com/blog/the-role-of-language-services-in-public-health-campaigns (accessed 3 May 2022).

72. (2015). *Language Access in Clear Communication*. National Institutes of Health (NIH). https://www.nih.gov/institutes-nih/nih-office-director/office-communications-public-liaison/clear-communication/language-access-clear-communication (accessed 3 May 2022).
73. Southwell, B.G., Niederdeppe, J., Cappella, J.N. et al. (2019). Misinformation as a misunderstood challenge to public health. *Am. J. Prev. Med.* 57 (2): 282–285.
74. U.S. Department of Health and Human Services. *Health Misinformation—Current Priorities of the U.S. Surgeon General*. 2021. https://www.hhs.gov/surgeongeneral/priorities/health-misinformation (accessed 30 April 2022).
75. Di Carlo, P., McDonnell, B., Vahapoglu, L. et al. (2022). Public health information for minority linguistic communities. *Bull. World Health Organ.* 100 (1): 78–80.
76. Castronuovo, C. (2022). *Evolving Covid Booster Guidelines Threaten to Widen Inequities*. Bloomberg Law News https://news.bloomberglaw.com/health-law-and-business/evolving-covid-booster-guidelines-threaten-to-widen-inequities (accessed 10 August 2023).
77. van der Linden, S. (2022). Misinformation: susceptibility, spread, and interventions to immunize the public. *Nat. Med.* 28 (3): 460–467.
78. O'Sullivan, P.B. and Carr, C.T. (2018). Masspersonal communication: a model bridging the mass-interpersonal divide. *New Media Soc.* 20 (3): 1161–1180.
79. Tam, L.T., Ho, H.X., Nguyen, D.P. et al. (2021). Receptivity of governmental communication and its effectiveness during COVID-19 pandemic emergency in Vietnam: a qualitative study. *Glob. J. Flex. Syst. Manag.* 22 (1): 45–64.
80. French, M. and Bazarova, N.N. (2017). Is anybody out there?: understanding masspersonal communication through expectations for response across social media platforms. *J. Comput.-Mediat. Commun.* 22 (6): 303–319.
81. Totenberg, N. and McCammon, S. (2022). *Supreme Court Overturns Roe v. Wade, Ending Right to Abortion Upheld for Decades*. NPR. https://www.npr.org/2022/06/24/1102305878/supreme-court-abortion-roe-v-wade-decision-overturn (accessed 6 July 2022).
82. Swift, T. (2022). *I'm Absolutely Terrified that this Is Where We Are*. Twitter, Inc https://twitter.com/taylorswift13/status/1540382753677627393?s=20&t=nnjXSh6iD3kw6zG4UNzVeA (accessed 8 May 2023).
83. Mirra, N., Morrell, E., and Filipiak, D. (2018). From digital consumption to digital invention: toward a new critical theory and practice of multiliteracies. *Theory Pract.* 57 (1): 12–19.
84. Hauge, C. and Reid, K. (2019). A production of survival: cancer politics and feminist media literacies. *Stud. Soc. Justice* 13 (1): 25.
85. Wee, V. (2017). Youth audiences and the media in the digital era: the intensification of multimedia engagement and interaction. *Cine J.* 57 (1): 133–139.
86. Pew Research Center. *News Habits & Media*. 2022. https://www.pewresearch.org/topic/news-habits-media
87. Kreps, G.L. (2020). The value of health communication scholarship: new directions for health communication inquiry. *Int. J. Nurs. Sci.* 7 (Suppl 1): S4–S7.

22 Health Information Seeking among Linguistically Diverse Populations in the United States

CHRISTINE SWOBODA, PRITI SINGH,
A. SUSANA RAMÍREZ, AND NALEEF FAREED

Introduction

Information seeking—defined as the conscious effort to acquire information [1]—may be undertaken to fulfill a goal, help with decision-making, improve understanding, or out of curiosity. With respect to health, individuals seek information to learn about diseases, health risks, prevention, treatment, and decision-making. Increasingly, the sources of health information are not doctors and nurses, but media including the Internet (websites, discussion boards, and social media) [2]. Information seeking from nonclinical sources can improve patient–clinician communication, increase patient self-efficacy, enhance engagement in decision-making, and promote health-enhancing behaviors [3–5]. Yet, disparities in health information seeking, along with the healthcare system's increased reliance on such patient behaviors, can exacerbate health disparities experienced by linguistically diverse population subgroups if individuals are not able to access or understand accurate health information. Focusing on the United States context, the goals of this chapter are to: synthesize what is known about health information seeking behaviors and outcomes, including disparities; analyze critical issues in health information seeking as they relate to linguistic minority populations; and present recommendations for research, education, and practice.

Historical development and theoretical framework

One of the earliest theoretical frameworks to describe why people use media is uses and gratifications. This theory postulates that people intentionally seek out media for their own purposes or gratifications, which may be cognitive, emotional, personal, social, or stress relief [6]. Introduced in the 1940s, the theory explains why people consume different types of media and was developed based on research seeking to define reasons for selection patterns (i.e., across media sources) so that these patterns

The Handbook of Language in Public Health and Healthcare, First Edition.
Edited by Pilar Ortega, Glenn Martínez, Maichou Lor, and A. Susana Ramírez.
© 2024 John Wiley & Sons, Inc. Published 2024 by John Wiley & Sons, Inc.

could be influenced. In a health context, people seek information not only to learn more about health conditions, but to feel social support, feel health-related empowerment, or for entertainment [3, 7].

A common critique of the uses and gratifications framework is that the theory implies all information seeking is active and is fulfilling a need, yet people are exposed to information that is relevant to their health while they are using media to fulfill other needs [8]. This "incidental" exposure has consequences as well: while information seeking involves actively looking for information to serve a purpose, information scanning is less purposeful acquisition of information that occurs during routine exposure. Health information scanning is more common than seeking, and scanning may have some positive effects on health-related knowledge and behaviors [9].

Research on information seeking has especially proliferated in the context of the intentional shift to a shared decision-making model in clinical care, which requires individuals (as patients) to obtain and make sense of health information [10]. Beyond the moral imperative of shared decision-making as a way to ensure patients' consent, people increasingly want information to help them feel they are making the best treatment decisions [11]. Some research has found evidence that shared decision-making can increase patient satisfaction with care, improve patient–physician communication, and improve adherence to treatment or recommendations, although there are disparities in who participates in shared decision-making [11]. Prior research indicates lower rates of shared decision-making among racial minorities, older patients, less educated patients, and those with low English proficiency [12, 13]. These racial, socioeconomic, and linguistic disparities in patient–provider communication and shared decision-making compound the gaps that exist in information seeking behaviors, even as the healthcare industry's intensifying focus on shared decision-making renders effective information seeking more essential (Figure 22.1).

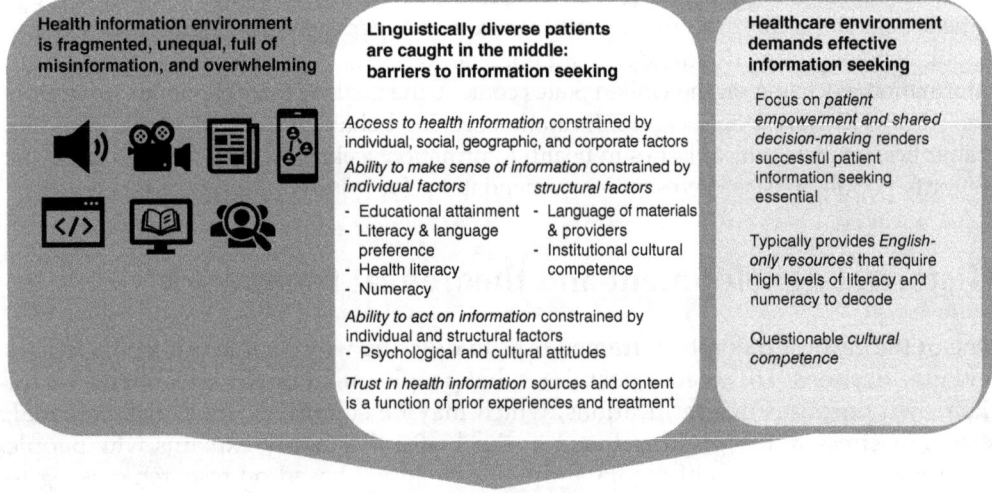

Figure 22.1 Conceptual framework to examine critical issues in health information seeking behaviors and outcomes among linguistically diverse populations.

Characterizing the health information seeker

An estimated 60%–80% of adults reported looking for health information from any source between 2007 and 2017, with an average of over 60% of those who seek going to nonclinical sources as their first source of health information [5]. Nonetheless, certain individual-level characteristics are persistently linked with information seeking behaviors: women and people with more education and higher incomes are more likely than men or people with low incomes and less education to seek any health information [2, 14, 15]. And while all information seekers are increasingly likely to turn to the Internet for health information, young people, more educated, higher income, and female individuals all report higher levels of health-related information seeking via the Internet [15].

Outcomes of health information seeking

Patient–clinician interaction outcomes

Health information seeking contributes to positive communication, psychosocial and psychological improvements, and health outcomes. Patients seeking health information may have improved communication with their physicians and be more satisfied with their care if they discuss information with their providers [4, 16, 17]. Those who seek health information participate more in medical decision-making, whereby enhanced decision-making behavior may be influenced by patients having increased knowledge regarding treatment options and by improved communication with providers [17].

While patient reports of information seeking are generally positive, provider perceptions of patient information seeking are mixed: providers feel concerned that patients may excessively worry, overutilize care, acquire incorrect information or material regarding unrelated conditions, and make visits less efficient due to extra questions, despite the pros of increased communication and engagement [16].

Psychosocial outcomes

Information seeking has positive effects on different aspects of psychosocial, psychological, and physical health. Patients who seek health information report feelings of empowerment, independence, and improved psychological well-being [18]. Online health information seekers have more medical visits, improved adherence, more medication compliance, and higher levels of self-care [5, 19]. Searching for medical information encourages asking questions to help with medical decision-making, increasing consultation with medical professionals, and enhancing patient–physician relationships [20].

Information seeking and health disparities

Despite the growing body of evidence for the positive outcomes of effective health information seeking, barriers in access to health information, as well as in the skills and resources necessary to make effective use of health information, mean that the positive outcomes experienced by those who seek health information are not experienced equally. There are racial disparities in trust of health information sources, with Black and Latino people trusting health information from doctors less and trusting health information from radio, Internet, television, and religious sources more relative to white people, potentially leading to exposure to less accurate information [21, 22]. Women seek health information and cancer information more than men and have higher perceived cancer risk, potentially leading to gender disparities in cancer screening and treatment [14]. Those with lower socioeconomic status and the uninsured also experience disparities in access to and trust in health information [23, 24]. Those with lower literacy or limited English ability may have trouble accessing or understanding health information written in English [25].

These health information access and seeking disparities can lead to poor understanding of health information, misinformation, improper, and inadequate healthcare. In prior research, feeling uncertain or confused about health information or seeing conflicting information has been linked to lower medication adherence [26]. To improve health disparities, it is important for individuals to have equitable access to accurate and understandable health information.

The role of trust in health information seeking source preferences

Trust in health information sources is an important determinant of use of those sources and can also explain some of the race- and ethnicity-based differences in health information seeking behaviors. Among all Americans, healthcare providers remain the most trusted source of health information, despite not being used as the first source of health information as often as web sources [27]. In contrast, while the Internet is the most common first source of health information, individuals may distrust the accuracy of information from the Internet [28]. Younger, more educated people with higher incomes and high levels of self-rated health, along with people identifying as white, report higher levels of trust in health information found online [28]. Trust in online health information is a major predictor of online information seeking [29], and thus trust in the information source helps to reinforce observed demographic differences in online information seeking behaviors [30].

But beyond the Internet, other nonclinical mediated sources are also important health information sources, especially for Black and Latino populations, and this is strongly associated with trust in those sources. Black and Latino populations report higher levels of trust in health information from the radio, the Internet, television, charitable organizations, and religious organizations, and lower trust in health professionals compared with white individuals [21]. Discrimination and historically worse treatment of ethnic and linguistic minorities by health professionals may have contributed to distrust in clinical sources [22, 31], while the ethnically and culturally targeted and linguistically concordant mediated sources of health information advertised within ethnic minority communities elicit trust by featuring influential members of the community and being available in other languages [25, 32]. These trust disparities may increase reliance on potentially less accurate or more biased sources like mass media, which could lead to misinformation and inappropriate health behaviors [33].

Critical issues in understanding health information seeking behaviors and outcomes of linguistic minority populations

While the US federal government recognizes English as the only national language, one-fifth—more than 66 million residents of the United States—speak a language other than English at home. Additionally, over 25 million people rate their English-speaking ability as less than "very well," and this group is referred to as "linguistic minorities" in the United States. Despite the diversity of languages spoken in the United States, neither the media nor the healthcare industries reflect that linguistic diversity. The lack of linguistic diversity in both health information sources and within healthcare present specific challenges to the health of linguistic minority populations: those who identify as a linguistic minority may experience difficulties accessing, understanding, trusting, and using health information.

In prior research, barriers related to language led to negative experiences regarding health information seeking, including frustration, difficulty understanding information, requiring a lot of effort, and concerns about information quality [34]. There is also limited access to quality health information because the majority of information on the Internet, including health information, is in English, and the most readily available health information for linguistic minorities is through the Internet [35, 36]. Outside of health information on the Internet, many doctor's offices and other medical facilities lack patient education materials in languages other than English, and materials in other languages may be written at high reading levels and less frequently updated than the English materials [37]. Conversely, a study by Villa Camacho regarding cancer education materials showed the opposite: Spanish-language content found online was written at lower literacy levels, albeit, a majority of websites lacked languages other than Spanish and English, and lacked diagrams and videos that could further improve comprehension [38].

Although many individuals discuss health information with their providers, language barriers may prevent linguistic minorities from having these discussions or having greater understanding of health information after doctor's visits. Linguistic differences make it difficult for non-English-speaking individuals to understand provider instructions, thus leading to feelings of frustration, prejudice, and unfamiliarity [39]. Commonly reported barriers by individuals with low English proficiency include difficulties communicating and interacting with providers, accessing interpreters, and addressing insurance concerns [40]. Many individuals who speak languages other than English feel discriminated against in healthcare settings and lack access to interpreters or language-concordant care [41]. These barriers to health information access and communication can exacerbate existing health disparities among linguistic minorities.

Proxy health information seeking

One strategy many linguistic minorities use to access health information that is not language-concordant is proxy seeking, where another person seeks information on the behalf of an individual and translates it to them. Proxy seekers are more likely to be women and younger ages [42]. There are many positive outcomes from proxy seeking, including both proxy seekers and those receiving information feeling better informed and more confident, more empowered to make change, and feeling supported [40]. There is risk of proxy seekers feeling anxious due to information overload, and tension when the seeker and the information receiver disagree, or the receiver ignores information. Despite the improved language and cultural concordance, using family as proxy seekers or translators could burden them, and lead to misinterpretation and confidentiality issues [13, 39, 42, 43].

Factors affecting health information seeking among linguistic minority populations

There are individual and structural factors that affect access to health information, ability to understand information, and the ability to act on information. Existing barriers that linguistically diverse patients have to interact with these factors to exacerbate health information disparities.

Individual factors

Many separate factors such as biological and personal attributes influence individuals' ability to seek and understand health information. Individual factors discussed below are interconnected factors that intersect with language and a person's identity, including sociodemographic factors, culture, and digital health literacy.

Sociodemographic factors

Age: Among linguistic minorities, those of school age are more likely to be bilingual and proficient in English, while a larger share of linguistic minority individuals are adults [44]. Many of the disparities experienced by older adults intersect with English-language proficiency. Since younger individuals are at the forefront of rapid technology adoption, they are more likely to use Internet and digital devices [45]. Younger individuals are also more likely to use Internet and digital devices [46], which is corroborated by research among non-English-speaking immigrants in the United States that reported greater use of the Internet for health information seeking among younger and more educated individuals [45].

Race and ethnicity: The majority of individuals in the United States who speak languages other than English at home are also races and ethnicities other than white [47]. Those who are racial and ethnic minorities often report poor communication with providers, fewer clinic visits, unfair treatment, and less trust in healthcare compared to their white counterparts [22, 48]. Health disparities such as unequal treatment and discrimination related to race and ethnicity and language barriers are associated with unequal access to healthcare and unequal health outcomes [31].

Gender: Gender differences also interact with disparities in health information seeking across linguistic minority populations. Some studies suggest that women have stronger social motives, engage in more Internet health information seeking, discuss health issues with others more often, and seek information more in general compared with men [2, 14].

Income: Individuals of lower socioeconomic status have lower odds of seeking and lower confidence in their ability to seek health-related information, less trust in doctors, and greater difficulty understanding information [24]. The complex interplay between socioeconomic status, race and ethnicity, and language exacerbates the barriers to health information seeking. In the United States, racial, ethnic, and linguistic minorities are overrepresented in deprived neighborhoods, for example, nearly 40% of Latinos in the United States live in communities of concentrated poverty; in nearly one-third of the households in these communities, English is not the primary language [49].

Education: Those with lower educational attainment have lower odds of seeking health information, lower confidence in ability to seek health information, lower trust of information from health professionals, and more trust in family or friends, television, government, and religious organizations compared to those with higher education levels [24]. Prior studies show less information seeking among linguistic and racial minorities with lower educational attainment, compounding the individual effects of education [45].

Cultural identity: Cultural identity refers to the interplay between factors including nationality, language, spiritual values, institutional systems, and lifestyles in a group. Linguistic minorities may share languages but have distinct cultural identities. Sociocultural factors that affect information seeking include values, norms, customs, morals and religious beliefs, taboos, perceptions, and preferences. Cultural barriers to information seeking often include feelings of being an outsider, lack of social support, and distrust of information sources [50]. Cultural beliefs may restrict information seeking for specific topics in certain groups; for example, beliefs exist across cultures regarding sexual and reproductive health that may reduce access to or uptake of information or services [51]. Cancer, in particular, is considered an inappropriate topic in some cultures [52, 53]. For example, in one study that examined cultural beliefs of immigrants on cancer, individuals from a particular cultural group regarded cancer as a "terrible emotional burden" and as a "death sentence" [52]. Such cultural beliefs make it difficult for survivors to discuss their cancer-related problems with others, including providers, challenging the effective delivery of care [52, 53]. These cultural restrictions accompanied by language barriers compound the effective delivery of care.

Digital health literacy: Health literacy consists of a set of skills necessary for people to obtain, process, and understand health information [33]. As health materials are increasingly online and Internet use is often necessary to obtain care, digital health literacy is important to achieve equitable care [54]. Expertise across all facets of literacy is needed for optimal eHealth usage, however, individuals with low English proficiency experience negative effects precipitated by the intersection of factors such as low socioeconomic status, discrimination, and less access to healthcare that can deter them from achieving skills in eHealth. Most online content is written in English, including health information [35, 36]. There are also many disparities regarding who has access to the Internet ("the digital divide") [55]. This disparity in ability to access or functionally use the Internet has health implications including reduced ability to communicate, find health information, and access healthcare [55]. Even linguistic minority individuals with greater access to the Internet may continue to face challenges in acquiring relevant, literacy-sensitive, and accurate health data from credible resources [33, 55]. Despite the availability of potentially useful health information online, being older, belonging to minority race and ethnicity groups, and having lower digital literacy were associated with trust in alternate means of information such as newspaper, television, and less credible Internet sources like social media and blogs, and lower trust of medical websites [15, 21, 33, 45].

Structural factors

Not only individual factors but also social, geographic, and societal factors interact to create health information seeking disparities among linguistic minorities. Many linguistic minorities live in family groups and in communities with heavy concentrations of minorities, socially interact with language-concordant peers, and are affected by neighborhood factors that influence health [44].

Social networks: Members of the same social network typically share the same language skills and background [43, 44, 56]. Individuals may rely on social networks for health information because friends and family can offer social support, share experiences, explain complex issues in a manner easy to understand, are often regarded as easy and quicker means to receive responses [56]. Personal social networks are often regarded as easier and quicker means to receive responses. Individuals seek support and help from personal networks to overcome feelings of inadequacy and frustration, especially among immigrant and minority communities. In addition, many immigrant families have unique family structures where parents and children have differing language abilities [44]. Many immigrant children learn English faster than their parents due to school and peers, and parents may rely on their children as translators [56].

Patient–clinician relationship: While patients still rely on doctors for health information, they are increasingly equipped with information from the Internet, which may influence their interaction with providers, either helping them become more collaborative or alternatively stoking distrust [4]. Despite looking up information online, many patients still value consultations with physicians and trust information from doctors more than the Internet [27]. In prior research, seeking health information from the Internet helped patients to better prepare for their visit, ask better questions, feel confident, and understand what physicians discussed with them [4]. On the other hand, some patients may self-diagnose or make medication decisions based on information gathered outside of healthcare settings [39]. Individuals with low English proficiency in the United States were more likely to report poor perceptions of patient–provider communication, less shared decision-making, and dissatisfaction with care when cared for by English-speaking providers [22, 31, 39, 48]. Conversely, in prior research, when patients were seen by language concordant physicians they reported better perceptions of care [31]. Providers, nonetheless, may often underuse professional interpretation services or utilize alternative modes of communication to interact with low English proficiency patients through smartphones, hand gestures, family members, and other nonprofessional interpreters [39, 41, 48].

Neighborhood factors: Linguistic minorities often live in areas with other members of their community, and some of these concentrated areas may be disadvantaged, like inner-city areas or farm communities [44, 57]. Research has shown that individuals living in areas with more neighborhood deprivation report poorer self-rated health, have higher prevalence of chronic diseases and that these deprived areas are often heavily segregated [58]. Neighborhood factors including, but not limited to safety, accessibility (to food and medical resources), walkability, and employment impact chronic disease outcomes [58]. Aspects such as substandard housing, poor air quality, crime, and barriers to accessing nutritious food influence health risk factors such as smoking, physical activity, diet, and ability to recover from stress [57, 58]. The onset of the COVID-19 pandemic shifted in-person visits to telemedicine, but there are substantial variations in telemedicine uptake between urban and rural areas and economically disadvantaged areas. Rural and inner-city areas experience shortages of health workers, as well as barriers to telehealth implementation such as connectivity issues, limitations in device ownership, language barriers, high costs, and electricity access [59]. Telehealth is convenient, but it is not easily accessible to people with limited English proficiency, who are more likely to live in poverty, often work service or construction jobs, and may be more at risk of exposure to COVID-19 [44, 60].

Government policies and healthcare

Broader societal factors include health, economic, educational, and social policies that contribute to inequities in health information seeking and health outcomes.

Policies guiding health insurance, costs of care, what kinds of care individuals receive, legality and approval of medications, and many other factors are decided on a large scale by state or national governments. Many individuals experience barriers to enrolling in health insurance and understanding their coverage, and in the United States, there are higher uninsured rates among those with limited English proficiency [61]. National health recommendations for preventive measures like vaccinations, screening tests, healthy food, and avoiding unhealthy behaviors change over time and may confuse citizens, especially when there are frequent changes like during the COVID-19 pandemic. Distrust of government may encourage the spreading of misinformation, which can lead to extra challenges for linguistic minorities, as they may have trouble understanding recommendations in addition to having to assess the truthfulness of claims from various sources [33, 62].

Implications for health information seeking among linguistic minorities

There is a complex interaction between language and individual, community, and societal factors that may put linguistic minorities at a distinct disadvantage in accessing adequate health information, and which may help to partially explain observed disparities in health behaviors and outcomes [63]. Many linguistic minority populations also experience disparities related to age, race, gender, socioeconomic status, and culture that compound to influence their ability to access, understand, and use health information [21, 24, 39, 45, 63]. It is often difficult for linguistic minorities to find appropriate health information on the Internet or in healthcare settings due to lack of non-English information [35, 36]. Linguistic minorities may rely on their social networks, family members, and inappropriate or inaccurate sources for health information when language-concordant information is not available to them [44, 56]. Interpersonal relationships between patients and providers are also affected by language barriers, and without language-concordant physicians or interpreters, understanding of health information may be limited and linguistic minorities may have worse perceptions of patient–provider communication [4, 39]. Additionally, linguistic minorities often live in neighborhoods that have concentrated populations of limited English proficiency individuals, so interventions to improve health information access may need to use community-based approaches to improve access and equity on a larger scale [57]. There are constantly shifting guidelines and national policies relating to health, both affecting what kinds of care are received and the content of behavioral health recommendations. Linguistic minorities may be at increased risk of misunderstanding health recommendations without specific interventions in place to ensure widespread information delivery [62, 64].

Recommendations for research

Despite copious research about the barriers in information seeking experienced by linguistic minorities, there are still opportunities for more areas of applied research, and for proposing approaches in which linguistically diverse audiences use information seeking to meet their health information needs. There is a lack of trend data over time to explore whether these barriers to health information seeking are stable or changing.

While trust in different information sources has been explored [21, 24, 27, 33], more data is necessary to identify exactly which are the most trusted sources within television, print, radio, and Internet sources and *how* they elicit trust. There is some research showing that linguistic minorities trust and use language-concordant information, which may more often come from television, radio, and interpersonal sources in the absence of appropriate Internet or print information [25, 43]. There are a lot of assumptions about the accuracy and reliability of nonstandard health information sources because of the variability, even though many of these sources may be useful and acceptable to large populations [65]. For example, there are many websites, social media, radio, and television sources that are accurate and accessible, but similar sources that spread misinformation may also appear legitimate [33, 65]. It is important for credible sources to correct misinformation and to have a presence on the Internet and social media to widen the audience receiving appropriate health information [66].

Although it is known that there are information and health disparities in linguistic minority populations, there is a dearth of research exploring the direct outcomes of lack of health information or misinformation and how this causes disparities – are those who have inadequate access behaving differently or experiencing poor outcomes directly due to the need for health information? For example, recent evidence indicates that during the COVID-19 pandemic, linguistic minorities and those with lower health literacy experienced more difficulty finding and understanding information about COVID-19, were less likely to rate social distancing as important, were more likely to endorse misinformation beliefs related to COVID-19 and vaccination, and were more likely to be hospitalized for COVID-19 [60]. Does providing information or correcting misinformation to linguistic and other minority populations improve outcomes? Prior research suggests that public health organizations and medical experts can fight misinformation by using social media and enlisting celebrities and influencers to promote accurate information and fight health myths [66]. Future research could bridge the gap by finding the mediators between information and outcomes and exploring the extent to which appropriate public health messaging affects behavior change.

Finally, research on assistive technology for health information is in its infancy. How do translation apps for health information sources, patient portals, and medical interactions affect patient–provider communication, behaviors, and health outcomes? There are some barriers to uptake of these technologies due to cost, learning curves, accuracy concerns, and the risk of mistranslations [67]. Do the benefits outweigh the concerns? There are many services available, but without research and uptake, disparities will remain.

Recommendations for practice

Recommendations to improve the reach, access, use, and effects of health information by linguistic minorities are presented below.

Technological solutions

Due to the increased reliance on the Internet for health information, linguistic minorities may need to use services that make understanding this information easier. Translational services such as Google Translator help with website navigation, which could help health information uptake from the Internet [67]. However, these sources have yet to be investigated from a health information seeking perspective.

Media

More interventions could focus on media literacy in high-risk linguistic minority populations. There is evidence that media literacy interventions are effective in a school setting, but not a lot of these interventions have been deployed in health or government settings or have focused on non-English media [68]. The misinformation and plethora of conflicting sources available during the COVID-19 pandemic renewed interest in importance of training the general population on how to be more critical of health media [69].

Targeting television, radio, and community resources to provide accurate health information in linguistic minority communities could improve health information uptake by providing information within trusted sources [3, 25]. Because language-concordant social media, web, television, and radio sources elicit trust and improve personal connection to the information provided, celebrities, and social media influencers that are highly regarded in linguistic minority communities could be encouraged to promote public health messages [68]. Healthcare systems can focus on inclusive web and print health information, along with increasing their online resources promoting accurate public health messaging [70, 71]. These changes are transformational and require long-term commitments from public and private organizations to invest in the health and well-being of individuals from linguistic minority communities.

Clinical interpretation and translation services

Most of the work to improve language-appropriate care has focused on language assistance and improving interpreter services in clinical settings. However, still many hospitals do not provide interpreters for patients who need them [72]. Strategies that can help overcome systemic barriers to language-appropriate patient-clinician communication include: incorporating multilingual patient experiences into user-centered design for patient-facing technology, improved language accessibility within patient portals, and increasing the use of mobile applications that help clinicians and patients communicate [72, 73].

Recommendations for policy

Within communities with high populations of linguistic minorities, funding and building infrastructure such as libraries and English teaching centers can help improve information access. Accreditation standards, like the patient-centered communication standards in the 2022 Comprehensive Accreditation Manual for Hospitals (CAMH) emphasize the importance of effective communication, cultural competence, and patient-centered care in providing safe care and holding healthcare facilities accountable for adhering to these standards should improve services for linguistic minority patients [74]. For health insurance organizations, although most have enrollment information in a few languages and services available to help interpret insurance applications, further expansion with more languages, phone numbers for assistance, and documentation of the use and need for language assistance can be further improved [75]. There is evidence that misunderstanding insurance leads to lower care utilization [61, 75], encouraging outreach to underinsured populations with cultural- and literacy-appropriate materials in multiple languages to increase insurance enrollment and care uptake.

Conclusion

Health information seeking behavior is linked to improvements in health outcomes, but disparities in information seeking disproportionately affect some subpopulations. Linguistic minorities experience significant difficulties accessing, understanding, and using health information, furthering health divides. There are significant intersections between language, sociodemographic, community, and societal factors that enable disparities to persist in linguistic minority populations. Interventions at the interpersonal, community, and government levels will be increasingly necessary to alleviate these disparities and provide more equitable information access.

Highlights

- Linguistic minorities face barriers to health information access and use that may exacerbate existing health disparities.
- Access to and the ability to understand and act on health information among linguistic minorities may be influenced by individual factors (e.g., age, race and ethnicity, gender, income, education, culture, and digital health literacy) and structural factors (e.g., social networks, patient–provider relationships, neighborhood factors, and government policies).
- Many ethnic and linguistic minority populations have higher levels of trust in non-clinical sources of health information like the radio, television, religious, and charitable organizations and lower trust in healthcare professionals due to discrimination and receiving care that is not linguistically or culturally concordant.
- The rise of shared decision-making in healthcare encourages health information seeking, but there is risk of misinformation, improper care, and anxiety among health information seekers who face linguistic and health literacy barriers.
- Targeted efforts must be made to disseminate accurate health information is that culturally and linguistically tailored to high-risk linguistic minority populations.

REFERENCES

1. Case, D.O. and Given, L.M. (2016). *Looking for Information: A Survey of Research on Information Seeking, Needs, and Behavior*, 4ee. Bingley, UK: Emerald.

2. Kelly, B., Hornik, R., Romantan, A. et al. (2010). Cancer information scanning and seeking in the general population. *J. Health Commun.* 15 (7): 734–753.

3. Ramírez, A.S., Freres, D., Martinez, L.S. et al. (2013). Information seeking from media and family/friends increases the likelihood of engaging in healthy lifestyle behaviors. *J. Health Commun.* 18 (5): 527–542.
4. Tan, S.S.L. and Goonawardene, N. (2017). Internet health information seeking and the patient-physician relationship: a systematic review. *J. Med. Internet Res.* 19 (1): e9.
5. Swoboda, C.M., Walker, D.M., and Huerta, T. (2021). Odds of meeting cancer prevention behavior recommendations by health information seeking behavior: a cross-sectional HINTS analysis. *J. Cancer Educ.* 36 (1): 56–64.
6. Ruggiero, T.E. (2000). Uses and gratifications theory in the 21st century. *Mass Commun. Soc.* 3 (1): 3–37.
7. Park, D.Y. and Goering, E.M. (2016). The health-related uses and gratifications of YouTube: motive, cognitive involvement, online activity, and sense of empowerment. *J. Consum. Health Internet* 20 (1–2): 52–70.
8. Sundar, S.S. and Limperos, A.M. (2013). Uses and Grats 2.0: new gratifications for new media. *J. Broadcast. Electron. Media* 57 (4): 504–525.
9. Hornik, R., Parvanta, S., Mello, S. et al. (2013). Effects of scanning (routine health information exposure) on cancer screening and prevention behaviors in the general population. *J. Health Commun.* 18 (12): 1422–1435.
10. Frosch, D.L. and Kaplan, R.M. (1999). Shared decision making in clinical medicine: past research and future directions. *Am. J. Prev. Med.* 17 (4): 285–294.
11. Chewning, B., Bylund, C.L., Shah, B. et al. (2012). Patient preferences for shared decisions: a systematic review. *Patient Educ. Couns.* 86 (1): 9–18.
12. Peek, M.E., Odoms-Young, A., Quinn, M.T. et al. (2010). Race and shared decision-making: perspectives of African-Americans with diabetes. *Soc. Sci. Med.* 71 (1): 1–9.
13. Kamara, D., Weil, J., Youngblom, J. et al. (2018). Cancer counseling of low-income limited English proficient Latina women using medical interpreters: implications for shared decision-making. *J. Genet. Couns.* 27 (1): 155–168.
14. Manierre, M.J. (2015). Gaps in knowledge: tracking and explaining gender differences in health information seeking. *Soc. Sci. Med.* 128: 151–158.
15. Jacobs, W., Amuta, A.O., and Jeon, K.C. (2017). Health information seeking in the digital age: an analysis of health information seeking behavior among US adults. Alvares C, ed. *Cogent Soc. Sci.* 3 (1): 1302785.
16. Luo, A., Qin, L., Yuan, Y. et al. (2022). The effect of online health information seeking on physician-patient relationships: systematic review. *J. Med. Internet Res.* 24 (2): e23354.
17. Asan, O., Yu, Z., and Crotty, B.H. (2021). How clinician-patient communication affects trust in health information sources: temporal trends from a national cross-sectional survey. Serrano K, editor. *PLoS One* 16 (2): e0247583.
18. Zhang, L., Jung, E.H., and Chen, Z. (2020). Modeling the pathway linking health information seeking to psychological well-being on WeChat. *Health Commun.* 35 (9): 1101–1112.
19. Thapa, D.K., Visentin, D.C., Kornhaber, R. et al. (2021). The influence of online health information on health decisions: a systematic review. *Patient Educ. Couns.* 104 (4): 770–784.
20. Chiu, Y.L., Tsai, C.C., and Liang, J.C. (2022). Laypeople's online health information search strategies and use for health-related problems: cross-sectional survey. *J. Med. Internet Res.* 24 (9): e29609.
21. Fareed, N., Swoboda, C.M., Jonnalagadda, P. et al. (2021). Differences between races in health information seeking and trust over time: evidence from a cross-sectional, pooled analyses of HINTS data. *Am. J. Health Promot.* 35 (1): 84–92.
22. Saha, S., Arbelaez, J.J., and Cooper, L.A. (2003). Patient–physician relationships and racial disparities in the quality of health care. *Am. J. Public Health* 93 (10): 1713–1719.
23. Lee, C.J., Ramírez, A.S., Lewis, N. et al. (2012). Looking beyond the internet: examining socioeconomic inequalities in

cancer information seeking among cancer patients. *Health Commun.* 27 (8): 806–817.
24. Fareed, N., Jonnalagadda, P., Swoboda, C.M. et al. (2021). Socioeconomic factors influence health information seeking and trust over time: evidence from a cross-sectional, pooled analyses of HINTS data. *Am. J. Health Promot.* 35 (8): 1084–1094.
25. Ramirez, A.S., Graff, K., Nelson, D. et al. (2015). Who seeks *Cita con El doctor*? Twelve years of Spanish-language radio program targeting U.S. Latinos. *Health Educ. Behav.* 42 (5): 611–620.
26. Alberti, T.L. and Crawford, S.L. (2020). Health information–seeking behaviors and adherence to urgent care discharge instructions. *J. Am. Assoc. Nurse Pract.* 32 (6): 438–446.
27. Swoboda, C.M., Van Hulle, J.M., McAlearney, A.S., and Huerta, T.R. (2018). Odds of talking to healthcare providers as the initial source of healthcare information: updated cross-sectional results from the health information National Trends Survey (HINTS). *BMC Fam. Pract.* 19 (1): 146.
28. Sbaffi, L. and Rowley, J. (2017). Trust and credibility in web-based health information: a review and agenda for future research. *J. Med. Internet Res.* 19 (6): e218.
29. Wang, X., Shi, J., and Kong, H. (2021). Online health information seeking: a review and meta-analysis. *Health Commun.* 36 (10): 1163–1175.
30. Arellano Carmona, K., Chittamuru, D., Kravitz, R.L. et al. (2022). Health information seeking from an intelligent web-based symptom checker: cross-sectional questionnaire study. *J. Med. Internet Res.* 24 (8): e36322.
31. Yeheskel, A. and Rawal, S. (2019). Exploring the 'patient experience' of individuals with limited English proficiency: a scoping review. *J. Immigr. Minor. Health* 21 (4): 853–878.
32. Estrada, E., Ramirez, A.S., Gamboa, S., and Amezola de Herrera, P. (2018). Development of a participatory health communication intervention: an ecological approach to reducing rural information inequality and health disparities. *J. Health Commun.* 23 (8): 773–782.
33. Chen, X., Hay, J.L., Waters, E.A. et al. (2018). Health literacy and use and trust in health information. *J. Health Commun.* 23 (8): 724–734.
34. Chu, J.N., Sarkar, U., Rivadeneira, N.A. et al. (2022). Impact of language preference and health literacy on health information-seeking experiences among a low-income, multilingual cohort. *Patient Educ. Couns.* 105 (5): 1268–1275.
35. Millar, R.J., Sahoo, S., Yamashita, T., and Cummins, P.A. (2020). Literacy skills, language use, and online health information seeking among Hispanic adults in the United States. *Patient Educ. Couns.* 103 (8): 1595–1600.
36. Web Technology Surveys. Historical trends in the usage statistics of content languages for websites. https://w3techs.com/technologies/history_overview/content_language (accessed 20 December 2022).
37. Novin, S.A., Huh, E.H., Bange, M.G. et al. (2019). Readability of Spanish-language patient education materials from http://RadiologyInfo.org. *J. Am. Coll. Radiol.* 16 (8): 1108–1113.
38. Villa Camacho, J.C., Pena, M.A., Flores, E.J. et al. (2021). Addressing linguistic barriers to care: evaluation of breast cancer online patient educational materials for Spanish-speaking patients. *J. Am. Coll. Radiol.* 18 (7): 919–926.
39. Pandey, M., Maina, R.G., Amoyaw, J. et al. (2021). Impacts of English language proficiency on healthcare access, use, and outcomes among immigrants: a qualitative study. *BMC Health Serv. Res.* 21 (1): 741.
40. Paternotte, E., van Dulmen, S., van der Lee, N. et al. (2015). Factors influencing intercultural doctor–patient communication: a realist review. *Patient Educ. Couns.* 98 (4): 420–445.
41. Butow, P.N., Sze, M., Dugal-Beri, P. et al. (2011). From inside the bubble: migrants' perceptions of communication with the cancer team. *Support. Care Cancer* 19 (2): 281–290.
42. El Sherif, R., Pluye, P., and Ibekwe, F. (2022). Contexts and outcomes of proxy online health information seeking: mixed studies review with framework synthesis. *J. Med. Internet Res.* 24 (6): e34345.

43. Ramirez, A.S., Leyva, B., Graff, K. et al. (2015). Seeking information on behalf of others: an analysis of calls to a Spanish-language radio health program. *Health Promot. Pract.* 16 (4): 501–509.
44. Batalova, J. and Zong, J. (2016). Language diversity and English proficiency in the United States. *Migr. Inf. Source* https://www.migrationpolicy.org/article/language-diversity-and-english-proficiency-united-states-2015.
45. Chae, S., Lee, Y.J., and Han, H.R. (2021). Sources of health information, technology access, and use among non–English-speaking immigrant women: descriptive correlational study. *J. Med. Internet Res.* 23 (10): e29155.
46. Onyeaka, H.K., Romero, P., Healy, B.C., and Celano, C.M. (2021). Age differences in the use of health information technology among adults in the United States: an analysis of the health information National Trends Survey. *J. Aging Health* 33 (1–2): 147–154.
47. US Census Bureau (2022). Language spoken at home and difficulty speaking English: Number of children ages 5–17 who speak a language other than English at home by language spoken and ability to speak English, and the percentages of those speaking a language other than English at home and those with difficulty speaking English by selected characteristics, selected years 1979–2019. America's Children: Key National Indicators of Well-Being, 2022. https://www.childstats.gov/americaschildren/tables/fam5.asp (accessed 10 August 2023).
48. Pérez-Stable, E.J. and El-Toukhy, S. (2018). Communicating with diverse patients: how patient and clinician factors affect disparities. *Patient Educ. Couns.* 101 (12): 2186–2194.
49. Meade, E. (2014). *Overview of Community Characteristics in Areas With Concentrated Poverty [Internet]*. Office of the Assistant Secretary for Planning and Evaluation. https://aspe.hhs.gov/reports/overview-community-characteristics-areas-concentrated-poverty (accessed 20 December 2022).
50. Savolainen, R. (2016). Approaches to socio-cultural barriers to information seeking. *Libr. Inf. Sci. Res.* 38 (1): 52–59.
51. Morales-Campos, D.Y., Snipes, S.A., Villarreal, E.K. et al. (2021). Cervical cancer, human papillomavirus (HPV), and HPV vaccination: exploring gendered perspectives, knowledge, attitudes, and cultural taboos among Mexican American adults. *Ethn. Health* 26 (2): 206–224.
52. Dohan, D. and Levintova, M. (2007). Barriers beyond words: cancer, culture, and translation in a community of Russian speakers. *J. Gen. Intern. Med.* 22 (S2): 300.
53. Daher, M. (2012). Cultural beliefs and values in cancer patients. *Ann. Oncol.* 23: iii66–iii69.
54. Smith, B. and Magnani, J.W. (2019). New technologies, new disparities: the intersection of electronic health and digital health literacy. *Int. J. Cardiol.* 292: 280–282.
55. Chesser, A., Burke, A., Reyes, J., and Rohrberg, T. (2016). Navigating the digital divide: a systematic review of eHealth literacy in underserved populations in the United States. *Inform. Health Soc. Care* 41 (1): 1–19.
56. Kim, W., Kreps, G.L., and Shin, C.N. (2015). The role of social support and social networks in health information–seeking behavior among Korean Americans: a qualitative study. *Int. J. Equity Health* 14 (1): 40.
57. Jargowsky, P.A. (2009). Immigrants and neighbourhoods of concentrated poverty: assimilation or stagnation? *J. Ethn. Migr. Stud.* 35 (7): 1129–1151.
58. White, K., Haas, J.S., and Williams, D.R. (2012). Elucidating the role of place in health care disparities: the example of racial/ethnic residential segregation. *Health Serv. Res.* 47 (3 Pt 2): 1278–1299.
59. Cherewka, A. (2020). The digital divide hits U.S. Immigrant households disproportionately during the COVID-19 pandemic. *Migr Inf Source*. https://www.migrationpolicy.org/article/digital-divide-hits-us-immigrant-households-during-covid-19 (accessed 20 December 2022).
60. Ingraham, N.E., Purcell, L.N., Karam, B.S. et al. (2021). Racial and ethnic disparities in hospital admissions from COVID-19:

determining the impact of neighborhood deprivation and primary language. *J. Gen. Intern. Med.* 36 (11): 3462–3470.

61. Foiles Sifuentes, A.M., Robledo Cornejo, M., Li, N.C. et al. (2020). The role of limited English proficiency and access to health insurance and health care in the affordable care act era. *Health Equity* 4 (1): 509–517.

62. Escoffery, C., Riehman, K., Watson, L. et al. (2019). Facilitators and barriers to the implementation of the HPV VACs (vaccinate adolescents against cancers) program: a consolidated framework for implementation research analysis. *Prev. Chronic Dis.* 16: 180406.

63. Sentell, T. and Braun, K.L. (2012). Low health literacy, limited English proficiency, and health status in Asians, Latinos, and other racial/ethnic groups in California. *J. Health Commun.* 17 (Suppl 3): 82–99.

64. Diamond, L.C., Jacobs, E.A., and Karliner, L. (2020). Providing equitable care to patients with limited dominant language proficiency amid the COVID-19 pandemic. *Patient Educ. Couns.* 103 (8): 1451–1452.

65. Kington, R.S., Arnesen, S., Chou, W.Y.S. et al. (2021). Identifying credible sources of health information in social media: principles and attributes. *NAM Perspect* https://nam.edu/identifying-credible-sources-of-health-information-in-social-media-principles-and-attributes (accessed 20 December 2022).

66. Bode, L. and Vraga, E.K. (2018). See something, say something: correction of global health misinformation on social media. *Health Commun.* 33 (9): 1131–1140.

67. Panayiotou, A., Gardner, A., Williams, S. et al. (2019). Language translation apps in health care settings: expert opinion. *JMIR Mhealth Uhealth* 7 (4): e11316.

68. Lim, S.S. and Tan, K.R. (2020). Front liners fighting fake news: global perspectives on mobilising young people as media literacy advocates. *J. Child. Media* 14 (4): 529–535.

69. Austin, E.W., Austin, B.W., Willoughby, J.F. et al. (2021). How media literacy and science media literacy predicted the adoption of protective behaviors amidst the COVID-19 pandemic. *J. Health Commun.* 26 (4): 239–252.

70. Collier, R. (2018). Containing health myths in the age of viral misinformation. *Can. Med. Assoc. J.* 190 (19): E578–E578.

71. Taira, B.R., Kim, K., and Mody, N. (2019). Hospital and health system–level interventions to improve care for limited English proficiency patients: a systematic review. *Jt. Comm. J. Qual. Patient Saf.* 45 (6): 446–458.

72. Schiaffino, M.K., Nara, A., and Mao, L. (2016). Language services in hospitals vary by ownership and location. *Health Aff.* 35 (8): 1399–1403.

73. Sezgin, E., Noritz, G., Hoffman, J., and Huang, Y. (2020). A medical translation assistant for non–English-speaking caregivers of children with special health care needs: proposal for a scalable and interoperable Mobile app. *JMIR Res Protoc.* 9 (10): e21038.

74. The Joint Commission (2022). *Comprehensive Accreditation Manual for Hospitals 2021*. Oakbrook Terrace, IL: Joint Commission Resources.

75. Chin, K.K. (2016). *HHS Must Improve Language Access To Make Meaningful Access A Reality*. Health Affairs Forefront.

23 Entertainment-Education as Linguistic Duality in Practice

SURUCHI SOOD AND
RACHAEL HAILESELASSE

Introduction

This chapter explores the dynamic relationship between linguistic diversity and entertainment-education strategies that promote health-related social and behavioral change (SBC). We begin with a brief review of the modern histories and definitions of both linguistic diversity and entertainment-education. We then describe the organic cross-influence between the two disciplines. Intervention examples from the field then illustrate current practices and provide overall guidance on ways to integrate linguistic diversity and entertainment-education.

Though linguistic diversity is more broadly the use of different languages, it includes language variation within culture and cultural variation within language, including but not limited to grammar, vocabulary, semantics, style, and nonverbal cues. As a health communication strategy designed to promote individual and social change, entertainment-education inherently influences language via a wide variety of media channels including audio, video, and visual arts. It is beyond the scope of this chapter and the authors' expertise to engage in debates of linguistic theory or complex linguistic terminologies or to provide a comprehensive overview of the theory and evidence within entertainment-education. However, some broad concepts are essential to understanding linguistic diversity and entertainment-education literature and the intersections between them.

Historical development and theoretical framework

History and theory of linguistic diversity

Language is how we can participate in what the United Nations Universal Declaration on Human Rights identifies as rights to "cultural life of the community, to enjoy the arts, and (to) share in scientific advancements and its benefits" [1–3]. The definitions and applications of linguistic diversity have evolved over time. Modern discourse is inextricable from the conquests, colonialism, and migration codified in language as a reflection of human identity. These include broader language families such as Afro–Asiatic or Indo–European, and also those we associate with nationalities such as Spanish, Chinese, or English despite the variances among each of these. Language use has always entailed a hierarchal system in which specific languages are deemed more sophisticated, pure, and essential to a high quality of life. Being a "good" citizen and enjoying the associated rights and privileges is often linked to national language proficiency [3]. A corporation's translation of materials and hiring of multilingual staff are perhaps more subtle forms of validating specific languages and associated opportunities. One can argue that language, vernacular, and accents signify one's identity and position even within communities and households. With this breadth of language practice in mind, social justice demands that practitioners address and understand common perceptions of language (and subsequent potential political conflicts) among lay language users vs. the understandings that linguists have about language [4].

Linguistics as a discipline draws from history, political science, anthropology, and language pedagogy. In recent decades, and across disciplines, there have been increasingly critical analyses of the concepts, power, and definitions of language diversity. It is difficult to imagine an industry, setting, or relationship that does not engage either implicit or explicit ideas about language. Immigration and citizenship requirements for language proficiency are structural settings where language is explicitly used to include and exclude individuals. English language instruction around the globe, especially in countries considered to be a part of the former British Empire, continues to standardize English as a competency for work and social opportunities. The dominance of English is tied to historical practice and the value of monolingualism [3]. This history has often been brutal, forcing communities to abandon the use of their languages and punishing those who did not. India is one of the most acute examples of the vestiges of English language monolingualism. Despite India's 448 individual living languages, 14 extinct languages, 22 scheduled national languages, and 99 nonscheduled languages, English, as a remnant of colonialism, remains one of the dominant languages of government and industry across the country [5]. Colonial definitions of language and identity continue to impact how we think about linguistic diversity. Africa, a continent of 54 recognized countries and approximately 2000 living languages is still referred to as either Anglophone, Lusophone, or Francophone, colonial language references that continue to obscure African native languages and epistemologies [6].

Social justice challenges the contemporary framing of language diversity around the changing patterns of immigration. For example, the United Kingdom and the United States have prided monolingualism as part of their colonial pasts. Yet, due to globalization and immigration, both the United Kingdom and the United States have recently had higher immigration rates from the global south against relatively homogeneous postcolonial populations that favored European immigration and the forced resettlement of indigenous people [7]. In the United States, the number of speakers of all top ten languages in continues to grow, with nearly 12% of the population speaking Spanish [8, 9]. Against this backdrop, responsible multilingual work entails recognizing the evolving nature of language and defining linguistic diversity in communications, content, and policy.

There are three fundamental systems of understanding linguistic diversity that likely inform how we think about language, whether we are conscious of them or not. First is *universalism*, the idea that languages share the same basic mechanics and purpose and that differences are innate to individual users [10]. A person with this perspective might think of linguistic diversity within regional dialects or vernacular within languages. Second, the **historical evolutionary perspective**, which emphasizes structural differences between languages (ordering of subjects and verbs) and language families, classifying language by geography and subsequent diffusion of languages through contact. Here one might see Spanish and Japanese as more linguistically different than Spanish and Italian. A more recent definition of linguistic diversity is *"practice-based."* A practice-based definition emphasizes linguistic diversity as a constantly emerging phenomenon based on everyday language use and exchange across social interactions. In this definition, language histories and cultures accumulate over time, belong to groups, and are constructed through individuals. [7] Because changes in daily language usage are not limited by what words are added formally into dictionaries, practice-based linguistic diversity acknowledges rapid changes to language in real time. An essential part of practice-based linguistic diversity is that of multilingualism. Multilingualism captures the everyday use of language in settings and among speakers using more than one language. It replaces bilingualism, a limited concept that often assumes that people use one language or the other. In reality, one may be thinking in one language, speaking in another, or speaking and thinking in a mix of languages. This results in informal references to multilingualism using terms like Spanglish as a mix of Spanish and English or Hinglish as a mix of Hindi and English. Multilingualism recognizes constant exchanges across languages, even within the same user or same group. It is, in a sense, a more ecological definition of linguistic diversity and includes settings such as migration, international work sites, regional variations, and industry-specific jargon as ecosystems of language. [11] This practical definition also encourages the reexamination of theories, histories, and definitions of languages through a social justice lens from individual exchanges to those across disciplines, communities, and countries. This practice-based definition of linguistic diversity aligns best with how entertainment-education works and what can be discerned as its underlying goal to facilitate the participation of all communities and individuals in their human rights to health and culture.

History and theory of entertainment-education

Entertainment-education is a health communication strategy that uses media to increase individual knowledge and change attitudes, beliefs, and behaviors to improve the human condition. Wang and Singhal (2021) offer the following definition: "Entertainment-education is a social and behavioral change communication (SBCC) strategy that leverages the power of storytelling in entertainment and wisdom from theories in different disciplines—with deliberate intention and collaborative efforts throughout the process of content production, program implementation, monitoring, and evaluation—to address critical issues in the real world and create enabling conditions for desirable and sustainable change across micro-, meso-, and macro-levels" [12]. Though entertainment-education began using channels like radio, TV, theater, and public service announcement, it has pivoted to using new and emerging media. Current entertainment-education ranges from streaming online videos to video games, interactive social media, and smartphone apps while still relying on the more traditional communication channels. Many entertainment-education interventions now include sharing content across multiple media channels and formats. For example, using posters can visually reinforce scenes and dialog from TV and radio shows, which then can be used to share shorter pieces of information and engage audiences on social media. This constitutes a method in entertainment-education called transmedia storytelling. The evolution of transmedia storytelling as a best practice in entertainment-education holds several unique advantages for bringing diverse people together and for reaching diverse audiences [13].

Early entertainment-education specialists borrowed from Aristotle's concepts of ethos, pathos, and logos when explaining the functions of language. Thus entertainment-education program design continues to be based on the understanding that appealing to the audience's feelings, sensibilities, identities, and cultural norms makes programmatic or technical content more palatable and therefore, easier to remember and incorporate into current behaviors [14]. Much entertainment-education literature is traditionally premised on Albert Bandura's social cognitive theory (SCT). As described in Chapters 21 and 26 of this volume, SCT emphasizes how humans learn by social modeling. We change our behavior when we observe new behavior and feel confident that we can adopt this new behavior. Behavioral change entails trial and maintenance of the new behavior [15]. A current example of behavioral modeling and the advancement of SCT in entertainment-education practice is gender-transformative theory. Gender transformative theory draws attention to how gender roles are socially constructed and encourages interventions to model healthy gender roles as alternatives to unhealthy ones [16]. A gender transformative approach is applied in entertainment-education to develop programs that model progressive gender identities. This is specifically true of entertainment-education work in sexual and reproductive health and domestic violence, where program content models nonviolence and male rejection of violent behaviors and provides cues to action for appropriate bystander behaviors.

Another foundational figure in entertainment-education, Paulo Freire, emphasized unequal power dynamics where researchers and communications experts often impose beliefs and behaviors on communities while failing to engage them in the creation of appropriate materials. Friere established the audience-centered approach that is now commonly referred to as community-based participatory research (CBPR).[17]. Public health practice encourages the use of CBPR within formative research, program monitoring, and program evaluation. In entertainment-education, fundamental CBPR concepts inform the best practices of making knowledge accessible to all and ensuring that knowledge from all communities and individuals is valued and included [18, 19]. The work of Mohan Dutta illustrates two key points when it comes to the use of language in communications research and practice in global settings. First, there are colonial vestiges of power in how language is studied and applied in global development efforts. Second, a decolonial approach to linguistics and language must critically interrogate whose knowledge, authorship, and power underlie language diversity [20].

Popular entertainment-education programs have been around for decades. Early examples include the BBC radio series *The Archers* in 1959, and the TV series *Simplemente María* in Peru, in 1969. In the 1970s, Miguel Sabido established himself as a foundational entertainment-education methodologist when he applied several theories, including Albert Bandura's SCT, to analyze *Simplemente María* and develop a series of Spanish-language telenovelas for Mexico and the Latin American markets [15]. The trajectory of entertainment-education programming around the world has differed significantly. In the global south, entertainment-education programs are developed and implemented as stand-alone health communication efforts to promote SBC. Entertainment-education has been used to promote several prosocial behaviors, including contraceptive use, condom promotion, anti-sexual violence, optimal maternal and child health (MCH) practices, and lifestyle choices such as diet and exercise [21]. While entertainment-education has emerged as a key public health communication strategy, more recent applications cover other development issues, including girls' education, gender, social norms, livelihood and income generation, and peacebuilding [22]. In the media-saturated markets of the global north, the more common use of entertainment-education is through the inclusion of accurate health and social messages within popular programs entertainment programs. The term social impact entertainment is currently used by some to describe these efforts [23]. Recent examples of United States TV-based programs that use entertainment-education include *Gray's Anatomy*, *Law and Order,* and *Scrubs* [24].

An early focus in entertainment-education was on answering the question, does entertainment-education work? Research associated with this question often relied on quantifiable, individual-level data. Once proof of its effectiveness was shown in a wide range of literature, across channels, formats, geography, and audiences, research attention shifted to explore how and why it worked. Academics and practitioners realized only through an understanding of the why and how could entertainment-education programs be replicated and sustained. Several current and prevalent models explaining how and why entertainment-education works include causal models that borrow from well-established social sciences (psychology, anthropology, and sociology) and the field of communication studies. Some SBC theories that function at the individual, interpersonal, community, organizational, and policy/social levels and help explain the entertainment-education process include the health belief model, stages of change, theory of planned behavior, and diffusion of innovations. Additionally, communication theories, including narrative theory and uses and gratifications, are often emphasized in entertainment-education [25]. Narrative theories explain how the intrinsic properties of storytelling change a person's knowledge, attitudes, and beliefs as a result of exposure to entertainment-education programs. Narrative persuasion is an umbrella term that comes from the field of communication and encompasses a set of theoretical constructs, including narrative transportation, narrative engagement, and identification with characters, among others [14, 26]. Such narrative engagement is critical in understanding the role of SCT, including vicarious learning, in entertainment-education.

Practice and evidence

The exchange between entertainment-education and linguistic diversity is rarely formal as there is little academic collaboration between linguists and entertainment-education practitioners. Based on a review of the literature, our personal experiences, and informal conversations with several colleagues, we hypothesize that entertainment-education influences linguistic diversity, and linguistic diversity influences entertainment-education. Examples of programs highlighting the correlations between linguistic diversity and entertainment-education and where each influences the other are listed in Table 23.1 and expanded upon in the section below. It is important to emphasize upfront that these examples are limited since there are likely many entertainment-education programs demonstrating these influences that we are unaware of. And there are likely additional relationships between entertainment-education and linguistic diversity than illustrated here.

Table 23.1 Descriptions of programs discussed in this chapter, with information related to audience and bidirectional influence of entertainment-education (EE) and linguistic diversity.

EE program and date	Target audience, location and language	Aim/goal	EE influence on linguistic diversity	Linguistic diversity influence on EE
Andar For a e Maningue Arriscado, 2009	Adults at risk of HIV, Mozambique, Portuguese	Discourage multiple sexual partnerships. Prevent HIV/STIs	Formative research resulted in the audience-generated phrase "Andar For" meaning "stepping outside" to be associated with a high-risk for HIV/STIs	Local phrasing informed the need to replace standard clinical terms associated with HIV and STIs, creating a culturally competent and acceptable program
Ashal Logne, 2002–2007	Pregnant women and their families, Nepal, Nepali	Encourage husbands and mothers-in-law to provide pre and postnatal support	Use of local Nepali phrasing as applied to new concepts of healthy gender norms. Associating "good husband" with nurturing, support of pregnant women	Local language impact on transcreation of a national campaign resulting in culturally relevant terminology and messaging
Culturally Sensitive Educational Videos (CSEV), 2020	Turkish and Moroccan–Dutch women aged 30–60, Netherlands, Turkish, Moroccan Arabic, Moroccan Berber, and Dutch	Promote testing participation for early detection and treatment of cervical cancer	Interdisciplinary collaboration on creating culturally appropriate and accessible messaging around cervical cancer screening. Use of language to transform stigma or taboo into cultural support for screening participation	Need for multilingual staff and messaging thus influencing multilingual videos to reach immigrant women via the multiple languages they use daily

Program, Years	Audience, Location, Languages	Goal		
East Los High, 2013–2017	Latinx Adolescents, United States, English, and Spanish	Foster positive SRH behaviors to improve women's health, decrease STI transmission, and promote family planning	Intentional use of narrative, various media types, and everyday multilingual use of Spanish, English and Spanglish in urban California settings resulted in new normative behavioral modeling	Intentional hiring of program staff who represent Latin-American communities and engagement with audiences result in the program's culture, language, and acceptability
Kyunki...Jeena Issi Ka Naam Hai, 2008–2011	Women aged 15-34 and their families, India, Hindi	Promote self-efficacy and behavioral change to decrease morbidity and mortality. Topics include sanitation, educating girls, safe motherhood, etc.	The audience relates to familiar social settings depicted in the TV series, including gender and caste-based discrimination. They then gain familiarity with health-related terms and concepts	Local language impact on transcreation of UNICEF *Facts for Life* book to local, primarily rural contexts
Main Kuch Bhi Kar Sakti Hoon, 2014–2019	Primarily rural families, India, Hindi	Empower community change toward a healthy, clean, and equitable society	Shaping new words from existing words to influence positive associations with previously stigmatized behaviors related to sexual and reproductive health (SRH)	Audience engagement through call-in program resulted in real-time interaction between audiences and programmers, influencing content and culture both in the program and in target communities
Mozaik, 1998–current[a]	School-aged children, Republic of North Macedonia, Macedonian, Albanian, Turkish, and Serbian	Contribute to interethnic peace by encouraging shared culture through school language immersion	Character modeling, and interactive learning of multiple languages to mitigate language-based discrimination	Circumstances demonstrate need for multilingualism, community collaboration, and the combination of languages in classroom instruction

(*Continued*)

Table 23.1 (Continued)

EE program and date	Target audience, location and language	Aim/goal	EE influence on linguistic diversity	Linguistic diversity influence on EE
mPulse Mobile Inc. Fotonovela text message campaign, 2020	Adult patients and members of health care companies, United States, English, and Spanish	Decrease COVID-19 transmission and encourage self-efficacy by following "simple steps" to "stay safe and healthy"	Fotonovelas originally targeted audiences in Latin America and adapted to multiple audiences in the United States with various literacy levels that require visual and simple language messaging. Inclusion of SMS mobile media messaging to share links and make fotonovelas accessible. Intentional effort to create shared culture and decrease isolation via shared narratives	Exposure to the program enriched COVID-19 lexicon of Spanish and English speakers across demographics. Continuity of messaging created shared behaviors among diverse audiences
Ouro Negro, 2014–current	Women aged 15–35 and their communities, Mozambique Portuguese, Changana, Sena, and Emakwa[b]	Improve children's health and development	Audience feedback in local languages explicitly identifies the need for diverse language content to reach audiences in the 40+ languages of Mozambique. De-emphasizing colonial influence via Portuguese language	Multilingual richness in Mozambique results in need for transcreated programs (UNICEF Facts for Life book) from national reach in Portuguese to 23 local languages
Ouro Negro's Access Without Barriers, 2020	Adolescents with deafness and their service providers, Mozambique, local sign languages	Improve access to information and positive SRH behaviors among adolescents with deafness	Expanding sign-language lexicons in multiple languages of Mozambique to include signs for SRH vocabulary	Unique local sign languages contribute to diversity of program need and content

Program	Audience	Goal	Cultural/Linguistic Approach	Notes
Sesame Workshop, 1970s–current	Children, all continents, 150+ countries, many languages	Fostering good health, learning, and kindness among children	Culturally appropriate puppet characters, names, and words are created to reach children where they are	Sesame is its own language of shared messaging and culture across many languages worldwide
SIAGA campaign, 1999–2004	Men, pregnant wives, families, midwives, and community groups	Increase pre and postnatal support within families to reduce maternal mortality	Introduction of new term SIAGA to mean "alert husband" as combination of three words in Bahasa language	Formative research to develop term SIAGA. Transcreation of national campaign to target rural province audiences
Suaahara Nepal Project, 2011–2016	New mothers aged 18–30 and their caretakers and husbands, 2013–2014, Nepal, Nepali, Awadi, Doteli	Improve maternal and early childhood nutrition	De-stigmatize and improve the use and accuracy of pregnancy-related terminology among families. Transforming gender identities via shared vocabularies	Data collected in rural Nepali dialects, translated into English program reports. Local influence on culturally appropriate program language and concepts
Tamale Lesson, 2012	Women Mexican American aged 25–45, Los Angeles County, United States, English with Spanish	Promote testing participation for early detection and treatment of cervical cancer	Audience is transported into video narrative by characters who feel familiar to people in their everyday lives and communities. Mixed use of English, Spanish, and cultural cues to enhance audience transportation	Generational differences in the use of SRH terminology, diversify the need for content across languages and age groups

[a] Latest information published in 2015 at https://www.sfcg.org/macedonia.
[b] These languages refer to those used by radio programs. Additional dubbed, rebroadcast, and other media channel programming has been adapted into many languages in Mozambique.

In our opinion, entertainment-education utilizes linguistic diversity within and among languages in at least two ways. First, entertainment education engages and alters linguistic context via narrative and storytelling. Second, entertainment-education experts intentionally create language by adding new lexicons and words to languages, expanding the use of existing words, and shaping the cultural acceptability of words and their connotations for audiences to accept messages and change behaviors. While entertainment-education influences linguistic diversity, the relationship is reciprocal. Linguistic diversity shapes the nature and implementation of entertainment-education work, from the need for linguistically diverse staff to translated materials, culturally adapted messaging, local language adaptations, or transcreation. Additionally, keen attention to linguistic diversity lies at the heart of formative research, process monitoring, and evaluation of entertainment-education.

Entertainment-education enriches linguistic diversity

Narrative and storytelling

Storytelling is the heart of entertainment-education. From TV to graphic art, music, radio, theater, social media, video games, dialog with the audience, and more, the use of entertainment to share informative health-based narratives is limitless. Entertainment-education scholars agree that the ability to model behaviors by creating stories that resonate with audiences is key to entertainment-education success. Early studies of entertainment-education explored the concept of parasocial interaction or the audience's development of a one-sided relationship with a fictional character. Over time, theorizing about parasocial interaction has been expanded to include audience involvement, identification, narrative engagement, and narrative transportation [27, 28]. A crucial element for fostering engagement is the creative use of verbal and nonverbal techniques to create highly immersive narratives that prompt the audiences to pay attention and generate mental imagery, transporting the audience into a world of a different time and space. The language and storylines within narratives influence individual behaviors and social and gender norms [29]. Narratives resonate particularly well with audience members who perceive the stories to be realistic and can identify and empathize with the narratives and characters utilized in entertainment-education based on existing similarities or desirable attributes [30, 31].

Empirical studies show that narrative-based interventions effectively reduce health disparities for historically marginalized minority populations and racial/ethnic groups with a rich storytelling tradition. An example of using culturally competent entertainment-education is "The Tamale Lesson," an 11-minute video produced by the University of Southern California to educate Mexican American women about cervical cancer prevention and detection (Figure 23.1). The fictional narrative film revolves around female family members preparing for a *Quinceañera* (15th birthday celebration), highlighting the cultural context of Mexican-American families. While preparing tamales for the celebration, the women discuss one character's abnormal Pap test and a positive human papillomavirus (HPV) test. During the ensuing conversation, 10 key facts about cervical cancer are discussed. Characters in the video use a chicken being prepared for the party meal to describe and demonstrate how simple a Pap test is conducted. The video ends with the women at a local clinic, where they go to be screened for cervical cancer [32, 33]. *The Tamale Lesson* integrated sexual and reproductive health terminology across

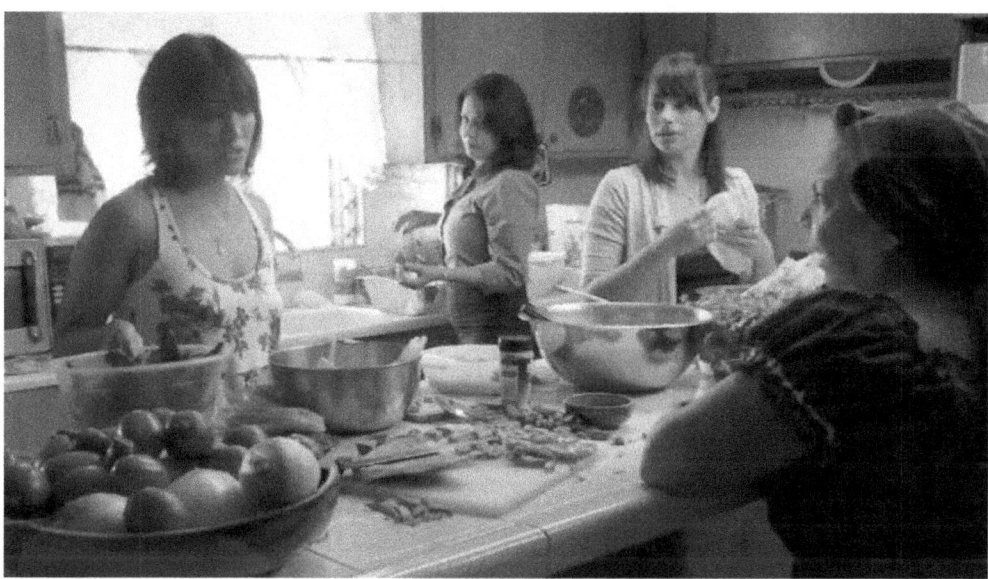

Figure 23.1 *The Tamale Lesson*. An intergenerational conversation about cervical cancer and HPV testing is woven into everyday life as a group of women cook traditional Latin American foods in preparation for a *Quinceañera* (15th birthday celebration) celebration. *Source: The Tamale Lesson*, University of Southern California.

generations with everyday analogies, quite literally from the kitchen, to address the sexually transmitted infection that causes cervical cancer and cervical cancer screening. The innovative use of imagery (women stuffing a chicken while discussing cervical cancer screening (Figure 23.2)) sticks with viewers, even if we only see the video once. *The Tamale Lesson*, therefore, directly engages the nexus of language and culture to confront the stigma associated with discussion around sexual and reproductive health.

Source credibility in entertainment-education

Source credibility is a term often used in communication literature to measure the extent to which audiences find a fictional source of information to be accurate and authentic. Several entertainment-education evaluations have concluded that relatability and source credibility promote entertainment-education effectiveness. One way entertainment-education practitioners make their programs relatable and reliable is by reflecting the verbal and nonverbal cues familiar to their audiences. In entertainment-education medical dramas, for example, the credibility of fictional doctors is enhanced by them wearing scrubs and by using medical terminology with each other. Successful entertainment-education TV programs based in the United States, such as *Gray's Anatomy* and *Scrubs*, serve as examples of this approach [34].

One example of the successful use of culturally aligned characters is Population Media Center's hit transmedia entertainment-education drama series *East Los High*, broadcast on Hulu from 2014 to 2017. The show is set in a fictional Los Angeles high school with episodes covering issues like family and partner violence, LGBTQ identity acceptance, and the prevention of sexually transmitted diseases. East Los High employed

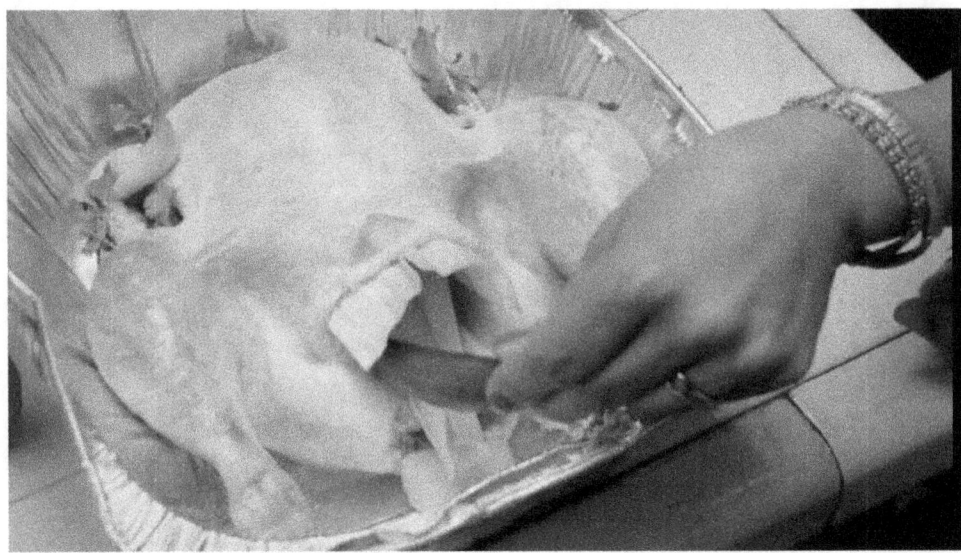

Figure 23.2 *The Tamale Lesson.* Characters innovatively use the foods they are preparing to demonstrate a Pap test to screen for cervical cancer. *Source: The Tamale Lesson*, University of Southern California.

cues to action, including integrating a Planned Parenthood widget within the narrative drama. The addition of character Vlogs where the real-life actors reprised their fictional characters to respond to audience concerns and questions and the creative use of Twitter and Facebook increased audience engagement with fictional characters, which motivated and empowered them to practice prosocial behaviors, resulting in a cumulative effect on shifting norms [13, 35]. East Los High demonstrated Latino engagement in the arts and health as means to support healthy and engaged lives. Accurate character development and relatable content promoted interest and pride in Latino culture and heritage among young viewers [13]. East Los High achieved cultural authenticity by including writers, producers, and staff from the target community. The show engaged audiences and community members to help contribute to program design as well as ongoing story and character development, thus increasing the validity and acceptability of messaging through an intentional application of language diversity across design and production. One evaluation of East Los High found that the collaborative team of producers, NGO partners, and researchers was able to leverage the full potential of digital and social media to create a story world, engage a critical mass of young and Latino audiences, and develop fan communities [36].

Some global examples of powerful storytelling are found in a TV drama and transmedia series in India, the Population Foundation of India's *"Main Kuch Bhi Kar Sakti Hoon" or "MKBKSH"* (I, a Woman Can Achieve Anything!), which promotes women's rights and community health. The now three-season program centers around a female medical doctor who models empowerment while serving her local village. Dr. Sneha confronts stigma-laden issues such as gender-based violence, open defecation, and the promotion of contraception use. The program addresses complex and taboo content via immersive storytelling and a direct audience engagement call-in component. The series includes dramatic plots and relatable characters, yet it reflects life and connects to the real issues of small-town life in India. *MKBKSH* has a prolific reach, including 183 original episodes, rebroadcasts on TV and radio, 1.7 million audience calls, a docuseries, social media stories, and more [26, 37].

Ouro Negro (Black Gold), a long-running radio drama from Mozambique, is another example of how programs contribute to linguistic diversity by creating narratives. Mozambique has some of the highest rates of child mortality, child marriage, and maternal mortality in the world. A thriving joint effort of UNICEF, the Mozambique Ministry of Health, PCI Media, Radio Mozambique, and Instituto de Comunicação Social *Ouro Negro* was launched in 2015 with funding and significant support from UNICEF Mozambique to address MCH issues. Using radio soap operas, public service announcements, social media live-streaming, and more, MCH narratives are inserted into fictionalized settings that reflect broader social, cultural, and economic issues in Mozambique (Figure 23.3). *Ouro Negro* contextualizes behavioral change through culturally aligned messaging, including information on maternal and child nutrition, sanitation, ending domestic violence, early marriages, HIV/AIDS prevention, and recently, COVID-19 prevention [38].

Rapid changes in how we communicate today demand even more attention to linguistic developments. For example, *Ouro Negro's* social media-based program Access Without Borders in Mozambique engaged local language and content area expertise to create sexual and reproductive health lexicons in sign languages to advance health information sharing across social media to audiences of diverse languages and abilities (Figure 23.4).

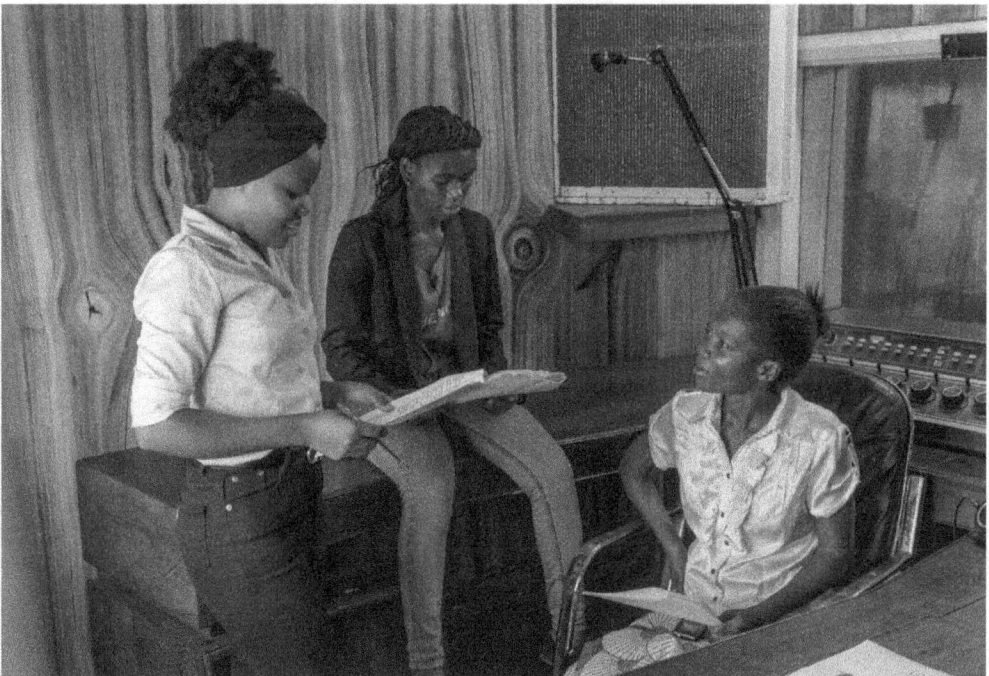

Figure 23.3 Ouro Negro producers and voice actors rehearse program stories that include accurate information related to common maternal and child health issues in Mozambique. *Source:* PCI Media.

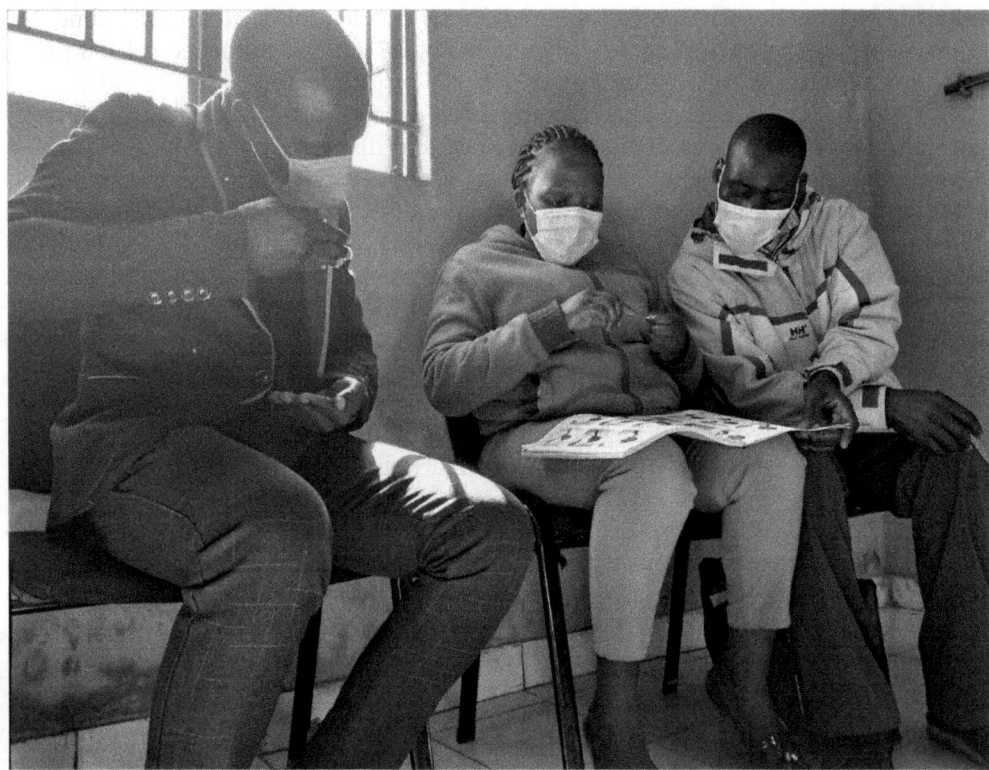

Figure 23.4 Access Without Borders works with local sign language in Mozambique to create signs for sexual and reproductive health content that can then be shared online via social media. *Source:* PCI Media.

Recreating language

The Sapir Whorf hypothesis, first advanced by Edward Sapir in 1929 and subsequently developed by Benjamin Whorf, proposed that language determines a native speaker's perception and categorization of experience and perceptions of reality [39]. Kincaid, Delate, Storey, and Figueroa argue that health communication programs take on a dialogic function by promoting a conversation between researchers/interventionists and community members [40].

Entertainment-education programs contribute to linguistic diversity by creating new words and expanding conceptualization of critical behaviors. This new application of familiar terms or the introduction of new terms to an audience can result in cultural and behavioral associations with these terms. The concept of "sticky messages" and markers is a relevant example of the contribution of entertainment-education to language. These are implemented in various ways, such as words that help explain something without complex descriptions or by providing mnemonics to enhance recall or "stickiness" of a message. Not all cultural markers are based on language. Instead, markers can be words, images, or characters that are easily remembered and associated with the health message [33]. Similarly, cues to action can be a simple prompt to act for the audience. Culturally aligned messages ensure that cues to action are communicated and contextualized specifically for intended audiences. Cultural alignment can be a nuanced creative process, going beyond spoken language to engage segmented audiences within languages. For example, the Vax Up Philly Parade in Philadelphia in 2021 used street art and music to encourage COVID-19 vaccination in young, urban populations [41]. Entertainment-education impacts linguistic diversity by giving new meaning to existing cultural categories and infusing existing words in a language with new meanings. There are many examples in the entertainment-education literature of creative language use.

An entertainment-education program in Mozambique used photo-based prompts to engage participants in discussions of normative sexual behaviors. Intending to decrease and prevent HIV/AIDS, researchers engaged community participants to learn how to talk about the issues. This resulted in the use of an existing euphemism in a novel way to refer to the risks of multiple-concurrent sexual partners and exposure to HIV/STIs *"Andar Fora e Maningue Arriscado"* or "stepping out is very risky" engaged "andar for a" or stepping out as a culturally competent way to describe multiple partner relationships while avoiding the imposition of foreign health terminology [42]. A multipronged SBC safe motherhood project in Indonesia combined three action words to create one overarching identity for a safe motherhood campaign. The term SIAGA was a combination of specific action verbs in Indonesian Bahasa: siap = transport, antar = to take or accompany, and jaga = standing guard. The term SIAGA in the local language translates into ALERT. This became the clarion call for safe motherhood in Indonesia. Husbands, midwives, communities, and villages were branded as being SIAGA or alert to position maternal and neonatal health as a public responsibility through ensuring transportation, a skilled attendant at birth, and donation of blood if required [43, 44].

Another way that entertainment-education promotes linguistic diversity is by changing the local language and connotations associated with specific behaviors and personality traits. MKBKSH provides an example of this. The Hindi language drama transformed use of the term *"nasbandhi,"* the colloquial term for vasectomy, by superimposing the use of the word *"mastbandhi"* meaning a practice that was related to enjoying sex without worrying about unintended pregnancy. This intentional language transformation is intended to shift the normative stigma associated with vasectomy.

Entertainment-education also showcases linguistic diversity by introducing new words to describe behaviors. One of the core objectives of a long-running TV drama from India, *"Kyunki Jeena Isi Ka Naam Hai"* (Because this is life), was to train community-level health workers and the public on good practices of infant and child feeding. The language used by experts to describe nutrition and diet involved discussing a balanced meal with adequate protein, carbohydrates, and fats. However, the creators had to develop accessible language for largely non- or low-literate audiences. During formative research, the creators came up with an idea of a *"tiranga"* (three-color) diet to describe good infant and child feeding practices. The term *"tiranga"* is used commonly in India to refer to the Indian flag, composed of three colors saffron, green, and white. *Kyunki...* popularized the term *"tiranga"* to refer to a diet rich in vitamins and minerals, including orange and red fruits and vegetables, leafy greens, and starches, such as rice and porridge, as being nutritionally sound for infant and child feeding.

Entertainment-education also contributes to language diversity by highlighting specific positive characteristics of a given person or behavior. For example, a large sexual and reproductive health project SUMATA, a partnership between the Government of Nepal and USAID, demonstrates the creation of a local language [45].

"*Ashal Logne*" "Good Husband" is a TV drama created as part of the larger SUMATA campaign. The title and content describe supportive husbands to transform the image of a typical Nepali man as supportive of sexual and reproductive health (SRH) through role modeling specific gender-transformative actions. The term *Ashal Logne* is synonymous with the health-related content of the show, thus reapplying local terminology to new concepts of what constitutes a good man. Another project in Nepal called *Suaahara* also integrated maternal health messaging and character modeling to create content for family and community members in Nepal, including husbands, mothers-in-law, and new mothers. The program consisted of a radio show, "*Bhanchhin Aama*" (Mother Knows Best), used to address improving the mother-in-law's influence on family nutrition, access to health information from female community health volunteers, medical treatment from clinicians, and the influence of traditional healers. Along with introducing new gender-associated terms and identities, *Suaahara* changed how local words were used. For example, in rural Nepal, hot and cold refer more to the energy than the temperatures of foods. This distinction needed to be made in content that provided cooking and nutritional advice (Figure 23.5). The program also used the opportunity to clarify popular local health-related lexicons, such as distinguishing that the word "vitamin" is not interchangeable with "nutrition" [46, 47].

One unique aspect of entertainment-education that sets it apart from other health communication strategies is its reliance on evidence. On this note, it is essential to highlight how entertainment-education utilizes language diversity across all stages of the

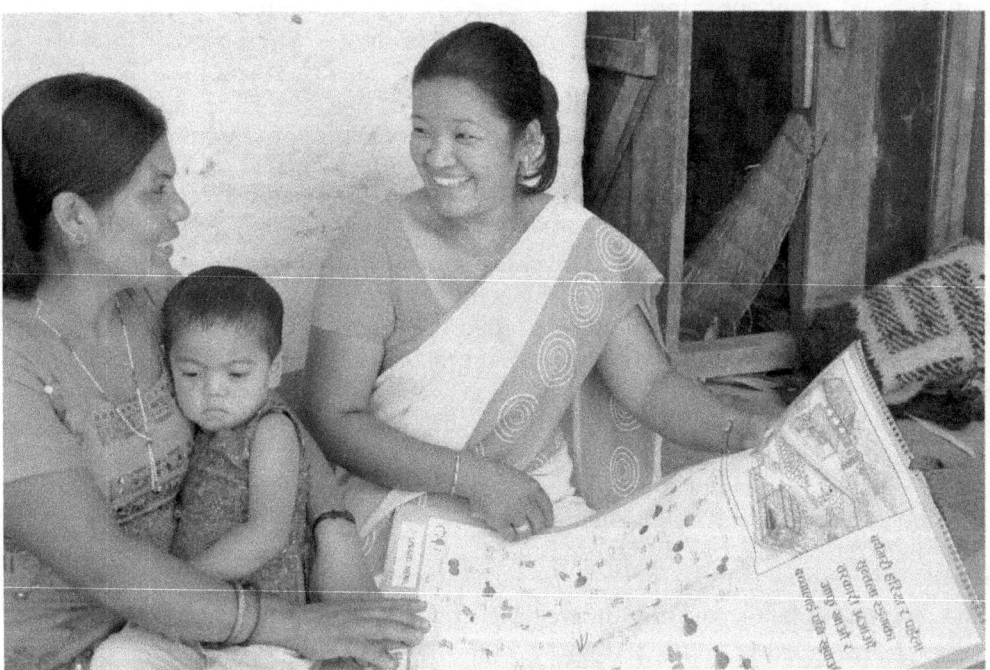

Figure 23.5 Suaahara. A female community health volunteer uses drawn images, pictographs, and text in local language to enhance nutrition-related lexicons used by families to improve maternal and child nutrition. *Source:* Valerie Caldas.

program cycle. Attention to linguistic diversity is beneficial to frame formative research and to pretest materials with audiences by providing an opportunity to converse with community members about issues of importance in current and future interventions. Formative research influences programming by emphasizing linguistic and cultural norms determined through collaboration with potential audiences. Process evaluation is used as a method to maintain this dialogue by gauging the proportion of the population that is being reached and engaged with entertainment-education content and that which is not. An added benefit of creating specific language within everyday terminology is that apart from being a strategic implementation strategy, sticky messages, and cultural markers can be utilized to examine encoded exposure to entertainment-education programming. Encoded exposure is a continuous measure of engagement with a program that suggests that a piece of the message is encoded in a person's memory [48]. Effective entertainment-education relies on audience reach and recall. Both reach and recall are critical to engagement which, in turn, helps entertainment-education meet its stated objectives. One way to robustly measure the direct contribution of entertainment-education to behavior and social change is through testing audience recall of newly introduced linguistically diverse content. In a media-saturated environment, the utilization of unique words and phrases, when recognized by audiences as representing specific places, people, and things, provides a strong justification for the direct and indirect effects of entertainment-education programming.

Linguistic diversity shapes entertainment-education

Linguistic diversity influences entertainment-education by prompting the need for audience specificity, employing local language, and impacting entertainment-education planning, program delivery, and monitoring and evaluation. One could argue that cultural adaptation, which includes linguistic diversity, always influences entertainment-education because successful sharing of health-related messages with lay audiences through entertaining media requires adaptation of content to reach segmented audiences, whether those audiences are across the globe or within a single city. Working in multilingual spaces adds attention to everyday communications that otherwise may be less considered or even ignored. For example, simple actions like greeting colleagues, recognizing important dates and holidays, and using gestures or cultural references are all means of communication. Interacting across diverse teams and disciplines allows one to reconsider the most basic semantics of daily communication. Entertainment-education programs need to be participatory, adapted, and tailored per context.

Linguistic diversity shapes how entertainment-education practitioners use language within and across programs by diversifying the use of different dialects and languages. Linguistic barriers are especially important to address when trying to reach disadvantaged audiences. Adapting programs to diverse audiences, languages, literacy levels, belief systems, social settings, and many other cultural elements requires much more than translating materials. Entertainment-education practitioners refer to the term *"transcreation"* to refer to cultural and language adaptations. The idea of transcreation comes from the use of audience segmentation strategies during formative research to identify ways to implement linguistically diverse programming by keeping linguistic variance among potential audiences in mind. Transcreation improves the reach and engagement with entertainment-education programming by reaching wider audiences.

A few explicit examples of entertainment-education work being shaped by linguistic diversity are as follows:

mPulse Inc.'s Fotonovela initiative providing accurate COVID-19 information is a timely example of the reciprocal nature of linguistic diversity and the influence of language and culture on messages and materials, and then the power of those messages and materials on modeled behaviors. This program was developed to reach health plan members and patients across the United States and was presented as a link within SMS text messages. The initiative leveraged Spanish and English language diversities and the need for accurate COVID-19 information using multilingual, multimedia strategies. Content included graphic illustrations of bumping elbows to replace handshakes and reenforcing new phrases like "stay home, save lives." The shared needs of Spanish and English speakers prompted the development of simple and engaging messages to reach across languages and literacy levels while providing support and fostering solidarity among participants. At the same time, they were social distancing to prevent the spread of the virus [49]. The program used fotonovelas to address "cultural and linguistic barriers" such as low literacy via low reader-level materials presented in a "light-hearted" graphic way. Fotonovelas were accessible via links sent by SMS. Storylines included vignettes "behind closed doors" during COVID-19 social distancing to illustrate coping mechanisms and the struggle to stay connected while staying healthy. Since the intervention used mobile phones, mPulse Mobile, Inc. was able to use natural language processing to recognize and respond to member questions [49] (Figure 23.6).

An example of entertainment-education's frequent emphasis on reaching minority communities comes from the Dutch National Institute for Public Health and Environment, which designed and evaluated a web-based culturally sensitive educational video (CSEV) to facilitate informed cervical cancer screening decisions among Turkish- and Moroccan-Dutch women aged 30 to 60 years. Each year in the Netherlands, 800 women are diagnosed with cervical cancer, and 200 women die from it [50]. The CSEV show how regional linguistic diversity based on migration patterns determines the need for transcreated entertainment-education programming. The motivations for women of Dutch origin to participate in cancer screening might differ from those of women of Moroccan or

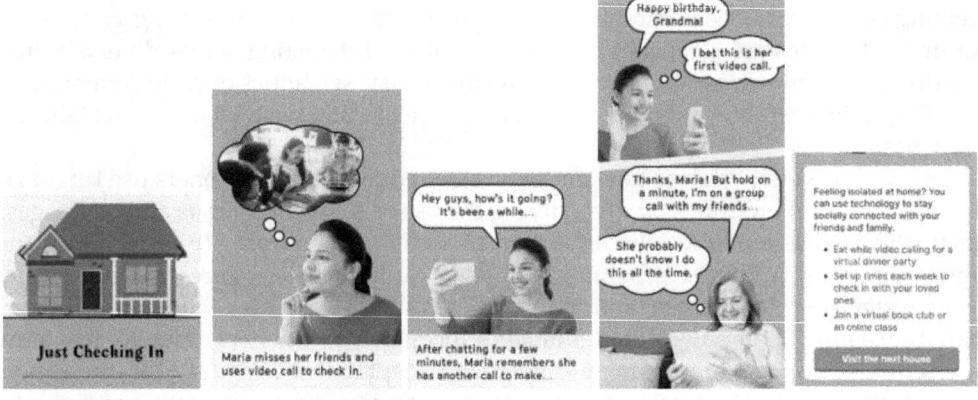

Figure 23.6 One narrative in the mPulse Mobile Inc. fotonovela "Stay Home Save Lives" uses humor, graphics, and simple language to engage audience across literacy competencies to promote maintaining social connection across generations while social distancing to reduce COVID-19 transmission. *Source:* mPulse Mobile Inc.

Turkish origin. The Dutch National Institute for Public Health and Environment used CSEVs produced in Turkish and Moroccan Arabic and Moroccan Berber languages, all subtitled in Dutch. This helped audiences via their multilingual realities with varying literacies and fluencies in multiple languages. Furthermore, the videos engage cultural cues, presenting cancer screening within a set of Muslim values to maintain women's health and be present for family members. The use of multiple languages can also forge new shared health-related languages (Figure 23.7) [51, 52].

Diverse localized languages in mountainous districts of Nepal shaped the work of *Suaahara* with data collection in local languages then being translated into English. *Suaahara's* sampling strategy was tailored (including complex logistics) to maximize an understanding of the diversity of practices, perceptions, and normative behaviors related to MCH, to create efficient content that reached as broad an audience as possible [46]. In Mozambique, *Ouro Negro* demonstrates another example of the richness of the relationship between entertainment-education and linguistic diversity within the boundaries of a single country. The program began broadcasting in Portuguese as the national language in Mozambique. However, community feedback resulted in transcreated programs broadcast by 55 radio stations in 23 local languages across 10 provinces. The program infuses each language with new terms and concepts related to health behaviors and outcomes. In addition to local language adaptations, *Ouro Negro* also responds to the demand for programming for deaf people through its social media component. Access Without Barriers, a program funded by the Government of Flanders, conducted resource mapping in Mozambique to reveal that deaf people use sign languages that are localized and unique from standardized sign languages. These local sign languages had limited SRH vocabulary. Access Without Borders trained youth peer

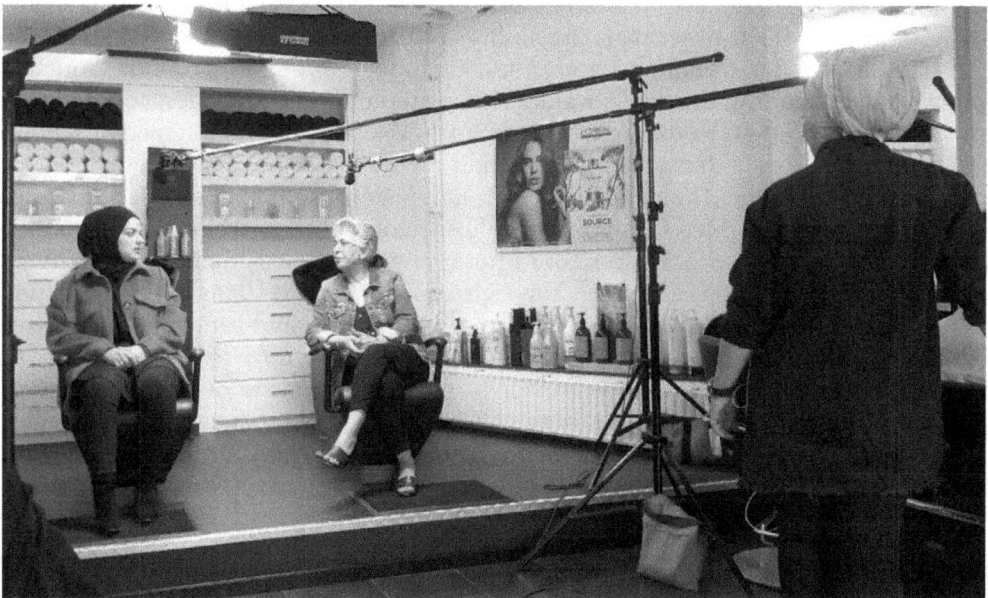

Figure 23.7 Filming Culturally Sensitive Educational Videos to facilitate informed cervical cancer screening decisions among Turkish- and Moroccan–Dutch women. Linguistic diversity via migration patterns influences the need and subsequent production of entertainment-education materials that engage culturally relevant cues and value systems. *Source:* Nora Hamdiui.

educators in local sign languages to help create SRH signs and teach them to deaf audiences. Videos of people using the new sign language can then be broadcast and posted online. Advancing the SRH lexicon among sign languages in Mozambique is now a critical part of Access Without Borders [53]. This aspect of Access Without Borders also serves as an example of how transcreation is often a community-led process from identifying challenges to creating their solutions.

The previous example of *Ouro Negro* illustrated transcreation within a country. However, linguistic diversity has also been leveraged on a global scale. For half a century, Sesame Workshop's international TV series has largely been premised on healthy self-image modeling across cultures for young children. Characters, names, and terms are developed to be culturally appropriate and easily identifiable markers of program messaging. This results in broadening content language and references across languages and regions. For example, in North America, a yellow bird called Big Bird is a central character. This same central character is more regionally identifiable as a green parrot, named *Abelardo* in the *Plaza Sésamo*, the Sesame Street adaptation in Mexico. Both characters model similar positive behaviors and promote the value of education and kindness in their respective languages. Additional regional versions of the program include *Galli Galli Sim Sim* in Hindi, *Hikayat Simsim* in Arabic, and *Sippuray Sumsum* in Hebrew, just to name a few. More than encouraging preliteracy and numeracy skills, and positive social role modeling, the program aims to share "a window into local culture" toward "humanizing the other and promoting pride and hope." With culturally relevant characters that share similar appearances and messages, the language of Sesame Workshop is arguably universal for children [54].

While most of the previous examples showcase language diversity as a way to reach multiple audiences, there is at least one example of an entertainment-education that promotes language assimilation among ethnically diverse audiences by encouraging multilingualism to weaken the ability to discriminate based on language. In 1997, The Search for Common Ground Organization (Common Ground) launched *Mozaik*, a longstanding education model with entertainment-education components, in what is now known as the Republic of North Macedonia. The interactive school-based program uses entertainment-education methods such as character modeling and interactive games. The concept of first language has often been used to foster ethnic segregation in Macedonia among those who speak Macedonian, Albanian, Turkish and Serbian. *Mozaik* aims to address language-based identities to actively address ethnolinguistic segregation through elementary-level language instruction and immersion across these languages, along with child-centered interactive approaches to overcome harmful stereotypes. Children who participate in *Mozaik* schools are multilingual and thus harder to target as speakers of one language or another. Children who participate in the Mozaik curriculum develop first-language competencies in multiple languages, challenging the association between identity and specific languages [55].

Recommendations and conclusions

There is no clear line between where and how entertainment-education influences linguistic diversity and where the reverse is true. In this chapter, we highlight the organic linkages between language diversity and entertainment-education by hypothesizing a bidirectional relationship. Entertainment-education impacts linguistic diversity by providing new ways to describe relationships, experiences, and actions, using abbreviations, shortcuts, mnemonics, and the introduction of new terminology. Principles from applied linguistics are utilized in entertainment-education through its careful attention to formative research and audience segmentation, as well as its reliance on culture-centric messaging and the use of narratives to enhance program reach and engagement.

In some ways, entertainment-education can be understood as the intentional engagement of diverse languages to create and convey content that encourages positive behavior and social change. Entertainment-education influences language by reframing its application in everyday reality through abbreviations, descriptions, mnemonics, or creating new terminology. Entertainment-education constitutes a field of practice that both drives the need for and results from international partnerships as sites where linguistic diversity is exercised, defined, and applied to understand and improve the human condition.

Collaboration between linguists and social and behavior change specialists can enrich and promote future innovation in both fields. Therefore, we see great value in formal collaborations between health communication experts and linguists, not merely as conjecture but of increasing relevance to both fields. An intentional and critical approach to the links between linguistic diversity and entertainment-education is relevant across all phases of health communication, program development, implementation, and evaluation. At the planning stage, some concrete steps toward multi-disciplinarity would be to extend the entertainment-education practice of identifying underlying theories and the program's theory of including language components. This will also aid in pre-identifying potential conflicts, barriers, or misunderstandings when working multilingually. Because entertainment-education is based on understanding audience cultural specificities, interventions should include a clear definition of how they operationalize language diversity. A more formal interplay between linguistic diversity and entertainment-education implementation can happen when entertainment-education programs intentionally focus on and document how they engage language via practitioners, intended audiences, and those who encounter programming. The potential impacts between language and entertainment-education should be also considered, not just from a design and implementation standpoint but also from the perspectives of formative research and monitoring and evaluation. Such examination of the bidirectional relationship, in theory, practice, and through empirical evidence can guide future theorizing, implementation, and evaluations of SBCC efforts and our understanding of linguistic diversity in the twenty-first century.

Highlights

- When possible, encourage intentional and/or formal collaborations between linguists and SBC specialists to build linguistic diversity evidence and understanding across disciplines.
- When planning programs, include the clear identification of underlying theories of how the use of linguistic diversity is important to a program and how the program will operationalize linguistic diversity throughout each phase of the program.
- When conducting formative research or designing, implementing, and evaluating programs, identify the ways that a program or SBC issue may be influencing language and ways in which language might influence programming. This can help mitigate misunderstandings as well as contribute to language-based outcomes that can be measured.

REFERENCES

1. United Nations. *Universal Declaration of Human Rights*. https://www.un.org/en/about-us/universal-declaration-of-human-rights; 1948.
2. Piller, I. (2016). *Linguistic Diversity and Participation*. New York: Oxford University Press.
3. Ricento, T. (2017). Conceptualizing language: linguistic theory and language policy. In: *Dynamics of Linguistic Diversity* (ed. H. Peukert and I. Gogolin). Amsterdam/Philadelphia, PA: John Benjamins Publishing Company.
4. Cooke, M. and Simpson, J. (2012). Discourses about linguistic diversity. In: *The Routledge Handbook of Multilingualism* (ed. M. Martin-Jones, A. Blackledge, and A. Creese). London: Routledge.
5. Kulkarni-Joshi, S. (2019). Linguistic history and language diversity in India: views and counterviews. *J. Biosci.* 44 (3): 1–10.
6. Ball, A.F. and Makoni, S. (2002). *Black Linguistics: Language, Society and Politics in Africa and the Americas*. Hoboken, NJ: Taylor & Francis Ltd.
7. Wei, L. (2018). Linguistic (super)diversity, post-multilingualism and translanguaging moments. In: *The Routledge Handbook of Language and Superdiversity. Routledge Handbooks in Applied Linguistics* (ed. A. Creese and A. Blackledge). Milton: Taylor and Francis.
8. Hugo Lopez, M. and Gonzalez-Barrera, A. (2013). *What Is the Future of Spanish in the United States?* Pew Research Center. https://www.pewresearch.org/fact-tank/2013/09/05/what-is-the-future-of-spanish-in-the-united-states (accessed 1 April 2022).
9. United States Census Bureau (2013). *Top Languages Other than English Spoken in 1980 and Changes in Relative Rank, 1990–2010*. United States Census Bureau. https://www.census.gov/dataviz/visualizations/045 (accessed 1 April 2022).
10. Chomsky, N. (1986). *Knowledge of Language Its Nature, Origin, and Use*. New York: Praeger.
11. Heugh, K. and Stroud, C. (2019). Diversities, affinities and diasporas: a southern lens and methodology for understanding multilingualisms. *Curr. Issues Lang. Plann.* 20 (1): 1–15.
12. Wang, H., Seth, A., Johri, M. et al. (2021). Communication infrastructure and community mobilization: the case of gram Vaani's COVID-19 response network for the marginalized in India. *J. Dev Commun.* 32 (2): 73.
13. Wang, H., Singhal, A., Quist, C. et al. (2019). Aligning the stars in East Los High: how authentic characters and storylines can translate into real-life changes through transmedia edutainment. *SEARCH J. Media Commun. Res.* 11: 1–22.
14. Gesser-Edelsburg, A. and Singhal, A. (2013). Enhancing the persuasive influence of entertainment-education events: rhetorical and aesthetic strategies for constructing narratives. *Crit. Arts* 27 (1): 56–74.
15. Bandura, A. (2004). Social cognitive theory for personal and social change by enabling media. In: *Entertainment-Education and Social Change: History, Research, and Practice* (ed. A. Singhal, M.J. Cody, E.M. Rogers, and M. Sabido), 75–96. Lawrence Erlbaum Associates, Inc.
16. De Vries, J.A. and van den Brink, M.C.L. (2016). Transformative gender interventions: linking theory and practice using the "bifocal approach". *Equal. Divers. Incl. Int. J.* 35 (7–8): 429–448.
17. Singhal, A., Cody, M.J., Rogers, E.M., and Sabido, M. (2004). *Entertainment-Education and Social Change: History, Research, and Practice*. Mahwah, NJ: Lawrence Erlbaum Associates, Inc., Publishers.
18. Bull S, Ezeanochie N. From Foucault to Freire through Facebook: toward an integrated theory of mHealth. *Health Educ. Behav.* 2016;43(4):399–a411.
19. Singhal, A.C., Michael, J., Rogers Everett, M., and Sabido, M. (2003). *Entertainment-Education and Social Change: History, Research, and Practice*. Mahwah, NJ: Taylor and Francis xxii-xxii p.

20. Dutta, M.J. (2020). Whiteness, internationalization, and erasure: decolonizing futures from the global south. *Commun. crit./Cult. Study* 17 (2): 228–235.
21. Sood, S., Shefner-Rogers, C., and Skinner, J. (2014). Health communication campaigns in developing countries. *J. Creat. Commun.* 9 (1): 67–84.
22. Storey, D. and Sood, S. (2013). Increasing equity, affirming the power of narrative and expanding dialogue: the evolution of entertainment education over two decades. *Crit. Arts* 27 (1): 9–35.
23. Riley Henderson, A., Sood, S., and Alarcon, K.C. (2017). *Entertainment-Education and Health and Risk Messaging*. Oxford University Press.
24. Suruchi, S., Amy Henderson, R., and Kristine Cecile, A. *Entertainment-Education and Health and Risk Messaging*. Oxford University Press.
25. Sood, S., Menard, T., and Witte, K. (2003). *The Theory Behind Entertainment-Education*, 117–149. Routledge.
26. Wang, H., Singhal, A., Muttreja, P. et al. (2020). The power of narrative persuasion: how an entertainment-education serial drama tackled open defecation and promoted contraceptive use in India. *J. Dev Commun.* 30 (2): 1.
27. Green, M.C. and Brock, T.C. (2000). The role of transportation in the persuasiveness of public narratives. *J. Pers. Soc. Psychol.* 79 (5): 701–721.
28. Green, M.C., Brock, T.C., and Kaufman, G.F. (2004). Understanding media enjoyment: the role of transportation into narrative worlds. *Commun. Theory* 14 (4): 311–327.
29. Riley, A.H., Rodrigues, F., and Sood, S. (2021). *Social Norms Theory and Measurement in Entertainment-Education: Insights from Case Studies in Four Countries – Chapter 11*. Springer International Publishing.
30. Murphy, S.T., Frank, L.B., Moran, M.B., and Patnoe-Woodley, P. (2011). Involved, transported, or emotional? Exploring the determinants of change in knowledge, attitudes, and behavior in entertainment-education. *J. Commun.* 61 (3): 407–431.
31. Moyer-Gusé, E. and Nabi, R.L. (2010). Explaining the effects of narrative in an entertainment television program: overcoming resistance to persuasion. *Hum. Commun. Res.* 36 (1): 26–52.
32. Frank, L.B., Murphy, S.T., Chatterjee, J.S. et al. (2015). Telling stories, saving lives: creating narrative health messages. *Health Commun.* 30 (2): 154–163.
33. Baezconde-Garbanati, L.A., Chatterjee, J.S., Frank, L.B. et al. (2014). Tamale lesson: a case study of a narrative health communication intervention. *J. Commun. Healthc.* 7 (2): 82–92.
34. Enayet, S. (2018). *What Makes for a Good Doctor? Analyzing the Physician-Patient Relationship in Grey's Anatomy and Scrubs*. The University of North Carolina at Chapel Hill University Libraries.
35. Population Media Center. *East Los High United States* 2022. https://www.populationmedia.org/projects/east-los-high (accessed 30 March 2022).
36. Wang, H., Xu, W., Saxton, G.D., and Singhal, A. (2019). Social media fandom for health promotion? Insights from east los high, a transmedia edutainment initiative. *SEARCH J. Media Commun. Res.* 11 (1): 1–16.
37. Population Foundation of India. *Main Kuch Bhi Kar Sakti Hoon* 2019. https://mkbksh.org (accessed 31 March 2022).
38. The Communication Initiative. *Black Gold (Ouro Negro) Radio Drama* 2015. https://www.comminit.com/edutain-africa/content/black-gold-ouro-negro-radio-drama (accessed 31 March 2022).
39. Whorf, B.L., Carroll, J.B., Levinson, S.C. et al. (2012). *Language, Thought, and Reality, Second Edition: Selected Writings of Benjamin Lee Whorf*. Cambridge, MA: MIT Press.
40. Kincaid, D.L., Delate, R., Storey, D., and Figueroa, M.E. (2012). Closing the gaps in practice and in theory. In: *Public Communication Campaigns* (ed. Ronald E. Rice and Charles K. Atkin). vol. 305, 305–319. Sage.
41. Dean, M.M. (2021). *"Let's have some fun": Vax Up Philly Parade Brings Vaccines and Free Ice Cream to People Where They Are*. The Philadelphia Inquirer. https://www.inquirer.com/news/vaxup-vaccination-paradephiladelphia-20210829.html.

42. Holman, E.S., Harbour, C.K., Azevedo Said, R.V., and Figueroa, M.E. (2016). Regarding realities: using photo-based projective techniques to elicit normative and alternative discourses on gender, relationships, and sexuality in Mozambique. *Glob. Public Health* 11 (5–6): 719–741.
43. Shefner-Rogers, C.L. and Sood, S. (2004). Involving husbands in safe motherhood: effects of the SUAMI SIAGA campaign in Indonesia. *J. Health Commun.* 9 (3): 233–258.
44. Kurniati, A., Chen, C.-M., Efendi, F. et al. (2017). Suami SIAGA: male engagement in maternal health in Indonesia. *Health Policy Plan.* 32 (8): 1203–1211.
45. The Compass for Social and Behavioral Change. Ashal Logne (Good Husband) Video on Safe Motherhood. Compass. https://www.thecompassforsbc.org/project-examples/ashal-logne-good-husband-video-safe-motherhood (accessed 31 March 2022).
46. USAID (2013). *Formative Research Report*. USAID.
47. The Compass for Social and Behavioral Change. Suaahara Nepal Project. USAID. https://www.thecompassforsbc.org/project-examples/suaahara-nepal-project.
48. Southwell, B. (2014). *Encoded Exposure and Aided Versus Unaided Awareness*, 401–403. Sage Publications.
49. Brar Prayaga, R. and Prayaga, R.S. (2020). Mobile Fotonovelas within a text message outreach: an innovative tool to build health literacy and influence behaviors in response to the COVID-19 pandemic. *JMIR Mhealth Uhealth* 8 (8): e19529-e.
50. The Netherlands National Institute for Public Health and the Environment Ministry of Health Welfare and Sport (2022). *Cervical Cancer Screening Programme*. National Institute for Public Health and the Environment Ministry of Health, Welfare and Sport. https://www.rivm.nl/en/cervical-cancer-screening-programme (accessed 31 March 2022).
51. Hamdiui, N., Bouman, M.P.A., Stein, M.L. et al. (2022). The development of a culturally sensitive educational video: how to facilitate informed decisions on cervical cancer screening among Turkish- and Moroccan-Dutch women. *Health Expect.* 25 (5): 2377–2385.
52. Hamdiui, N., Stein, M.L., van Steenbergen, J. et al. (2022). Evaluation of a web-based culturally sensitive educational video to facilitate informed cervical cancer screening decisions among Turkish- and Moroccan-Dutch women aged 30 to 60 years: randomized intervention study. *J. Med. Internet Res.* 24: e35962.
53. PCI Media. *Progress Report for the First Half February-August 2020*. 2020.
54. Cole, C.F. and Lee, J.H. (2016). *The Sesame Effect: The Global Impact of the Longest Street in the World*. London: Routledge.
55. Search for Common Ground. *Macedonia 2020*. https://www.sfcg.org/macedonia (accessed 31 March 2022).

24 Graphic Medicine and Visual Communication Techniques for Public Health and Healthcare in Linguistically Diverse Settings

MK CZERWIEC, Q. JANE ZHAO, ISA ÁLVAREZ, AND PILAR ORTEGA

Introduction to graphic medicine

The artistic and expressive medium of comics is defined by work that is "an art and literary form that deals with the arrangement of pictures or images and words to narrate a story or dramatize an idea" [1, 2]. The term "graphic novel" is used interchangeably with "comic." Comics that take as their subject health, healthcare, illness, disability, and caregiving have come to be known as *graphic medicine*. The author/artist who generates graphic medicine work can be anyone with a perspective on health or healthcare in the broadest sense. This includes clinicians such as physicians, nurses, therapists, and other health professionals who can generate graphic medicine work by applying their professional expertise or lived experience to providing healthcare services. But graphic medicine can also be produced by professional artists who collaborate with clinicians and public health experts to develop materials for educational, advocacy, community-building, or therapeutic purposes. Nonfiction long-form comics created by patients and/or their caregivers to tell the story of an illness, ailment, or pain (*pathos*) from the author/artist's lived experience are called *graphic pathographies* [3].

The field of graphic medicine is relatively new and rapidly growing. The 2015 *Graphic Medicine Manifesto* established the field's theoretical, ethical, and practical underpinnings [1]. Central to these underpinnings is the power of comics to transcend traditional boundaries, those between patient and healthcare professional, between the academic and the practical, and between the visual and the textual.

The Handbook of Language in Public Health and Healthcare, First Edition.
Edited by Pilar Ortega, Glenn Martínez, Maichou Lor, and A. Susana Ramírez.
© 2024 John Wiley & Sons, Inc. Published 2024 by John Wiley & Sons, Inc.

Comics have been employed as educational interventions in public health, with upticks in their use documented during epidemics and pandemics [4]. This is because the efficiency of the comic medium, given a stepwise combination of image and text, makes comics effective educational interventions when the content to be learned is important, there is much to be learned, and the learner is under stress [5]. The informational card on airplanes demonstrating emergency evacuation procedures is an example. It is most frequently wordless, which allows it to transcend literacy and language. Additionally, comics can have an immediacy and accessibility, both in reading and creating. With basic drawing skills and supplies, a comic can be created, reproduced, and distributed relatively quickly, efficiently, and inexpensively, both in print and online. All of these features of comics explain their frequent use in times of crisis.

In what follows, we present a historical and theoretical perspective on the use of comics in health. We then analyze critical issues in graphic medicine as they relate to linguistically diverse populations. Finally, we present recommendations for education and clinical practice that draw from the principles of graphic medicine.

Historical roots of graphic medicine

It is an intensely human quality to story our experience, to begin to understand our world through these structures. Storytelling techniques have been used for healing purposes for as long as history is recorded.

Storying health: history of medicine, sociopolitical movements, and zines

Healthcare professionals have long struggled with the balance of the art and science of medicine and healthcare. From the context of Western medicine, physicians have historically approached patients in a "detached, yet interested" manner [6]. Given an emphasis on scientific knowledge and the biomedical model in medical education, the human side, aspects of medicine related to emotion, compassion, and empathy were oftentimes not taught and even discouraged [7]. Yet, healthcare has always been intensely human, as patients, their loved ones, and their surrounding clinicians are forced to confront the mortality of bodies and navigate the healthcare system [8].

Sociopolitical movements and events of the 1960s–1990s such as Second Wave Feminism, Roe v. Wade, the Stonewall riots, the reproductive rights movement, and the HIV/AIDS epidemic mobilized community activists toward healthcare advocacy. Many of these movements focused on expanding rights for marginalized individuals, creating spaces for individuals to be informed and empowered (i.e., the Jane Collective [9], ACT UP [10], and the Black Panther Party [11]), which frequently meant broaching topics considered too taboo by mainstream media [12]. Production of zines, or smaller comics, specifically, allowed for cheap, reproducible, timely content to be easily distributed and shared among different social circles. Zines offered a means for communication with individuals normally excluded in the media, increasing connections and an overall sense of community [12]. In fact, many zines produced around this time ("Abortion Eve," "Tits and Clits," and many AIDS education comics, to name a few) centered on health topics, making this information more accessible and easier to understand [13], and supporting a humanistic approach to health and healthcare. In what follows, we will describe the development of storytelling through the lens of narrative medicine and subsequently through the emergence of the field of graphic medicine.

Medical education, the medical humanities, and the emergence of narrative medicine

Movements from the 1960–1990s also led to a shift in the physician–patient relationship. The concept of patient-centered interaction was developed to address concerns about patients' lack of satisfaction with care that ignored psychosocial issues to focus solely on biomedical topics. Patient-centered care encourages physicians to seek out the patient's perspective, making it easier for the patient to communicate with the physician as well as for the physician to better understand the patient. This approach significantly improved medical compliance and patient satisfaction [14]. As physicians gained a better understanding of this patient-centered approach, narrative medicine further emphasized the importance of the physician–patient relationship by focusing on the experiences and stories of the patient [15]. Other studies emphasized the importance of narrative in medicine, highlighting the AIDS epidemic and the role narrative played in bringing attention to the movement and a collective duty to take action, mentioning the research that focused on AIDS patients and their stories and experiences [16].

The establishment of the field and discipline of *narrative medicine* has helped pave the way to strengthen relationships between the health humanities – encompassing philosophy, history, sociology, anthropology, literature, and others – and the practice of modern medicine. Complaints from patients in the latter half of the twentieth century frequently cite the disconnection and increased digitization of medicine and healthcare [17]. Narrative medicine and the health humanities more broadly can be seen as a response by healthcare professionals and patients alike to improve communication and the clinical encounter, integrate tools from the humanities, and to rescue medicine from the ails of depersonalization.

The term "narrative medicine"[1] was coined in 2000 by Dr. Rita Charon, a general internist and literary scholar. With the conviction that knowing how stories worked would improve her clinical practice, Dr. Charon first applied the tools of literary analysis and the study of narrative theory in the healthcare setting [18]. Charon and colleagues developed the conceptual framework of narrative medicine—attention, representation, and affiliation—to train the next generation of effective healthcare professionals [19]. Over the years, narrative medicine has incorporated approaches and methods from the humanities (literary theory, narratology, creative writing, phenomenology, aesthetic theory, and cultural studies) and clinical practice (primary care, bioethics, qualitative methods, and psychoanalysis).

The practice of narrative medicine involves two main components: (1) the reading and discussion of text in all its forms (fiction, poetry, memoir, nonfiction, essay, film, music, podcast, and comics), and (2) reflective writing. In a narrative medicine workshop, participants are presented with a text and through facilitated discussion learn perspectives regarding the practice of healthcare and medicine, as well as about themselves and other participants (self and other). Students are also presented with a prompt and asked to write for a short, timed duration. It is recognized that the act of writing itself and seeing one's writing on a page allows the author to gain access to knowledge that would have otherwise remained unarticulated, inaccessible, and effectively "useless" [20]. Putting the practice together, practitioners of narrative medicine begin cultivating the skills of close reading, attentive listening, and witnessing.

Questions regarding the benefits and impact of narrative medicine arose with the emergence of the field. Early studies demonstrated the ability for practitioners of narrative medicine to build stronger therapeutic relationships with their patients and increased trainee empathy, techniques which were fostered through the close reading of fiction, as well as exercises in reflective and creative writing [20]. In Taiwan's largest teaching hospital, participants in a narrative medicine program were highly satisfied and engaged; more interestingly, their empathy scores increased immediately after the program, and this increase was sustained for one and a half years [21].

Studies have consistently found positive effects of narrative medicine skills on the development of medical students and residents' professional identity, peer relationships, and empathy, as well as on the delivery of patient-centered care [22–24]. Narrative medicine has also offered its practitioners enhanced skills in professional ethics, narrative humility, and structural competency [25]. These ask the practitioner to navigate and discern complex and nuanced clinical encounters, paying attention to sociopolitical power within an often inequitable and hierarchical system. The uptake of narrative medicine and the health humanities more generally within the healthcare system has fostered the space and milieu where graphic medicine now intersects and thrives.

What graphic medicine offers to story healthcare

Graphic medicine enhances the practice of storytelling for health by adding the sequential and the visual nature of comics, thereby expanding educational and therapeutic possibilities. In what follows, we review the unique characteristics of graphic medicine and how they add to public health and healthcare storytelling.

Medium. Comics have the ability to create a special bond between the reader and artist. For example, thought bubbles and word balloons are able to evoke an intimacy with the reader as the reader is witness to someone else's thoughts and feelings [26]. Simplifying an image offers the ability to focus on specific details that the artist wants the reader to see, influencing the message the artist conveys [27]. There is also the work the reader has to do to add meaning and life to the book, integrating a piece of the reader into the story. This is especially seen in work that discusses that which is socially stigmatized. Graphic novels about the trauma of miscarriage, for example, are able to convey the various emotional states through "verbal-visual affordances" (i.e., facial expressions, postures, and handwriting), offering the artist a form of expression and self-reflection as well as offering the reader an intimate look into the experiences of others, destigmatizing the shame and fear that often come with taboo topics [28].

Persuasion. Simply put, persuasion refers to a resource's ability to convince the user of something, such as to take an action that they may have been previously unlikely to do (e.g., convincing a woman to get a mammogram). Dual coding theory (DCT) highlights the importance of visual learning and imagery, specifically that imaging and verbal associative processes played major roles in comprehension, learning, and memory [29]. Studies showed that "vivid information," or material that includes pictures, narratives, and specific examples, is more persuasive when it comes to health communication than nonvivid information, specifically STD and skin cancer awareness [30]. Health communication research has shown a positive effect when narratives focus on healthy behaviors, first-person perspectives, and relatable characters [31, 32].

Thus, individuals are more likely to relate to characters who look like them, speak like them, and share a common cultural and linguistic connection. For more on narrative persuasion, refer to Chapters 3, 21, and 23 in this volume.

Data visualization. Graphic medicine has the ability to communicate data-driven stories to a wider audience. "Data comics" look at graphic medicine to humanize data visualization [33]. Data comics share data in a way that goes beyond solely addressing numerical information, but also conveying this information in a manner that uses the emotional impact of narrative work. Patients prefer visual simplicity and familiarity when looking at quantitative information, increasing their ability to understand [32].

Reach and impact. Graphic medicine has the ability to reach a diverse audience given the medium's flexibility. A review of health literature showed that patients prefer pictures that were linked with narratives and emotional responses, and this was especially true for patients with low literacy skills [33]. In another study, emergency department patients who were assigned to view cartoon illustration instructions were more likely to read and understand the instructions [34]. Since graphic medicine combines the emotional aspect of storytelling with the visual aspect of art, it can reach populations that are normally excluded from public health messaging.

Medical education. Graphic medicine can enhance medical education in that it allows for self-reflection and promotes wellness of trainees. Using graphic medicine curricula has demonstrated increases in overall empathy, connection with patients, and self-efficacy to communicate with empathy and understanding [35].

The trend toward the increased use of comics in healthcare is an international one, and not limited to the English language. We now turn our attention to specific examples of graphic medicine that illustrate the development of this emerging and proliferating field.

Graphic medicine and the HIV/AIDS crisis

The usefulness of comics as a powerful, accessible, and effective educational intervention in public health was evident during the AIDS crisis years, roughly 1981–2000. Public health departments, along with not-for-profit, grass-roots aid organizations created and distributed comics to provide clear messaging about HIV. The goals of these comics were to provide information to reduce HIV transmission and manage AIDS [36]. So many comics were created during this time and for these purposes that cataloging them today is considered impossible since most are lost to history [37]. One exception, perhaps due to its sexually explicit drawings and inclusion in the American legislative discourse, is the Safer Sex series of comics by the educational outreach branch of the Gay Men's Health Crisis in New York City[2] [38].

Another well-archived and well-remembered example of the use of comics during the AIDS crisis is the New York City Health Department's comic *Decisión* [39]. Produced by the New York City Department of Health and funded by the federal government to reach Spanish- and English-speaking subway riders, this comic ran for more than a decade and on more than 6000 train cars. The Spanish-language version, *La Decisión*, serialized the story of Marisol, a Latina struggling with her boyfriend, Julio, over using a condom, and watching friends die of AIDS [40]. The series employed a conventional black and white comic style combined with a heavily dramatic romantic subplot, a strategy typical in the Latin American telenovelas (soap operas) familiar to the target audience and which have also been leveraged for health education (see Chapter 23).

While the *Decisión* comic was widely discussed, remembered, and written about [41], no formal study of its efficacy as a public health education intervention was conducted. However, other studies of AIDS education comic books have found positive outcomes on sexual knowledge, attitudes, and beliefs [42, 43]. The studies that have assessed the impact of AIDS prevention comics highlight the ability of graphic medicine comics to educate and, ultimately, impact the behavior of individuals, especially among high-risk populations.

Modern era of graphic medicine

In this section, we describe two main themes in the modern era of graphic medicine: humanizing medicine and public health.

Humanizing medicine through comics

The recent growth in graphic medicine may in part respond to initiatives in medicine that call for the *humanization* of healthcare professionals to foster a wellness-oriented workplace environment that can reduce burnout and job dissatisfaction and improve professional identity formation [44–46]. Humanism has been defined as a historical philosophical movement that prioritizes human interests, values, and dignity; when applied to the practice of medicine, it is often referred to as "humanism in medicine" [46]. The ultimate goal of graphic medicine is to use comics to create understanding, community, and support humanistic care that recognizes the complex needs of patients, families, and caregivers.

Major medical journals, including the *Annals of Internal Medicine*, the *Journal of the American Medical Association* (JAMA), and the *New England Journal of Medicine* have begun including medically themed comics in their publications. Comics are not included in these journals as comic relief for therapeutic purposes. They are carefully commissioned or chosen from submissions in response to a call [47] in order to convey aspects of patients' experience of care provided [48], to detail a physician's personal story [49], or to share a case study [50]. The inclusion and increased number of active calls for graphic medicine content in academic journals are significant because academic discourse has historically been rigid in the types of materials that are considered appropriate for clinicians and scientists to advance health, research, and healthcare practice. The fact that journals are actively seeking graphic medicine supports the validity of comics and other visual representations as methods to portray health, illness, and the unique perspectives of patients and clinicians.

A unique application of graphic medicine has been as a tool used by healthcare professionals to portray their experiences in the healthcare workplace. On the other side of the stethoscope, graphic medicine has also been used by patients and nonprofessional caregivers. Comics have thereby expanded the focus of healthcare beyond illness alone and to encompass complex issues such as healthcare relationships (e.g., the doctor–patient relationship, the patient–caregiver relationship, etc.), as well as the identities, attitudes, feelings, and experiences of individuals beyond their ailments and professional identities [51]. Quite simply, people are more than just patients, patients are more than individuals with ailments, and doctors are more than people who treat ailments. Graphic medicine is a tool that helps to illuminate the complexity of individuals' identities and experiences.

Through the sequential use of images that portray emotion and include often ignored lived experiences of illness, graphic medicine can include the humanistic in the medical. In other words, the ideas of humanistic and values-based medicine remind physicians of the value of their patients as people needing compassion and care [52].

Graphic medicine for improving public health

The role of graphic medicine in humanizing healthcare and improving its accessibility to the general population is especially salient in the realm of public health.

One salient example is *No Ordinary Flu*, an eerily prescient comic created in 2008 by Meredith Li-Vollmer of the King County Public Health Department and Seattle-based cartoonist David Lasky [53]. Telling the story of the 1918 influenza outbreak, Li-Vollmer and Lasky demonstrated what a public health lockdown might look like in the Seattle area and provided recommendations for good practices for staying healthy. The intention was to "help people visualize and mentally rehearse a possible public health crisis that was then hard for most people to fathom" [54].

Although originally created in English, the *No Ordinary Flu* comic book was simultaneously published in 22 languages, all versions of which are publicly available for download at no cost. Figure 24.1 displays a sample page from the Korean version of the comic alongside the English original. The translation illustrates some of the challenges of adapting comics to multiple languages, including differences in how numerals or names may be displayed, whether the target audience will feel represented when looking at the physical features of the characters in the images, and challenges around adapting words or text embedded within the images themselves (e.g., the word "flu" on the television screen on the sample displayed).

Fast forward to March 2020, when the scenes depicted in *No Ordinary Flu* became reality in Seattle and worldwide. Immediately, other educational comics relating to COVID-19 emerged online, were shared on social media, and employed by websites that had not previously featured comics, such as National Public Radio [55]. Volunteers at http://graphicmedicine.org, aware of the loss of AIDS/HIV comics to history, began work to archive and organize COVID-19 comics as they emerged so that they would be readily available to patients and practitioners [56]. At the time of this writing, unique visits to the educational category of COVID-19 comics outpace those to any other pages on the site. While data are not available as to who the viewers are and why they are accessing the page, the high utilization speaks to the value of accessible and comprehensible public health resources during a crisis.

The power of the medium to increase reach was evidence during a pandemic: physician and cartoonist Mónica Lalanda created the comic *Síntomas Coronavirus* (Figure 24.2) and posted it to her social media channels, where it was cataloged with educational comics. A request came through the website's email form to reprint the comic for use in a meat packing plant. The requester wrote, "The CDC only gives pictorials of the 3 symptoms, not the additional ones! This would be hugely beneficial for us. In some locations, 31 languages are spoken, and pictures speak a thousand words."[3]

The dramatic rise in creation and consumption of health-related comics during the COVID-19 pandemic demonstrated the readiness of the field to step up and perform the many jobs that graphic medicine is well suited to do. Given the international impact of the COVID-19 pandemic, Callender and colleagues described the use of graphic medicine to synthesize, contextualize, and make visible "the invisible paths of contagion" [57].

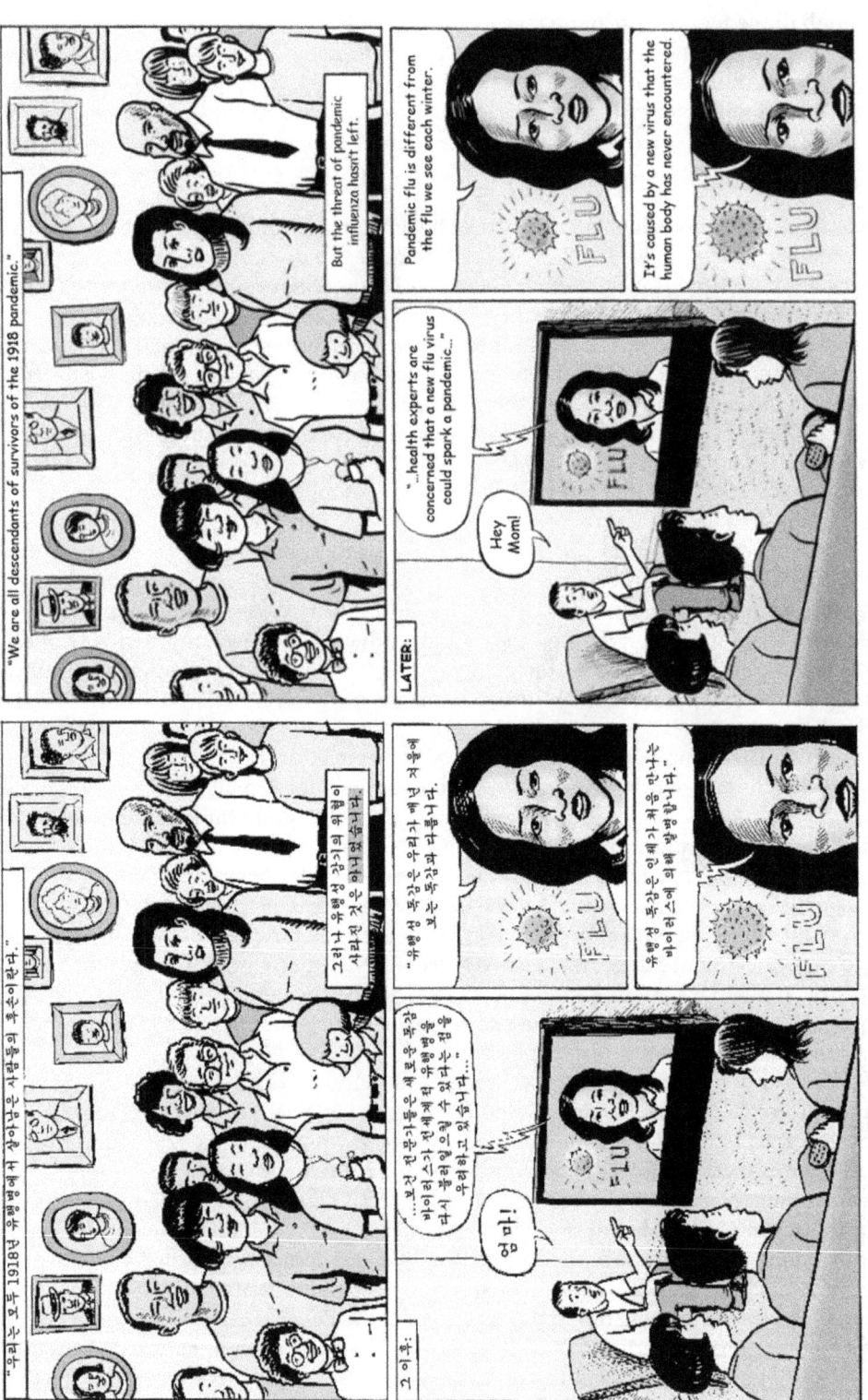

Figure 24.1 Image from Korean translation (left) and original English version of *No Ordinary Flu*, David Lasky and Meredith Li-Vollmer, 2008. *Source:* Reproduced with permission from Meredith Li-Vollmer.

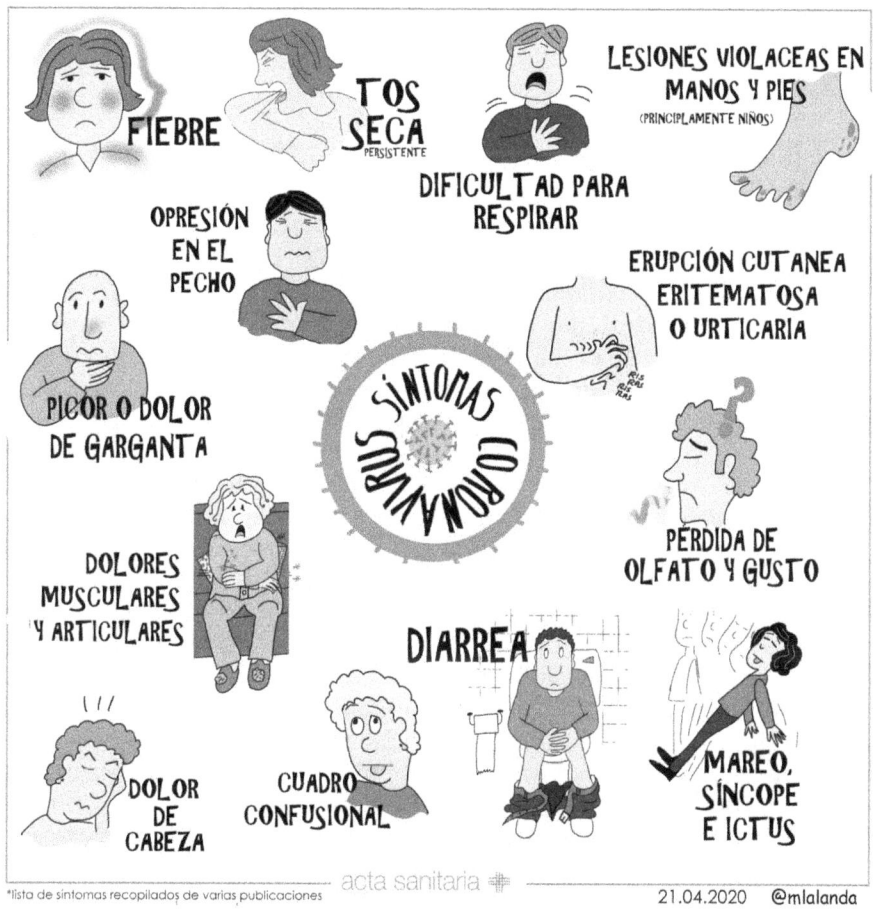

Figure 24.2 Síntomas Coronavirus, Mónica Lalanda, 2020. *Source:* Reproduced with permission from Mónica Lalanda.

Yet despite these and similar anecdotes, the impact of graphic medicine on preventive behaviors among populations is unknown. Future research should evaluate the effectiveness of graphic medicine approaches to urgent health communication in times of crises such as pandemics (see also Chapter 26).

Beyond infectious diseases and pandemics, graphic medicine has been used to address chronic illness prevention and treatment, and in this area, there are promising scientific results demonstrating the potential for graphic medicine to improve public health.

Fotonovelas, or photo comics stylized after Latin American comics, have specifically been successfully used to communicate about a diverse set of topics specifically with Latinx populations. Fotonovelas trace their roots to Mexican and Colombian comics; as such, they have been effective at fortifying social connections and reaching diverse audiences, and specifically, as a means of communicating with low-income, low-literacy, and predominantly rural communities about reproductive health, feminist theory, and empowerment, coinciding with other entertainment education approaches [58, 59] (also see Chapter 23). Fotonovelas have been used in the United States to communicate with Spanish-speaking Hispanic communities about highly stigmatized issues from infectious disease to mental health [60–62]. Fotonovelas continue to empower community to take actions leading to health and social improvements [63, 64].

Critical issues in applying graphic medicine in linguistically diverse settings

Graphic medicine presents an opportunity to make health information more accessible to patients. Throughout the world, immigrant populations face difficulties in accessing health information and healthcare when their language preferences and practices differ from the dominant language of the place where they live. We refer to settings in which multiple languages may be spoken as "linguistically diverse." Even in linguistically diverse settings, a particular language is typically used as the main language of instruction for healthcare professionals. For example, the United States is home to speakers of over 350 languages, and over 25 million individuals report having limited English proficiency (LEP), defined as speaking English less than very well [65]. The United States health professions education takes place in English as the dominant language of instruction, assessment, and certification for clinicians, and public health information is not consistently disseminated in non-English languages. As a result, the US patients who preferentially communicate in a non-English language are subject to inequitable access to healthcare services, poor understanding of health information including informed consent for procedures, and reduced quality of care due to pervasive systemic barriers that marginalize individuals who have limited proficiency in the dominant language [66–69].

In what follows, we describe the use of graphic medicine to address challenges in public health communication for linguistically diverse populations, patient–clinician communication in nondominant languages, and multilingual clinician well-being and burnout.

Using graphic medicine for public health communication among linguistically diverse populations

Public health interventions frequently use visual tools to communicate important health information or promote specific health behaviors, such as vaccination, preventive health screening exams, or instructions for using a medical device. Graphic medicine's utility to public health is intrinsically tied to the linguistic simplicity and flexibility of this medium for health communication [70].

Linguistically diverse communities are seldom monolingual; for example, hybrid, spontaneous use of language is frequent and there may also be generational and family specific differences in linguistic practices [71]. Viewed from this multilingual lens, Li-Vollmer's assertion [70] regarding the wealth of meaning carried by images can be understood to extend to improving health communication beyond the (theoretical) bounds of a single named language (the monolingual perspective). In this sense, graphic medicine and other forms of visual art for healthcare purposes are well suited to address a multilingual perspective on communication by reducing reliance on rigid linguistic standards (and on words in general) and by reinforcing health concepts in a visual format that can be understood by individuals with diverse linguistic practices (Figure 24.3).

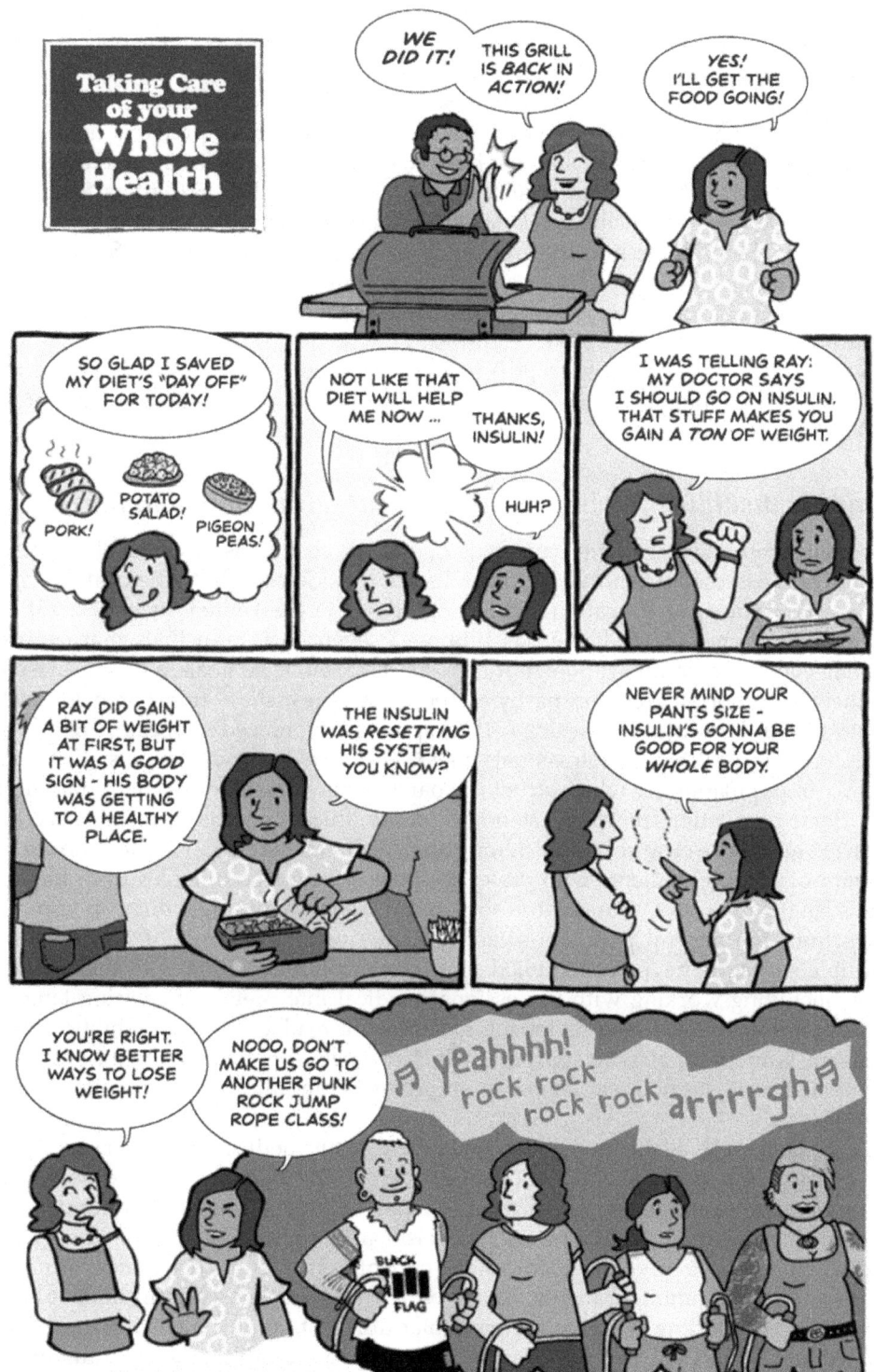

Figure 24.3 Image from diabetes self-management education and support program: Suzie and Ray, Cathy Leamy, 2016. *Source:* Reproduced with permission from Massachusetts General Hospital.

Despite the growth in comics that address public health concerns on a global scale, public health information from official sources such as government healthcare institutions has not always equitably addressed the linguistic diversity of their country's population. For example, in the United States, Spanish is the second most common language spoken, comprising over 60% of individuals who prefer a non-English language [65]. By comparison, all other languages each comprise a considerably smaller percentage of the LEP population (6% or less). Although the US Centers for Disease Control (CDC) website includes *selected* information in Spanish, not *all* information is provided in Spanish despite the frequency of this language in the US population, presenting some potential concerns regarding equity of health communication for Spanish-speaking individuals with LEP. For example, the COVID-19 infographic regarding common symptoms (https://www.cdc.gov/coronavirus/2019-ncov/downloads/COVID19-symptoms.pdf) is only provided in English yet is linked from the Spanish webpage (https://espanol.cdc.gov/coronavirus/2019-ncov/symptoms-testing/symptoms.html) (see Figure 24.4).

Graphic medicine for improving patient–clinician communication

Effective communication with patients is one of the core skills in which clinicians are trained and assessed. Communication skills are considered core to medical education standards by medical education accrediting bodies in the United States [72, 73]. The National Academy of Medicine has proposed seven basic principles that comprise patient–clinician communication: mutual respect, harmonized goals, a supportive environment, appropriate decision partners, the right information, transparency and full disclosure, and continuous learning [74]. Despite the recognized importance of communication skills, healthcare professionals may lack clinical communication skills training specific to populations in which structural barriers may preclude effective communication. Some populations in which "standard" communication techniques may need to be adjusted to achieve clear communication about health include: individuals who are deaf or hard-of-hearing, patients who prefer to speak a language different from the clinician's language skillset, those whose sociocultural experiences may differ in important ways from the general population, and patients with low levels of health literacy. Multiple strategies have been studied to improve communication with these populations, including working with professional medical interpreters, increasing language education for clinicians, and reviewing materials for readability and usability. Graphic medicine is another potential approach, which can be complementary to the previously mentioned well-studied strategies to improve communication with marginalized populations.

Some data are available to demonstrate how graphic medicine has been successfully used to improve patient–clinician communication. For example, in an observational study of an educational comic designed to increase patient–physician communication through an electronic health record, Alkreishi and colleagues showed the greatest improvement in patient engagement among patients who identified as African American or Hispanic, and among patients who reported a lower level of educational attainment [75]. This finding points to the particular utility of graphic medicine strategies to engage individuals who may be less likely to feel comfortable or to fully understand health information with other more "standard" methods of communication. Standard clinical communication typically includes verbal communication with health

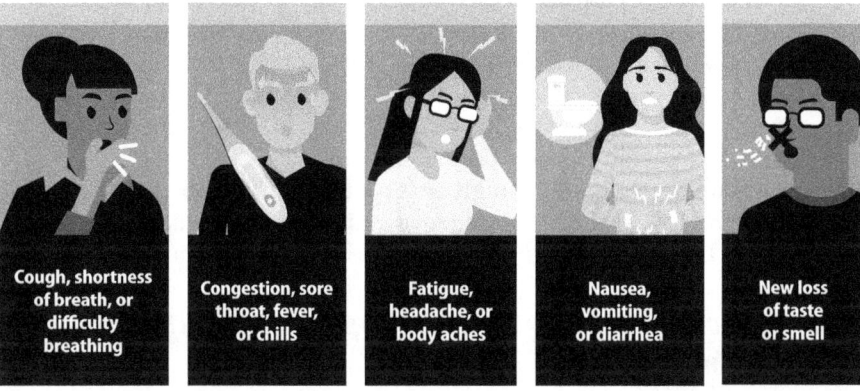

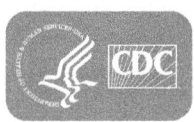

Figure 24.4 English-only public health infographic about COVID-19 symptoms accessible from both Spanish and English links of the United States Centers of Disease Control and Prevention's website. *Source:* CDC (Centers for Disease Control and Prevention) / https://www.cdc.gov/coronavirus/2019-ncov/downloads/COVID19-symptoms.pdf / last accessed 8 May 2023.

professional staff, which is often fraught with medical jargon and written instructions regarding treatments, medications, or diagnosis, and which may not always be available or accurate in patients' preferred language. Hence, graphic medicine is an opportunity to communicate important health concepts more clearly and in a more person-centered fashion that is less reliant on complex terminology or lengthy instructions. Furthermore, when interacting with clinicians after an appointment, the electronic health portals often allow patients to access their health information, such as lab results, or exchange written messages with their clinician, yet these features may be inaccessible to linguistically diverse groups if their clinicians are not able to respond to messages in their language. Given the recent growth in electronic communication, including telemedicine, graphic medicine may be a helpful strategy to increase participation of marginalized groups in electronic health portals (Figure 24.5).

Graphic medicine is being increasingly incorporated and studied at various stages of medical education as a strategy to improve patient-centered communication skills, improve student clinician wellness, and reduce health-professional burnout [75–77].

Graphic medicine as a strategy for improving multilingual clinician wellness

Multilingual clinicians face ethical dilemmas related to use of language in their day-to-day practice. For example, they must decide whether their language skills are adequate for explaining a particular diagnosis, treatment, or procedure with a patient or whether they should obtain a medical interpreter. For some, the decision may be fraught with difficulty, particularly when their language skills are limited. For example, in the United States, Spanish is spoken at home by nearly 66 million people and is by far the most common non-English language [65]. More than half of medical residency applicants (53.2%) report speaking Spanish, but less than a quarter (21%) report their Spanish level to be advanced or higher [66]. This suggests that a majority of US medical students and resident physicians have some skills in the language yet likely also have significant limitations during complex health conversations with patients. Data show that clinicians and clinicians-in-training often underutilize professional interpreters due to complex reasons, including difficulty accessing interpreters and the sense that they are able to "get by" with their own skills [50, 51]. Oftentimes, multilingual individuals are also asked by other members of the healthcare team to use their non-English skills in patient care. This can put multilingual clinicians and trainees in a difficult position since they may not want to disappoint their supervisors or colleagues, yet they may sometimes feel that their skills are insufficient for the communication task at hand [52]. Thus, multilingual clinicians must often play a dual role in using their language skills to assist the healthcare team in addition to providing direct patient care.

These challenges unique to multilingual clinicians may endanger their sense of professional fulfillment and wellness, factors that have been identified as important to physician health, work productivity, and quality of care [52]. Given the multiple ethical dilemmas that multilingual clinicians may face regarding their language skills, opportunities to share their personal stories through graphic medicine may be valuable for improving identity formation among trainees, increasing clinician professional fulfillment, and fostering a sense of community among multilingual clinicians with shared experiences.

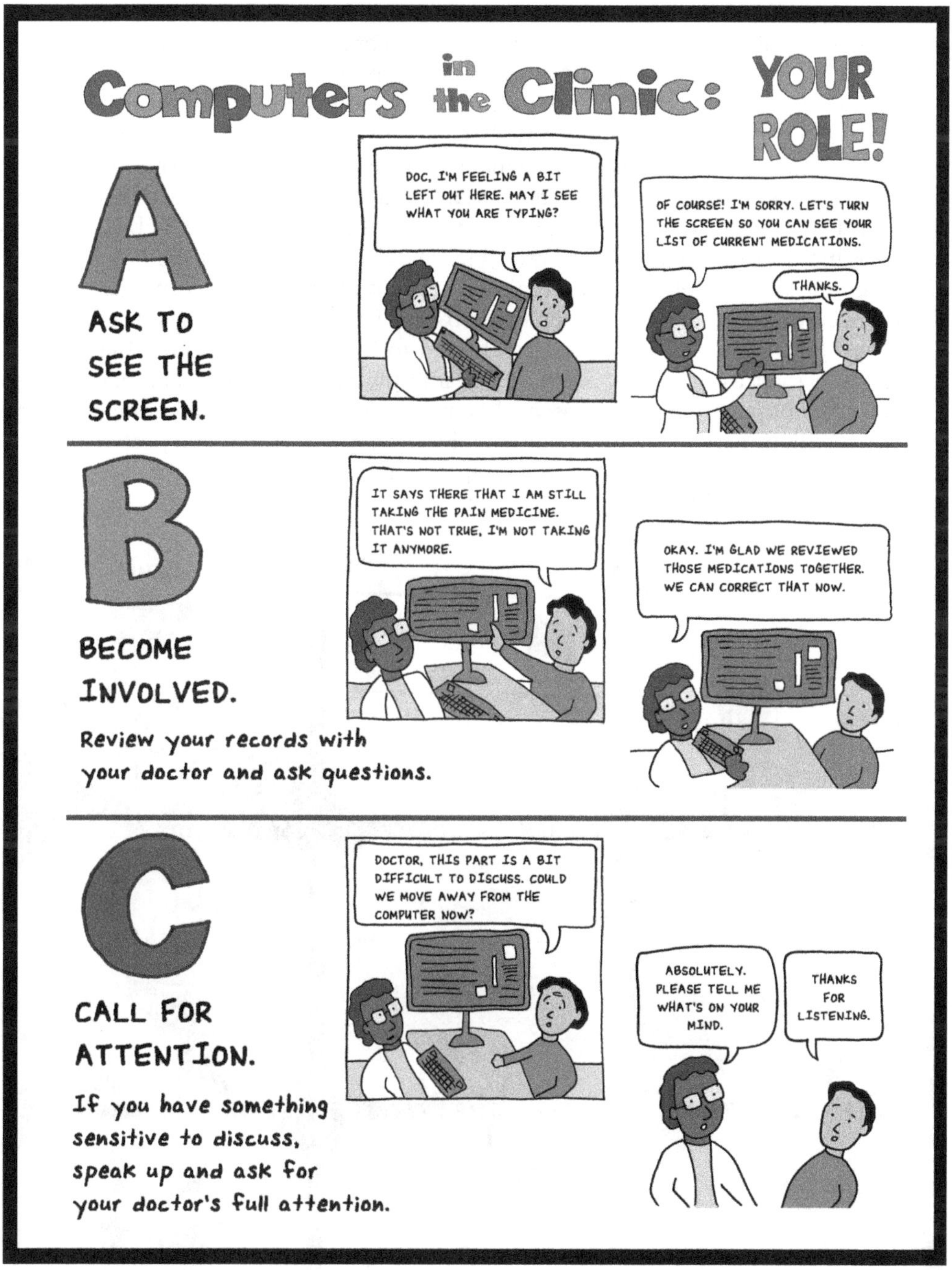

©2016 Alkureishi ML, Czerwiec MK, Arora V, Lee WW

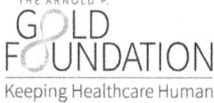

Figure 24.5 Comic to improve patient–clinician communication through an electronic health record. *Source:* Reproduced with permission from MK Czerwiec (Chapter Contributor).

Graphic medicine has played an important role in humanizing medicine, from the perspective of patients as well as that of clinicians. For some, comics have been used to critique problems such as structural or systemic barriers present in the healthcare system [78]. Clinician authors have used graphic medicine in a cathartic capacity to share a lived experience that others can also relate to and may help them process complex or stressful aspects of their professional responsibilities, such as a comic by Caplow "The Weekly Road to Burnout in Primary Care" that focuses on a physician's progressive journey through worsening stages of burnout as the weekdays go by [72]. Ortega's comic "Which Doctor Shall I Be Today?" (Figure 24.6) was first published on the cover of the journal *Academic Medicine* and is aimed at exploring the intersectionality of a physician's multiple identities, the personal and the professional, including cross-linguistic challenges [73]. Some of the challenges alluded to in this comic include the author's personal experiences in serving as an ad hoc interpreter for a family member during a medical appointment and the apparent dissonance between thinking in one or several languages and professional work in another. By sharing a personal perspective on multilingualism, comics such as these may help normalize and amplify the lived experiences of an increasingly diverse healthcare professional workforce.

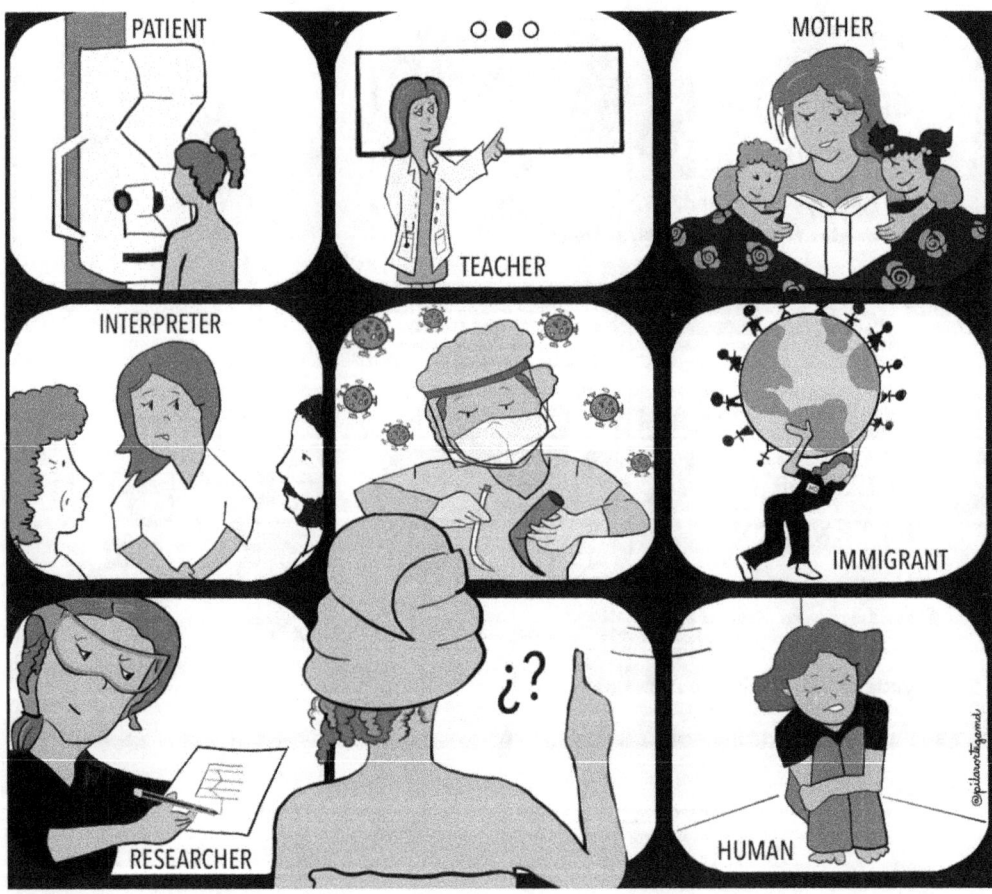

Figure 24.6 "Which doctor shall I be today," Pilar Ortega, 2022. *Source:* Reproduced with permission from Pilar Ortega (Chapter Contributor).

Recommendations for incorporating graphic medicine in education and clinical practice

Graphic medicine as a tool for medical education

Graphic medicine is gaining momentum as an educational tool for clinicians in training [79, 80]. Multiple educational resources for teaching about graphic medicine are available. One source is the graphic medicine exhibition available through the National Library of Medicine [81], which includes a collection of graphic medicine publications as well as two educational resources to lead a graphic medicine educational intervention: one focused on junior high and high school mental health, and another focused on university and health professions students using graphic medicine to communicate stories about healthcare and illness. These two examples demonstrate how graphic medicine can be incorporated in teaching health concepts and could be adapted and evaluated among physician/health professional trainees. For instance, as part of his course Graphic Storytelling and Medical Narratives at the Pennsylvania State College of Medicine, Dr. Michael Green curates a collection of graphic stories created by his medical students, showing that students with a breadth of creative "talent" can tell stories through drawings [50].

Thus, existing graphic medicine educational resources could be integrated into medical education in a way that explicitly incorporates the experiences of linguistically diverse communities and of the clinicians who care for them. For instance, an activity in a medical Spanish classroom might be having students draw an experience they had with a Spanish-speaking patient. The drawing process can help students process an experience in a new way. Furthermore, public health infographics from different countries and in different languages could be examined during a medical language course. Discussion points can include: variations in language use that might be observed in one Spanish-speaking country or region as compared to another; how the information is visually organized; the types of pictures or graphics that are used; and how the infographic compares to an English (or other language) infographic about the same topic.

Graphic medicine tools for clinical practice in linguistically diverse settings

An important but largely unexplored application of graphic medical education tools is their potential use for improving healthcare for linguistically diverse populations. Given that graphic medicine resources are, by definition, visual in nature, the visual aspects of the resources may be applicable across linguistic differences. One such approach involves the cultural and linguistic adaptation of available graphic medicine materials targeting a specific linguistic population. Golden et al. employed this strategy in creating the "Communicating the External Beam Radiotherapy Experience (CEBRE) en español," a series of graphic narrative pamphlets that are intended for clinicians to explain radiation oncology treatment to patients [82]. While these guides were originally created in English, an interdisciplinary team including translators, physicians, and information designers collaborated on creating a Spanish version of these resources.

It should be noted that even when graphic medicine materials are primarily visual, it is essential for both textual and visual components to be relevant, appropriate, and accurate to the target population. Textual components should be translated professionally and reviewed for readability and usability to ensure relevance for the patient population for whom they are intended. Visual elements should also be inclusive enough that patients feel represented by them. For example, diversity can be manifested through varied physical features such as skin color, height, weight, and age. Other social factors that can be depicted graphically to improve inclusive representation of specific communities include type of clothing worn, presence of family members during medical visits, languages spoken, and disability status.

Recommendations for research

Future graphic medicine research should focus on advancing the science of health communication by collecting evidence of effectiveness and usability by target populations. Given that comics can reach diverse audiences, public health communication should focus on presenting visuals and narratives that better prepare communities for public health crises [83] (see also Chapter 26). A better understanding of the role of visual misinformation and narratives would also help public health officials in improving the information they produce to counteract mis- or disinformation, particularly among populations with nondominant language preferences. Research efforts should specifically evaluate graphic medicine tools among linguistically diverse communities to determine how such strategies may help build trust, empowerment, and health knowledge.

Including community members as participants in research about graphic medicine may also benefit the linguistic and cultural appropriateness of the content, particularly considering that language practices may change over time and need to be adapted to ensure usability. Similarly, graphic medicine content used for medical educational purposes should incorporate patient perspectives to ensure that educational initiatives that claim to be patient-centered actually address the needs and authentic linguistic practices of the community.

The burgeoning field of graphic medicine is slowly beginning to transform medicine into a more supportive, understanding, and diverse profession. Incorporating graphic medicine in the medical curriculum, in particular, has led to increased knowledge of cultural issues, confidence, and preparedness among practitioners, and greater knowledge surrounding health equity [80, 84, 85]. Broader topics such as healing from trauma, social justice, and fighting against sexual violence are starting to make their way into graphic medicine as well [78, 86]. For patients, graphic medicine has served as a means of increasing health literacy among underserved communities. This was especially the case during the COVID-19 pandemic [83], including increased technological awareness, which allowed patients to better engage with their healthcare team during outpatient visits [87]. For patients and practitioners alike, graphic medicine serves as a form of reflection, providing a safe space to share intimate truths of their experience [71, 88]. This should come as no surprise given its accessibility, both in distribution of content and connection within academic and health institutions [89]. With that said, it is important that librarians, educators, scholars, and creators highlight underrepresented voices within the field and play their part to further diversify graphic medicine and evaluate their use. To ensure effectiveness, research should analyze data about who the users/readers are, how the graphic medicine materials are being used, and whether they are effective at meeting their aims of improving health and wellbeing. Moving forward, it is imperative that graphic medicine comics are vetted by a panel of healthcare professionals and patients to ensure that factual, usable, and comprehensible information is conveyed rather than scientific misinformation to drive a political message. With healthcare being so intertwined with politics in the United States, it is imperative that we use appropriate scientific data to ensure that we are spreading a message of reform in support of basic human rights for those being marginalized.

Conclusion

Graphic medicine is the use of comics, sequential images, often incorporating text, to describe, analyze, and disseminate themes around health, healthcare, illness, disability, and caregiving. Graphic medicine has become an important means for expressing and voicing healthcare experience, transcending language boundaries, and humanizing healthcare. In order to achieve effective and equitable health communication with linguistically diverse populations, clinicians, medical centers, educators, and healthcare systems must think beyond the dominant language. By applying visuals, reducing and simplifying text, and centering humanism, graphic medicine achieves what language alone does not. Public health, medical/health professions education, and clinician–patient interactions represent valuable opportunities to apply graphic medicine to improve communication with patients who have historically been marginalized due to the languages they speak.

Highlights

- Graphic medicine, comics on broad and diverse health themes, is an effective strategy for communicating with linguistically diverse populations and increasing equity in access to healthcare information, services, and education.
- Graphic medicine can be used as a tool for improved public health messaging, medical education, patient–clinician communication, and clinician wellness.
- Graphic medicine can be seen as part of a long tradition of humanism in medicine, best characterized by the emergence of the field of narrative medicine, a response by clinicians and patients alike to shift the practice of medicine away from deep depersonalization within medicine.
- Increasing recognition has come to graphic medicine from leading journals publishing graphic medicine content to increasing roles and functions of graphic medicine within public health, patient education, and in linguistically diverse populations.
- Additional research is needed to evaluate effectiveness and usability and better understand the readership of graphic medicine resources and educational initiatives.

NOTES

1 Not to be confused with *narrative-based medicine*, coined one year earlier by Greenhalgh and Hurwitz to describe "what happens between the healthcare professional and the patient: from the collection of information about events before the disease, to how the disease displayed, with focus on psychological, social, and ontological themes." That same year, the British Medical Journal ran a special five-part series on five facets of narrative based medicine, from why study narrative to its place in ethics to its tension with evidence-based medicine. Similar and overlapping, Greenhalgh and Hurwitz also give attention to the individual patient and

their healthcare providers, framing sickness and health within cultural context to better understand power and the relationships between various players. But this is where similarities end, as Greenhalgh and Hurwitz's narrative medicine does not draw as much from the humanities and the social sciences, nor does Charon and colleagues' narrative medicine draw as much from qualitative research in the social sciences.

2 Evidence of the educational impact of these comics unfortunately is not documented, but American Senator Jesse Helms did photocopy one issue and distribute it to members of Congress, erroneously claiming that their creation was funded by tax dollars. This act of political theater resulted in the 1988 Appropriations bill prohibiting the Federal Centers for Disease Control from funding AIDS programs that "promote, encourage or condone homosexual activities."

3 Personal correspondence with author MK Czerwiec, 2020. The name of the author of the correspondence is omitted to protect their identity.

REFERENCES

1. Czerwiec, M.K., Williams, I., Squier, S.M. et al. (2015). *Graphic Medicine Manifesto*. Pennsylvania State University Press.
2. Green, M.J. and Myers, K.R. (2010). Graphic medicine: use of comics in medical education and patient care. *BMJ* 340 (mar03 2): c863.
3. Squier, S.M. and Krüger-Fürhoff, I.M. (2020). *PathoGraphics: Narrative, Aesthetics, Contention, Community*. Penn State Press.
4. Noe, M.N. and Levin, L.L. (2020). Mapping the use of comics in health education: a scoping review of the graphic medicine literature. *Graph. Med.* 24. https://www.graphicmedicine.org/mapping-comics-health-education/ (accessed 14 August 2023).
5. Crawford, P., Brown, B.J., and Charise, A. (2020). *The Routledge Companion to Health Humanities*. London: Routledge.
6. Starr, P. (2017). *The Social Transformation of American Medicine: The Rise of a Sovereign Profession and the Making of a Vast Industry*. Hachette UK.
7. Dobkin, P.L. (2020). Art of medicine, art as medicine, and art for medical education. *Can. Med. Educ. J.* 11 (6): e172.
8. Downie, R.S. (1991). Literature and medicine. *J. Med. Ethics* 17 (2): 93–98.
9. Horwitz, R. (2017). The Jane Collective (1969–1973). In: *Embryo Project Encyclopedia (2017-08-07)*. ISSN: 1940-5030 http://embryo.asu.edu/handle/10776/12969 (accessed 14 August 2023).
10. Gill-Peterson, J. (2013). Haunting the queer spaces of AIDS: remembering ACT UP/New York and an ethics for an endemic. *GLQ J. Lesbian Gay Stud.* 19 (3): 279–300.
11. Jones, C.E. (1998). *The Black Panther Party (Reconsidered)*. Black Classic Press.
12. Ramdarshan, B.M. (2017). Why diverse zines matter: a case study of the people of color zines project. *Publ. Res. Q.* 33: 215–228.
13. McGovern, M. and Eve, M.P. (2019). Information labour and shame in farmer and Chevli's abortion eve. *Comics Grid J. Comics Scholarsh.* 9 (1): 1–6.
14. Stewart, M.A. (1984). What is a successful doctor-patient interview? A study of interactions and outcomes. *Soc. Sci. Med.* 19 (2): 167–175.
15. Charon, R. (1986). To render the lives of patients. *Lit. Med.* 5 (1): 58–74.
16. Clark, J.M. and Paivio, A. (1991). Dual coding theory and education. *Educ. Psychol. Rev.* 3: 149–210.
17. Block, L.G. and Keller, P.A. (1997). Effects of self-efficacy and vividness on the persuasiveness of health communications. *J. Consum. Psychol.* 6 (1): 31–54.
18. Hydén, L.C. (1997). Illness and narrative. *Sociol. Health Illn.* 19 (1): 48–69.
19. Halpern, J. (2001). *From Detached Concern to Empathy: Humanizing Medical Practice*. Oxford University Press.
20. Charon, R. (2008). *Narrative Medicine: Honoring the Stories of Illness*. Oxford University Press.

21. Charon, R., DasGupta, S., and Hermann, N. (2017). *The Principles and Practice of Narrative Medicine*. Oxford University Press.
22. DasGupta, S. and Charon, R. (2004). Personal illness narratives: using reflective writing to teach empathy. *Acad. Med.* 79 (4): 351–356.
23. Chen, P.J., Huang, C.D., and Yeh, S.J. (2017). Impact of a narrative medicine programme on healthcare providers' empathy scores over time. *BMC Med. Educ.* 17: 1–8.
24. Arntfield, S.L., Slesar, K., Dickson, J., and Charon, R. (2013). Narrative medicine as a means of training medical students toward residency competencies. *Patient Educ. Couns.* 91 (3): 280–286.
25. DasGupta, S., Meyer, D., Calero-Breckheimer, A. et al. (2006). Teaching cultural competency through narrative medicine: intersections of classroom and community. *Teach. Learn. Med.* 18 (1): 14–17.
26. Milota, M.M., van Thiel, G.J.M.W., and van Delden, J.J.M. (2019). Narrative medicine as a medical education tool: a systematic review. *Med. Teach.* 41 (7): 802–810.
27. Remein, C.D., Childs, E., Pasco, J.C. et al. (2020). Content and outcomes of narrative medicine programmes: a systematic review of the literature through 2019. *BMJ Open* 10 (1): e031568.
28. Versaci, R. (2007). *This Book Contains Graphic Language: Comics as Literature*. Continuum International Publishing Group.
29. McCloud, S. (1993). *Understanding Comics: The Invisible Art*, vol. 7, 4. Northampton, MA: Tundra Pub.
30. Venkatesan, S. and Murali, C. (2022). "It just went wrong, as bodies are prone to do": graphic medicine and the trauma of miscarriage. In: *The Medical/Health Humanities-Politics, Programs, and Pedagogies* (ed. T. Jones and K. Pachucki), 251–263. Springer.
31. Alamalhodaei, A., Alberda, A.P., and Feigenbaum, A. (2020). Humanizing data through 'data comics': an introduction to graphic medicine and graphic social science. In: *Data Visualization in Society* (ed. M. Engebretsen and H. Kennedy), 347. Amsterdam University Press.
32. Ancker, J.S., Senathirajah, Y., Kukafka, R., and Starren, J.B. (2006). Design features of graphs in health risk communication: a systematic review. *J. Am. Med. Inform. Assoc.* 13 (6): 608–618.
33. Houts, P.S., Doak, C.C., Doak, L.G., and Loscalzo, M.J. (2006). The role of pictures in improving health communication: a review of research on attention, comprehension, recall, and adherence. *Patient Educ. Couns.* 61 (2): 173–190.
34. Delp, C. and Jones, J. (1996). Communicating information to patients: the use of cartoon illustrations to improve comprehension of instructions. *Acad. Emerg. Med.* 3 (3): 264–270.
35. Ronan, L.K. and Czerwiec, M.K. (2020). A novel graphic medicine curriculum for resident physicians: boosting empathy and communication through comics. *J. Med. Humanit.* 41 (4): 573–578.
36. Czerwiec, M.K. (2018). Representing AIDS in comics. *AMA J. Ethics* 20 (2): 199–205.
37. Rifas, L. (1991). AIDS educational comics. *Ref. Serv. Rev.* 19: 81–87.
38. U.S. National Library of Medicine (2014). *Safer Sex Comix #8, 1987 – Surviving and Thriving: AIDS, Politics, and Culture*. U.S. National Library of Medicine.
39. Barron, J. (1993). *AIDS Message in a Subway Comic Strip: New York City Health Agency Teaches About the Disease in a Soap with a Sober Focus*. New York Times.
40. U.S. National Library of Medicine (2014). *La Decisión I*. New York City Department of Health, 1990.
41. United Press International Inc (1994). *Julio & Marisol: AIDS Drama Unfolds*. United Press International Inc.
42. Gillies, P.A., Stork, A., and Bretman, M. (1990). Streetwize UK: a controlled trial of an AIDS education comic. *Health Educ. Res.* 5 (1): 27–33.
43. Milleliri, J.M., Krentel, A., and Rey, J.L. (2003). Sensitisation about condom use in Gabon (1999): evaluation of the impact of a comic book. *Sante* 13 (4): 253–264.
44. (2015). Of science, humanism, and medicine. *JAMA* 314 (7): 734.

45. Rabinowitz, D.G. (2021). On the arts and humanities in medical education. *Philos. Ethics Humanit. Med.* 16 (1): 1–5.
46. Shapiro, J., McMullin, J., Miotto, G. et al. (2022). Medical students' creation of original poetry, comics, and masks to explore professional identity formation. In: *The Medical/Health Humanities-Politics, Programs, and Pedagogies* (ed. T. Jones and K. Pachucki), 91–113. Springer.
47. Comic Nurse (2013). Call for Work: Comics and the Annals of Internal Medicine. Blog Post. https://www.graphicmedicine.org/call-for-work-comics-and-the-annals-of-internal-medicine/ (accessed 5 September 2022).
48. Councilor, K.C. (2017). Annals graphic medicine – dear doctor I. *Ann. Intern. Med.* 167 (5): W36–W40.
49. Schor, J., Koscal, N., and Knoper, K. (2021). Revival. *N. Engl. J. Med.* 385: 1925–1927.
50. Green, M.J. and Rieck, R. (2013). Annals graphic medicine – missed it. *Ann. Intern. Med.* 158 (5_Part_1): 357–361.
51. Nazario, R.J. (2009). Medical humanities as tools for the teaching of patient-centered care. *J. Hosp. Med.* 4 (8): 512–514.
52. Little, J.M. (2002). Humanistic medicine or values-based medicine... what's in a name? *Med. J. Aust.* 177 (6): 319–321.
53. Li-Vollmer, M. and Lasky, D. (2022). *No Ordinary Flu*. Seattle and King County Advanced Practice Center – Public Health.
54. Li-Vollmer, M. (2022). *Graphic Public Health: A Comics Anthology and Road Map*, vol. 25. Penn State Press.
55. Gharib, M. (2020). *11 Original NPR Comics That Brought Joy, Hope and Help During the Pandemic*. NPR.
56. Jaggers, A. (2021). COVID-19 Comics. Blog Post. https://www.graphicmedicine.org/covid-19-comics/ (accessed 5 September 2022).
57. Callender, B., Obuobi, S., Czerwiec, M.K., and Williams, I. (2020). COVID-19, comics, and the visual culture of contagion. *Lancet* 396 (10257): 1061–1063.
58. Carrillo, L. and Lyson, T.A. (1983). The "fotonovela" as a cultural bridge for Hispanic women in the United States. *J. Pop. Cult.* 17 (3): 59.
59. Flora, C.B. and Flora, J.L. (1978). The fotonovela as a tool for class and cultural domination. *Lat. Am. Perspect.* 5 (1): 134–150.
60. Unger, J.B., Cabassa, L.J., Molina, G.B. et al. (2013). Evaluation of a fotonovela to increase depression knowledge and reduce stigma among Hispanic adults. *J. Immigr. Minor. Health* 15: 398–406.
61. Grigsby, T.J., Unger, J.B., Molina, G.B., and Baron, M. (2017). Evaluation of an audio-visual Novela to improve beliefs, attitudes and knowledge toward dementia: a mixed-methods approach. *Clin. Gerontol.* 40 (2): 130–138.
62. Kopelowicz, A., Lopez, S.R., Molina, G.B. et al. (2023). Evaluation of an audio-visual novela to improve COVID-19 knowledge and safe practices among Spanish-speaking individuals with schizophrenia. *J. Immigr. Minor. Health* 25: 889–898.
63. Zhou, M., Ramírez, A.S., Chittamuru, D. et al. (2023). Testing the effectiveness of narrative messages using critical health communication. *J. Commun. Healthc.* 15: 1–8.
64. Unger, J.B., Soto, D.W., Rendon, A.D. et al. (2019). Empowering hispanic multiunit housing residents to advocate for smokefree policies: a randomized controlled trial of a culturally tailored Fotonovela intervention. *Health Equity* 3 (1): 198–204.
65. U.S. Census Bureau (2019). *American Community Survey, Language Spoken at Home Data Table*. U.S. Census Bureau.
66. Diamond, L., Grbic, D., Genoff, M. et al. (2014). Non–English-language proficiency of applicants to US residency programs. *JAMA* 312 (22): 2405–2407.
67. Schenker, Y., Pérez-Stable, E.J., Nickleach, D., and Karliner, L.S. (2011). Patterns of interpreter use for hospitalized patients with limited English proficiency. *J. Gen. Intern. Med.* 26: 712–717.
68. Hsieh, E. (2015). Not just "getting by": factors influencing providers' choice of interpreters. *J. Gen. Intern. Med.* 30: 75–82.
69. Vela, M.B., Fritz, C., Press, V.G., and Girotti, J. (2016). Medical students' experiences and perspectives on

interpreting for LEP patients at two US medical schools. *J. Racial Ethn. Health Disparities* 3: 245–249.
70. Agarwal, S.D., Pabo, E., Rozenblum, R., and Sherritt, K.M. (2020). Professional dissonance and burnout in primary care: a qualitative study. *JAMA Intern. Med.* 180 (3): 395–401.
71. Venkatesan, S. and Murali, C. (2019). Graphic medicine and the critique of contemporary US healthcare. *J. Med. Humanit.* 43: 27–42.
72. Caplow, J. (2020). Annals graphic medicine-the weekly road to burnout in primary care. *Ann. Intern. Med.* 173 (3): W55–W56.
73. Ortega, P. (2022). Artist's statement: which doctor shall I be today? *Acad. Med.* 97 (3): 356.
74. LCME (2021). *Functions and Structure of a Medical School Standards for Accreditation of Medical Education Programs Leading to the MD Degree*. Association of American Medical Colleges, American Medical Association.
75. Alkureishi, M.A., Johnson, T., Nichols, J. et al. (2021). Impact of an educational comic to enhance patient-physician–electronic health record engagement: prospective observational study. *JMIR Hum. Factors* 8 (2): e25054.
76. Paget, L., Han, P., Nedza, S. et al. (2011). *Patient-Clinician Communication: Basic Principles and Expectations. NAM Perspectives*. Discussion Paper. Washington, DC: National Academy of Medicine.
77. Sammer, C.E., Lykens, K., Singh, K.P. et al. (2010). What is patient safety culture? A review of the literature. *J. Nurs. Scholarsh.* 42 (2): 156–165.
78. Donovan, C. and Ustundag, E. (2017). Graphic narratives, trauma and social justice. *Stud. Soc. Justice* 11 (2): 221–237.
79. Pieper, C. and Homobono, A. (2000). Comic as an education method for diabetic patients and general population. *Diabetes Res. Clin. Pract.* 50: 31.
80. Lesińska-Sawicka, M. (2023). Using graphic medicine in teaching multicultural nursing: a quasi-experimental study. *BMC Med. Educ.* 23 (1): 255.
81. U.S. National Library of Medicine (2018). *Graphic Medicine: Ill-Conceived and Well-drawn*. U.S. National Library of Medicine.
82. Radiation Oncology Education Collaborative Study Group. Communicating the External Beam Radiotherapy Experience (CEBRE) en Español. https://roecsg.org/cebre-en-espanol/ (accessed 5 April 2022).
83. Zhao, X., Feigenbaum, A., and McDavitt, S. (2021). Feasibility of comics in health communication: public responses to graphic medicine on Instagram during the COVID-19 pandemic. *J. Vis. Polit. Commun.* 9 (1): 9–28.
84. Humphrey, A. (2022). Graphic medicine and health professional education: an internship comic book case study. *Focus Health Prof. Educ. Multi-Discip. J.* 23 (2): 1–20.
85. Chin, M.H., Orlov, N.M., Callender, B.C. et al. (2022). Improvisational and standup comedy, graphic medicine, and theatre of the oppressed to teach advancing health equity. *Acad. Med.* 97 (12): 1732–1737.
86. Yousri, S. (2022). Graphic medicine as a wake-up call to stand against female genital mutilation in Egypt. *QSci. Context.* 2022 (3): 36.
87. Nichols, J.W., Johnson, T., Lee, W.W. et al. (2019). Connecting the dots: evaluating the impact of graphic medicine to empower patient-centered technology use. *Pediatrics* 144 (2_MeetingAbstract): 232.
88. Raphael, L.S. and Rowell, M. (2018). How should we judge the ethics of illustrations in graphic medicine novels? *AMA J. Ethics* 20 (2): 176–187.
89. Farthing, A. and Priego, E. (2016). Graphic medicine' as a mental health information resource: insights from comics producers. *Comics Grid J. Comics Scholarsh.* 6 (3): 1–23.

25 Social Media and Health in Linguistically Diverse Communities: An Examination of Overlooked Populations and Understudied Platforms

ANNA GAYSYNSKY, KATHRYN HELEY, AND WEN-YING SYLVIA CHOU

Introduction

The use of social media—defined as any digital technology that enables users to create and share content or participate in social networking [1]—has increased significantly over the past two decades. In 2021, over 72% of American adults reported using social media platforms such as YouTube, Facebook, Instagram, Twitter, and TikTok [2]. Social media use can have both positive and negative impacts on health. For example, platforms make it easy to find and share health information [3], connect with others to exchange social support [4], and deliver health promotion interventions [5]. However, these benefits may not be equitably distributed, as groups may have differential access to social media and some may lack the skills needed to successfully navigate information on these platforms. Social media can also negatively affect health, for example, through the promotion or normalization of behaviors like self-harm [6] and tobacco use [7], and by amplifying poor-quality health information or misinformation [8].

Although a substantial body of literature examining the role of social media in health has emerged in recent years, much of this research has focused on (1) platforms popular in Western countries, and (2) English language posts on those platforms. Consequently, we have limited knowledge regarding social media use among diaspora communities who may use platforms popular in their home countries (e.g., WeChat and Vkontakte) or people who predominantly engage with non-English-language content on social media. In this chapter, we consider the health impacts of social media use among linguistically diverse communities in the United States, which we define broadly as any

---

The Handbook of Language in Public Health and Healthcare, First Edition.
Edited by Pilar Ortega, Glenn Martínez, Maichou Lor, and A. Susana Ramírez.
© 2024 John Wiley & Sons, Inc. Published 2024 by John Wiley & Sons, Inc.

group living in the United States that speaks or uses a language other than English, including, among others, those with limited English proficiency, bilingual/multilingual individuals, and immigrant populations [9]. Linguistically diverse communities in the United States face unique communication barriers that can exacerbate health inequities [10], making it vital to understand communication and media use patterns in these communities, including how their social media experiences may differ from those of individuals belonging to the dominant linguistic culture in the United States. We limit our analysis to US-based communities to make the discussion more focused and actionable, as differences in the social media platforms used, the larger media and policy environments, and the healthcare contexts of other countries make it difficult to draw generalizable conclusions or make meaningful comparisons. Additionally, we focus on the United States for a practical reason: while not extensive, most of the available research regarding social media use in linguistically minoritized communities has been conducted in the United States.

Importance of examining social media use among linguistically diverse communities

The lack of social media research focused on linguistically diverse communities is problematic for several reasons. First, with over 300 languages spoken, the United States is one of the most linguistically diverse countries in the world [11], and linguistically diverse communities represent a significant proportion of the population. United States Census Bureau data suggest that approximately 21.7% of the country's population speaks a language other than English at home, and 1 in 12 United States residents speaks English less than "very well" [12].

Second, certain members of linguistically diverse communities are uniquely vulnerable to negative health and communication outcomes. For example, limited English proficiency has been recognized as an important driver of health disparities [13]. Individuals with limited English proficiency may face barriers to accessing health care and understanding health information [14]. In health emergencies, they are among the most vulnerable, with a lack of information disseminated in languages other than English, low health literacy, cultural barriers, limited access to health care, and other forms of social disadvantage contributing to excess morbidity and mortality [15]. Anecdotal evidence suggests that many individuals with limited English proficiency suffered from miscommunication and a lack of health information early in the COVID-19 pandemic—particularly where public agencies did not prioritize the translation of materials and guidance about COVID-19 [16]—and that the lack of language-concordant information about COVID-19 from reputable sources may have left members of immigrant communities more susceptible to misinformation circulating on social media [17]. Because some linguistically diverse communities may have less access to resources and fewer alternative sources of accurate information [18, 19], the potential benefits, as well as the potential risks, of social media use, may be greater for these groups.

Third, understanding social media use patterns in linguistically diverse communities is essential for designing health promotion efforts that meet their needs. The limited research that exists on this topic indicates that these communities use social media for a variety of reasons, including staying connected to family and friends in their countries of origin [20] and obtaining health information [21, 22]. Social media could therefore be a promising way to reach these populations, but nuances and patterns of use must be considered for these efforts to be truly effective. For example, a study examining the experiences of Chinese American adolescents with health information on social networking sites found that they use sites popular with American adolescents (e.g., Facebook, Twitter, Instagram, and Snapchat) as well as sites originating in China (e.g., QQ, WeChat, and Weibo) and encounter health information regarding a variety of topics on these sites, including culturally specific health information based on traditional Chinese medicine [21]. Based on these findings, the authors suggest that to successfully reach immigrant groups, culturally tailored, language-concordant messages should be disseminated through the various platforms used by the target population [21]. Although disseminating culturally appropriate messages in channels preferred by the intended audience is a longstanding principle of effective health communication, the ease of transnational—and thus also multilingual—information flows, means that health communicators must consider non-US-based social networks in addition to platforms that are widely used by the general US population.

Additional studies point to the importance of considering factors such as acculturation (the process of adapting to a new culture), nativity (place of birth), and cultural identity (how individuals define themselves in relation to the cultural groups to which they belong) in understanding platform preference and social media use in linguistically diverse communities. For example, a study examining Latinx adolescents' social media utilization found differences by acculturation, with use of YouTube and Instagram increasing over the study period, particularly among more acculturated youth [23]. Similarly, a qualitative interview study conducted with Chinese and Vietnamese young adults found differences in platform use based on nativity: compared to those born in the United States (22.2%), a much higher proportion of those born outside the United States (66.7%) used WeChat, while those born in the United States reported higher rates of Snapchat and Instagram use [24].

More work is clearly needed to better understand the impact of social media use on the health and well-being of linguistically diverse populations and to identify ways to leverage social media to promote the health of these communities while protecting them from harm. To that end, this chapter considers the potential risks and benefits of social media use for those in the United States who speak a language other than English and proposes a set of future directions for research and practice.

Critical issues and topics

Social media has the potential to benefit linguistically diverse communities by increasing access to health information, creating opportunities for the exchange of social support, and enabling the implementation of low-cost health promotion interventions. However, social media use can also expose individuals to harm-promoting content, misinformation, hate speech, or discriminatory language. Evidence suggests that social media platforms dedicate fewer resources to content moderation in languages other than English, which leaves individuals who speak these languages more vulnerable to problematic content and threatens to further exacerbate health disparities.

Benefits of social media for linguistically diverse communities

Health information access

Individuals who speak languages other than English face barriers to accessing health information [25, 26], and research suggests that social media can be an effective tool for disseminating health information to linguistically diverse communities. Several initiatives conducted during the COVID-19 pandemic illustrate the utility of social media for reaching linguistically diverse communities during public health emergencies. For example, an effort spearheaded by the Ironbound Initiative aimed to disseminate information to Latinx immigrants in Newark, New Jersey through social media during the pandemic, as relevant information was "seldom disseminated in Spanish and even less frequently in Portuguese" [25]. The initiative provided general in-language medical guidance through the organization's Instagram and Facebook accounts as well as more individualized guidance through WhatsApp to community members who needed support navigating a COVID-19 diagnosis [25]. Another initiative focused on Spanish-speaking cattle feed yard workers, a population that faces unique occupational safety and health risks, has limited access to healthcare and social services, and contends with significant challenges related to language barriers [27, 28]. Due to COVID-19 social distancing requirements, the Central States Center for Agricultural Safety and Health had to rely on social media to reach these vulnerable workers during the pandemic, instead of more traditional face-to-face outreach [27]. Responding to the need for reliable, trusted information on COVID-19 prevention in the community, the organization developed two Spanish-language infographics and disseminated them through boosted Facebook posts and by asking individuals that regularly engage with these workers (e.g., staff from the migrant education program and bilingual Extension professionals) to share the posts [27]. These infographics reached over 54 000 people and garnered nearly 3000 engagements, whereas an English-language COVID-19 post from the organization that was also boosted during the same period received far less engagement, indicating that there is a receptive audience and a need for Spanish-language safety and health information on social media [27].

In addition to disseminating information to vulnerable communities during a public health emergency, social media can also be a useful tool for providing prevention, treatment, and chronic disease management education to linguistically diverse communities. For example, a recent study explored the utility of using a YouTube video in Cantonese to provide health information about palliative care to Chinese speakers in the United States [29]. The video garnered 1594 views over the span of five years, demonstrating the viability of this approach [29]. A study by Lam and Woo [30], which tested Facebook ads as a method to promote an educational YouTube video about fall prevention to Chinese-speaking adults, provides further support for the feasibility of reaching Chinese speakers through social media. The results of the study suggest that Facebook may be a promising tool for health education outreach in this population due to its ability to directly target ads to the desired group (i.e., older Chinese adults) at relatively low cost (the total cost of running the advertisement for 48 hours was $6.82, the advertisement received a total of 1087 impressions, and there were 121 clicks on the YouTube video link, for a click-through rate of 11.13% and a cost per link click of $0.06). Although these studies demonstrate the feasibility of reaching this population through social media, additional research is needed to assess whether these approaches are ultimately effective in changing behavior and improving health outcomes.

A different approach to information dissemination via social media that leverages some of the unique features of these platforms is illustrated by a study from Bonnevie and colleagues [31], which assessed the feasibility of promoting flu vaccination to African American and Hispanic populations through social media influencers (individuals who have built a credible reputation and a sizeable following on social media). The researchers posited that influencers could successfully communicate health information, as they already use the language and style of speech of the target audience [31]. As part of the campaign, micro-influencers (those who had between 500 and 10 000 followers and were popular with members of the target communities) were asked to choose from a set of vetted messages about flu vaccination and create their own original, user-generated content in either English or Spanish. Overall, the campaign was successful at increasing vaccination in the target communities, but it is particularly notable that Spanish-language posts were found to have especially high engagement rates, with 20 000 engagements across a potential reach of 1.5 million (compared to 50 000 engagements across a potential reach of 8.4 million for English-language posts). The authors suggest that the higher rate of engagement may be due to the fact that Spanish-speaking individuals are less accustomed to seeing health information presented in their native language and in a style that resonates with them and are therefore more motivated to engage with the influencer content [31].

Although the use of influencers is still relatively limited in public health practice, research is beginning to show their health promotion potential, as they are able to achieve high levels of engagement from target audiences [31]. Micro-influencers, especially, could be effective messengers as they may be perceived as trusted friends or aspirational peers rather than celebrities [31]. In contrast to more traditional approaches to health communication, where content is created by experts and social media simply serves as a channel for dissemination, approaches that involve collaboration with influencers who already have an established audience in the target community can enable health messaging to be tailored and disseminated to linguistically diverse populations in a more organic way.

Intervention delivery

Social media platforms also present opportunities for delivering health interventions to linguistically diverse populations, thereby giving groups who may face barriers to participating in traditional in-person programs a chance to benefit. A study by Chalela et al. [32] offers an illustrative example: the research team built a Facebook chat application ("Quitxt") designed to provide a linguistically and culturally appropriate smoking cessation service for Spanish-speaking young adults in South Texas—a group that is generally underserved and has limited access to traditional cessation services. Over 2300 young adult Spanish-speaking cigarette smokers responded to Facebook ads for the Quitxt service between December 30, 2019, and January 8, 2020. After setting a quit date, Quitxt participants received daily messages appropriate to their phase of the cessation process from the service. Of the 926 individuals who were ready to "quit tomorrow," 11.3% reported being tobacco free at the one-week follow-up, and 3.1% reported the same at the four-week follow-up. Among the 947 enrollees who set a quit date within two weeks, 2.8% reported being tobacco free at one-week follow-up, and 1.3% reported being tobacco free at four weeks. These results suggest that social media chat applications may help prompt quit attempts and achieve short-term cessation among young adult Spanish-speaking smokers. In addition, results showing that the Quitxt messenger chat was well received and generated high levels of enrollment (particularly among Spanish-speaking young adult males) indicates that the service meets a need for smoking cessation services in this population [32].

Although the Quitxt service was entirely digital, social media can also help enhance more traditional, in-person interventions that serve linguistically diverse populations.

For example, the Avance Center for the Advancement of Immigrant/Refugee Health used social media to increase engagement with "Adelante," a primary prevention program designed to address factors contributing to substance use, risky sexual behavior, and interpersonal violence among Latinx immigrant adolescents in Langley Park, Maryland [33]. An analysis of the "Adelante" Facebook page, which served as a social media extension of in-person programming, showed that there was higher engagement with posts that were either bilingual or in Spanish, and this supported the importance of using a mixed-language strategy for the content, as most of the participants were immigrant youth and there was diversity within the target population in terms of primary language spoken [33]. Based on their results, the authors recommended that programs targeting youth include social media efforts that intersect with in-person programming in order to enhance engagement and reach those in the broader community who may face barriers to participation in traditional health programs (e.g., recently arrived immigrants) [33].

Research participation

In addition to increasing access to health promotion programs, social media can also facilitate greater participation in research by members of linguistically diverse communities who are often underrepresented in studies. For example, Martinez and colleagues [34] explored the potential of using social media, in addition to more traditional outreach (e.g., distributing recruitment materials through community-based organizations) to enroll gay Latino couples into an HIV intervention adaptation study – noting that relatively little research had been conducted on social media use among primarily Spanish-speaking Latino men who have sex with men. Based on their experience, the authors conclude that culturally appropriate outreach efforts on social media can be an effective way to recruit members of this "hard to reach" population [34].

Working with other linguistically diverse populations similarly demonstrates the potential utility of social media to support recruitment efforts. For example, a 2019 study found that encouraging African immigrant women to use WhatsApp to share information about a community-based cancer prevention study improved recruitment yield because it leveraged preexisting social bonds and fit into existing information-sharing norms within the community, as the target population already used WhatsApp to disseminate news and health information [35]. A study exploring the feasibility of using Facebook ads in English, simplified Chinese, traditional Chinese, Korean, and Spanish to recruit cancer survivors for psychosocial research also found the Facebook campaign to be a feasible recruitment strategy [36].

Social support and social capital

Social media use can also benefit members of linguistically diverse communities by enabling the exchange of social support and the provision of social capital, both of which are associated with better health outcomes [37, 38]. A 2018 interview study conducted with both recent and long-term immigrants showed that social media platforms can help immigrants address a range of needs (e.g., financial, cultural, and settlement) [39]. Participants reported that they used private groups on WeChat and WhatsApp, as well as public groups (e.g., on Facebook), to connect with individuals who share their cultural or ethnic background and that these groups helped them form connections and access information and resources such as used goods and transportation assistance. Several participants highlighted the fact that resources were easily exchanged within these groups because there were no language barriers [39]. Social media platforms like Facebook also facilitated immigrants' connection to the larger communities in which they lived – mainly by providing information about events that afforded them opportunities for offline social encounters. This finding is significant, as research shows that such engagement builds connections to the native-born population and helps immigrants thrive in a new country [39].

Social media can also increase resilience in immigrant communities, as demonstrated by a survey study examining the use of WeChat groups by Chinese–Americans in Houston, Texas to disseminate disaster relief information and coordinate recovery activities after Hurricane Harvey in 2017 [40]. Respondents reported using the groups to share and receive hurricane-related information, obtain or offer resources and aid (e.g., childcare, recommendations for specific services), and provide comfort to group members who suffered due to the hurricane [40]. The dynamics of user interactions and group formation on platforms like WeChat allow users to build social connections and mobilize social capital, which can be vital for immigrants and other marginalized communities who may otherwise face barriers to accessing the kinds of social capital that are most functional in natural disaster situations [40].

Finally, social media can also be a way for both minority groups and the broader community to engage in activism, express solidarity, and fight against prejudice [41]. For example, during the COVID-19 pandemic, hashtags like #IAmNotAVirus sought to counter racist rhetoric and support Asian communities that have been stigmatized and unfairly blamed for spreading or causing COVID-19 [42]. Notably, versions of this hashtag exist in several languages (e.g., #NoSoyUnVirus, #JeNeSuisPasUnVirus), enabling the campaign to have a global reach and allowing linguistically diverse communities to participate, express solidarity, and receive support.

Risks of social media for linguistically diverse communities

Promotion of harmful behaviors

In contrast to noted benefits, social media use can also entail risks for members of linguistically diverse communities. One concern is that content on social media may promote behaviors that are detrimental to health. A mixed-methods study examining how Russian speakers on Instagram discuss orthorexia nervosa, an eating disorder characterized by a pathological fixation on healthy eating, is illustrative [43]. The study highlights the dual effect of Instagram, noting that the platform has the potential to both trigger the onset of eating disorders (e.g., by promoting specific diets, unrealistic beauty ideals) and support recovery (e.g., by raising awareness of eating disorders and disseminating recovery advice [43]). The authors note that the popularity of dieting for health purposes is growing on Russian-language social media, with content about "healthy lifestyle" and "correct eating" proliferating on platforms like Instagram [43]. Individuals interacting with Russian language posts on social media platforms may therefore be increasingly exposed to content that promotes harmful eating patterns.

An analysis of pro-anorexia Tumblr posts containing Spanish in their hashtags or captions suggests that individuals interacting with Spanish-language content on social media platforms might encounter similar issues [44]. The authors note that although

Hispanic individuals use social media platforms like Tumblr at high rates, there is a gap in the literature around Spanish-language content in the pro-anorexia community online, as well as a lack of awareness regarding pro-anorexia terms in Spanish, which can hinder efforts to address the problem in this community [44]. The analysis highlights some of the "hidden hashtags" used by Spanish language speakers on Tumblr to evade restrictions imposed by social media platforms (such as #princesasanaymia). Studies suggest that platform content moderation efforts on this topic are flawed even for English-language content, as users often attempt to circumvent restrictions by using alternative spellings for keywords or hashtags [45], requiring platforms to regularly update their algorithms to keep pace [46]. However, if researchers and platforms are paying less attention to pro-anorexia terms in languages other than English, users from those language communities are likely to be even less protected from exposure to harm-promoting content than English speakers.

Exposure to misinformation

Linguistically diverse communities similarly lack adequate protection against misinformation. Recent reports suggest that the quality of misinformation monitoring and moderation on social media platforms is worse for non-English-language content, which may put users who speak other languages at greater risk of misinformation exposure [47, 48]. For instance, an investigation from *The Wall Street Journal* highlights the "language gap" on Facebook, noting that the company's internal documents suggest that it does not have enough employees who speak relevant languages to adequately monitor harmful content in those languages and that despite Facebook's content moderation and enforcement strategy relying on artificial-intelligence systems, the platform failed to build classifiers that could identify and/or remove problematic posts in many languages that are used on the site [47]. Furthermore, even when moderators and classifiers ostensibly exist for a given language, Facebook may not have sufficient resources dedicated to moderating all the dialects of that language. For example, Arabic is spoken by millions of Facebook users, but most of the platform's Arabic-language content reviewers speak Moroccan Arabic and are often unable to properly monitor content in other dialects [47]. Facebook's algorithms similarly fall short when it comes to handling different dialects [47]. Although much of the discourse on this topic tend to focus on the negative consequences that can occur in developing countries when platforms fail to act on false information in non-English languages, it should be noted that many individuals with ties to those countries who reside in the United States can also be exposed to, and therefore harmed by, foreign language misinformation that platforms fail to identify and remove.

Studies show that a substantial amount of health misinformation is circulating on social media platforms in languages other than English. For example, an analysis of the most viewed Spanish language YouTube videos about flu vaccines identified misinformation in 19% of the videos in the sample, with videos suggesting that flu vaccines are not safe, claiming that the vaccines are ineffective and just a way for pharmaceutical companies to make money, promoting alternatives remedies, or suggesting that the vaccines actually spread the flu [49]. Similarly, an analysis conducted in December 2020 examining Spanish language tweets containing the hashtag/phrase "yo no me vacuno" (I do not get vaccinated) identified a high proportion of anti-vaccine tweets (31%) and conspiracy theory tweets (17%) that discussed adverse effects, indicated that COVID-19 vaccines were ineffective, suggested that vaccination campaigns were a government effort to help the pharmaceutical industry increase profits, promoted alternative treatments, and even suggested that COVID-19 vaccines would manipulate the human genetic code [50]. These findings are particularly concerning given that Hispanic populations in the United States have high rates of social media use [22], which may increase their likelihood of exposure.

In addition to studies documenting a substantial amount of Spanish-language misinformation on social media, a qualitative study by Rivera and colleagues [22] shows that Spanish speakers in the United States are interacting with health misinformation on these platforms and that this exposure could be influencing their health-related decisions. In this study, 20 Latinx Facebook users were interviewed about the cancer-related information they had engaged with on Facebook over the previous year. In addition to finding that the majority of participants engaged with content in Spanish, the researchers observed that much of the content participants engaged with came from unreliable sources, featured sensationalist titles, and promoted natural remedies that have little empirical support [22]. Although many of the participants did not necessarily believe the curative claims of these posts, and advice to eat certain traditional foods is unlikely to be particularly detrimental even if the claims about their health benefits are not evidence-based, the study did highlight potentially more serious harms that might result from exposure to cancer-related misinformation. For example, a woman who had previously been adherent to screening recommendations reported canceling her mammography appointment after seeing a video on Facebook claiming that mammograms cause cancer [22].

This research suggests that exposure to health misinformation among linguistically diverse communities is occurring and that it has the potential to cause serious adverse consequences. What makes this situation, especially concerning is that in addition to being less protected against misinformation on social media, these communities may also lack access to sources of credible information in their native language. A recent article on misinformation in the Vietnamese–American community noted that in the absence of credible news channels that broadcast in Vietnamese, many people (particularly those who are older and have limited English proficiency) turn to Vietnamese-language YouTube channels and Facebook live streams that often contain misinformation [18]. Although there have been some efforts to address misinformation in this community—including a volunteer-led project to fact-check misinformation called "Viet Fact Check" and an effort to translate news articles from reputable media outlets into Vietnamese—these initiatives often operate on a smaller scale and face significant challenges, such as harassment from those who spread misinformation [18]. Similarly, Chinese Americans with limited English proficiency have few media options available to them, and may therefore rely on WeChat microblogging spaces (or "outlets") for news, where they are in danger of coming across misinformation [51]. Again, the modest Chinese-language fact-checking efforts that exist on this platform are largely volunteer-led and likely insufficient given that WeChat has over 1.2 billion users [52]. Thus, linguistically diverse communities are both more vulnerable to misinformation and have fewer resources available to mitigate its harms.

Another major challenge to addressing misinformation in linguistically diverse communities is that much of the dissemination occurs via private messaging apps (e.g., WhatsApp), which diaspora communities rely on more heavily than the general US population, using them to stay in touch with loved ones in their country of origin as well as members of their community in the United States [53]. Misinformation might originate on social media platforms like Facebook or YouTube but subsequently moves to closed groups, which are harder to monitor and harder to intervene in [52, 54], particularly if messages are encrypted. In addition, any warning labels that might be applied to misinformation on platforms like Facebook or Twitter do not travel with the post when it is shared on messaging apps [52], allowing misinformation to have a second life in chat groups, even after it has supposedly been "addressed" on other platforms. The social context and particular features of messaging apps may increase their ability to effectively spread misinformation. For example, groups in these apps are largely built around existing, trusted networks and relationships, which could lead users to apply less scrutiny to information being shared in these spaces [52]. Additionally, the way these apps are designed deemphasizes the source of the content, making fact-checking more difficult, and leading users to make judgments regarding the credibility of information based on the trustworthiness of the person who shared the information, rather than by scrutinizing the source of the information or considering evidence supporting the claim [55].

Amplification of hate speech and discriminatory language

In addition to hosting content that promotes harmful health behaviors or propagates unverified health claims, social media can also negatively impact members of linguistically marginalized communities by serving as a channel for hateful or discriminatory speech [42]. Social media can therefore harm members of targeted communities directly by exposing them to distressing content (particularly if they also speak English), or indirectly, by normalizing discrimination and abuse, which could spill over into real-world hostility against members of these vulnerable groups [56]. A time series analysis conducted during the 2016 election found that increased negative sentiment toward Hispanics on Twitter was followed one week later by an increase in reported daily worry among Hispanic individuals in a national poll [56]. Although the data used in the study represent population-level aggregates (and therefore causality cannot be inferred), the results do point to an association between these phenomena that needs to be further explored. Even if content on social media simply reflects discriminatory offline attitudes and behaviors, rather than causing them, monitoring social media content could be useful as an early warning system for shifts in real-world sentiment that might threaten vulnerable communities [56].

However, the possibility that social media platforms may be shaping antagonistic attitudes toward immigrants and other linguistically diverse communities by creating spaces where xenophobic, racist, and nationalistic discourse can flourish [57] is particularly concerning and warrants greater attention. A survey conducted during the COVID-19 pandemic provides some support for the notion that social media use among Caucasian (white) Americans is associated with prejudice toward other groups. The study found that white Americans who did not use social media on a daily basis were less likely to perceive Chinese people as a "symbolic threat" than those who used Facebook daily and that the more white individuals felt that their preferred social media site is fair, accurate, present the facts, and is concerned about the public, the more likely they were to believe that Chinese people pose a symbolic and realistic threat [41].

To date, most studies on hate speech and discrimination online have focused on racial discrimination or anti-immigrant sentiment, rather than content targeting linguistically diverse communities specifically, but in many cases speaking a language other than

English intersects with characteristics such as immigration status, religious affiliation, and race, which makes these communities vulnerable to the negative effects of discrimination based on many different factors. More research is therefore needed to establish whether and how linguistically diverse communities are being harmed by discriminatory or hateful social media content, and whether this content is exacerbating discrimination and negative sentiment against these groups in the real world.

Recommendations for practice and research

Practice

The issues discussed in the previous section point to a number of practical measures that could be taken to help ensure that social media promotes equity and improves the health and well-being of linguistically diverse communities. First, more resources need to be devoted to moderating potentially harmful content in languages other than English on these platforms. This is particularly important because linguistically diverse communities might not have as many high-quality sources of information or services available to them in their native language and may therefore rely on social media to a greater extent. Dedicated content moderation teams composed of people who are familiar with the language, culture, history, and context of these communities (and are therefore capable of understanding the nuances and implied meanings of posts) could be particularly effective [18]. Beyond expanding content moderation capacity, ensuring clarity, transparency, and equitable application of content moderation policies across different languages will also be critical.

Community-based efforts are also needed. For example, public health practitioners and health care professionals could partner with community organizations and trusted local leaders to disseminate accurate, culturally appropriate information to the target population [52]. Digital literacy interventions that train community members to recognize false information and encourage the use of trustworthy sources could also help reduce vulnerability to misinformation and other harmful content in linguistically diverse communities. Additionally, supporting fact-checking efforts and high-quality journalism in these communities could help mitigate harm from exposure to problematic social media content. Existing fact-checking efforts in these communities are generally small and volunteer-led and are likely insufficient to fully address the existing need. In addition to bolstering these language-specific efforts, partnerships with larger fact-checking organizations to translate their work into additional languages could make these services more accessible to members of linguistically diverse communities.

Ethnic media and other institutions serving linguistically diverse communities can also contribute to these efforts by providing their audiences with high-quality information and debunking falsehoods, such as when Chinese-language media outlets based in New York stopped a rumor that was spreading about COVID-19 at a local supermarket by reporting on a news conference that was held to provide accurate information to the community [58]. However, as people increasingly get their news from social media rather than traditional media [58], interventions delivered through social media platforms are needed to complement traditional media efforts. For example, in-language YouTube videos that correct rumors and provide accurate information about a health topic are more likely to reach individuals who are already watching videos about that topic on the platform.

Finally, it is important to acknowledge that social media use can benefit linguistically diverse populations, and more efforts are needed to leverage social media's potential to improve health and well-being in these communities. Several studies have shown that social media can be used to reach hard-to-reach populations [34] and deliver health promotion interventions to linguistically diverse populations who may face barriers to participating in other types of programs [32]. As linguistically diverse communities are traditionally underserved, how best to leverage social media to provide education, services, and resources to these populations deserves further attention.

Research

There are several research gaps that will need to be addressed to advance knowledge regarding the impact of social media on linguistically diverse populations and to inform strategies for mitigating harm and increasing benefit from social media use in these communities. First, there is a need for improved surveillance of the information ecosystems that linguistically diverse communities are situated in. Surveys, interviews, content analyses, and other methods can enable better understanding of how social media is used in these communities and inform efforts to mitigate harm and promote health on these platforms. Increasing the linguistic diversity of research teams, collaborating with researchers from other countries, and partnering with diaspora communities themselves can help increase research capacity to monitor and analyze social media content in languages other than English, and on the specific platforms that are used by linguistically diverse communities.

Second, there is a need to use the knowledge gained from communication surveillance efforts and observational research to develop and test social media interventions for linguistically diverse populations. Researchers need to identify effective ways to combat misinformation in these communities and test effective dissemination strategies to ensure that accurate information reaches groups that may be uniquely vulnerable because of language and health access barriers. Understanding how and why these communities use social media could also enhance community-based outreach and recruitment efforts, thereby facilitating research that tests both online and offline interventions with linguistically diverse populations. It is also important to ensure that any advances in social media research and intervention equitably benefit non-English-speaking populations. For instance, if efforts to automatically detect individuals experiencing health problems like depression or suicidal ideation on social media only focus on English-language posts [59], speakers of other languages may not equally benefit from any ensuing interventions that are developed based on this work.

Finally, there is a need to consider a broad range of linguistically diverse communities to ensure no groups are overlooked. For example, although this chapter has mostly focused on communities that utilize spoken languages other than English, it is important to note that individuals who rely on sign language to communicate constitute a relatively large, and largely overlooked, linguistic community. Additional social media research and intervention efforts focused on this population are needed, as the limited studies that exist on deaf/hard-of-hearing adults suggest that they face more barriers to accessing information, and are more likely to use social media for news, than those who are hearing [60]. Researchers have noted that the multimodal delivery capabilities of social media platforms like YouTube could improve health information access for deaf users, but that further efforts are needed to make content on these platforms useful for individuals who mainly rely on American Sign Language (ASL) [61]. Additionally, there are many research gaps concerning the use and impact of social media in this community that need to be addressed. For example, we are unaware of any studies that have specifically looked at misinformation content in ASL or exposure to misinformation among ASL users; therefore, the scale of the problem in this community is currently unknown.

Conclusion

Members of linguistically diverse communities often face barriers to accessing resources, health information, and services through traditional channels, which both suggest that they may stand to substantially benefit from social media use and that they may be uniquely vulnerable to the negative impacts of social media. However, as the focus of most social media research to date has been on English-language content on platforms that are most popular in Western countries, little is currently known about how populations that speak languages other than English use social media, or how this use impacts their health. The limited research that exists on social media use among immigrant populations in the United States suggests that these platforms can be successfully leveraged to recruit individuals for research, disseminate health-related information, and deliver health promotion interventions; however, additional research on use patterns and preferences of different language groups will likely be necessary to make these efforts truly effective. More work is needed to understand the preferred platforms of different groups, why and how these platforms are used for health-related communication and decision-making, the types of information being shared, and the impact of social media use on the well-being of these populations.

Concerningly, evidence also suggests that linguistically diverse communities may be less protected against harmful content on social media due to inadequate moderation efforts in languages other than English, highlighting the need to mount interventions to protect these users and mitigate the impacts of exposure at the population level. More work is needed to identify successful strategies for reaching linguistically diverse groups with high-quality health information through social media or through partnerships with trusted community organizations, and greater efforts to monitor hate speech and discriminatory language on social media are needed to ensure that resources to mitigate harm can be rapidly deployed when necessary [56].

Highlights

- Because linguistically diverse communities in the United States face barriers to accessing health information, resources, and services through traditional channels, the potential benefits (as well as the potential risks) of social media use may be greater for these groups.
- Social media has the potential to benefit linguistically diverse communities by increasing access to health information, creating opportunities for the exchange of social support, and enabling the implementation of low-cost health promotion interventions; however, social media can also expose individuals from these communities to harm-promoting content, misinformation, and hate speech.

- Several measures could be taken to protect linguistically diverse communities from harm related to social media use, such as improving content moderation in languages other than English on social media platforms, implementing digital literacy interventions that train individuals to recognize false information, and supporting fact-checking efforts, high-quality journalism, and health communication efforts in these communities.
- The focus of social media research to date has been on English-language content on platforms that are popular in Western countries, and consequently little is known about how populations that speak languages other than English use social media, or how this use impacts their health.
- There is a need for improved surveillance of the information ecosystems that linguistically diverse communities are situated in, as well as a need to develop and test social media interventions specifically for these populations.

REFERENCES

1. Chou, W.-Y.S., Gaysynsky, A., Trivedi, N., and Vanderpool, R.C. (2021). Using social media for health: national data from HINTS 2019. *J. Health Commun.* 26 (3): 184–193.
2. Pew Research Center. 2021 Social Media Fact Sheet 2021 https://www.pewresearch.org/internet/fact-sheet/social-media.
3. Paige, S.R., Stellefson, M., Chaney, B.H., and Alber, J.M. (2015). Pinterest as a resource for health information on chronic obstructive pulmonary disease (COPD): a social media content analysis. *Am. J. Health Educ.* 46 (4): 241–251.
4. Gavrila, V., Garrity, A., Hirschfeld, E. et al. (2019). Peer support through a diabetes social media community. *J. Diabetes Sci. Technol.* 13 (3): 493–497.
5. Chou, W.-Y., Prestin, A., Lyons, C., and Wen, K.-Y. (2013). Web 2.0 for health promotion: reviewing the current evidence. *Am. J. Public Health* 103 (1): e9–e18.
6. Arendt, F., Scherr, S., and Romer, D. (2019). Effects of exposure to self-harm on social media: evidence from a two-wave panel study among young adults. *New Media Soc.* 21 (11–12): 2422–2442.
7. Albarracin, D., Romer, D., Jones, C. et al. (2018). Misleading claims about tobacco products in YouTube videos: experimental effects of misinformation on unhealthy attitudes. *J. Med. Internet Res.* 20 (6): e229.
8. Suarez-Lledo, V. and Alvarez-Galvez, J. (2021). Prevalence of health misinformation on social media: systematic review. *J. Med. Internet Res.* 23 (1): e17187.
9. Attrill, S., Lincoln, M., and McAllister, S. (2017). Culturally and linguistically diverse students in speech–language pathology courses: a platform for culturally responsive services. *Int. J. Speech Lang. Pathol.* 19 (3): 309–321.
10. Ortega, P., Martínez, G., and Diamond, L. (2020). Language and health equity during COVID-19: lessons and opportunities. *J. Health Care Poor Underserved* 31 (4): 1530–1535.
11. Ang, C. (2021). *Ranked: The Countries with the most Linguistic Diversity*. World Economic Forum https://www.weforum.org/agenda/2021/03/these-are-the-top-ten-countries-for-linguistic-diversity.
12. U.S. Census Bureau. 2021 *Why We Ask Questions About... Language Spoken at Home* 2021 https://www.census.gov/acs/www/about/why-we-ask-each-question/language.
13. Espinoza, J. and Derrington, S. (2021). How should clinicians respond to language barriers that exacerbate health inequity? *AMA J. Ethics* 23 (2): 109–116.
14. Healthy People 2030 (n.d.). *Language and Literacy: Office of Disease Prevention and*

Health Promotion. U.S. Department of Health and Human Services. https://health.gov/healthypeople/objectives-and-data/social-determinants-health/literature-summaries/language-and-literacy (accessed 14 August 2023).

15. D'Ambrosio, L., Huang, C.E., and Kwan-Gett, T.S. (2014). Evidence-based communications strategies: NWPERLC response to training on effectively reaching limited English-speaking (LEP) populations in emergencies. *J. Public Health Manag. Pract.* 20: S101–S106.

16. Velasquez, D., Uppal, N., and Perez, N. (2020). *Equitable Access to Health Information for Non-English Speakers Amidst the Novel Coronavirus Pandemic.* Health Affairs Blog.

17. Ross, J., Diaz, C.M., and Starrels, J.L. (2020). The disproportionate burden of COVID-19 for immigrants in the Bronx, New York. *JAMA Intern. Med.* 180 (8): 1043–1044.

18. Lý, J.K. (2021). *Young Vietnamese Americans Say Their Parents Are Falling Prey To Conspiracy Videos*. BuzzFeed News https://www.buzzfeednews.com/article/katejohnston2/vietnamese-american-youtube-misinformation-covid-vaccine.

19. Chen, X., Acosta, S., and Barry, A.E. (2016). Evaluating the accuracy of Google translate for diabetes education material. *JMIR Diab.* 1 (1): e5848.

20. Hong, Y.A., Juon, H.-S., and Chou, W.-Y.S. (2021). Social media apps used by immigrants in the United States: challenges and opportunities for public health research and practice. *Mhealth* 7: 52.

21. Zhang, N., Teti, M., Stanfield, K., and Campo, S. (2017). Sharing for health: a study of Chinese adolescents' experiences and perspectives on using social network sites to share health information. *J. Transcult. Nurs.* 28 (4): 423–429.

22. Rivera, Y.M., Moran, M.B., Thrul, J. et al. (2021). When engagement leads to action: understanding the impact of Cancer (Mis) information among Latino/a Facebook users. *Health Commun.* 37: 1–13.

23. Landry, M., Vyas, A., Turner, M. et al. (2015). Evaluation of social media utilization by Latino adolescents: implications for mobile health interventions. *JMIR Mhealth Uhealth* 3 (3): e4374.

24. Cohen, C., Alber, J.M., Bleakley, A. et al. (2019). Social media for hepatitis B awareness: young adult and community leader perspectives. *Health Promot. Pract.* 20 (4): 573–584.

25. Behbahani, S., Smith, C.A., Carvalho, M. et al. (2020). Vulnerable immigrant populations in the New York metropolitan area and COVID-19: lessons learned in the epicenter of the crisis. *Acad. Med.* 95: 1827–1830.

26. Shu, S. and Woo, B.K. (2020). Digital media as a proponent for healthy aging in the older Chinese American population: longitudinal analysis. *JMIR Aging* 3 (1): e20321.

27. Ramos, A.K., Duysen, E., Carvajal-Suarez, M., and Trinidad, N. (2020). Virtual outreach: using social media to reach spanish-speaking agricultural workers during the COVID-19 pandemic. *J. Agromedicine* 25 (4): 353–356.

28. Palacios, E.E. and Sexsmith, K. (2020). *Occupational Justice for Latinx Livestock Workers in the Eastern United States. Latinx Farmworkers in the Eastern United States,* 107–131. Springer.

29. Kuang, W. and Woo, B.K. (2021). Disseminating palliative care education to Chinese Americans through social media. *Int. Psychogeriatr.* 33 (8): 843–844.

30. Lam, N.H. and Woo, B.K. (2018). Digital media recruitment for fall prevention among older Chinese-American individuals: observational, cross-sectional study. *JMIR Aging* 1 (2): e11772.

31. Bonnevie, E., Rosenberg, S.D., Kummeth, C. et al. (2020). Using social media influencers to increase knowledge and positive attitudes toward the flu vaccine. *PLoS One* 15 (10): e0240828.

32. Chalela, P., McAlister, A.L., Akopian, D. et al. (2021). Facebook chat application to prompt and assist smoking cessation among Spanish-speaking young adults in South Texas. *Health Promot. Pract.* 23: 378–381. 15248399211026263.

33. Andrade, E.L., Evans, W.D., Barrett, N. et al. (2018). Strategies to increase latino

34. Martinez, O., Wu, E., Shultz, A.Z. et al. (2014). Still a hard-to-reach population? Using social media to recruit Latino gay couples for an HIV intervention adaptation study. *J. Med. Internet Res.* 16 (4): e113.
35. Cudjoe, J., Turkson-Ocran, R.-A., Ezeigwe, A.K. et al. (2019). Recruiting African immigrant women for community-based cancer prevention studies: lessons learned from the AfroPap study. *J. Community Health* 44 (5): 1019–1026.
36. Tsai, W., Zavala, D., and Gomez, S. (2019). Using the Facebook advertisement platform to recruit Chinese, Korean, and Latinx cancer survivors for psychosocial research: web-based survey study. *J. Med. Internet Res.* 21 (1): e11571.
37. Ehsan, A., Klaas, H.S., Bastianen, A., and Spini, D. (2019). Social capital and health: a systematic review of systematic reviews. *SSM Popul. Health* 8: 100425.
38. Holt-Lunstad, J. and Uchino, B.N. (2015). Social support and health. In: *Health Behavior: Theory, Research and Practice* (ed. K. Glanz, B.K. Rimer, and K. Viswanath), 183–204. John Wiley & Sons.
39. Hsiao, J.C.-Y. and Dillahunt, T.R. (2018). Technology to support immigrant access to social capital and adaptation to a new country. *Proc. ACM Hum. Comput. Interact.* 2 (CSCW): 1–21.
40. Chu, H. and Yang, J.Z. (2020). Building disaster resilience using social messaging networks: the WeChat community in Houston, Texas, during hurricane Harvey. *Disasters* 44 (4): 726–752.
41. Croucher, S.M., Nguyen, T., and Rahmani, D. (2020). Prejudice toward Asian Americans in the COVID-19 pandemic: the effects of social media use in the United States. *Front. Commun.* 5: 39.
42. Chou, W.-Y.S. and Gaysynsky, A. (2021). Racism and xenophobia in a pandemic: interactions of online and offline worlds. *Am. J. Public Health* 111 (5): 773–775.
43. Zemlyanskaya, Y., Valente, M., and Syurina, E.V. (2021). Orthorexia nervosa and instagram: exploring the Russian-speaking conversation around# орторексия. *Eat. Weight Disord.*, Bulimia and Obesity 27: 1–10.
44. Elrod, K. and Dykeman, C. (2019). A Corpus linguistic analysis of pro-anorexia public Tumblr posts written in Spanish. *PsyArXiv* https://doi.org/10.31234/osf.io/q24p7.
45. Chancellor, S., Pater, J.A., Clear, T. et al. (ed.) (2016). # thyghgapp: Instagram content moderation and lexical variation in pro-eating disorder communities. In: *Proceedings of the 19th ACM Conference on Computer-Supported Cooperative Work & Social Computing*.
46. Subedar, A. and Whalley, J. (2018). *Instagram Tightens Eating Disorder Filters After BBC Investigation*. BBC News https://www.bbc.com/news/blogs-trending-46505704.
47. Scheck, J., Purnell, N., and Horwitz, J. (2021). Facebook employees flag drug cartels and human traffickers. The Company's response is weak, documents show. *Wall Street J.* https://www.wsj.com/articles/facebook-drug-cartels-human-traffickers-response-is-weak-documents-11631812953.
48. AVAAZ (2020). *How Facebook Can Flatten the Curve of the Coronavirus Infodemic*. AVAAZ https://secure.avaaz.org/campaign/en/facebook_coronavirus_misinformation/ (accessed 14 August 2023).
49. Hernández-García, I. and Giménez-Júlvez, T. (2021). YouTube as a source of influenza vaccine information in Spanish. *Int. J. Environ. Res. Public Health* 18 (2): 727.
50. Herrera-Peco, I., Jiménez-Gómez, B., Romero Magdalena, C.S. et al. (2021). Antivaccine movement and COVID-19 negationism: a content analysis of Spanish-written messages on twitter. *Vaccine* 9 (6): 656.
51. Fang, J. (2021). *Social Media Sites Popular With Asian Americans Have a Big Misinformation Problem*. PRISM https://prismreports.org/2021/05/26/social-media-sites-often-used-by-asian-americans-have-a-big-problem-with-right-wing-misinformation.
52. Zhang, S. and Chan, E. (2020). *It's Crucial to Understand How Misinformation Flows Through Diaspora Communities*. First Draft.

53. Gursky, J., Riedl, M.J., and Woolley, S. (2021). *The Disinformation Threat to Diaspora Communities in Encrypted Chat Apps*. Brookings TechStream https://www.brookings.edu/techstream/the-disinformation-threat-to-diaspora-communities-in-encrypted-chat-apps.
54. Valencia, S. (2021). *Misinformation Online is Bad in English. But it's Far Worse in Spanish*. The Washington Post https://www.washingtonpost.com/outlook/2021/10/28/misinformation-spanish-facebook-social-media.
55. Guo, E. (2017). *How WeChat Spreads Rumors, Reaffirms Bias, and Helped Elect Trump*. Wired.
56. Hswen, Y., Qin, Q., Williams, D.R. et al. (2020). Online negative sentiment towards Mexicans and Hispanics and impact on mental well-being: a time-series analysis of social media data during the 2016 United States presidential election. *Heliyon* 6 (9): e04910.
57. Ekman, M. (2019). Anti-immigration and racist discourse in social media. *Eur. J. Commun.* 34 (6): 606–618.
58. Fuchs, C. (2020). *How Chinese-Language Media in U.S. are Debunking WeChat Coronavirus Misinformation*. NBC News https://www.nbcnews.com/news/asian-america/how-chinese-language-media-u-s-are-debunking-wechat-coronavirus-n1156621.
59. Leis, A., Ronzano, F., Mayer, M.A. et al. (2019). Detecting signs of depression in tweets in Spanish: behavioral and linguistic analysis. *J. Med. Internet Res.* 21 (6): e14199.
60. Panko, T.L., Contreras, J., Postl, D. et al. (2021). The deaf Community's experiences navigating COVID-19 pandemic information. *Health Lit. Res. Pract.* 5 (2): e162–e170.
61. Kushalnagar, P. and Kushalnagar, R. (2018). Health-related information seeking among deaf adults: findings from the 2017 Health Information National Trends Survey in American Sign Language (HINTS-ASL). In: *eHealth: Current Evidence, Promises, Perils and Future Directions*. Emerald Publishing Limited.

26 Urgent Communication During Public Health Crises: Reaching Linguistically Diverse Populations

VICTORIA LEDFORD, A. SUSANA RAMÍREZ, AND XIAOLI NAN

Introduction

In May 2020, residents of South Korea glanced at their cellphones to find a COVID-19 emergency alert mandating COVID-19 testing and quarantine for patrons of certain LGBTQ+ friendly clubs (Figure 26.1) [1]. Though intended to promote health and safety, the message quickly garnered backlash from LGBTQ+ advocates who argued that this type of messaging could compromise the anonymity and safety of LGBTQ+ people in South Korea and might discourage COVID-19 testing or disclosure [3]. These fears were affirmed as LGBTQ+ people living in South Korea during the pandemic shared in interviews the importance of anonymous testing for safety among an already marginalized group. As advocates shared their frustrations with the government's location-specific messaging, the crisis communication message changed and listed more general affected locations rather than specific clubs. One person aptly described the root of the government's crisis communication failure and resolution: "At the beginning, the government mentioned specific clubs with specific dates. Then, they realized that some people feel uncomfortable [acknowledging that they had been at a gay club]. Instead, they called it the Itaewon neighborhood and expanded the period. Some people, who had been afraid, got tested" [2]. Unfortunately, this is neither the first nor the last time that a public health agency has or will get it wrong. Such communication requires urgency – and to communicate effectively during urgent health communication crises, we must look to our world's past and present.

One of the largest health crises to face the world in the 20th and 21st centuries, the COVID-19 pandemic has killed more than 6.2 million people, with approximately 505 million cases of the disease on record as of July 2022 [4]. Like the waves of virus

---

The Handbook of Language in Public Health and Healthcare, First Edition.
Edited by Pilar Ortega, Glenn Martínez, Maichou Lor, and A. Susana Ramírez.
© 2024 John Wiley & Sons, Inc. Published 2024 by John Wiley & Sons, Inc.

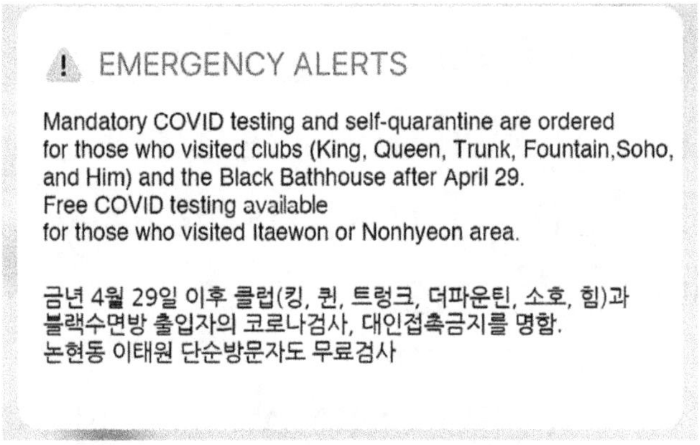

> ⚠ EMERGENCY ALERTS
>
> Mandatory COVID testing and self-quarantine are ordered for those who visited clubs (King, Queen, Trunk, Fountain, Soho, and Him) and the Black Bathhouse after April 29.
> Free COVID testing available for those who visited Itaewon or Nonhyeon area.
>
> 금년 4월 29일 이후 클럽(킹, 퀸, 트렁크, 더파운틴, 소호, 힘)과 블랙수면방 출입자의 코로나검사, 대인접촉금지를 명함.
> 논현동 이태원 단순방문자도 무료검사

Figure 26.1 South Korean Emergency COVID-19 Alert [1, 2].

variants that continue to emerge, so too have waves of crisis communication ebbed and flowed during the pandemic. Throughout this crisis, the World Health Organization (WHO) and the United States Centers for Disease Control and Prevention (CDC), along with country, state, and local health agencies have consistently needed to share timely health information related to disease transmission and symptoms, testing and contact tracing, and vaccination.

COVID-19 was not the first and will not be the last public health crisis that requires effective communication to manage; nonetheless, the unique context, duration, and scale of this pandemic offer a useful example of how communication theory and research can contribute to effective public health crisis mitigation. Using the COVID-19 pandemic as a primary example, in this chapter, we describe the challenges and strategies that health actors (e.g., medical personnel, health agencies, policymakers, and individuals) may face and use when communicating urgent information in public health crises. We first define the role of communication in public health crises, then examine the pitfalls of poor health crisis communication, offer insight into how theory can be used to guide effective crisis communication, discuss critical issues and topics, and offer recommendations for future research and practice. In each section, we offer implications for communicating with linguistically diverse communities during health crises.

Characteristics of public health crises

Public health crises require clear and effective communication, and breakdowns in communication can hinder effective responses. For example, the emergency alert in South Korea introducing this chapter emphasizes the importance of inclusive communication that considers the experiences of marginalized communities and potential negative effects even well-intentioned communication can create. The United States' response to the COVID-19 pandemic has also been criticized for its lack of urgency and its initial undermining of the risk associated with the disease [5]. In this section, we define characteristics of public health crises and describe how these characteristics affect communication strategies and their impact.

Public health emergencies, or crises, are distinct from everyday issues in that their "scale, timing, or unpredictability threaten to overwhelm routine capabilities" [6]. Crises necessitate urgent responses: communicators must share pertinent information for crisis mitigation in the hopes that the rest of us *do something* with that information. In short, communicators must consider three key elements when communicating about a public health crisis: (1) scale; (2) urgency or timing; and (3) information exchange and the potential for misinformation. Below, we describe each of these with examples from the COVID-19 pandemic.

Scale

A public health issue becomes a crisis in part because the scale of the issue is so large that the public health system cannot adequately care for all of those affected [7]. For example, COVID-19 was declared a pandemic, "an event in which a disease spreads across several countries and affects a large number of people," just three months after the first case [8, 9]. One indicator that influenced health policy change and crisis response throughout that pandemic was the number of intensive care unit (ICU) or inpatient beds available at hospitals. In addition to influencing lockdown or masking policies, this metric indicated the extent to which the pandemic stretched hospitals' capacities to uphold their standard of care for other health issues. In March 2020, the Italian Society of Anesthesia, Analgesia, Resuscitation, and Intensive Care released guidelines for physicians to use for prioritizing and rationing care [10]. Recommendations included: "When the availability of resources is overwhelmed by their need, a decision to deny access to one or more life-sustaining therapies, solely based on the principle of distributive justice, may ultimately be justified" [10]. Such a painstaking decision demonstrates why scale is an important metric for defining and responding to a public health crisis: When a crisis strikes, it is large enough to overwhelm the capacity of existing structures that can adequately address the problem.

Urgency

A second characteristic of public health crises is the necessity for urgent action – whether on the part of affected individuals (e.g., wearing masks to reduce exposure to airborne viruses), policymakers (e.g., mandating lockdowns to reduce the spread of disease), or other actors (e.g., employers allowing remote work). Regardless of the action and actor, the timeliness of response is a critical component during public health crises.

During the COVID-19 pandemic, the WHO and CDC activated emergency management processes within days following the identification of the disease [8]. However, the speed of recommended actions was uneven across countries and localities. For example, in anticipation of viral spread in early stages of the pandemic, South Korea's CDC implemented widespread drive-through COVID-19 testing, testing over 290 000 people within seven weeks of identification of the virus in South Korea. In contrast, the United States, a country with more than six times the population of South Korea [11, 12], tested only 60,000 people in the same time period [13]. Disparities in the timing of actions no doubt contributed to differential outcomes across geographies and populations.

Information exchange and the potential for misinformation

A final characteristic of public health crises is the need for governments, organizations, and citizens to exchange accurate and relevant information. Combined with the scale of the issue and the urgency of action, information exchange engenders an environment where misinformation can spread quickly and easily, undermining public health efforts.

The importance of urgent, actionable communication is clear from the United States CDC's Crisis and Emergency Risk Communication's webpage: "The right message at the right time from the right person can save lives" [14]. Yet during urgent health crises, scientific uncertainty about the disease itself creates an ever-changing information landscape. Often, at the outset of public health crises, essential information about the severity, mode of transmission, prevention strategies, and treatment options are unknown. Even as scientists race to answer these questions, officials must maintain open and regular channels of communication with their publics. Such communication is fraught with tensions: When the right message is unknown (e.g., will masks protect against COVID-19 infection?) or shared at the wrong time (e.g., the message that masks are effective in preventing COVID-19 infection was communicated after the opposing message was originally released due to mask shortages), communication itself can contribute to poor crisis management.

It is also important to recognize that official communication about public health crises occurs within a complex media environment. In the context of COVID-19, WHO and CDC messaging existed alongside news articles with titles that emphasized scientific uncertainty: "How long is COVID infectious? What scientists know so far," "COVID-19 vaccines: time to talk about the uncertainties," and "'Mix of science and politics' leading to people's uncertainty about the COVID-19 vaccine, NIH director says" [15–17]. The unknowns about viral origin, spread, and treatment led organizations to share varying degrees of information as the crisis unfolded, but the contradictory or delayed sharing of information may have contributed to online mis- and disinformation.

Even before COVID-19 was formally recognized as a pandemic by the WHO, WHO staff were addressing a corresponding pandemic: one of the spread of false information, dubbed an "infodemic" [18]. Thus, a key element in the third defining characteristic of a modern public health crisis—information exchange—is the potential for misinformation, whether intentional or not, and its impact on health behaviors and outcomes [19]. The COVID-19 pandemic was accompanied by mis- (false information unintentionally shared) and disinformation (false information intentionally created for the purpose of deception) across information sources, particularly social media. Research on COVID-19 misinformation has documented the spread of false information in large quantities on Twitter, YouTube, and Facebook [20–22]. We discuss the impacts of mis- and disinformation on health outcomes further in later sections of this chapter as well as in Chapter 25 of this volume.

Understanding the role of public health organizations in times of crises

Communicating during a public health crisis

Effective public communication by responsible agencies during crises requires recognizing the characteristics of a health crisis as they develop clear and actionable strategies for risk mitigation to the public [23]. To communicate such information effectively during a crisis, the WHO [24] advises organizations to:

- **Plan for an emergency before it occurs.** Planning includes clearly defining responsibilities for the next crisis, carefully considering the needs of and seeking input from diverse communities, establishing multiple channels for communication, training organizational members for rapid response, preparing communication materials in advance, and creating infrastructure for evaluating the effectiveness of messages.
- **Conduct research that evaluates which methods can best assess emergency risk communication interventions.** As communicators use multiple methods to study the effectiveness of risk communication strategies (e.g., focus groups, interviews, surveys, etc.), they should also dedicate resources to analyzing which methodologies and mechanisms can be most effective for such use in a rapid response environment.
- **Leverage social media for accurate and effective information sharing.** This includes pairing social media messages with traditional media, using social media to correct misinformation, and training and employing people to leverage social media for relationship building and information distribution.
- **Communicate risk clearly, consistently, and quickly.** When sharing information about risk, organizations should ensure risk is explained in easily understandable terms, avoiding jargon that can prevent people from engaging in health behaviors. Furthermore, messages should be specific and realistic, asking people to engage in behaviors they have the capacity to engage in. Health actors should also communicate quickly and distribute consistent information across multiple information sources. Both of these strategies can mitigate the potential for misinformation and rumor spread [24].

Communicating risk when the science is unclear

A key challenge during a public health crisis is communicating clearly and efficiently during situations of scientific uncertainty. This uncertainty may pertain to the most effective disease prevention behaviors (e.g., wearing a mask, and if so, what kind of mask), the nature of the disease and its transmission (e.g., understanding viral composition and transmission of new viruses), or the magnitude of risk and impact (e.g., consequences of climate change). Research suggests communicators can effectively communicate scientific uncertainty by acknowledging the uncertainty and implementing strategies to mitigate it [25–27]. Normalizing the nature of scientific uncertainty can reduce people's feelings of ambiguity about uncertain information [25]. Beyond these strategies for communicating scientific uncertainty, communicators can also employ communication theories to craft their crisis responses.

Organizational responsibility and situational crisis communication theory

An essential component of effective public health communication is trust in the messenger, so understanding and identifying trusted messengers for specific target audiences is paramount. For example, in one study assessing the effect of trust on COVID-19 vaccination intentions, researchers found that, among Native Hawaiian and Pacific Islander people, those who reported high levels of trust in official information sources were more likely to be vaccinated than those who had higher trust in unofficial sources [28]. During times of public health crises, organizations responsible for messaging about risk and mitigation strategies serve as messengers with valuable yet fragile reputations. Maintaining public trust must be a core value.

Situational crisis communication theory (SCCT) offers a framework for considering how organizations might protect their reputation during the management of a crisis [29]. In the context of a public health crisis like COVID-19, organizations like the CDC or the WHO may bear the brunt of communicating about the health crisis because they have some governing power or influence over the public health issue and response. Because a public health crisis affects most of society—and its effective mitigation requires participation from organizations across sectors—SCCT also can be used to consider potential reputational crises experienced by organizations who need to communicate operational or procedural changes to their stakeholders based on a *public health* crisis. In addition, public health crises may often necessitate organizational crisis responses, as "the first priority in any crisis is to protect stakeholders from harm, not to protect the reputation." [29, p. 165]. For example, in the first year of the COVID-19 pandemic, when there was widespread support for prevention and mitigation strategies, workers in the industries most directly affected by the travel bans and quarantine orders were considered public health heroes. When restaurants were shut down, national media provided advice on how people could help workers and keep businesses afloat [30]. However, as the pandemic lingered, and once emergency orders were lifted, organizations that opted to implement mitigation policies such as masking or vaccination faced reputational crises as a result of, or related to, their pandemic policies or communication. For example, in April 2022, when the federal government lifted the face-mask requirement for airlines, Delta Airlines responded with a statement that "We are relieved to see the United States mask mandate lift to facilitate global travel as COVID-19 has transitioned to an ordinary seasonal virus." After quick public backlash—the virus was still killing hundreds daily—the airline updated its statement and replaced its reference to COVID-19 as "ordinary seasonal virus" with language calling it a "more manageable respiratory virus" [31].

According to SCCT, response to a reputational crisis should match the amount of responsibility attributed to the organization for the crisis. Organizational response strategies fall into three categories: *deny, diminish, or rebuild* [29]. Response strategies that *deny* aim to distance the organization from any connection to or culpability for the crisis and may be used when organizational responsibility is negligible, as in the case of a rumor. For example, an organization might attack the accuser, deny the crisis altogether, or scapegoat someone else. Consider furniture company Wayfair's response to the false rumor circulated in 2020 that the organization and its products were associated with child trafficking: Given the conspiratorial and false claims, Wayfair appropriately denied the allegations [32].

Strategies that *diminish* seek to minimize the effect of the crisis (i.e., the crisis is not that severe) or the organization's role in the crisis (i.e., it is not the organization's fault) and should be used when there is low or minimal organizational responsibility. An organization might excuse its role or blame by appealing to its good intent, or might use justification to downplay the harm of the crisis. Delta's revised statement about the COVID-19 pandemic illustrates how diminishing can be used to minimize the effect of the crisis: When they revised their statement calling COVID-19 an "ordinary season virus" to a "more manageable respiratory virus," the organization did not admit culpability or issue an apology but instead made a minimal edit to their statement to downplay the role of that communication failure.

Finally, corresponding to the highest level of perceived organizational responsibility are strategies that *rebuild*. These strategies involve an organization's acceptance of responsibility and attempt to build rapport with stakeholders, through compensation, financial or otherwise, or an explicit apology for the crisis. The CDC demonstrated this strategy in August 2022 when then-Director Rochelle Wallensky admitted the organization's errors in navigating the pandemic: "For 75 years, CDC and public health have been preparing for COVID-19, and in our big moment, our performance did not reliably meet expectations" [33]. Wallensky's admission of responsibility was followed by an action plan to restructure the organization.

While these three strategy areas (deny, diminish, and rebuild) are the primary ways an organization can respond to a crisis, organizations may also wish to *bolster* their primary response by reminding people of the organization's past good works, ingratiating stakeholders with praise or continued reminders, or insinuating the organization itself is a victim of the crisis, too. These strategies offer possibilities for an organization's reputational repair. For example, as universities responded to the 2020 pandemic onset, several reaffirmed their commitment to education, reminding their stakeholders that the institution highly valued education and their decisions to shift to online learning were challenging calls that no one wanted to have to make – these universities bolstered their responses by depicting themselves as victims of the pandemic in addition to reaffirming the good of their institution (e.g., an excellent education).

In summary, SCCT can support organizations during public health crises by shedding light on and prompting reflection into elements of crisis responsibility and response. In the following section, we describe the causes and consequences of poor communication in public health crises.

When communication goes wrong: causes and consequences of poor communication in public health crises

South Korea's stigmatizing emergency alerts, the United States contradictory messages surrounding the effectiveness of mask-wearing, and the WHO's delayed communication of COVID-19 as a serious global health emergency [34] all undoubtedly worsened the harms of the pandemic. In what follows, we consider two key areas of study—news framing and misinformation—that can help us understand the causes of, consequences to, and solutions for poor communication during a health crisis.

News framing effects

As described in Chapter 21, framing is one of the most commonly used theories to explain the impact of mass media on people's perceptions. News framing specifically focuses on the lens through which mass media portray particular issues in the news. News frames present audiences with a schema, or system for understanding, for interpreting journalistic reporting [35]. Framing can shape an audience's attitudes and behaviors because of a two-way relationship between a journalist's frame and the audience's frame of reference. In other words, audiences think in schema, and media frames activate those existing schemas [36].

During crises, news media often provide us not only with what to think about news content but also *how* to think. Substantial framing research has been conducted about mass media portrayals of public health crises; much of this research uses content analysis, a method that systematically analyzes news coverage of a topic, to decipher framing. For example, a content analysis of global news media coverage early in the COVID-19 pandemic revealed that the most common frame used in global news stories was a "human interest" frame [37]. Another study compared *New York Times* coverage of three different health issues: mad cow disease, West Nile virus, and the avian flu during the late 1990s and early 2000s; across all three disease outbreak coverages, the most common frames were action, which emphasized actions individuals could take against a disease, and consequence, which discussed the impact of the disease on people or society [38]. The other major finding was that media coverage of each of these public health crises largely centered around crisis *events* such as government actions or a change in infection rates.

How we think about the problem, in turn, shapes how we think the problem can be solved. To that end, research has examined the ways that news frames affect public opinion and decision-making. News articles and other media channels may emphasize individual responsibility for a health issue or condition, or they may emphasize collective or societal responsibility. For example, in a systematic review of responsibility frames in the health context, researchers found consistent evidence that messages emphasizing societal responsibility for health led to greater support for relevant public health policies [39]. In the context of COVID-19, messages that emphasized the benefits of social distancing on communities rather than only on individuals led people to express more desire to help other people [40]. Messages emphasizing personal health risks (compared to economic and collective health risks) that come from a virologist as opposed to a (nonexpert) influencer can also positively affect people's intentions to get the COVID-19 vaccine [41]. Figure 26.2. provides an example of framing used by an organization during the COVID-19 pandemic to encourage COVID-19 vaccination.

Two key takeaways from news framing research are that (1) news framing often unintentionally leads to negative health attitudes or behaviors and (2) societal responsibility messages offer promising frames for action, though those frames may be dependent on individual and contextual factors. Furthermore, it is important to consider that news frames are linguistic markers that often require cultural and contextual interpretation. As such, framing effects may be differentially pronounced for members who may not have as strong of cultural or contextual basis for interpretation. Similarly, news outlets who communicate with linguistic minorities in their primary language may adopt similar or different framing strategies that may or may not carry the same meaning or context in another language. As such, health journalists seeking to promote consistent messaging among linguistically diverse communities may consider publishing parallel information in multiple languages.

Misinformation effects

Misinformation has plagued the COVID-19 information landscape, from questions about the origin of the virus itself to the efficacy of the vaccine. Research has documented the widespread existence of misinformation related to the pandemic, especially across social media (see Chapter 25). A practical implication of misinformation is that it takes up space that could otherwise be used for useful, actionable health communication. Moreover, misinformation has real and significant consequences for individuals'

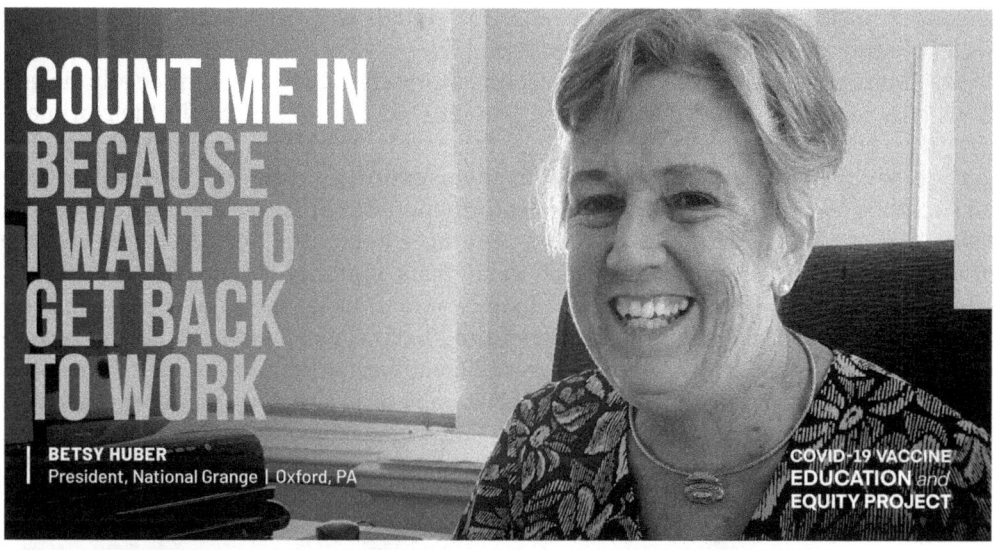
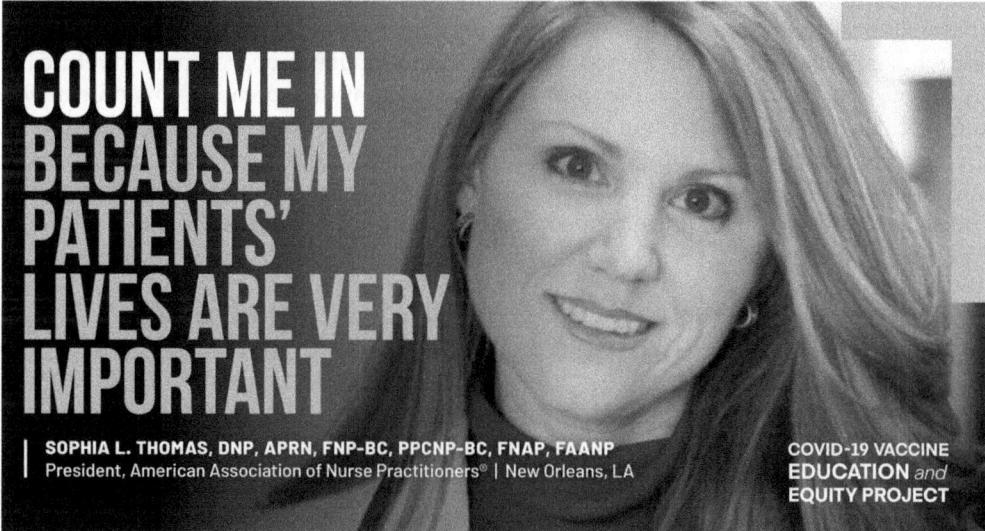

Figure 26.2 These images, part of the COVID-19 Vaccine Education and Equity Project [42] depict different frames at work in their communication strategy. Both messages aim to persuade individuals to obtain the COVID-19 vaccine but use different reasons, expressed as frames, for doing so. The top image emphasizes an economic frame by appealing to people's desire to "get back to work," whereas the bottom image emphasizes a more humanistic frame through its focus on the importance of "patients' lives." These images illustrate how frames used in news media can intentionally in health communication campaigns. Neither message is inherently "better" – but one may be more effective among a particular segment of the target audience. *Source:* COVID-19 Vaccine Education and Equity Project [42].

and the public's health. Research has suggested that people more exposed to misinformation about COVID-19 prevention behaviors were more likely to engage in unrelated behaviors (e.g., eating garlic) and simultaneously less likely to engage in evidence-based prevention behaviors like social distancing [43]. Exposure to misinformation can also engender mistrust in the institutions and individuals in whom trust is required for society to function, including the media itself [19].

For linguistically diverse populations, misinformation may have especially deleterious effects: communities may be most likely to trust news sources in their primary language, and linguistic minorities may be targeted by misinformation attacks for that very reason. For example, Spanish-language misinformation about COVID-19 spread on Facebook just as English-language misinformation, but Spanish-language posts have taken longer to be flagged or taken down than those in English [44]. Moreover, because of the generally lower levels of outreach in linguistic minority languages, underserved linguistically diverse populations may look to leaders or to message sources in their country of origin for relevant information during a crisis, which may not always be reliable, accurate, or relevant (also see Chapters 22 on information seeking and 25 on social media). Organizations must work in tandem to release accurate health information and combat misinformation in the multiple languages spoken by their constituent communities.

In light of mis- or disinformation prevalence, health communicators should consider strategies for combatting misinformation. One strategy, "pre-bunking," is based on inoculation theory, which suggests that we can inoculate people against arguments by giving them a small "dose" of an argument before they are ever exposed to the argument itself, but supplemented with a strong counterargument that prepares them to refute the argument [45]. *Pre-bunking* works to preempt or prevent the spread of misinformation and predicts that if an individual is given an argument or incorrect message along with a counterargument to refute or debunk it, the individual's susceptibility to false information will be minimized [46]. Other proposed strategies include bolstering health and science literacy and equipping people to correct misinformation [47].

Applying communication theory to develop effective communication in public health crises

Despite the potential for communication pitfalls to exacerbate public health crises, well-executed communication also plays an essential role in mitigating these failures. Health communication efforts guided by theories are more likely to be successful than those without similar grounding [48]. In the following section, we describe selected communication theories relevant to public health crises. First, we consider how framing might be intentionally applied to design public health messages and training for institutional spokespersons. We then describe two major theoretical frameworks for understanding how people make decisions about engaging in health behaviors, and how these theories may be applied to design messages to maximize impact on specific audiences.

Applying framing theory to the design of crisis response messages

Health communicators can use framing to intentionally motivate positive attitudes or behavior change, selecting among evidence-based frames that lead to prosocial or proactive health outcomes for both policy support and individual behavior change.

Societal frames may be especially useful for promoting support of policies that respond to crises. For example, emphasizing a collective responsibility to mitigate the spread of COVID-19 might be more useful for garnering policy support – and adherence to the policies – than messages that frame health behaviors as individual choices with individual consequences [49]; see Box 26.1.

Humanistic frames, which provide personal stories and emphasize the people affected by an issue, have been shown to increase engagement and positive attitudes toward the

---

Box 26.1 Case Study.

From "We take care of each other" to "You do you": New York City's Shifting Framing of Responsibility for Ending the COVID-19 Pandemic

New York City was an initial epicenter of COVID-19 infection in the United States, and consequently, one of the first localities to implement mitigation strategies [50]. By mid-2020, as part of a comprehensive plan to reopen society safely after weeks of stay-at-home orders, the city had implemented a mask mandate requiring masks on all public transport [51]. To support this policy, the Metropolitan Transport Authority (MTA) developed what would become an award-winning communication campaign, featuring clean graphics and a modern font against the MTA's signature bright yellow background.

The set of messages that launched in April 2020 and ran through mid-2022 featured educational messages instructing people not only that wearing a face covering was the law but also how to properly wear a face covering (A). The messages were simple, but they cleverly leveraged two important dimensions of public health communication: first, they used *framing* that spoke to the collective nature of infectious disease mitigation: the tagline "Stop the spread. Wear a mask." referenced the need to protect others. More directly stated, one message showed two masked people and appealed to the reciprocity needed to transcend the pandemic: "I take care of you. You take care of me." (B). These messages appealed to the sense of collective action – the spirit of "we're in this together" that characterized the early stage of the pandemic.

The second important characteristic was the use of *normative appeals* [52]: in a single message (C), they managed to convey both descriptive norms (that most people do the proscribed behavior) and injunctive norms (that people want you to do the behavior). Later, messages in this campaign emphasized respect for others displayed when wearing masks appropriately (D). This campaign was largely a success, which rates of mask adherence on public transport around 90% through 2021 [53].

But messaging alone can only do so much: even as this campaign was updating posters with seasonally appropriate and comedic versions, the larger culture surrounding the campaign was shifting and responding to concerted campaigns against not only masking but other COVID mitigation efforts. By mid-2022, reflecting the increased political polarization of the era, public health agencies around the country, from the federal government to individual counties, had essentially abandoned mandates of any type in favor of relatively weak guidance that left masking, social distancing, staying home, vaccination, and other mitigation strategies up to individuals. In New York City, masking rates on public transportation plunged and in early September 2022, Governor Kathy Hochul lifted all mask mandates. The new MTA slogan reflected an individualist approach to public health crisis mitigation: "You do you." (E) (Figure 26.3).

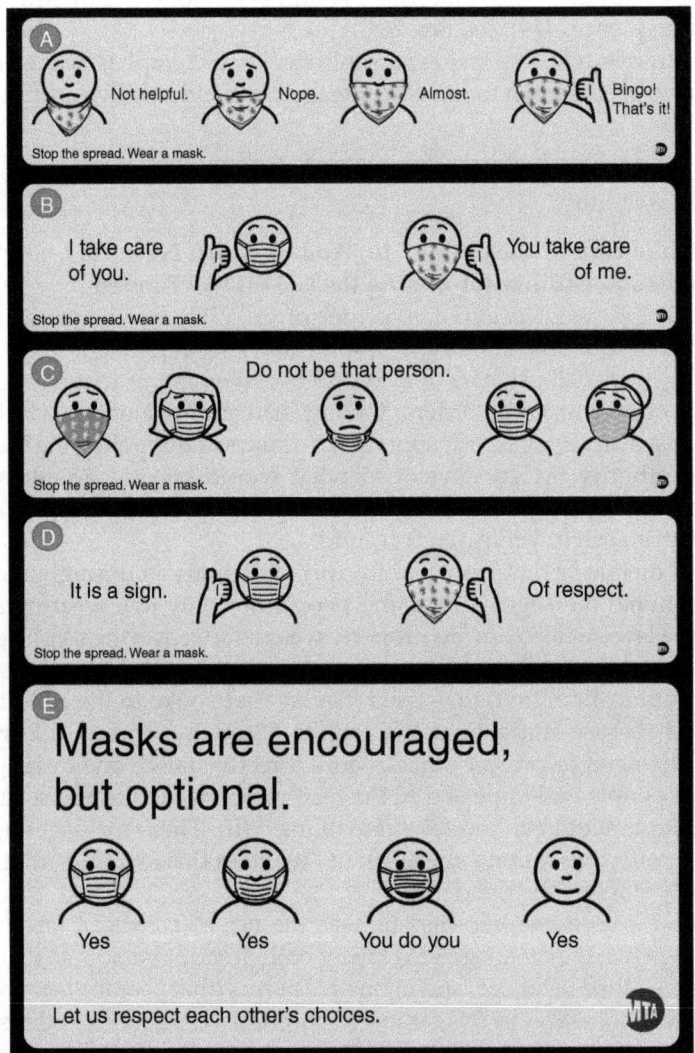

Figure 26.3 Evolution of the New York Metropolitan Transportation Agency's Messaging About Masks During the COVID-19 Pandemic, April 2020–September 2022.

relevant health solution [54]. For example, a study analyzing the role of influenza news framing on flu vaccine uptake between 2011 and 2018 found that emphasizing illness and death associated with the flu (i.e., consequence framing that increased the perceived severity of the issue) was consistently associated with greater vaccine uptake [55].

Beyond considering the use of specific frames in the design of health communication campaigns, public health actors responsible for communicating about crises should consider how they frame the issue in their interactions with news media and the public. Lessons from effective health and crisis communication should be utilized. Spokesperson training should include primers on effectively communicating scientific uncertainty, health risks, and crisis mitigation strategies. In addition, spokespeople should receive training on the sharing of health narratives so that they can adequately frame health issues with humanistic frames.

These same principles ring true for communicating with linguistically diverse populations, with the additional caveat that specific cultural factors that may make message factors more or less persuasive must also be considered [56].

Applying the health belief model to design effective messages during public health crises

The health belief model was developed in the mid-twentieth century by US Public Health Services psychologists who were concerned that people largely did not participate in disease detection and prevention programs, despite their growing availability and significance in preventing serious illness [57]. According to the health belief model, an individual will engage in a health-protective behavior (e.g., wearing a mask or obtaining a vaccine) if they hold a certain set of beliefs (Table 26.1) and there is a cue that motivates action. When an individual perceives themselves as susceptible to an illness that is severe (the two components of perceived risk), they have confidence in their ability to perform the behavior to avert the illness (i.e., self-efficacy), and they can see the benefits of performing that behavior and perceive few barriers to such action, the health belief model argues that they will be motivated to engage in the health-protective action, particularly when a cue to such action is present. Of course, individual-level factors (e.g., age, gender, and ethnicity) may modify or change the way these variables work [57].

Work grounded in the health belief model suggests that in crises, communicators should maximize the perceived benefits of engaging in a health-protective behavior and simultaneously minimize the perceived barriers to performing the behavior. Health communication campaigns may highlight benefits of behavior by providing explicit arguments in favor of the behavior or by highlighting how an individual's peers positively view that behavior [57]. Campaigns may minimize barriers through a host of tactics from providing directions and easy-to-use assistance for engaging in the behavior to correcting misinformation [57].

Table 26.1 Health Belief Model Constructs.

Belief	Description
Perceived susceptibility	Beliefs about an individual's vulnerability to a risk or likelihood of contracting an illness
Perceived severity	Beliefs about the intensity of the consequences of an illness or risk
Perceived benefits	Beliefs about the advantages of engaging in a behavior to mitigate an illness or risk
Perceived barriers	Beliefs about the disadvantages of engaging in a behavior to mitigate an illness or risk
Self-efficacy	Beliefs about one's confidence in their ability to perform the behavior needed to mitigate an illness or risk

When applying the health belief model to design messages for linguistically diverse populations, it is crucial to consider and collect information on all beliefs in the model to understand where belief-based differences may emerge. For example, research on colorectal cancer screening beliefs found that Spanish-monolingual Latinos differentially perceived barriers and susceptibility to colorectal cancer and screening compared with white, English-speaking individuals [58]. This work, however, generally conflates ethnicity and attendant life experiences with language preference [59, 60]. Little research has explored these differences across health behaviors, and more work is needed to support linguistic minorities during crises.

Applying the integrative model of behavioral prediction to crisis communication

Underlying the integrative model of behavioral prediction is the idea that an individual's intention to perform a behavior is the most significant predictor of actual behavior. Three overarching factors directly predict an individual's behavioral intentions: their attitudes toward the behavior, perceived norms surrounding the behavior, and their agency over performing the behavior. Each of these determinants of behavioral intention is based on associated beliefs (see Figure 26.4). Attitudes can be both experiential (i.e., feelings about performing a behavior) and instrumental (i.e., perceived advantages and disadvantages of performing a behavior) and are directly influenced by associated beliefs about the behavior. Perceived norms, which consist of injunctive and descriptive norms, follow a similar pattern. Injunctive norms are perceived norms surrounding what an individual thinks others would believe about them performing a behavior, and descriptive norms concern perceived norms surrounding the others in an individual's life who might also perform the behavior. Finally, perceived control and self-efficacy correspond to an individual's ability to perform a behavior and their confidence in performing that behavior, respectively.

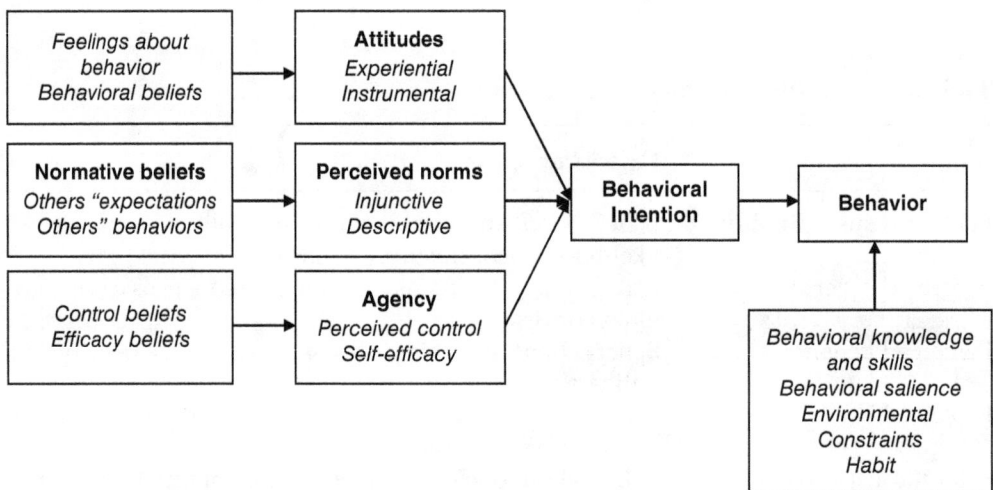

Figure 26.4 The Integrative Model of Behavioral Prediction.

Research on the integrative model has primarily sought to identify the most salient predictors of behavioral intention, adjusting and readjusting the model when relevant to a health context. For example, one study examined predictors of two key health-protective behaviors during the COVID-19 pandemic: (1) wearing a health-protective face covering or mask and (2) physical distancing [61]. Results of the study affirmed the positive relationship between attitudes toward the behaviors and behavioral intentions but suggested differential effects of efficacy and perceived norms based on the behavior. Self-efficacy to physically distance was associated with physical distancing intentions, but mask-wearing self-efficacy was not associated with intentions to wear masks. Alternatively, perceived norms were positively associated with mask-wearing intentions but not with physical distancing intentions. The authors also found that societal and personal perceived risk of COVID-19 were predictive of these three central variables, with personal risk exhibiting a negative relationship to attitudes, perceived norms, and self-efficacy but societal risk exhibiting positive relationships. Though seemingly contradictory, these results suggest the importance of analyzing the unique behavioral context for particular health behaviors. For example, perceived norms and behavioral control for wearing a mask and distancing may vary greatly due to the environmental constraints associated with these behaviors [61]. This research has found the importance of attitudes and subjective norms in predicting behavioral intentions to get the COVID-19 vaccine [62].

Achieving linguistic and cultural competencies in message design and dissemination: targeting and tailoring strategies for linguistically diverse populations

Theories of behavior change should guide how public health actors design maximally effective messages for specific audiences and with specific outcomes in mind. Two important strategies for operationalizing behavioral predictors in message design that are especially useful for linguistically diverse populations are message targeting and tailoring. *Targeting* describes the process of identifying a specific audience group based on audience characteristics; *tailoring* describes the efforts to customize a message to a higher degree of individual specificity [63]. Among linguistically diverse communities, this targeting involves not only translating information into the relevant language of the community but also appealing to cultural characteristics through visually representing the community, including demographic-level statistics and making cultural references, among other strategies. One study that examined cultural targeting of cardiovascular health messages found that Asian American participants, mostly from Pakistan or India, expressed a strong aversion to direct/blunt risk communication messages about the health issue (i.e., these participants negatively reacted to a message about risk factors in their specific community) [64]. This type of communication preference reveals how message targeting can be effective and ineffective. In another study, researchers developed and analyzed the implementation of a *Salud iTu (Health-E You)* a mobile health application that provided custom user-based sexual health information to Latinx adolescents who could also choose to receive information in English or Spanish [65]. Tailoring and targeting message strategies can be best accomplished through multi-methodological and multi-staged approaches to audience analysis and message development and may utilize a combination of qualitative (e.g., focus groups, interviews, and expert advice) and quantitative (e.g., surveys and experiments) methods [66].

How crises exacerbate health disparities

A public health crisis can exacerbate existing health disparities, as evidenced prominently during the COVID-19 pandemic: Black, Latino, and Asian US residents were more likely to become infected with COVID-19, to experience more severe symptoms requiring hospitalization, and to die from the disease [67]. Disparities are centrally caused by structural racism and systemic failures, yet health communicators can be complicit in perpetuating these systems that blame the individual rather than the structural issue [68]. For example, communication interventions predominantly center on individual-level behavior change, a paradigm that obscures the structural and environmental barriers that limit certain people's abilities to engage in healthy (or healthier) behaviors. Similarly, news reporting often focuses on individual-level actions or failures, rather than on societal structures or causes [69, 70]. The urge to focus on individual-level behaviors is particularly strong in a time of crisis: wear a mask, get vaccinated. The communication strategies we suggest above can improve the efficacy of messaging around these individual behaviors. However, the ultimate solution to public health crises is structural change that addresses the systemic, political, and other factors. For example, during the COVID-19 pandemic, more people wore masks in public when there were laws or policies requiring such, as compared to when mask-wearing was a voluntary behavior.

A recent study also suggests that communicating health disparities may be a message strategy best suited for cultural targeting. In a study of white US adults, researchers found that emphasizing health disparities reduced perceived fear of COVID-19 in addition to reducing empathy and support for safety precautions [71]. This complex relationship of health disparities and communication should prompt more health communication research about the role of identity in influencing message effects. Second, in addition to changing the framing of health communication to focus on social determinants of health, another key takeaway for health communication research and practice is to proactively consider health disparities when examining resource distribution and information sharing.

Recommendations for research and practice: toward multilingual theory building

An important challenge documented in research broadly and within the discipline of communication specifically is the applicability of research findings and recommendations across cultures and contexts. This challenge may be exacerbated by differences in language, which is why social scientists often seek to replicate theories, studies, or measures in more than one language. However, researchers should work toward building theory that integrates multilingual perspectives proactively rather than relying on sequential studies. Proactive theory building could support health communicators during times of crisis; that way, researchers can enter the next public health crisis with more insights for how to communicate with linguistic minorities. Such a theoretical shift will ultimately promote effective health communication practice.

Conclusion

The COVID-19 pandemic is neither the only current (ongoing as of October 2023) nor the last public health crisis our world will face. While each health crisis brings with it contextual nuance, the public health needs (e.g., clear, quick, and accurate communication and resource distribution) remain the same. Theory-driven research accompanied by community-oriented practice is necessary strategies for mitigating health disparities, inequities which are frequently exacerbated by health crises, and the communication failures during these crises.

Highlights

- Public health crises are characterized by their scale, need for urgent action, and importance of accurate information exchange.
- Effective public health crisis communication involves proactive planning prior to a crisis, research-informed risk communication strategies, a social media plan, and communication that is clear, consistent, and quick.
- Theories like the situational crisis communication theory, framing theory, the health belief model, and the integrative model of behavioral prediction can be used by practitioners to create effective public health crisis communication.
- Communicating inclusively during health crises requires communicators to target and tailor messages for linguistically diverse audiences, ensuring that information is not only translated into languages of different audience members but also that messages utilize culturally relevant and appropriate messaging strategies.

REFERENCES

1. Ministry of the Interior and Safety. *Disaster Alerts* 2021. https://www.safekorea.go.kr/idsiSFK/neo/sfk/cs/sfc/dis/disasterMsgList.jsp?menuSeq=679
2. Lim, J.R., Jun, H., and Ledford, V. (2022). LGBTQ+ Individuals' intersectional stigma experiences during COVID-19 outbreaks: effective risk communication to motivate testing, tracing, and treatment. *PxyArXiv* https://doi.org/10.31234/osf.io/2nbmj.
3. Cha, S. and Smith, J. (2020). *South Korea Tracks New Coronavirus Outbreak in Seoul nightclubs*. Reuters. https://www.reuters.com/article/uk-health-coronavirus-southkorea-idUKKBN22K0SX (accessed 7 April 2022).
4. COVID-19 Map. Johns Hopkins Coronavirus Resource Center. https://coronavirus.jhu.edu/map.html (accessed 19 April 2022)
5. Sauer, M.A., Truelove, S., Gerste, A.K., and Limaye, R.J. (2021). A failure to communicate? How public messaging has strained the COVID-19 response in the United States. *Health Secur.* 19 (1): 65–74.
6. Nelson, C., Lurie, N., Wasserman, J., and Zakowski, S. (2007). Conceptualizing and defining public health emergency preparedness. *Am. J. Public Health* 97 (Suppl 1): S9–S11.
7. London, A.J. (2016). *Research in a Public Health Crisis: The Integrative Approach to Managing the Moral Tensions*. Oxford University Press. https://academic.oup.com/book/24612/chapter/187920549 (accessed 7 August 2022).

8. CDC (2022). *CDC Museum COVID-19 Timeline*. Centers for Disease Control and Prevention. https://www.cdc.gov/museum/timeline/covid19.html (accessed 7 August 2022).
9. CDC (2020). *Coronavirus Disease 2019 (COVID-19)*. Centers for Disease Control and Prevention. https://www.cdc.gov/coronavirus/2019-ncov/science/about-epidemiology/identifying-source-outbreak.html (accessed 7 August 2022).
10. Craxì, L., Vergano, M., Savulescu, J., and Wilkinson, D. (2020). Rationing in a pandemic: lessons from Italy. *Asian Bioeth. Rev.* 12 (3): 325–330.
11. The World Bank. *Population, Total - Korea, Rep. | Data*. 2022. https://data.worldbank.org/indicator/SP.POP.TOTL?locations=KR (accessed 16 September 2022).
12. United States Census Bureau. *U.S. and World Population Clock*. 2022. https://www.census.gov/popclock (accessed 16 September 2022).
13. *Special Report: How Korea Trounced U.S. in Race to Test People for Coronavirus*. Reuters. https://www.reuters.com/article/us-health-coronavirus-testing-specialrep/special-report-how-korea-trounced-u-s-in-race-to-test-people-for-coronavirus-idUSKBN2153BW?utm_medium=Social&utm_source=twitter (accessed 7 August 2022).
14. (2018). *Crisis & Emergency Risk Communication (CERC)*. CDC. https://emergency.cdc.gov/cerc (accessed 13 July 2022).
15. Adam, D. (2022). How long is COVID infectious? What scientists know so far. *Nature* 608 (7921): 16–17.
16. COVID-19 vaccines: time to talk about the uncertainties. https://www.nature.com/articles/d41586-020-02944-8 (accessed 7 August 2022).
17. Covid vaccine "Mix of science and politics" leading to uncertainty, NIH director says | CNN. https://www.cnn.com/2020/09/16/health/us-coronavirus-wednesday/index.html (accessed 7 August 2022).
18. W.H.O. Fights a Pandemic Besides Coronavirus: An 'Infodemic' - The New York Times. https://www.nytimes.com/2020/02/06/health/coronavirus-misinformation-social-media.html (accessed 7 August 2022)
19. Schillinger, D., Chittamuru, D., and Ramírez, A.S. (2020). From "Infodemics" to health promotion: a novel framework for the role of social media in public health. *Am. J. Public Health* 110 (9): 1393–1396.
20. Knuutila, A., Herasimenka, A., Au, H. et al. (2020). *Covid-Related Misinformation on YouTube*, 7. Oxford Internet Institute https://canucklaw.ca/wp-content/uploads/2020/09/covid.related.misinformation.on_.youtube.pdf.
21. Kouzy, R., Jaoude, J.A., Kraitem, A. et al. (2020). Coronavirus goes viral: quantifying the COVID-19 misinformation epidemic on Twitter. *Cureus* 12 (3): e7255. https://www.cureus.com/articles/28976-coronavirus-goes-viral-quantifying-the-covid-19-misinformation-epidemic-on-twitter (accessed 21 April 2022).
22. Obiała, J., Obiała, K., Mańczak, M. et al. (2021). COVID-19 misinformation: accuracy of articles about coronavirus prevention mostly shared on social media. *Health Policy Technol.* 10 (1): 182–186.
23. Glik, D.C. (2007). Risk communication for public health emergencies. *Annu. Rev. Public Health* 28 (1): 33–54.
24. WHO (2018). *Communicating Risk in Public Health Emergencies: A WHO Guideline for Emergency Risk Communication (ERC) Policy and Practice*. https://www.who.int/publications-detail-redirect/9789241550208 (accessed 7 August 2022).
25. Han, P.K.J., Scharnetzki, E., Scherer, A.M. et al. (2021). Communicating scientific uncertainty about the COVID-19 pandemic: online experimental study of an uncertainty-normalizing strategy. *J. Med. Internet Res.* 23 (4): e27832.
26. Retzbach, A. and Maier, M. (2015). Communicating scientific uncertainty: media effects on public engagement with science. *Commun. Res.* 42 (3): 429–456.
27. Wegwarth, O., Wagner, G.G., Spies, C., and Hertwig, R. (2020). Assessment of German public attitudes toward health communications with varying degrees of scientific uncertainty regarding

COVID-19. *JAMA Netw. Open* 3 (12): e2032335.
28. Juarez, R., Phankitnirundorn, K., Okihiro, M., and Maunakea, A.K. (2022). Opposing role of trust as a modifier of COVID-19 vaccine uptake in an indigenous population. *Vaccines* 10 (6): 968.
29. Coombs, W.T. (2007). Protecting organization reputations during a crisis: the development and application of situational crisis communication theory. *Corp. Reput. Rev.* 10 (3): 163–176.
30. Sager, J. (2020). Serve your servers: how to help restaurant workers during Coronavirus pandemic. *Parade* https://parade.com/1009905/jessicasager/how-to-help-restaurants-coronavirus.
31. *Delta no longer calls COVID an 'ordinary, seasonal virus'*. NPR. https://www.npr.org/2022/04/19/1093543895/delta-mask-mandate-seasonal (accessed 13 July 2022).
32. (2020). *Wayfair: The False Conspiracy about a Furniture Firm and Child Trafficking*. BBC News. https://www.bbc.com/news/world-53416247 (accessed 16 September 2022).
33. Kimball, S. (2022). *CDC Director Walensky to Reorganize Agency After Admitting Covid Pandemic Response Fell Short*. CNBC. https://www.cnbc.com/2022/08/17/cdc-admits-covid-response-fell-short-launches-reorganization.html (accessed 16 September 2022).
34. Maxmen, A. (2021). How the World Failed to Curb COVID. *Nature*. https://www.nature.com/articles/d41586-021-01284-5 (accessed 7 August 2022).
35. Gamson, W.A. and Modigliani, A. (1989). Media discourse and public opinion on nuclear power: a constructionist approach. *Am. J. Soc.* 95 (1): 1–37.
36. Scheufele, D.A. and Tewksbury, D. (2007). Framing, agenda setting, and priming: the evolution of three media effects models: models of media effects. *J. Commun.* 57 (1): 9–20.
37. Ogbodo, J.N., Onwe, E.C., Chukwu, J. et al. (2020). Communicating health crisis: a content analysis of global media framing of COVID-19. *Health Promot. Perspect.* 10(3): 257–269.
38. Shih, T.J., Wijaya, R., and Brossard, D. (2008). Media coverage of public health epidemics: linking framing and issue attention cycle toward an integrated theory of print news coverage of epidemics. *Mass Commun. Soc.* 11 (2): 141–160.
39. Temmann, L.J., Wiedicke, A., Schaller, S. et al. (2021). A systematic review of responsibility frames and their effects in the health context. *J. Health Commun.* 26 (12): 828–838.
40. Ceylan, M. and Hayran, C. (2021). Message framing effects on individuals' social distancing and helping behavior during the COVID-19 pandemic. *Front. Psychol.* 12. https://www.frontiersin.org/articles/10.3389/fpsyg.2021.579164 (accessed 8 August 2022).
41. Betta, S., Castellini, G., Acampora, M., and Barello, S. (2022). The effect of message framing on COVID-19 vaccintion intentions among the younger age population groups: results from an experimental study in the Italian context. *Vaccines* 10: 559.
42. COVID-19 Vaccine Education and Equity Project. COVID-19 Vaccine Resources. COVID-19 Vaccine Education and Equity Project. https://covidvaccineproject.org/resources (accessed 12 July 2022).
43. Kim, H.K. and Tandoc, E.C. (2022). Consequences of online misinformation on COVID-19: two potential pathways and disparity by eHealth literacy. *Front. Psychol.* 13. https://www.frontiersin.org/articles/10.3389/fpsyg.2022.783909.
44. Perspective | Misinformation online is bad in English. But it's far worse in Spanish. Washington Post. 2021. https://www.washingtonpost.com/outlook/2021/10/28/misinformation-spanish-facebook-social-media (accessed 8 August 2022)
45. McGuire, W.J. (1961). The effectiveness of supportive and refutational defenses in immunizing and restoring beliefs against persuasion. *Sociometry* 24 (2): 184–197.
46. Lewandowsky, S. and van der Linden, S. (2021). Countering misinformation and fake news through inoculation and prebunking. *Eur. Rev. Soc. Psychol.* 32 (2): 348–384.

47. Vraga, E.K., Tully, M., and Bode, L. (2020). Empowering users to respond to misinformation about Covid-19. *Media Commun.* 8 (2): 475–479.
48. Fishbein, M. and Cappella, J. (2006). The role of theory in developing effective health communications. *J. Commun.* 56 (s1): S1–S17.
49. Cannon, J.S., Farkouh, E.K., Winett, L.B. et al. (2022). Perceptions of arguments in support of policies to reduce sugary drink consumption among low-income white, black and Latinx parents of young children. *Am. J. Health Promot.* 36 (1): 84–93.
50. CDC COVID-19 Response Team, Bialek, S., Bowen, V. et al. (2020). Geographic differences in COVID-19 cases, deaths, and incidence — United States, February 12–April 7, 2020. *MMWR Morb. Mortal. Wkly Rep.* 69 (15): 465–471.
51. MTA Headquarters. *MTA Launches 'Keep Them Covered' Campaign as New Yorkers Now Required to Wear Face Coverings While Riding Public Transportation.* 2020 April 18. https://www.mta.info/press-release/mta-headquarters/mta-launches-'keep-them-covered'-campaign-new-yorkers-now-required.
52. Cialdini, R.B., Demaine, L.J., Sagarin, B.J. et al. (2006). Managing social norms for persuasive impact. *Soc. Influ.* 1 (1): 3–15.
53. MTA Headquarters. *Subway and Bus Mask Compliance Statistics, May 2020–April 2022.* https://new.mta.info/safety-and-security/nyct-mask-compliance (accessed 9 September 2022).
54. Hong, H. (2013). The effects of human interest framing in television news coverage of medical advances. *Health Commun.* 28 (5): 452–460.
55. Xu, Z., Ellis, L., and Laffidy, M. (2022). News frames and news exposure predicting flu vaccination uptake: evidence from U.S. newspapers, 2011-2018 using computational methods. *Health Commun.* 37 (1): 74–82.
56. Ramírez, A.S., Willis, G., and Rutten, L.F. (2017). Understanding Spanish-language response in a national health communication survey: implications for health communication research. *J. Health Commun.* 22 (5): 442–450.
57. Skinner, C.S., Tiro, J., and Champion, V.L. (2015). The health belief model. In: *Health Behavior: Theory, Research, and Practice*, 5the, 75–94. San Francisco: Jossey-Bass.
58. Brenner, A.T., Ko, L.K., Janz, N. et al. (2015). Race/ethnicity and primary language: health beliefs about colorectal cancer screening in a diverse, low-income population. *J. Health Care Poor Underserved* 26 (3): 824–838.
59. Ramírez, A.S. (2013). Effects of ethnic targeting on the perceived effectiveness of cancer prevention messages among Latinas and non-Hispanic white women. *J. Health Commun.* 18 (10): 1256–1273.
60. Ramírez, A.S. and Arellano-Carmona, K. (2018). Beyond fatalism: information overload as a mechanism to understand health disparities. *Soc. Sci. Med.* 219: 11–18.
61. Duong, H., Nguyen, H., Julian McFarlane, S., and Nguyen, L. (2020). Risk perception and COVID-19 preventive behaviors: application of the integrative model of behavioral prediction. *Soc. Sci. J.* 1–13.
62. Ezati Rad, R., Kahnouji, K., Mohseni, S. et al. (2022). Predicting the COVID-19 vaccine receive intention based on the theory of reasoned action in the south of Iran. *BMC Public Health* 22 (1): 229.
63. Davis, R. and Resnicow, K. (2012). The cultural variance framework for tailoring health messages. In: *Health Communication Message Design: Theory and Practice* (ed. H. Cho), 115–135. Thousand Oaks: Sage.
64. Kandula, N.R., Khurana, N.R., Makoul, G. et al. (2012). A community and culture-centered approach to developing effective cardiovascular health messages. *J. Gen. Intern. Med.* 27 (10): 1308–1316.
65. Tebb, K.P., Leng Trieu, S., Rico, R. et al. (2019). A mobile health contraception decision support intervention for Latina adolescents: implementation evaluation for use in school-based health centers. *JMIR Mhealth Uhealth* 7 (3): e11163.
66. Hornik, R. and Woolf, K.D. (1999). Using cross-sectional surveys to plan message strategies. *Soc. Mark. Q.* 5 (2): 34–41.
67. Lopez, L. III, Hart, L.H. III, and Katz, M.H. (2021). Racial and ethnic health disparities related to COVID-19. *JAMA* 325 (8): 719–720.

68. Hull, S., Stevens, R., and Cobb, J. (2020). Masks are the new condoms: health communication, intersectionality and racial equity in COVID-times. *Health Commun.* 35 (14): 1740–1742.
69. Nagler, R.H., Bigman, C.A., Ramanadhan, S. et al. (2016). Prevalence and framing of health disparities in local print news: implications for multilevel interventions to address cancer inequalities. *Cancer Epidemiol. Biomarkers Prev.* 25 (4): 603–612.
70. Turchi, J. and Melton-Fant, C. (2022). Media framing of COVID-19 racial disparities: lessons from Memphis, Tennessee. *Sociol. Race Ethn.* 8 (3): 355–369.
71. Skinner-Dorkenoo, A.L., Sarmal, A., Rogbeer, K.G. et al. (2022). Highlighting COVID-19 racial disparities can reduce support for safety precautions among white U.S. residents. *Soc. Sci. Med.* 301: 114951.

Glossary

Ad hoc interpreter: A person who is asked to serve as an interpreter because they happen to be there, but they have generally not been trained as an interpreter, nor is interpreting part of their official or compensated role. Also known as untrained interpreter. Despite multiple federal, state, and hospital regulations prohibiting ad hoc interpreting, it remains in common practice. Family members and hospital clinical or non-clinical staff are commonly asked to serve as ad hoc interpreters. Research has consistently shown evidence that this practice increases medical errors and endangers patient safety. For more, see Chapters 6 and 7.

Applied linguistics: A field of study commonly defined in one of two ways: (1) the study of learning and teaching another language; and (2) the application of language and linguistics to practical problems.

Bilingualism: A conceptualization of those who speak two languages, using one language or the other. This term has been replaced with multilingualism to emphasize that speaking two or more languages is an asset greater than the precise sum of its parts. See *multilingualism*.

Cross-linguistic communication skills: The communication skillset needed by a clinician to effectively communicate with patients across languages. In some prior literature, this is also known as *global linguistic competence*. However, given the multiple meanings of global linguistic skills in the language literature (the term *global* can be understood to mean either international or generalized), we use the term cross-linguistic communication skills to refer to the skillset required for healthcare communication with linguistically diverse patient populations.

Cultural humility: A lifelong process and commitment to self-reflection and analysis, to repair power imbalances in the clinician-patient relationship, and to develop mutually beneficial, non-paternalistic advocacy partnerships with individuals and communities. In some circumstances, the concept of cultural humility has gained attention to avoid a check-box approach to gaining *cultural competency* skills. Cultural humility does not end since it requires constant re-evaluation and self-reflection in a spirit of mutual respect and highlights the importance of understanding all cultural backgrounds as complex, heterogeneous, and equally valuable.

Disinformation: False information intentionally created and disseminated for the purpose of deception. See also *misinformation* for discussion on the impact on linguistically diverse populations and public health implications. For more, see Chapters 22, 25, and 26.

Dual role interpreter: Individual who takes on two different roles simultaneously, where one of those roles is to serve as a medical interpreter. Usually, it is a clinician or healthcare professional (e.g. a nurse, a technician, a registration clerk) who is identified as multilingual and officially tasked with interpreting responsibilities. The National Council on Interpreting in Health Care, Inc. defines dual role interpreter as "staff member in a health care facility whose primary responsibility is not medical interpreting but in addition to regular duties works for the facility as a medical interpreter." While offering the benefit of using the skills of existing bilingual staff to improve care, the appropriateness of having dual role interpreters is controversial as there may be variations in the training required of dual role interpreters. Also, each of the two roles (e.g. clinician vs. interpreter) has distinct goals in a medical encounter, which can sometimes be in conflict with each other. Sometimes also known as *dual role staff*. For more, see Chapter 7.

Edutainment: See *entertainment education*.

Entertainment-education: A communication strategy that uses principles from storytelling and narrative theory typically disseminated via media to increase individual knowledge and change attitudes, beliefs, and behaviors to improve the human condition. Also known as *EE* or *edutainment*. For more, see Chapter 23.

Health equity: Achieved when every individual has the opportunity to reach their full potential and no individual is disadvantaged from achieving this potential because of social position or other socially determined circumstances.

Health literacy: The set of functional, interactive, and critical thinking skills that enable an individual to find, understand, assess, and use information to support health-related decisions and actions and to navigate the health environment. Health literacy is generally operationalized as the degree to which individuals have the capacity to obtain, process, and understand basic health information and services needed to make appropriate health decisions. For more, see Chapter 8.

Healthcare: A term used to describe the prevention, diagnosis, treatment, and management of illness and the preservation of mental and physical well-being through the services offered by the medical, nursing, and allied health professions. Healthcare includes the provision of primary care, secondary care, and tertiary care, as well as public health services.

Heritage speaker: A person who learned a language at home while living in a place where a different language was the dominant language taught in school. Heritage speakers enter medical education with a pre-existing linguistic skillset in the heritage language developed throughout their lives, at home or in their communities, naturalistically (i.e. as opposed to through instruction), and with little (if any) educational support and representation in the school system. For more, see Chapter 16.

Interpreter: Person who changes spoken or signed words from one language into another. They interpret words and phrases to facilitate communication between individuals or groups who do not share a common language. There are processes to train and separate processes to certify as a professional medical interpreter.

Interpreters may serve distinct roles that are theorized in various models. For example, the Cross Cultural Health Care Program, one of the first and leading training programs for healthcare interpreters, proposed four interpreter roles: (1) *Conduit*, the default role, involves rendering in one language literally what has been said in the other without any additions, omissions, editing, or polishing; (2) *Clarifier* is a role interpreters assume when they adjust speakers' register, interject their explanations, describe terms that have no linguistic equivalent, or check for understanding when necessary; (3) A *cultural broker* provides a necessary cultural framework for understanding the message being interpreted; (4) An *advocate* works on behalf of the patient outside the bounds of an interpreted interview, ensuring the patients' quality of care in addition to quality of communication. While various models use different nomenclature to describe the roles, there is agreement that interpreters serve multiple and distinct roles in the healthcare system. For more, see Part 2.

Interpreter-mediated interaction: A healthcare visit in which the clinician and patient are language-discordant and the communication between them is mediated by an interpreter. Also known as *interpreter-mediated encounter*. For more, see Chapters 6 and 7.

Interpreting: The act of converting spoken words in one language into another. This is conducted by a medical interpreter, who is proficient in both languages. Also see the definition of *medical interpreter* and Chapters 6 and 7.

Language-appropriate care: When patients receive care in a language they understand, they are receiving language-appropriate care. In healthcare contexts, this can generally be accomplished in one of two principal ways: (1) *language-concordant care* (when the patient and the clinician communicate directly in the same language) or (2) *interpreter-mediated care* (when a professional interpreter is present during a language-discordant patient–clinician interaction). See *language-concordant clinician* and *interpreter-mediated interaction* for more information.

Language assessment: The evaluation of language proficiency, which may vary by context and domain (see *language proficiency*). Assessment may be done for formative (educational feedback, progress checks, etc.) or summative (final evaluation, certification, credentialing, etc.) purposes. For more, see Chapters 12 and 13.

Language barrier: Term to be avoided. Typically, this term is used to refer to barriers to health and healthcare access that patients experience when they have limited proficiency in the dominant language. However, it positions language as the reason why their health or healthcare access is poor and inadvertently blames the patient rather than the system for poor access or outcomes. Instead, we recommend using *structural barriers to language-appropriate care* or *systemic barriers to language-appropriate care*.

Language concordance: When the patient and the clinician are able to communicate directly in the patient's preferred language, the encounter is said to be language-concordant. See *language-concordant clinician*. For more, see Chapters 10, 11, and 14.

Language-concordant clinician: Relative to a patient or population with a particular language preference, a language-concordant clinician is a clinician who is able to provide language-concordant care. It is important to note that the term language-concordant clinician must be contextualized within a particular linguistic group; in other words, language concordance is necessarily relational. One cannot determine whether language concordance is present unless one knows the language of both/all parties involved in the communication or encounter in question. For more, see Chapters 10, 11, and 14.

Language discordance: When the patient and the clinician are not able to communicate directly in the patient's preferred language, the encounter is said to be language-discordant. An interpreter-mediated encounter is a way to provide *language-appropriate care* during a language-discordant encounter.

Language equity: A component of health equity that is achieved when a patient is able to communicate and access healthcare using their preferred language and without structural barriers. For more, see Chapter 20.

Language for healthcare purposes: A relatively new field of research and teaching within the broader discipline of Language for Specific Purposes (LSP), which began in the 1960s in the United Kingdom. For more, see Chapter 15.

Language for specific purposes: Field of language education and research that addresses the needs of learners for learning and using language for use in their job, training, or profession.

Language proficiency: The level at which an individual is able to use a language or what an individual is able to do with a language; it may refer to their overall proficiency in using a language across all domains (speaking, listening, reading, and writing) or can be specific with respect to a particular domain. Additionally, the context of language use can be specified or unspecified; for example, *medical language proficiency* refers to an individual's ability to use a language in a medical context across all domains. By contrast, *medical oral language proficiency* refers more specifically to an individual's ability to use a language in a medical context for verbal communication (speaking and listening domains). There are multiple strategies available for evaluating language proficiency. Health systems sometimes treat language proficiency as binary, which is problematic because proficiency may vary depending on the contextual nuances of a situation and the individuals involved.

Limited English proficiency: Term used by the United States federal government to refer to individuals who report speaking English less than "very well" in the United States Census questionnaire and commonly abbreviated as LEP. If an individual reports speaking English less than "very well," they are understood to not speak English as their primary language and to have a limited ability to read, speak, write, or understand English. This term is commonly used in the United States in the context of English being the dominant language. This is problematic because it focuses on deficits rather than assets of individuals who prefer to communicate in languages besides English. Additionally, it does not capture individuals who are multilingual and do not report a single primary language nor individuals who may prefer one language in certain contexts and a different language in others. Instead, the term *non-English language preference* is recommended.

Linguistic capital: A type of *cultural capital* that refers to the scholarly and social skills that are captured when individuals have proficiency in multiple languages. This term captures that language skills are valuable and should be viewed as an asset in healthcare and other professional sectors.

Linguistic humility: A component of *cultural humility*, linguistic humility refers to an awareness that language is fluid, dynamic, and heterogeneous (even among speakers of the same named-language) and that a single individual may not know everything about a given language or its use. This is important for language learning in medical contexts to avoid falling into traps where one may think one is communicating effectively but may actually be using a term differently than the other interlocutor may understand it, or vice versa. Being linguistically humble for a clinician would mean being cognizant of the patient's linguistic practices, mirroring the patient's language (as possible and appropriate), checking in frequently with the patient to ensure understanding, and remaining attentive to potential sources of miscommunication.

Linguistic marginalization: Commonly recognized as a major structural or systemic barrier to access to health services and health information based on having a language preference that differs from the dominant language in a particular setting. By extension, individuals with non-dominant language preferences are sometimes referred to as being a part of a *linguistically marginalized, linguistically minoritized*, or *linguistic minority* group. Also referred to as *linguistic minoritization*.

Linguistically diverse population: A population in which multiple languages are represented.

Linguistically minoritized population: A population that preferentially communicates in a language different from the dominant language in a particular setting. Also known as *linguistically marginalized* or *linguistic minority* groups or populations. The term *minoritized* is typically preferred over *minority*, since *minoritized* emphasizes that a population need not be a numerical minority to be marginalized due to what is perceived to be the dominant or normalized culture, language, or practice. See *linguistic marginalization*.

Medical language education: Educational field in which a clinician or aspiring clinician learns a language for use in medical contexts, primarily for patient–clinician communication. Most published literature focuses on medical Spanish education in the United States, and students are typically either *second language learners* or *heritage speakers* of the language who wish to enhance their skills in a given language to perform their healthcare job responsibilities. See *medical Spanish*. For more, see Chapter 18.

Medical Spanish: Field of study that encompasses the use of Spanish in medical and healthcare contexts. Primarily, this field has been used to demarcate the use of Spanish in medical settings for clinician communication with Spanish-speaking patients in a medical environment in which Spanish is not the dominant language. The primary growth in the field has been in the United States, where there is a large Spanish-speaking population but a small subset of clinicians who are proficient in Spanish. Common synonyms include *healthcare Spanish, Spanish for healthcare purposes*, or *Spanish for medical professionals*, among others. Medical Spanish is an interdisciplinary area of research and education in which both healthcare professionals and language professionals have shaped the field's development. For more, see Chapters 17 and 19.

Misinformation: False information unintentionally shared, typically via news and social media. Misinformation is distinguished from disinformation primarily with respect to intent. Exposure to mis- and disinformation can have direct negative effects on population health; for example, through encouragement of unsafe behaviors. Potentially more significant, however, are the indirect effects, mediated through the mistrust engendered by mis- and disinformation in the institutions and individuals in whom trust is required for society to function, including public health officials, the democratic process, and the media. *Linguistic minority* populations are especially susceptible to exposure to mis- and disinformation given the paradoxical role of media in such communities: On the one hand, ethnic media are a highly trusted news source through which bad actors may deliberately target linguistic minority populations for misinformation. On the other hand, because of the generally lower levels of official outreach in linguistic minority languages, linguistically diverse populations often turn to media and sources from their countries of origin, but these may not be reliable, accurate, or relevant for their context. For more, see Chapters 22, 25, and 26.

Model of Bilingual Health Communication: A communicative model that explains how interpersonal dynamics can shape the process and content of interpreter-mediated interactions in cross-cultural care. The model was developed in 2017 by Hsieh. For more, see Chapter 7.

Multilingual clinician: Clinician who is able to perform their healthcare responsibilities in more than one language. This is not to be confused with a medical interpreter. Multilingual clinicians are able to provide language-concordant care, and their clinical roles, responsibilities, and training (e.g., as a physician, nurse, physical therapist, etc.) *do not* include medical interpreting.

Multilingualism: The ability to speak, read, write, and/or understand more than one language; an individual's proficiency in each language can vary. Multilingual individuals often spontaneously incorporate linguistic elements (words, grammatical structures, sounds, gestures) from multiple languages and cultures into their day-to-day linguistic practices. For more, see Chapter 16.

Non-English language preference: An individual who prefers a language other than English, where English is the dominant language, can be said to have a non-English language preference. This term has been proposed by Ortega, Martínez, and Shin as a more accurate and inclusive alternative to the term limited English proficiency. More broadly, can be referred to as *non-dominant language preference*.

Patient-clinician communication: Communication between a patient and a clinician. Creating and maintaining effective patient-clinician communication is defined as creating a good interpersonal relationship and facilitating the exchange of information. Ideally, patient–clinician communication should be patient-centered, meaning that the patient's values, preferences, and needs are prioritized in order to enhance comprehension, engagement, satisfaction, and effectiveness that positively impact health and wellbeing.

Second language acquisition: Situated within applied linguistics, second language acquisition (SLA) encompasses a broad area of study, focusing on how another language (L2) is acquired in the classroom, as well as in non-instructed, naturalistic contexts. For more, see Chapter 15.

Social determinants of health: The conditions in the environments where people are born, live, learn, work, play, worship, and age that affect a wide range of health, functioning, and quality-of-life outcomes and risks. Social determinants of health (SDOH) have a major impact on people's health, well-being, and quality of life. Examples of SDOH include safe housing, transportation, and neighborhoods; racism, discrimination, and violence; education, job opportunities, and income; access to nutritious foods and physical activity opportunities; polluted air and water; and language and literacy skills. SDOH also contributes to wide health disparities and inequities. For example, people who do not have access to grocery stores with healthy foods are less likely to have good nutrition; this lack of access raises their risk of health conditions like heart disease, diabetes, and obesity – and even lowers their life expectancy relative to people who do have access to healthy foods (Definition from the US Department of Health and Human Services).

Language preference outside of the dominant language in which healthcare is typically provided in a given location is a social determinant of health.

Standardized patients: Individuals who are trained to play the role of a patient in a simulated medical encounter. The use of standardized patients is a common practice for communication and other clinical skills training and assessment. For more, see Chapter 19.

Structural determinants of health: The elements of the healthcare system or institution that present obstacles or create barriers to individuals accessing healthcare or achieving their best health. Also known as *systemic determinants of health, systemic barriers,* or *structural barriers to care.*

Transcreation: The cultural and linguistic adaptation of communication, based on the idea of reaching across different segments of a larger audience, to improve program engagement and appeal. For more, see Chapter 23.

Translanguaging: The complex processes of meaning and sense-making engaged in by multilingual individuals during communication. Translanguaging may involve spontaneously combining multiple languages or linguistic practices. For more, see Chapter 16.

Translation: The process of taking written material in one language and converting it into another. See *translator*. For more, see Chapter 8.

Translator: An individual who converts text from one written language to another. There is a process for obtaining training and certification to become a professional translator; certification is specific and unidirectional. For example, a person can be certified in English-to-Spanish translation, but not in Spanish-to-English translation. Individuals can further develop expertise in medical or healthcare translation, specifically. For medical translation of patient-facing materials, it is often necessary to not only translate but also culturally adapt materials to ensure usability by the intended patient population. For more, see Chapter 8.

Transmedia: The use of multiple media channels, such as television, posters, and social media, as part of a comprehensive storytelling method where each media channel is used to reinforce messaging from the other. For more, see Chapter 23.

Index

ACA. *See* Affordable Care Act of 2010 (ACA)
Accreditation Council for Graduate Medical Education (ACGME), 331
ACGME. *See* Accreditation Council for Graduate Medical Education (ACGME)
Acquisition, 286
ACTFL. *See* American Council on the Teaching of Foreign Languages (ACTFL)
Active construction process, 12
ADC. *See* Anal Dysplasia Clinic-MidWest (ADC)
Address language concordance research, 258
Ad hoc interpreters, 3, 34, 107, 126, 255, 259, 270, 309, 311, 312
Adult learners, 4
  education, 10
  population, 4
Advocacy groups, 248
Affordable Care Act of 2010 (ACA), 103–105, 123, 128, 235, 257
Agenda-setting theory, 410–411
AIDS pandemic, 49, 50
Alcoholism, in Guatemala, 64–68
ALTA Language Services, 181, 283
American agricultural industry, 264
American Council on the Teaching of Foreign Languages (ACTFL), 282–283
American Sign Language (ASL), 387, 505
Anal cancer prevention (case study), 68–73
Anal Dysplasia Clinic-MidWest (ADC), 69, 70
  boundary objects, 73
  patient intake form, 71
Applied linguistics, 12, 404
  comprehension models, 14
  conversation analysis (CA), 79–81
  definitions, 77, 281
  empirical research, 77, 78
  expertise of, 12
  in HL measurement, 17. *See also* Health literacy (HL)
  interactional sociolinguistics (IS). *See* Interactional sociolinguistics (IS)
  and key terms, 281–282
  leadership roles in, 17
  methodologies, 89
  perspectives, 18
  provider-patient interaction. *See* Provider-patient interaction
  public health and, 78
  research, 78
  and translation studies, 87
Appropriate authorship, 358
Argumentative text genres, 140
Argument-based validation approach, 215
Arturo's health history, 194–201
ASL. *See* American Sign Language (ASL)
Aspirational capital, 393

The Handbook of Language in Public Health and Healthcare, First Edition.
Edited by Pilar Ortega, Glenn Martínez, Maichou Lor, and A. Susana Ramírez.
© 2024 John Wiley & Sons, Inc. Published 2024 by John Wiley & Sons, Inc.

Assessing clinician language skills. *See also* Language assessment
  IELTS, 216–217
  key considerations, 218–227
  for language professional purposes, 216–218
  methodological consideration, 221
  Occupational English Test (OET), 216–218
  overview, 215
  scoring performance, 219–220
  standard setting, 220–223
  test development, 218–219
Assessment
  CCLA ALTA, 356
  clinical skills training and, 338
  formative, 355
  language. *See* Language assessment
  language proficiency, 362
  learner, 339
  of learner medical Spanish skills, 338–339
  LSP, 289
  with patients, 337
  proficiency, 327
  skill, 292
  standardized proficiency, 269
Assistive technology, 438
Asylum seekers, 145
Audience analysis, 415–416
Audiolingual Method, 285
Australian CMIs, 148
Authentic language assessments, 219
Auto-reported proficiency, 260

Back-translation method, 87, 138, 139, 271
Basic/functional health literacy, 155
"Beasts," 65
Benchmarking language proficiency, 355, 357
"Berlitz Method," 285
BHC model. *See* Bilingual Health Communication (BHC) model
Bilingual/biliterate populations, 11
Bilingual Fluency Assessment, 237
Bilingual Health Communication (BHC) model, 118, 120–128
  bilingual medical professionals, 123–125
  nonprofessional interpreters, 126–128
  professional interpreters, 121–123
Bilingualism, 86, 291
  individual level, 238–239
  organizational level, 239
  professional approach to, 231, 238–240
  as professional competency, 248
  research, 191
  in Spanish, 313
  systemic level, 239–240
  trainees, 248
Bilingual medical employees, 124–125
Bilingual medical professionals, 123–125
  bilingual medical employees, 124–125
  bilingual providers, 123–124
Bilingual providers, 123–124
Bilingual qualification system, 240–246
Bi-/multilingual communication, 307
Biomedicalization, 69, 72
Biomedical surveillance, 73
Biopsychosocial model, 47
Black and Latino populations, 432
Black Cadejo, 66
Blogs, 410
"Bobo Doll Experiment," 413
Bordering theory, 59, 60, 73
Boundaries/Border
  between humans and animals, 64–68
  of life and death, 60–64
  sex/gender and sexuality, 68–73
Boundary objects, 69, 70, 73
Boundary work, 69
Bridging communications gaps, 146

CA. *See* Conversation analysis (CA)
CAI. *See* Comunicación y Habilidades Interpersonales (CAI)
CALD. *See* Culturally and linguistically diverse (CALD)
CAMH. *See* Comprehensive Accreditation Manual for Hospitals (CAMH)
Canadian English Language Benchmark Assessment for Nurses (CELBAN), 234
CanopyCredential, 241
Case-based learning, 379–380
CBPR. *See* Community-based participatory research (CBPR)
CCHI. *See* Certification Commission for Healthcare Interpreters (CCHI)
CCLA. *See* Clinician Cultural and Linguistic Assessment (CCLA)

CCLA-S. *See* Clinician Cultural and Linguistic Assessment-Spanish (CCLA-S)
CEBRE. *See* Communicating the External Beam Radiotherapy Experience (CEBRE)
CEFR. *See* Common European Framework of Reference for Languages (CEFR)
CELBAN. *See* Canadian English Language Benchmark Assessment for Nurses (CELBAN)
Center for Open Educational Resources and Language Learning, 283
Center for Open Resources in Language Learning, 289
Centers for Disease Control and Prevention (CDC), 158
Certification Commission for Healthcare Interpreters (CCHI), 107
Certified interpreters, 388
Cervical cancer, 69
Chance interpreters, 127
Charter for Professionalism for Healthcare Organizations, 232
Cisgender, 70
CIS scale. *See* Communication and Interpersonal Skills (CIS) scale
CLAS. *See* National Standards for Culturally and Linguistically Appropriate Services (CLAS)
Classroom methods, 337
CLC. *See* Culture and language coach (CLC)
"Clean India" campaign, 416
CLEE. *See* Clinical Language Equity Education (CLEE)
CLIL approach. *See* Content and language integrated learning (CLIL) approach
Clinical communication skills training, 182
   case-based learning, 379–380
   conceptual framework for, 370
   graduate programs, 373
   and interpersonal communication training, 378–379
   issues and topics in, 370–376
   medical languages and advocacy, 376
   medical school programs, 373–375
   in minoritized languages, 374, 383
   non-physician healthcare professionals, 376
   oral communication, 371
   patient-centered, 374
   physicians-in-practice, 375–376
   resident physician training programs, 375
   simulation training, 379–380
   undergraduate programs, 372–373
Clinical Language Equity Education (CLEE), 389, 390–393, 394, 395, 396–397
Clinical learning environment, 312
Clinician Cultural and Linguistic Assessment (CCLA), 236, 283–284, 328, 356
Clinician Cultural and Linguistic Assessment-Spanish (CCLA-S), 341
Clinician-patient language concordance, 182
CMI. *See* Consumer Medicine Information (CMI)
Codeswitching, 192
Coding systems, 79
Collaborative communication, 288
Collaborative translanguaging, 28
Colloquialisms, 36
Comics, 469, 470, 472
Comics, genre of, 51–52
Common European Framework of Reference for Languages (CEFR), 283, 374
Communicating the External Beam Radiotherapy Experience (CEBRE), 485
Communication, 25. *See also* Healthcare communication
   English speakers, 26
   in healthcare, 16, 84
   interpreter-mediated, 311–312
   inter-professional, 218
   intra-professional, 218
   language discordance, 310
   mass media, 11
   medical professional, 218
   with minoritized language speakers, 34
   mode of, 54
   patient-centered, 31, 35, 311
   patient–clinician, 256
   with patients through medical text genres, 138–143
   in public health crises, 520–525
   skills training, 277
   sociolinguistics in healthcare, 25–29
Communication and Interpersonal Skills (CIS) scale, 339
Communication assistance, 235

Communication theory, 415
"Communicative activity," 140
Communicative affordances, 2, 44, 54, 55
Communicative competence
  activities, 288
  goal of, 188
  model, 286
  notion of, 287
Communicative effectiveness, 53
Communicative/interactive health literacy, 155
Communicative language teaching, 286–288
Communicative practices, 59–61, 63
Communicative repertoires, 27
Community-based participatory research (CBPR), 447
Community-based practitioners, 18
Community cultural wealth model, 389, 393
Community engagement, 381
Community voices, 381
Compensating QBS program, 245–246
Comprehension models, 14–15
Comprehensive Accreditation Manual for Hospitals (CAMH), 439
Computer-based interpretation modalities, 103
Computer technology, 101
Comunicación y Habilidades Interpersonales (CAI), 339
Concept-metaphor, 65
"Conditional effects era," 415
Conduit model, 117, 311
Consumer Medicine Information (CMI), 141, 148
Consumption model, 421
Content and language integrated learning (CLIL) approach, 15
"Contextualization cues," 82
Contextual learning, 331
Continuing education (CE), 165, 245
Contract interpreters, 121–122
Contrastive Analysis, 285
Conversational data, 80
Conversation analysis (CA), 79–81
  goal of, 79
  and intercultural communication, 80–81
  and interpreting, 81
  miscommunication, 80
  "streams" of, 80
Corpora, 78, 86

COVID-19
  misinformation, 514
  news on Twitter, 33
  Síntomas Coronavirus, 475, 477
  social media use. *See* Social media
  sociolinguistics and, 28–29
  South Korean Emergency Alert, 512
  supports health literacy, 163
  vaccination messaging, 419
  Vaccine Education and Equity Project, 519
  by World Health Organization (WHO), 410
Credentialing application, 108
Critical health literacy, 7, 155
Cross Cultural Health Care Program (CCHCP), 118
Cross-cultural medicine, 340
Cross-language research methods, 109–110
Crosslinguistic healthcare communication skills, 326–328, 336
  teaching, 340
Crosslinguistic OT, 259
CSEV. *See* Culturally sensitive educational video (CSEV)
Cultivation analysis, 413–414
Cultural and Linguistic Competence Policy Assessment, 164
Cultural and linguistic competencies, 33, 261
Cultural beliefs, 435
"Cultural brokers," 326
Cultural competency, 310
  framework, 73
Cultural differences, 145
Cultural humility, 73, 261, 337, 371
  training, 370
Cultural identity, 435
Cultural Indicators Project, 413–414
Culturally and linguistically diverse (CALD), 264
Culturally diverse communities, 308
Culturally relevant occupational therapy, 259
Culturally sensitive educational video (CSEV), 462
Culture, 270, 337
Culture and language coach (CLC), 375
Curricula and teaching methods, 288

Data collection process, 110
Data comics, 473

Data gathering, 376–377
Data visualization, 473
DCT. *See* Dual coding theory (DCT)
Declaration of Helsinki, 141
Deconstructing language proficiency, 190–191
De facto measure of language, 16
"Deliteracization of Spanish," 11
Determinologization, 148
Didactic LHP resources, 290
Diet-release disease, 36
Diffusion of innovations theory (DoI), 416
Digital age, risk communication in, 31–32
Digital divide, 419
Digital health, 161–162
Digital health literacy, 435
Digital literacy, 503
Digital media, 407
Direct mechanisms, LEP, 256
Direct Method, 285
  of language acquisition, 288
Discrete languages, 192
Discrimination, 256, 432
Diversity, 327
  of language and messages, 417
  linguistic. *See* Linguistic diversity
Diversity, and multilingualism, 306–307
Doctor-patient interactions, 46–47, 78–79, 375
Doctor's Stories (Hunter), 48
Documentation, of language-related data, 108
Document Design principles, 147
DoI. *See* Diffusion of innovations theory (DoI)
Domain description inference, 225–226
Dominant language, 215, 231
  face barriers, 143
  proficiency, 233
  proficiency policy, 234
"Dominicanisms," 27
Dual coding theory (DCT), 473
Dual-role interpreters, 125, 326, 327
Dutch medical curriculum, 310

Ebola epidemic, 358
ECFMG. *See* Educational Council for Foreign Medical Graduates; Education Commission for Foreign Medical Graduates (ECFMG)
Education, 111, 435
  faculty development, 394–398
  healthcare, 277
  of healthcare professionals, 307
  in medical Spanish education, 340–341
Educational Council for Foreign Medical Graduates (ECFMG), 234
Educational linguistics, 17
Education Commission for Foreign Medical Graduates (ECFMG), 240
eHealth Literacy Scale (eHEALS), 162
"El Cadejo," 66
Electronic health (eHealth), 108, 161, 162
Electronic medical record (EMR), 70, 72
Emergency Medicaid, 62
Emergency Medical Treatment and Active Labor Act (EMTALA) regulations, 61
Emotional support and protection, 28
Empathy, 52, 312
Empowerment, 14–15, 32, 88
EMR. *See* Electronic medical record (EMR)
EMTALA regulations. *See* Emergency Medical Treatment and Active Labor Act (EMTALA) regulations
End-stage renal disease (ESRD), 59, 61, 62
Enforcement of Section 1557, 236
Engel's biopsychosocial model, 47
English-as-a-Second-Language (ESL), 11, 86, 89, 190
English for specific purposes (ESP), 241, 369
English-language media, 411
English language skills, 227
English-medium tertiary program, 217
English-Spanish interpreter, 30
English-Spanish language, 147
English speakers, 26, 30
"English-speaking majority," 190
Entertainment-education strategies, 404, 416, 445
  audience and bidirectional influence of, 450–453
  enriches linguistic diversity, 454–464
  history and theory of, 447–449
  linguistic diversity and, 445
  in Mozambique, 459
  narrative and storytelling, 454–455
  narrative theories, 449
  practice and evidence, 449–454
  programs, 448
  recreating language, 458–461
  source credibility in, 455–458

Equivalence-based approach, 139
Errors, types of, 144
ESL. *See* English-as-a-Second-Language (ESL)
ESP. *See* English for specific purposes (ESP)
Essentialized language codes, 192
Ethical listening, 294
Ethnic media, 503
Ethnic minority communities, 259, 432
Ethnic/racial minority participants, 145
European Medicines Agency, 141
European PILs, 141
European Union (EU) law, 140
Evaluation tools, 378
Evidence-based causal model, 158
Exclusionary violence, 61
Executive Order 13166, 102
"Extractive research," 358

Facebook, 500, 502
Face social determinants, 387
Face-to-face interaction, 192
Fact sheets for patients (FSP), 140
Faculty development
  in Clinical Language Equity Education, 389, 390–393, 396–397
  clinical practice, 394–398
  community cultural wealth, 393–394
  education, 394–398
  overview, 387–389
  research, 394–398
  terminology for, 389
  theoretical framework, 389–394
False-fluency, 338
Familial capital, 389
Familismo, 34, 338
Family interpreters, 126, 128
Fatalism, 414
Federal and state government, 247
Federal Plain Language Guidelines, 158
Federal policies, 257
Feedback, 338, 379
Figurative language, 53
Flesch–Kincaid formula, 148
Fluency, 180
Formal language assessments, 26, 103, 111, 181
Formal *vs.* informal registers, 318
Formative assessment, 355
Formative research, 415–416

Fossilization, 286
Fotonovelas, 477
Framing, mass media, 411–413
Framing theory, 520–523
FSP. *See* Fact sheets for patients (FSP)
Functional HL, 7

Gender differences, 434
"Gender Identity," 70
Gender transformative approach, 447
General language proficiency test, 216–218
General Medical Council (GMC), 217
Genesis, of illness narratives, 44–45
Gerbner, George, 413
German-as-a-second-language, 9
Global health engagement, language learning to, 357–360
"Global linguistic competence," 326
Global mass media campaigns, 416
Glycated hemoglobin levels, 184
Glycemic control, 183
GMC. *See* General Medical Council (GMC)
Google Translator, 439
Government policies, 437
Graduate programs, in healthcare, 373, 388
Grammar, 290
Graphic medicine, 404, 469
  for clinical practice, 485–486
  emergence of narrative medicine, 471–472
  historical roots of, 470–478
  in linguistically diverse settings, 478–484
  medical education, 471–472
  medical humanities, 471–472
  modern era of, 474–478
  for patient-clinician communication, 480–482
  research, 486–487
  sociopolitical movements, 470–471
  to storytelling, 472–473
  as tool for medical education, 485
  zines, 470–471
Graphic pathographies/novels, 44, 45, 50–54, 469
Guatemala, indigeneity and alcoholism in, 64–68

Harvard Medical School (HMS), 350. *see also* HMS Medical language program
HCW. *See* Healthcare workers (HCW)

Health belief model, 523–524
Healthcare communication, 16, 36, 80
   intercultural communication in, 80–81
   sociolinguistics in, 25–29
   target language use domain of, 225
   test tasks and, 226
Healthcare education, 277
Healthcare practitioners, 34
Healthcare professionals, 211, 232–233
   interpreter-mediated communication, 311–312
   language test for, 222
Healthcare systems, 236–237, 387, 439
Healthcare translation, 137
   for asylum seekers and refugees, 145
   challenges of, 143–146
   impacted populations, 142–143
   intralingual translation, 137, 138, 148–149
   medical and, 138
   models for, 138–139
   package information leaflets (PIL), 140–141, 147–148
   practices and recommendations, 146–149
   process-oriented research in, 138
   studies, 138
   text genres, 140–142
   theoretical framework, 138–139
Healthcare workers (HCW), 185, 186, 236, 308, 376, 387
Health disparities, 431–432, 526
Health equity, 2, 233, 248, 362
   in medical education, 394
Health Equity Accreditation, 237
Health/Healthcare
   critical issues in, 418–419
   definition of, 5
   delivery, 120
   graduate programs in, 373
   health and, 60
   and healthcare, 60
   intercultural communication in, 80–81, 308–310
   interpreters. *See* Interpreters, in healthcare
   language access in, 30–31
   language concordance. *See* Language concordance
   Latinxs in. *See* Latinxs
   linguistics of, 17, 18
   mass media and, 409–418. *See also* Mass media
   messaging, 33–34
   minoritized groups in, 372
   organizations, 103, 107
   perspectives on, 5–8
   social determinant of, 1
   sociolinguistics of mobility in, 36–37
   structural inequities in, 109
   workers, 258
Health information seeking (HIS), 417–418. *See also* Linguistic minority populations
   characterizing, 431
   critical issues in, 430, 433–434
   decision-making renders, 430
   factors affecting, 434–437
   and health disparities, 431–432
   outcomes of, 431
   patient-clinician interaction outcomes, 431
   patient-physician communication, 430
   policy, 439–440
   practice, 438–439
   proxy, 433–434
   psychosocial outcomes, 431
   research, 438
   research on, 430
   social media, 495–497
   source preferences, trust in, 432
   theoretical frameworks, 429–432
"Health insurance," 33
Health literacy (HL), 2, 4, 143
   basic/functional, 155
   communication strategies, 162
   communicative/interactive, 155
   concept, 84, 86
   conceptual frameworks, 158–160
   conceptual models, 85
   critical, 155
   critical issues and topics, 160–163
   definitions, 155
   digital health, 161–162
   education, 163–165
   framework, 7
   and health outcomes, 156
   historical development, 157–160
   history, 83–85
   initiatives, 157–158
   integrated model of, 158, 160

Health literacy (HL) *(cont'd)*
　languages in, 7–8
　learning, 4
　levels, 8–10
　limited, 155
　limited eHealth literacy and, 161–162
　and literacy-oriented category, 47
　low, 36, 97, 83
　measurement, 160–161
　in multilingual communities, 89
　and multilingualism, 85–86, 91
　national assessment of, 157
　as "national priority," 84
　non-English measures, 86
　operationalizing, 84–85
　organizational, 155
　patient-provider interaction and, 77
　personal, 155
　and plain language, 98, 88
　public health emergencies, 162–163
　recognition of, 157
　research and practice, 155, 163–165
　reviews of, 161
　scholarship, 87
　skills, 84
　theoretical framework, 157–160
　trans-approach to, 317
　trans-perspective on, 317
　and written documents, 86–88
"Health literacy load analysis," 87
"Health literacy solid facts," 9
Health Literacy Universal Precautions Toolkit, 164
Health misinformation, 419
Health outcomes, 156
Health professional language assessment, 176
Health professions, 107–108
Health systems, 185–186
Healthy People 2010, 158
Healthy People 2020, 158
Healthy People 2030, 158
Heritage speakers, 305, 313, 318
　as locally appropriate model, 318–319
Heterogeneous ethnic group, 325
HHS. *See* United States Department of Health and Human Services
Higher-scale language resources, 26
HIS. *See* Health information Seeking (HIS)
Hispanic/Latinx populations, 325, 337, 342

Historical evolutionary perspective, 447
HL. *See* Health literacy (HL)
HMS. *See* Harvard Medical School (HMS)
HMS Medical language program, 350–357
　current scope, 351–353
　curriculum development and innovation, 351
　formalization, 356
　goal of, 351
　history, 350–351
　language assessment, 355–356
　longitudinal learning and maintenance, 356–357
　timeline of, 351
　virtual platforms, 354–355
Hospital interpreters, 121–122
HPV. *See* Human papillomavirus (HPV)
HRSA. *See* United States. Health Resources and Services Administration (HRSA)
Humanism, 312
"Humanism in medicine," 474
Humanitarian ethics, 64
Human–nonhuman border, 64, 66
Human papillomavirus (HPV), 69
Humans *vs.* animals, 64–68
"Hypodermic needle" effect, 409

ICD. *See* Informed consent document (ICD)
ICFs. *See* Informed consent forms (ICFs)
IELTS. *See* International English Language Testing System (IELTS)
IHCAI. *See* International Health Central American Institute (IHCAI)
Illness narratives, 44
　concept of, 47
　cultural and linguistic interactive aspects of, 46
　expressive modes of, 55
　in face-to-face interactions, 50
　genesis of, 44–45
　graphic pathographies/novels, 50–54
　Kleinman's notion of, 45–47
　modes of expression, 44
　oral and written versions, 45–50
　as pathographies, 49
　patients', 48
　as patient's explanatory model, 46
　publication, 54

Illness Narratives: Suffering, Healing, and the Human Condition (Kleinman), 45
ILR. *See* Interagency Language Roundtable (ILR)
Immigrants, 4
  Latinxs, 31
  women, 10
Incentives QBS program, 245–246
Incorrect patient education, 107
Indigeneity, in Guatemala, 64–68
Indirect mechanisms, LEP, 256
Individual clinician language, 238–239
Individual factors, 434
Individual orientation, 28
Individual trait, 4
Infectious disease pandemics, 404
Informal interpreters, 126
Information dissemination strategies, 163
Information exchange, 514
Informed consent document (ICD), 141–142
Informed consent forms (ICFs), 137, 141–142
In-person communication, 370
In-person interpreting practice, 107
In-person professional interpreters, 121–122, 124
Instant written translation, 146
Instructor recruitment and qualifications, 361
Instructor training, in SLA and LSP, 290–291
Instrument's translation, 110
Integrated model of health literacy, 158, 160
Integrating socioculture, in medical Spanish education, 337–338
Integrative model of behavioral prediction, 524–525
Intensive language learning, 353
Interactional sociolinguistics (IS), 79, 81–82
  and intercultural communication, 82–85
  perspective, 82
Interaction analysis systems, 79
Interactive HL, 7
Interagency Language Roundtable (ILR), 283, 329, 362
Intercultural communication, 80–81, 305, 308–310, 310
  conversation analysis and, 80–81
  interactional sociolinguistics (IS), 82–83
  in medical curriculum, 310–312
Interdisciplinary collaboration, 4

Interdisciplinary team, 258–263
Intergeneric translation, 148
Interlanguage, 286–287
Intermediate language, 370
International English Language Testing System (IELTS), 216–217, 222, 234
International Health Central American Institute (IHCAI), 352
International migrations, 97
International public health, 156
Internet, 432, 435–436
Internet, 433
Interpersonal communication training, 378–379
Interpreter-as-conduit model, 117
Interpreter-mediated interactions, 98, 120
  BHC model, 120
  effectiveness and appropriateness, 120–121
  professional practices in, 311
Interpreter roles
  advocate, 118
  BHC model, 120–128
  clarifier, 118
  conduit, 118
  cultural broker, 118
  investigation of, 119
  performances, 120
  professional interpreters, 121–123
  typologies of, 118, 119, 120
Interpreters, in healthcare, 81, 326. *See also* Interpreter roles
  and clinician, 336
  cross-language research methods, 109–110
  diversity of, 120–128
  documentation of, 108
  educational standardization for, 107
  family interpreters, 128
  industry, 106
  labor market of, 106
  performance evaluation, 106
  poor quality, 107
  professional, 255
  qualified, 257
  regulation and training, 106–107
  shaping providers' choice of, 127
  subcategories of, 127
  trained, 255
  types of, 121
  wages for, 106

Interpreter-mediated communication, 311–312
Inter-professional communication, 218
Interprofessional education (IPE), 311, 332
Intervention delivery, 497–498
Interviewees, 66, 67
Intralingual translation, 137, 138, 148–149
Intra-professional communication, 218
IS. *See* Interactional sociolinguistics (IS)

Javed's internship, 211
JCAHO. *See* Joint Commission on Accreditation of Healthcare Organizations (JCAHO)
Job-specific language proficiency, 232
Joint Commission, 237, 327
Joint Commission on Accreditation of Healthcare Organizations (JCAHO), 387–388

Kaiser Permanente system, 183, 185, 237, 259
Kleinman, Arthur, 45–47
Komen Tissue Bank (KTB), 417
Krashen's Natural Approach, 286
KTB. *See* Komen Tissue Bank (KTB)
"Kyunki Jeena Isi Ka Naam Hai", 459

Language. *See also specific types*
  capacity in health professions, 107–108
  competence, 103
  complexity, 14–15
  development, 9
  discrete, 192
  of exclusionary healthcare policies, 63
  in healthcare, 3
    re-thinking six myths, 8–17
    written communication, 10–11
  health literacy and, 1
  in health literacy research, 7–8
  instructors, 371
  Latinx health and, 30–33
  learning, 4
  levels of instruction, 360
  of medicine, 314
  modes, 283
  named, 192
  native/national, 264
  in occupational therapy (OT), 259
  perspectives on, 5–8
  skills of learners, 9
  as social determinant of health, 5–6
  and sociolinguistics, 33
  teaching and learning, 4
Language acceptance, concept of, 35
Language access
  advocacy, 238
  component for, 103
  and health equity, 248
  policies and laws in United States., 102–106
  services implementation, 109
Language acquisition theories, 77, 285–286
Language-appropriate care, 256, 257, 261
Language assessment, 355–356
  for professional purposes, 215–227
    authenticity in, 219
    for clinicians, 222
    distinct features, 215
    for professional purposes, 215, 218–219
    revisions/refinement of, 225
    validity of, 223–227
Language assistance, 235
Language barriers, 126, 258, 308, 433
  experiences, 101, 120
  health outcomes associated with, 106
  impact of, 183
  and language concordance, 263
"Language capability," 360
Language concordance, 6, 106, 363
  actual, 212
  address, 258
  adequate, 264
  aspects of, 258
  benefits, 182
  care, 257, 326
  challenges, 258
  and clinical care, 181–182
  and clinical outcomes, 183
  clinician-patient, 182
  conceptual framework, 181
  data, 193
  definitions, 180, 184
  doctor-patient, 375
  education and training, 184–185
  effects of, 189
  field of, 269–271
  fundamental notion, 271
  healthcare, 179–180, 189, 255–258

health systems and clinicians, 185–186
impact of, 181
in interdisciplinary team, 258–263
language-appropriate care, 261
language barriers and, 263
measurement, 180, 267–269
missing elements in, 262–263
notion of, 318
occasioned membership category, 193–209
and patient behaviors, 182
in patient care, 259
and patient experience of care, 182
practical applications, 176
primary care into surgical fields, 264–267
proficiency level, 184
quality of care and outcomes, 269
race/ethnicity, 175–176
research in, 175, 258, 263–264, 264, 269, 271
using professional interpreters, 261
Language-concordant care, 175, 433
Language discordance, 30, 98, 101, 143, 308
 access policies and laws in United States., 102–106
 addressing, 102, 106–110
 best practices for, 129
 communication, 310
 definitions, 102
 effects of, 261
 experiences, 101, 120
 historical overview, 102–106
 during hospitalization, 101
 language diversity and, 102
 physicians, 183
 and poor-quality interpretation, 107
Language diversity, 102, 306, 446
Language equity, 394
Language for Health Purposes (LHP), 282, 288–289
 curricular design, 291–292
 didactic resources, 290
 educational levels, 294–297
 focus and research, 297
 instructor training, 290–291
 National Association of Medical Spanish, 292
 proficiency levels, 293–294
Language for specific purposes (LSP), 289, 367, 368

Language learning, 211, 282, 286, 349, 371, 378
 to global health engagement, 357–360
 to health equity, 362
 virtual learning environment for, 361–362
Language-minoritized patients, 35, 36
Language pedagogy, 367
Language proficiency, 77, 84, 176, 190, 282–285, 358
 assessment, 216, 362
 benchmarking, 355, 357
 in clinical practice, 233
 components of, 216
 deconstructing, 190–191
 development, 372
 frameworks, 284
 levels of clinicians, 269
 nondominant language. *See* Nondominant languages
 second language acquisition (SLA), 282–285
 self-awareness of, 327–328
 unified measurement of, 269
Language resources, 26
 higher-scale, 26
 lower-scale, 26
Language-sensitive health communication frameworks, 15
Language training, 356
Latinxs, 30–33
 and Black participants, 34
 clinical interactions, 32
 community, 37
 immigrant, 31
 language access, 30–31
 non-English speaking, 30
 patient experiences, 31
 promoting local language, 32–33
 risk communication in digital age, 31–32
 Spanish-speaking, 30, 31, 34
 in United States, 30
Lay sexual identity categories, 72
LCME. *See* Liaison Committee of Medical Education (LCME)
Leaders, in medical education, 388
League of Latin American Citizens (LULAC) organization, 328
Learner medical Spanish skills, 338–339
Learning resources, 333
LEP. *See* Limited English proficiency

LGBTQ+ people, 69, 70
LHP. *See* Language for Health Purposes (LHP)
Liaison Committee of Medical Education (LCME), 327
License/credentialing application, 108
Licensed independent practitioners, 240
Lifelong learning process, 4
Lifeworld-system continuum, 119
Limited eHealth literacy, 161–162
Limited English proficiency (LEP), 6, 97, 90, 91, 103, 157, 164, 179, 190, 235, 239, 255, 349
  concentrated populations, 437
  patients with, 256, 258, 350
  Spanish speakers with, 326
  in United States, 256
Limited health literacy, 155, 156, 256
  prevalence of, 156
Limited language proficiency, 124, 143
Linguistically diverse populations, 233, 316, 326–330, 429
  community cultural wealth in, 393
  crosslinguistic healthcare communication skills, 326–328
  medical Spanish education, 328–330
  public health communication, 478–480
  social media in. *See* Social media
  standards of care for, 388
  targeting and tailoring strategies, 525
Linguistic capital, 388, 389
Linguistic competence, 327
Linguistic diversity, 340, 388, 404, 433, 445
  audience and bidirectional influence of, 450–453
  entertainment-education and. *See* Entertainment-education strategies
  historical evolutionary perspective, 447
  history and theory of, 445–447
  of patient populations, 349
  practice-based definition, 447
"Linguistic minorities," 433–434
Linguistic minority populations, 419. *See also* Health information Seeking (HIS)
  behaviors and outcomes of, 433–434
  clinical interpretation and translation services, 439
  government policies and healthcare, 437
  implications for, 437
  individual factors, 434
  neighborhood factors, 436
  sociodemographic factors, 434–435
  structural factors, 436–437
"Linguistic minority status," 7
Linguistic practices
  case studies, 60–73
  communicative and, 60
  in health/care documents, 60
  theoretical framework, 59–60
Linguistics of healthcare, 17. *See also* Sociolinguistics
"Linguistic turn," 44–45, 47
Literacy, attributions, 16–17
Literalization, of metaphors, 53
"Literary/literature approach," 48
Local language, 32–33, 37
Logico-scientific mode, 43
Longitudinal learning, 356
Lower-scale language resources, 26
Low health literacy, 36, 97
"Low-skilled" myth, 8–10
LSP. *See* Language for Specific Purposes (LSP)
LULAC organization. *See* League of Latin American Citizens (LULAC) organization

Machine translation (MT), 147
"*Main Kuch Bhi Kar Sakti Hoon*" ("*MKBKSH*"), 456, 459
Marginalized/minoritized groups, 137
Marketing, of QBS program, 246
Mass communication, 403
Mass media, 403, 407
  agenda-setting theory, 410–411
  communication, 11
  coverage of health, 412
  critical issues in, 418–419
  cultivation analysis, 413–414
  effects, 409–414
  framing, 411–413
  health campaign efforts, 415–417
  health communication, 415
  health information seeking, 417–418
  health interventions, 415–417
  research and practice, 420–423
  social cognitive theory, 413

Masspersonal Model of Communication (MMoC), 420–421, 423
McCluhan, Marshall, 417
Meaningful access, 102, 235
"Meaningful linguistic access," 257
Meaning-making process, 52
"Mean world syndrome," 414
Media. *See* Social media
Mediated communication campaigns, 415
Medicaid threshold languages, 185
Medical curriculum, intercultural communication in, 310–312
Medical history, 72
Medical humanities, 471–472
Medical interpreter, 291
Medical language education, 277–279, 306, 367
  clinical learning environment, 312
  communication skills. *See* Clinical communication skills training
  conduit model of, 311
  courses, 379
  curricula and teaching methods, 288
  evaluation tools, 378
  faculty development in. *See* Faculty development
  graphic medicine tool, 485
  health equity in, 394
  historical development of, 368–370
  intercultural communication, 310–312
  interdisciplinary nature of, 371
  interpreter-mediated communication, 311–312
  limited English proficiency, 370
  with linguistically diverse populations, 328
  in non-English languages, 350
  pedagogy, 288
  perception of skills (self-evaluation), 377
  possibilities for, 313
  recommendations for, 360–362
  and research, 339–341, 376–383
  service learning, 380–381
  standardization in, 369
  study abroad programs, 382
  teaching tools, 377–378
  training, 185
  transformation, framework for, 313–319
  type of student, 377
  uniformity in, 369
  virtual education, 382–383
Medical language proficiency, 103
Medical language program
  aligning curricula across languages, 361
  curricula and teaching methods, 288
  at Harvard Medical School (HMS), 350–357
  instructor recruitment and qualifications, 361
Medical languages and advocacy, 376
"Medical language" teaching, epistemologies of, 314–317
Medical professional communication, 218
Medical school programs, 373–375
Medical Spanish education, 278, 328–330
  assessment of learner, 338–339
  education in, 340–341
  guiding principles for, 330–331
  integrating sociocultural context in, 337–338
  physical examination, 336
  research in, 339–340
  for residents, 332
  structure of, 330
  targeting, 333–338
  targeting resident and practicing physicians, 331–333
  in United States, 326, 330
Medical Spanish textbooks, 32–33, 333
Medical Spanish training, 124
Medical text genres, 138–143
Medical translation, 137
Medication adherence, 182
Medication Guide (MG), 141
MELAB. *See* Michigan English Language Assessment Battery (MELAB)
Memoirs
  as illness narratives, 48
  as "pathographies," 44
Metaphors, literalization of, 53
MG. *See* Medication Guide (MG)
Michigan English Language Assessment Battery (MELAB), 222
Micro-level language, 25
"Micro-linguistic" level, 81
Migrants, 143
Minoritized groups, 3, 270
Minoritized languages, 87–88, 376, 383
  speakers, 34, 36
Miscommunication, 325

Misinformation, 419
  effects, 518
  potential for, 514
Mixed-methods research, 83, 87, 88, 419
"MKBKSH". *See* "Main Kuch Bhi Kar Sakti Hoon" ("MKBKSH")
MMoC. *See* Masspersonal Model of Communication (MMoC)
Mobility, sociolinguistics of, 26–27, 35–37, 38
Model of Bilingual Health Communication, 118, 120–128
Mode of communication, 54
"Moderate effects era," 415
"Monolingual bias," 13
Monolingualism, 316
Monolingual language, 209
Monolingual orientation, 191
Movimiento Pro Salud program, 328
Mozaik, 464
mPulse Mobile Inc., 462
MT. *See* Machine translation (MT)
Multilingual communication, 231
Multilingual healthcare consultations, 190
Multilingualism, 84, 191, 447
  bilingualism and, 86
  diversity and, 306–307
  in healthcare, 14
  health literacy and, 85–86, 90
  language and, 305
  in professional practice, 191–193
  translanguaging, 307–308
Multilingual practices, 306
Multilingual repertoires, 27
Multilingual theory building, 526
"Multilingual turn," 13–14, 18, 307
Multiliteracies model, 317, 423
Multisector/multistakeholder approach, 157

"nacer por abajo", 32
Named languages, 192
NAMS. *See* National Association of Medical Spanish (NAMS)
"Narrative competence," 50
Narrative engagement, 449
Narrative medicine, emergence of, 471–472
Narrative mode of knowledge, 43
"Narrative turn," 43–45, 47
National Academy of Medicine, 480

National Action Plan to Improve Health Literacy, 157, 164
National Assessment of Adult Literacy, 156
National Association of Medical Spanish (NAMS), 249, 292, 329, 339, 368
National Committee for Quality Assurance (NCQA), 237
National Council for Interpreting in Healthcare (NCIHC), 107
National professional organization, 107
National Service-Learning Clearinghouse, 380
National Standards for Culturally and Linguistically Appropriate Services (CLAS), 103, 164, 234–235, 257
Native/national languages, 264
Native speakers, 291
Natural disasters, 163
Navigational capital, 389
NCIHC. *See* National Council for Interpreting in Healthcare (NCIHC)
NCQA. *See* National Committee for Quality Assurance (NCQA)
Neighborhood factors, 436
NELP. *See* Non-English language preference (NELP)
Nondominant languages
  health equity, 233
  job-specific proficiency in, 232
  and limitations, 327–328
  practices, 318
  professional communication skills training in, 278
  "professionalization" of, 231
  professional training in, 245
  proficiency in, 271
  proficiency policy, 234–236
  skills, 231, 248
  standardization and regulation of, 231
  validation of, 269
Non-English language preference (NELP), 179, 184, 191, 269, 325, 326
Non-English languages
  medical language education in, 350
  populations, 389
  proficiency, 260
  speaking Latinxs, 30
  in United States, 161, 255

Nonequivalent interpretations, 128
Nonfiction long-form comics, 469
"Non-linguistic" language, 78
Nonliterate language, 11
Non-physician healthcare professionals, 376
Nonprofessional interpreters, 126–128
Normative monolingualism, 191
Not-for-profit organization, 327
Nurse–patient relationship, 258

Obama, Michelle, 421
Objective Structured Clinical Examinations (OSCE), 287, 355, 362
Observational skills, in graphic medicine, 52
Occasioned membership category, 193–209
Occupational English Test (OET), 216–218, 220, 226
Occupational therapy (OT), 259
OET. *See* Occupational English Test (OET)
Office of Scholarly Engagement, 351, 354
Online resources, 290, 333
On-the-spot written translation, 146
OPI. *See* Oral proficiency interview (OPI)
Oral communication, 371
Oral language skills, 241
Oral proficiency interview (OPI), 282, 332
Oral versions, of illness narratives, 45–50
Organizational health literacy, 155
Organizational-level statistics, 107
Organizational policy, 240–241
Organizational responsibility, 515–516
Organization for Economic Co-operation and Development, 156
Organ system-based approach, 331
OSCE. *See* Objective Structured Clinical Examinations (OSCE)
Ouro Negro (Black Gold), 457, 464
Overgeneralization, 286
Over-the-counter (OTC) medicines, 148

Package information leaflets (PIL), 140–141, 145
  patient comprehension, 147
  recommendations for, 147–148
Passive audiences, 409
Passive conduit, 117

Pathographies, 44
  elements, 55
  and graphic pathographies, 54
  illness narratives as, 49
Patient (information) brochures, 140
Patient-centered communication, 31, 35, 311, 471
Patient-clinician relationship, 256, 436
  graphic medicine for, 480–482
Patient Instructions for Use (PIFU), 141
Patient intake form, 70, 71
Patient-nurse relationship, 258
Patient Package Insert (PPI), 141
Patient-physician communication, 430
Patient Protection and Affordable Care Act (ACA) of 2010. *See* Affordable Care Act of 2010 (ACA)
Patients
  communication needs, 258
  comprehension of PILs, 147
  decision-making process, 148
  experience of care, 31, 182
  explanatory model, 46
  healthcare translation for. *See* Healthcare translation
  health information seeking, 431
  with LEP, 256, 258
  with limited English proficiency (LEP), 256, 258, 350
Patient's preferred language, 108, 175, 186, 215, 232, 255–256, 259, 269, 326
Pearson Test of English (PTE), 222
Pediatric resident physician, 375
Performativity, 59, 60
Personal health literacy, 155
Personalismo, 36, 334, 336
Personal smartphones, 121
Physical examination, 336
Physician education, 291
Physician–patient relationship, 471
Physicians-in-practice, 375–376
Physiotherapy educators, 219
PIFU. *See* Patient Instructions for Use (PIFU)
PIL. *See* Package information leaflets (PIL)
Plain language, 2, 14, 86–87, 137
  approach, 31–32
  guidelines, 86
  health literacy and, 98

Plain language (cont'd)
  initiatives, 158
  principles, 162
  principles of, 86
  protocols and translation, 78
  tools, 165
  use of, 86
Plain Language Medical Dictionary, 165
Plain Writing Act of 2010, 84, 86, 158, 164
Podcasts, 410
Poor-quality interpretation, 107
Population health, 327
Positive washback, 219
PPI. *See* Patient Package Insert (PPI)
Practice, recommendations for, 111
PRIME-LC program, 211
Proactive theory building, 526
Procedural validity, 223
Process-oriented research, 138
Professional interpreters, 121–123, 255, 259, 260, 261, 270, 309, 310
  hospital, 121–122
  in-person, 121–122, 124
  medical, 325, 328
  technology-based, 121–122
Professionalism, 232–233
Professionalization
  of bilingualism, 238–240
  of nondominant language, 231
Professional purposes, language assessment for, 216–218
Promotion, of QBS program, 246
Promotoras, 33
Provider-patient interaction, 77, 78, 93, 120
  applied linguistic approaches in, 79–81
  historical context, 78–79
  interpreters in, 129
  linguistic disparities in, 430
  situational challenges in, 120
Proxy health information seeking, 433–434
Psychiatric resident physician, 375
Psychosocial outcomes, 431
PTE. *See* Pearson Test of English (PTE)
Public health, 78
  communication, 478–480
  emergencies, 162–163
  mediated interventions for, 403

Public health crises, 512–514
  communicating during, 514–517
  effective communication in, 520–525
  framing theory to, 520–523
  health belief model to, 523–524
  information exchange, 514
  integrative model of behavioral prediction, 524–525
  misinformation effects, 518
  news framing effects, 517–518
  organizational responsibility, 515–516
  potential for misinformation, 514
  situational crisis communication theory, 515–516
Publicly-funded programs, 10
Public social media, 420

QBS program. *See* Qualified bilingual staff (QBS) program
Quackery medical advertisement, 409
"Qualified bilingual providers," 327, 328
Qualified bilingual staff (QBS) program, 236–237, 239, 284
  accrediting bodies, 247
  assessment of, 241–244
  elements of, 240–246
  federal and state government, 247
  incentives and compensation for, 245–246
  marketing and promotion of, 246
  organizational policy, 240–241
  in organizational policy, 249
  policy and practice, 246–250
  post-qualification expectations, 245
"Qualified interpreter," 257
Quality assessment methods, 138
Quality translation, 143
Quasi-experimental research designs, 183, 184
Queer and trans people, 69–70
Questionable language, 215

Race/ethnicity
  concordance, 175–176
  language and, 318
  minority group, 30
Rapid Estimate of Adult Literacy in Medicine (REALM), 160
Readability formulas, 148

REALM. *See* Rapid Estimate of Adult Literacy in Medicine (REALM)
Reconstructing Illness (Hawkins), 44
Recovering Bodies (Couser), 44
Recruitment of medical language, 361
Refugees, 145
   adults, 4
   and immigrant women, 10
   migrants and, 143
   women, 143
Regulatory agencies, 257
Reparative reading, 49
Representational mediacy, 52
Republic of North Macedonia, 464
Research, 110–111
   applied linguistics, 78
   bilingualism, 191
   cross-language methods, 109–110
   faculty development, 394–398
   graphic medicine, 486–487
   health literacy, 155, 163–165
   language concordance, 175, 258, 263–264, 264
   LHP programs, 293–294
   mass media, 420–423
   in medical Spanish education, 339–340
   mixed-methods, 83
   process-oriented, 138
   quasi-experimental designs, 183, 184
   sociolinguistics, 2
Resident physicians, 331–332, 375
   training programs, 375
Resistance capital, 393
Reuland's guiding principles, 330–331, 341
RIAS. *See* Roter Interaction Analysis System (RIAS)
Risk communication, 31–32
Robert Wood Johnson Foundation, 233
Roter Interaction Analysis System (RIAS), 79
Rural Mexican Spanish, 32
Russian-language social media, 499

SBC. *See* Social and behavioral change (SBC)
SBCC strategy. *See* Social and behavioral change communication (SBCC) strategy
Scale, public health emergencies, 513
SCCT. *See* Situational crisis communication theory (SCCT)

SCT. *See* Social cognitive theory (SCT)
SDOH. *See* Social determinant of health (SDOH)
Second language acquisition (SLA), 191, 282
   ALTA Spanish, 329
   communicative language instruction, 287
   communicative language teaching, 286–288
   curricula and teaching methods, 288
   didactic LHP resources, 290
   for healthcare purposes, 282
   language acquisition theories, 285–286
   language proficiency, 282–285
Seguro médico, "health insurance" as, 33
Self-assessment, 285, 293, 297, 374, 377
   of proficiency, 285
   reliance on, 293
Self-awareness, of language proficiency, 327–328
Self-efficacy, 413, 525
Self-evaluation, 377
"Self-qualification," 236
Semi-structured interviews, 52, 62
"Sensation-seeking," 415
Service learning, 337, 380–381
Sex/gender, 68–73
Sexuality, 68–73
Sexual orientation, 72
SHDPP. *See* Stanford Heart Disease Prevention Program (SHDPP)
Signaling devices, 86
Simple Measure of Gobbledygook (SMOG), 148
Simplemente María (TV series), 447
Síntomas Coronavirus, 475, 477
Situational crisis communication theory (SCCT), 515–516
Skilled language, 9
Skilled translator, 144
SLA. *See* Second language acquisition (SLA)
SMOG. *See* Simple Measure of Gobbledygook (SMOG)
SmPCs. *See* Summary of Product Characteristics (SmPCs)
Social and behavioral change (SBC), 445
Social and behavioral change communication (SBCC) strategy, 447
Social capital, 393
Social cognitive theory (SCT), 413, 448

Social determinant of health (SDOH), 1, 281
  language as, 5–6
  prominent role of, 6
  WHO Commission on, 6
Social media, 412, 493
  exposure to misinformation, 500–502
  harmful behaviors, 499–500
  health information access, 495–497
  intervention delivery, 497–498
  issues and topics, 495
  platforms, 407
  for practice and research, 503–505
  research participation, 498
  social support and social capital, 498–499
  transnational and trans-language
    power of, 413
  use linguistically diverse communities,
    494–495
Social networks, 436
Sociocultural theory, 286
Sociodemographic factors, 434–435
Socioeconomic status, 434
Sociolinguistics
  and COVID-19, 28–29
  in healthcare communication, 25–29
  of illness narratives, 44–45
  language and, 33
  of mobility, 26–27, 35, 36–37, 38
  perspectives, 31, 38
  recommendations, 33–37
    clinician and interpreter training, 35
    improving interpretative encounters, 34
    time allotted to minoritized patients, 36
  research, 2
  translanguaging, 27–28
Sociopolitical movements, 470–471
Source credibility, 455–458
Source text (ST), 138
South Korean Emergency Alert, 512
SP. *See* Standardized patient (SP)
Spanglish, 335
Spanish-English bilingual patients, 11
Spanish language, 30, 180
  instruction in United States schools, 32
  interactions, 192
  learners' needs and readiness by, 334
  medical textbooks, 32–33
  proficiency, 259
  pronunciation and grammatical
    accuracy, 201
  social marketing campaigns in, 33
Spanish monolinguals, 30, 36
Spanish-speaking Latinxs, 30, 31, 34
Speech Act Theory, 87
Stakeholder collaboration, 35
Standardized evaluation, 293
Standardized interpretation process, 110
Standardized language assessments, 328
Standardized language test, 227
Standardized patient (SP), 378
Stanford Heart Disease Prevention Program
  (SHDPP), 415
"Sticky messages," concept of, 458
Stigma, 256
Storytelling, 454–455, 472–473
Structural inequities, in healthcare, 109
Structuralist language, 307
Structural simplification, 141
Student-centered assessments, 287
Study abroad programs, 382
Suaahara, 460, 463
Summary of Product Characteristics
  (SmPCs), 141
Summative feedback, 287
Superdiversity, 306, 307
Survey instrument translation, 109, 110
Switching PCPs, 184
System-wide certification system, 249

Tamale Lesson, The, 454–456
Target language (TL), 138, 316, 334, 353,
  378, 382
Target texts, 138–139
Task-Based Language Teaching (TBLT), 331
Task-Based Learning, 289
TBLT. *See* Task-Based Language Teaching
  (TBLT)
Teach-back method, 12
Teaching tools, 377–378
Technology-based professional interpreters,
  121–122
Telehealth, 437
Telenovelas, 416
Telephone interpreting services, 121
Terminological lacunae, 145
Test construct, 216

Test developers, 219, 228
Test of English as a Foreign Language (TOEFL), 222, 234
Test tasks mirror language, 223
Text genres, 140–142
  fact sheets for patients (FSP), 140
  informed consent form (ICF), 141–142
  package information leaflets (PIL), 140–141
'Threat to research rigor,' 109–110
Title VI of the Civil Rights Act of 1964, 102, 235, 257, 387
TOEFL. *See* Test of English as a Foreign Language (TOEFL)
Total Physical Response (TPR), 288
Traditional Grammar-Translation Method, 285
Traditional translation, 271
Training
  clinical skills education, 370–376
  for clinical trainees, 261
  in cross-language research methods, 109–110
  in cultural and linguistic skills, 327
  cultural humility, 370
  healthcare interpreters, 35, 106–107
  of healthcare professionals, 307
  implications for, 210–211
  language concordance, 184–185
  as language instructor, 291
  medical Spanish education in, 326
  medical Spanish program, 337
  physical examination, 336
  simulation, 379–380
Transcreation, 461
Transformation, framework for, 313–319
Trans-ing boundaries, 317–318
Translanguaging, 27–28, 37, 206–209, 278, 293–294
  cornerstones of, 315–316
  curricular politization, 316
  heritage language education, 313
  heritage speakers, 313
  in medical language pedagogy, 278
  "medical language" teaching, 314–317
  multilingualism, 307–308
  notion of, 305
  in professional practice, 191–193
  transliteracy, 317
  VAME and, 319

Translational services, 439
Translation quality assessment methods, 138
Translingual orientation, 316
Transliteracy, 317
Trump administration, 157
"Turn-by-turn" analysis, 79
Twitter, 412, 423, 456, 493, 502, 514
Two-way information gap, 287

Undergraduate medical language programs, 372–373, 388
Undocumented immigrants, 61, 63, 64
United Nations Universal Declaration on Human Rights, 445
United States
  Hispanic/Latinx population in, 342
  hospital accreditor, 103
  language access policies and laws in, 102–106
  language concordance research, 263–264
  Latinxs in, 30
  limited English proficiency in, 256
  medical Spanish education in, 278, 326
  non-English language in, 161, 255
  population with non-English language, 179
  racial/ethnic minority group in, 30
  Spanish speakers in, 33, 37
  undocumented immigrants in, 64
United States Medical Licensing Examination (USMLE), 216, 339
Universalism, 447
Untrained interpreters, 126
Urgent communication, 511–527
  public health crises. *See* Public health crises
United States Department of Health and Human Services (HHS), 5, 6
United States Health Resources and Services Administration (HRSA), 317
United States–Mexico borderlands, deservingness in, 60–64
USMLE. *See* United States Medical Licensing Examination (USMLE)
United States practitioners, 27

Vagrancy Law, 67
Validation framework, 223–224
Validity, of language assessments, 223–227

Value-Added Medical Education (VAME), 312
Value community orientation/collectivism, 28
VAME. *See* Value-Added Medical Education (VAME)
Vibrant religious community, 193
Vicarious learning, concepts of, 413
Video remote interpreting (VRI), 122
Viet Fact Check, 501
Vietnamese–American community, 501
Virtual education, 382–383
Virtual learning environment, 361–362
Vocabulary, 290, 292, 334
VRI. *See* Video remote interpreting (VRI)

Wages, for healthcare interpreters, 106
WeChat, 499, 501
Western biomedical ideology, 128
White Cadejo, 66
WHO. *See* World Health Organization (WHO)

Women
 health information seeking, 432
 immigrant, 10
 refugee, 143
World Health Organization (WHO), 5, 6, 155, 410
Written communication, 10–11, 164, 370
Written documents, 86–88
 health documents, 87–88
 minoritized languages, 87–88
 plain language, 86–87
Written healthcare communication, 140
Written translation, 143
Written versions, of illness narratives, 45–50

YouTube, 502

Zines, 470–471
Zone of Proximal Development (ZPD), 286
ZPD. *See* Zone of Proximal Development (ZPD)

Printed in the USA
CPSIA information can be obtained
at www.ICGtesting.com
CBHW081306140524
8289CB00003B/48